THIRD EDITION

Neuroscience for the Study of Communicative Disorders

Subhash C. Bhatnagar, PhD

Neurolinguistics Laboratory
Speech Pathology and Audiology Department
Marquette University

Wolters Kluwer | Lippincott Williams & Wilkins
Health
Philadelphia · Baltimore · New York · London
Buenos Aires · Hong Kong · Sydney · Tokyo

Acquisitions Editor: Peter Sabatini
Managing Editor: Andrea M. Klingler
Marketing Manager: Allison M. Noplock
Production Editor: Sally Anne Glover
Designer: Stephen Druding
Compositor: Circle Graphics, Inc.

Third Edition
Copyright © 2008, 2002, 1995 Lippincott Williams & Wilkins, a Wolters Kluwer business.

351 West Camden Street   530 Walnut Street
Baltimore, MD 21201   Philadelphia, PA 19106

Printed in the Peoples Republic of China

09   10   11   12   13   14
8   7   6   5   4   3   2

Library of Congress Cataloging-in-Publication Data

Bhatnagar, Subhash Chandra.
  Neuroscience for the study of communicative disorders / Subhash C.
Bhatnagar. — 3rd ed.
      p. ; cm.
  Includes bibliographical references and index.
  ISBN-13: 978-1-60547-661-2
  1. Communicative disorders—Pathophysiology.   2. Neurosciences.   I. Title.
  [DNLM: 1. Central Nervous System—anatomy & histology.   2. Central Nervous System—
physiology.   3. Communication Disorders—physiopathology.   WL 300 B575n 2008]
  RC423.B53 2008
  612.8—dc22

2007006804

DISCLAIMER

Care has been taken to confirm the accuracy of the information present and to describe generally accepted practices. However, the authors, editors, and publisher are not responsible for errors or omissions or for any consequences from application of the information in this book and make no warranty, expressed or implied, with respect to the currency, completeness, or accuracy of the contents of the publication. Application of this information in a particular situation remains the professional responsibility of the practitioner; the clinical treatments described and recommended may not be considered absolute and universal recommendations.

The authors, editors, and publisher have exerted every effort to ensure that drug selection and dosage set forth in this text are in accordance with the current recommendations and practice at the time of publication. However, in view of ongoing research, changes in government regulations, and the constant flow of information relating to drug therapy and drug reactions, the reader is urged to check the package insert for each drug for any change in indications and dosage and for added warnings and precautions. This is particularly important when the recommended agent is a new or infrequently employed drug.

Some drugs and medical devices presented in this publication have Food and Drug Administration (FDA) clearance for limited use in restricted research settings. It is the responsibility of the health care provider to ascertain the FDA status of each drug or device planned for use in their clinical practice.

To purchase additional copies of this book, call our customer service department at (800) 638-3030 or fax orders to (301) 223-2320. International customers should call (301) 223-2300.

Visit Lippincott Williams & Wilkins on the Internet: http://www.lww.com. Lippincott Williams & Wilkins customer service representatives are available from 8:30 am to 6:00 pm, EST.

Vidya Dadati Vinayam. Vinayat
Yati Patratam. Patra Dhanamapnoti
Yatra Dhanam Yatah Sukham.
(Knowledge gives humility and modesty,
which bring ability for valued judgment.
A person with value-based
judgment attains prosperity, which
brings happiness.)
—Sanskrit saying from *Panchatantra,*
Stories of Wisdom.

In memory of
My late father, Shri. Chiranji L. Bhatnagar,
who nurtured and inspired me
and
My late friend and colleague,
Orlando J. Andy, who mentored me in
the applications of the neurosurgical
techniques to human behavior
and
My late teacher, Mary B. Mann, who
provided me with the opportunity to
teach neuroscience when I was a
graduate student.

Foreword

I am once again honored by Subhash Bhatnagar's asking me to write the foreword to this third edition of his text *Neuroscience for the Study of Communicative Disorders*. Dr. Bhatnagar continues to be responsive to the needs of students of human communication and its disorders in terms of providing a most relevant and readable text. Just as important, Dr. Bhatnagar has updated the text to meet the standards of the rapidly evolving world of neuroscience to ensure that students will have access to the most current information as possible. This is a breathtaking endeavor.

The essence of *Neuroscience for the Study of Communicative Disorders*, 3rd edition, with its commitment to improving the learning process, has been enhanced. This new edition builds on the success of the earlier editions and shares their responsiveness to student needs and ways to meet those needs. Further, it encourages teachers who use the book as the text for their courses to adapt it to their own specialized needs. More case studies, a more substantive glossary, and insights into the specialized professional language of the medical profession are provided. In these ways, this text provides more inroads into the arcane world of those aspects of neuroscience that relate to human problems.

Students of human communication and its disorders will quickly feel at home with this book. It speaks to them about issues in neuroscience that are basic to adult neurogenic disorders and provides the necessary background for understanding early development and how and why it goes astray—critical for principled clinical intervention for a range of disorders from autism to craniofacial disorders. The problem-solving skills that are encouraged and taught in this book, the carefully crafted review questions, and the direction provided by its learning objectives all offer crucial guidance for students.

This book's earlier editions have become the gold standard for teaching neuroscience to students of human communication disorders. They have raised the bar in the profession's teaching of one of its most important basic scientific foundations. This latest edition will clearly move that important tradition along.

Audrey L. Holland, PhD
Regents' Professor Emerita
University of Arizona
Tucson, Arizona

My conviction—shared by my late friend, colleague, and co-author, Orlando J. Andy, MD—has been that neuroscience can be simplified; learning neurologic concepts need not evoke dread in the hearts of students. We followed this reasoning so that students from behavioral sciences could find the study of neuroscience to be a challenging and purposeful experience. The information presented was essential, contextual, relevant to human behavior, and devoid of trivial encyclopedic detail. Two earlier editions of the book, which exemplified this vision, received encouraging feedback from students and faculty from various universities in the United States and abroad, thus vindicating our decision to integrate visual and clinical approaches to promote analytical thinking.

In this 3rd edition of *Neuroscience for the Study of Communicative Disorders*, I have endeavored to enhance the effectiveness of the material and the interactive, visual-analytic approach to learning and teaching. Although neuroscience consistently has been simplified, a flavor of the subject's comprehensiveness is retained lest students lose a sense of its inherent complexity. In some ways, this book conforms to Albert Einstein's famous aphorism: "Make everything as simple as possible but not simpler."

FEATURES AND ORGANIZATION

This new edition continues to promote the learning of simplified neuroscience, but now students have access to many additional analytic, visual, and informational tools to facilitate their learning. A step-by-step approach introduces vocabulary, factual information, neurologic concepts, and clinical applications for developing the reader's knowledge base. Concise descriptions of technical issues are presented in the context of their relevance to human behavior. With the revision of a great number of existing figures and the inclusion of new images, the visual approach to learning has been strengthened. Structures and neuronal pathways are now illustrated in multiple figures and from different orientations so that their familiarity can facilitate an analytic approach to brain functions and problem solving. Important clinical information is highlighted in boxes throughout the text. Neurologic reasoning is emphasized by making

students participate interactively in solving clinical problems. The emphasis on reasoning skills is further enhanced by the addition of practical case studies with solutions. Multiple-choice questions have been used to create an online question bank for evaluating students' consolidated knowledge.

Some of the prominent highlights of the revised text are the following:

- Substantially revised chapters to promote student learning
- Quiz questions at the conclusion of each chapter
- Addition of 50 interactive case studies to promote problem solving
- Addition or revision of approximately 70 figures to promote visual learning
- Inclusion of 18 figures for the online exercises
- Addition of 18 summary tables to consolidate students' learning
- Rewritten neuroimaging section to cover advances in diagnostic MRI (functional MRI, diffusion-weighted MRI, perfusion MRI, diffusion-tensor imaging, MRI spectroscopy)
- Updated discussion of cellular biology and neuro-embryology, including neuronal pruning and synapse establishment in the developing brain and the physiology of neoplasm
- Updated discussion of consciousness
- Addition of more than 50 medical abbreviations
- Addition of more than 400 new terms and definitions to the glossary
- Development of an online question bank with more than 450 multiple-choice and objective questions (along with answers) to facilitate student evaluation

Some details inherent to neuroscience may not be central to some instructors' teaching goals. Course instructors are, therefore, encouraged to reorganize the information to meet their teaching needs and control the coverage and depth of the material in accordance to individual courses. The bulleted "Learning Objectives" are designed to help instructors reprioritize the book's content.

Subhash C. Bhatnagar

Acknowledgments

I am indebted to many of my colleagues who have helped me in the preparation of this book:

Audrey L. Holland, PhD, Regents' Professor at the University of Arizona, for agreeing to write the foreword for this edition, as she did for the previous two editions of the book. I have been privileged to have her support and cherished friendship ever since I was a graduate student.

Duane E. Haines, PhD, from the Department of Anatomy at the University of Mississippi Medical Center, Jackson, who is an established and prolific neuroscience author. I am grateful to him for his encouragement and support throughout preparation of this and earlier editions. He has been generous in providing many brain images and has allowed me to freely use many serial brain dissections from his publication *Neuroanatomy: An Atlas of Structures, Sections, and Systems*.

Robin L. Curtis, PhD, formerly from the Department of Cell Biology, Neurobiology, and Anatomy at the Medical College of Wisconsin, for his thoughtful critique on a large number of the chapters in the text. His comments have helped me further simplify the presentation of many complex issues concerning sensorimotor topics.

Alexandru Barboi, MD, from the Department of Neurology, Medical College of Wisconsin, for reviewing neurologic case studies and other clinical information. His comments have helped me ensure the correctness of many important clinical concepts.

Howard Kirshner, MD, from the Department of Neurology, Vanderbilt College of Medicine, for his help with technical neurologic issues. I also thank him for writing the chapter on higher functions and for providing the PET images.

Varun K. Saxena, MD, from the Center for Neurological Disorders, Milwaukee, for many discussions and for filling in the gaps in my knowledge of neuroscience.

Lotfi Hacein-Bay, MD, from the Department of Radiology at Loyola Medical Center, Chicago. His comments have improved the presentation of the section on neuroimaging in Chapter 20. I also thank him for his encouragement and consistent support.

George T. Mandybur, MD, from the Department of Neurosurgery, University of Cincinnati College of Medicine. His assistance with therapeutic issues dealing with neurosurgery is appreciated.

Michelle Mynlieff, PhD, from the Department of Biological Sciences at Marquettte University, for her assistance in rewriting the chapter on cellular physiology and neurotransmitters.

Madhuri Behari, MD, from the Department of Neurology, All India Institute of Medical Sciences, New Delhi, India, for her help in clarifying many neurologic concepts and clinical issues contained in Chapter 20.

Kunwar P. Bhatnagar, PhD, from the Department of Anatomical Sciences and Neurobiology, University of Louisville School of Medicine, Louisville, for his encouragement and for writing the chapter on neuroembryology.

I thank Xu Li, MD, PhD, from Ohio University, Athens; William Mustain, PhD, from the University of Mississippi Medical Center, Jackson; and Edward W. Korabic, PhD, from Marquette University, for their comments on selected information.

I thank Ms. Martha Jerme, health science librarian from Marquette University, for her assistance in searching for references.

I also thank the independent reviewers (Martha A. Boose, PhD, from the college of St. Rose, Mary Jo German, PhD, from Ball State University, Jenis M. Jarecki-Liu from Clariton University of Pennsylvania, and John W. Oller, PhD, from the University of Louisiana at Lafayette) for their comments and valuable suggestions.

I also thank Dr. Brooke Hallowell from Ohio University for her enthusiasm and encouraging support for this book and its earlier editions.

I would like to graciously acknowledge the assistance of my graduate students, who have helped diligently with various phases of the book. I thank Julie Polzin, MS CCC-SLP, and Teresa Schwartz, MS CCC-SLP, for their assistance in the early phases of manuscript preparation. I thank Ashley Bohanan for her help in the final stage of the book. I am especially thankful for the impeccable work of Maria Fratangelo, MS CCC-SLP, who worked closely with me for 2 years. Her talent has added to the consistency in formatting the text, tables, and figures; I also acknowledge her help in the preparation of the online review questions.

Finally, I thank Priti, my wife and my best friend; I also thank my sons, Manav and Gaurav. The encouragement and emotional support of my family were most inspiring to me. Without their understanding and cooperation, this book and this edition could not have become realities.

Contents

Foreword v
Preface vii
Acknowledgments ix

CHAPTER 1

Essential Concepts and Principles of Neuroscience 1

Relationship between Neuroscience and Speech-Language-Hearing Pathology 1

Scope of Neuroscience 3

Principles Governing Functional Organization of the Human Brain 6

Orientation to Basic Terminology 8

Gross Structures of the Central Nervous System 14

Functional Classification of the Nervous System 15

Cellular Organization (Cytoarchitecture) and Brodmann Areas 16

Techniques for Solving Problems When Learning Neuroscience 18

Clinical Considerations 24

Summary 24

Quiz Questions 25

Technical Terms 26

CHAPTER 2

Gross Anatomy of the Central Nervous System 27

Structures of the Central and Peripheral Nervous Systems 27

Primary Divisions of the Brain 29

Gross Structures of the Brain 30

Ventricles 60

Medullary Centers in the Brain 61

Meninges of the Brain 65

Meninges of the Spinal Cord 70

Cranial Nerves 71

Autonomic Nervous System 75

Lesion Localization 77

Clinical Considerations 78

Summary 80

Quiz Questions 81

Technical Terms 81

CHAPTER 3

Internal Anatomy of the Central Nervous System 82

Anatomic Orientation Landmarks 82

Spinal Cord in Cross-Sections 84

Brainstem in Transverse Sections 86

Forebrain in Coronal Sections 101

Forebrain in Horizontal Sections 108

Summary 113

Quiz Questions 113

Technical Terms 113

CHAPTER 4

Development of the Central Nervous System 114

Human Chromosomes, Genes, and Cell Division 114

Early Human Development 116

The Central Nervous System 119

Clinical Concerns 125

Summary 129

Quiz Questions 129

Technical Terms 130

CHAPTER 5

Basic Physiology of Nerve Cells 131

Neuron 131

Central and Peripheral Nervous Systems 134

Neuronal Pruning and Synapse Establishment in the Brain 135

Nerve Impulse 137

Neuronal Responses to Brain Injuries 139

Neurotransmitters 143

Clinical Concerns 147

Clinical Considerations 149

Summary 150

Quiz Questions 150

Technical Terms 151

CHAPTER 6

Diencephalon: Thalamus and Associated Structures 152

Gross Anatomy of the Diencephalon 152

Thalamus 152

Functional Classification of the Thalamic Nuclei 160

Epithalamus 160
Subthalamus 160
Hypothalamus 161
Cognitive Functions of the Thalamus 161
Thalamic Syndrome 161
Clinical Considerations 162
Summary 163
Quiz Questions 163
Technical Terms 163

CHAPTER 7

Somatosensory System 164

Somatosensation 164
Innervation Pattern 166
Anatomic Division of the Somatosensory System 166
Trigeminal Nerve 176
Unconscious Proprioception 180
Lesion Localization—Rule 3: Spinal Central Gray Lesion 182
Clinical Considerations 182
Summary 184
Quiz Questions 184
Technical Terms 184

CHAPTER 8

Visual System 185

Anatomy of the Eye 185
Vascular Supply of the Retina 190
Photochemistry of Retina 191
Optical Mechanism 192
Central Visual Pathways 195
Visual Cortex Development 197
Visual Reflexes 197
Clinical Concerns 200
Lesion Localization—Rule 4: Visual Pathway Lesion 205
Clinical Considerations 205
Summary 206
Quiz Questions 206
Technical Terms 207

CHAPTER 9

Auditory System 208

Sound, Properties, and Measurements 208
Anatomy and Physiology 209
Central Auditory Pathways 214
Auditory Reflexes 219
Vascular Supply to the Auditory Mechanism 219
Distinctive Properties of Auditory System 219
Clinical Concerns 221
Clinical Considerations 224
Summary 226

Quiz Questions 226
Technical Terms 226

CHAPTER 10

Vestibular System 227

Anatomy of the Vestibular System 227
Neural Mechanism for Controlling Eye Movements 232
Physiology of Equilibrium 233
Clinical Concerns 234
Clinical Diagnostic Tests 235
Clinical Considerations 236
Summary 237
Quiz Questions 237
Technical Terms 237

CHAPTER 11

Motor System 1: Spinal Cord 238

Spinal Preparation 238
Innervation Pattern 238
Gross Anatomy of the Spinal Cord 239
Tracts of the Spinal Cord 240
Motor Nuclei of the Spinal Cord 245
Motor Functions of the Spinal Cord 245
Spinal Reflexes 248
Neurotransmitters 252
Clinical Concerns 252
Lesion Localization 256
Clinical Considerations 257
Summary 259
Quiz Questions 259
Technical Terms 259

CHAPTER 12

Motor System 2: Cerebellum 260

Innervation Pattern 261
Cerebellar Anatomy 261
Cerebellar Cortex 266
Motor Learning 268
Clinical Concerns 268
Clinical Considerations 270
Summary 271
Quiz Questions 271
Technical Terms 271

CHAPTER 13

Motor System 3: Brainstem and Basal Ganglia 272

Brainstem Motor Mechanism 272

Basal Ganglia 274
Clinical Concerns 280
Clinical Considerations 286
Summary 288
Quiz Questions 288
Technical Terms 288

CHAPTER 14

Motor System 4: Motor Cortex **289**

Anatomy of Motor Cortex 289
Innervation Pattern 290
Clinical Terms 291
Descending Pathways 291
Clinical Concerns 293
Lesion Localization 296
Clinical Considerations 297
Summary 299
Quiz Questions 299
Technical Terms 299

CHAPTER 15

Synopsis of Cranial Nerves **300**

Functional Classification of Cranial Nerves 301
Branchial Origin of Speech-Related Muscles 302
Cranial Nerves and the Autonomic Nervous System 306
Cranial Nerve Nuclei 306
Pathways 308
Innervation Pattern 309
Cranial Nerves and Their Sensorimotor Functions 310
Function-Based Cranial Nerve Combinations 342
Clinical Concerns 343
Common Cranial Nerve Syndromes 344
Clinical Considerations 347
Summary 351
Quiz Questions 351
Technical Terms 352

CHAPTER 16

Axial-Limbic Brain: Autonomic Nervous System, Limbic System, Hypothalamus, and Reticular Formation **353**

Autonomic Nervous System 353
Limbic System 360
Hypothalamus 364
Reticular Formation 369
Clinical Considerations 375
Summary 376
Quiz Questions 377
Technical Terms 377

CHAPTER 17

Survey of the Cerebrovascular System **378**

Vascular Network 378
Selective Vulnerability to Anoxia 389
Risk Factors 390
Venous Sinus System 391
Regulation of Cerebral Blood Flow 391
Treatment of Vascular Diseases 393
Blood–Brain Barrier 395
Lesion Localization—Rule 10: Vascular System Disorder 395
Clinical Considerations 396
Summary 397
Quiz Questions 398
Technical Terms 398

CHAPTER 18

Survey of the Ventricles and Cerebrospinal Fluid **399**

Choroid Plexus 399
Cerebrospinal Fluid Circulation 399
Absorption of the Cerebrospinal Fluid 400
Clinical Concerns 401
Clinical Considerations 403
Summary 404
Quiz Questions 404
Technical Terms 404

CHAPTER 19

Cerebral Cortex: Higher Mental Functions . .**405**

Methods of Study 405
Functional Localization in the Brain 405
Disorders of Cortical Functions 408
Clinical Considerations 417
Summary 420
Quiz Questions 420
Technical Terms 420

CHAPTER 20

Diagnostic Techniques and Neurologic Concepts **421**

Brain Imaging 421
Advances in MRI 427
Additional Imaging Techniques 430
Sodium Amytal Infusion for Assessing Cerebral Dominance . . .431
Electroencephalography 434
Electromyography 436
Evoked Potentials 437

Dichotic Listening 439

Lumbar Puncture 440

Neurosurgical Procedures 440

Genetic Inheritance 442

Specific Neurologic Disorders 444

Summary 449

Quiz Questions 449

Technical Terms 450

Glossary   451

Suggested Readings   479

Figure and Table Credits   483

Index   487

Essential Concepts and Principles of Neuroscience

LEARNING OBJECTIVES

After studying this chapter, students of speech-language-pathology and human behavior should be able to:

- Describe the subject matter of neuroscience and speech-language-hearing pathology

- Discuss the relationship between neuroscience and speech-language-hearing pathology

- Explain the rationale for learning neuroscience

- Discuss the benefits of neuroscience training

- Describe the scope of the major branches of neuroscience

- Explain the components of a neurologic examination

- Describe common neurologic diseases that have clinical relevance to students of human behavior

- Explain the basic principles that govern human brain function

- Define technical terms used for directional reference, brain section planes, and anatomic structures

- Describe the major structures of the central nervous system and describe their functions

- Discuss the functional components that are used to categorize the functions of the nervous system

- Discuss common hurdles encountered when learning neuroscience and outline strategies for overcoming them

- Discuss the architectural layers of the cerebral cortex and the function of each layer

- Describe the functions of important Brodmann areas commonly used in cognitive neurology

- Appreciate the rationale underlying neurologic rules used for localizing lesions in the nervous system

- Display a level of comfort with the technical tools used in applying neuroscience to human behavior

- Appreciate the rationale for using technical concepts for solving neurologic problems

RELATIONSHIP BETWEEN NEUROSCIENCE AND SPEECH-LANGUAGE-HEARING PATHOLOGY

Speech-language-hearing pathology and neuroscience are closely related disciplines. A well-developed and adequately connected neuronal organization of the brain serves as the prerequisite for the acquisition of language and other higher mental functions, which are also clinically used to evaluate the brain's structural integrity. This brain–behavior relationship was underscored over a century ago by the observations of Paul Broca and Carl Wernicke on the localization of specific expressive and receptive language functions in particular areas of the human brain. After examining a series of patients who had no motor problems with the speech muscles, who could understand spoken language, but who could not speak, Broca proposed in 1861 that we speak with the left hemisphere. An examination of the brains of such patients during autopsy revealed a lesion in the lower posterior frontal region (a region now called the area of Broca). Wernicke in 1876 described a different type of aphasia (language disorder) caused by impaired auditory comprehension instead of impaired expression. He related this type of aphasia to a lesion in the left posterior temporal lobe, a different area from the one described by Broca. These observations of Broca and Wernicke significantly enhanced our knowledge of the brain–behavior relationship. In doing so, they established the groundwork for modern neurolinguistic studies, in which other language functions were assigned to different brain regions and their interactive connections. Language and speech disturbances have since become sensitive indicators of structural and physiologic impairment in the brain.

Phylogenetically, the evolution of the brain is progressively linear, reaching its highest level in humans (*Homo sapiens*), in whom the brain is not merely a scaled-up version of its primitive forms. Rather its structural advancement reflects an enormously increased cellular complexity (in terms of cellular density and synaptic connectivity), and the brain regions serving specific functions grow at different rates. Owing to this variable rate of cellular growth, the neocortex (six-layered cellular organization) occupies a large percentage of the **cerebral cortex**, which has a great architectural (cellular aggregates) complexity found only in the human brain. Thicker in appearance and highly laminated compared to other primates, the human brain is only 2% of the body weight, but it is uniquely equipped to analyze and synthesize information in past, present, and future contexts. Through its biologic interaction with the environment, the human brain also generates substrates for consciousness; cognition (attention, memory, and decision making); symbolic communication; learning; knowledge; personality; emotions; thoughts; creative ability; imagination; and skilled sensorimotor functions.

Domain of Neuroscience

The goal of neuroscience is to identify and explain the mechanisms the brain uses to acquire and regulate higher mental functions and to produce both basic and skilled actions. The biologic basis of such functions interfaces with both the cellular activities and the mind, the seat of consciousness and mental processes. The scope of neuroscience includes the study of the anatomic structures, cellular functions, and physiologic processes of the nervous system. Neuroscience provides a foundation for the study of normal anatomy and physiology of the brain, making it possible for clinicians to identify sites of structural and functional abnormalities in patients exhibiting altered functions. Site of a lesion is indicated by sensory, motor, cognitive, and behavioral changes, all of which reflect the involvement of one or more specific areas of the brain. Neuroscience is indispensable for understanding the physiologic relationships among speech, language, gestures, and cognition.

Domain of Speech-Language-Hearing Pathology

Speech-language-hearing pathology deals with the normal mental processes and disorders (developmental and acquired) of human cognition, language, and speech. Speech-language-hearing pathologists receive comprehensive training in normal development and in abnormal aspects of human communicative processes, including clinical assessment and therapeutic management of such communication disorders. With an extensive background in the physiology and psychology of communication, speech-language-hearing pathologists are also trained to undertake or assist in the neurolinguistic assessment of the behavioral effects of neurologic injury and to pursue research in brain–behavior relationships.

Need for Training in Neuroscience

An understanding of both the development and clinical nature of communicative disorders necessitates a functionally adequate background in neuroscience. Recent advances in medical care have generally increased longevity, prolonging the life span of many patients. This care has required comprehensive interdisciplinary rehabilitative intervention, especially in the field of speech-language-hearing pathology. Furthermore, there is an ever-increasing number of patients

with cognitive and communicative disorders, resulting from **head trauma, vascular accidents, embryologic malformations, degenerative conditions, senility, tumors, epilepsy,** and a variety of **congenital and acquired organic disorders** (Box 1-1). Such patients require special rehabilitative intervention, which demands not only the interaction of speech-language-hearing pathology with neuroscience but also clinicians trained in **neuroanatomy, neurophysiology,** and **neurology.** The application of training in neuroscience is not restricted to adult patients with neurologic conditions; neuroscience is also important in the treatment and understanding of communicative disorders across the spectrum of ages and disorders. Training in neuroscience can be integrated throughout the speech-language-hearing curriculum. However, because of its comprehensiveness and complexity, neuroscience is best studied as a separate course taken at the beginning of graduate-level academic and clinical training.

Nature of Training in Neuroscience

A well-trained professional in communicative disorders and human behavior must obtain a working knowledge of neuroanatomy, neurophysiology, and neurology. Knowledge of how nerve cells communicate, how their axons serve as pathways for transmitting information to other cortical or subcortical regions, and at what point they cross the midline provides a basis for understanding the neurologic correlates of higher mental functions and sensorimotor behavior. Training in neuroscience facilitates a grasp of the neurolinguistic properties of the human brain and provides clini-

---

BOX 1-1

Neurologic Disorders in the United States

More than 20% (about 50 million people) of the U.S. population is estimated to have some form of chronic or acquired neurologic disorder; roughly 15 million of these individuals have either a developmental or an acquired communicative–cognitive disorder (Castro 2004). Because of increasing longevity and a rapidly lowering average age for cerebral pathology, stroke not only constitutes the cause of > 50% of cases of brain dysfunction but has become the leading cause of aphasia and the third leading cause of death and disability in adults. Stroke affects 600,000–700,000 people each year. Furthermore, as the number of people living into their 80s and beyond increases, so have the challenges and demands for supportive and rehabilitative services for dementia and other disorders. Specialists in speech-language-hearing pathology provide valuable care for these patients.

cians in communicative disorders with a broader and better understanding of the origin of illness, the sensorimotor pathways, and the structural properties and potentials of the brain. This understanding helps us appreciate the rationale underlying neurologic management and contributes to a more effectively structured and realistic rehabilitation program for communication disorders.

The prevailing attitude that there is a simpler version of neuroscience related to hearing, speech, language, and mental functions is not accurate. The fundamental sensorimotor rules that apply to locomotion also apply to complex skills in speaking. Similarly, the mental processes in the brain are represented by their combined elementary operations. Thus, some depth of discussion is unavoidable in learning neuroscience. However, students of behavioral science need not undergo the extensive training in neuroscience generally given to neurologists and neurosurgeons. Audiologists, speech-language pathologists, psychologists, and neurolinguists need basic familiarity with the functional and anatomic organization of the nervous system, including the cerebral cortex, the subcortical structures, and the spinal cord.

Benefits of Training in Neuroscience

On a technical level, familiarity with the fundamentals of neuroscience does more than provide professionals in behavioral science, such as speech-language-hearing pathologists, with an understanding of the origins of medical conditions associated with communicative disorders. Training also enables these clinicians and researchers to appreciate the signs and symptoms associated with abnormalities of subcortical and cortical areas, to comprehend the principles of differential diagnosis, and to interpret neuroimaging. Such skills facilitate the recognition of clinically significant symptoms—covert and overt—and the detection of life-threatening conditions associated with a variety of cortical and subcortical pathologic processes.

Students of communicative disorders and human behavior trained in neuroscience have an improved ability to provide effective and realistic clinical services. Their background in neuroscience makes them creative partners on a diagnostic team and helps forge a constructive working relationship with medical colleagues from a variety of disciplines (neurology, neurosurgery, radiology, pediatrics, and physiatry). Clinicians trained in neuroscience are able to appreciate the rationale of neurologic diagnoses, follow scientific literature, understand complex medical terminology, help solve neurologic problems, and promote neurolinguistic research; thus, they have a broad view of their profession.

SCOPE OF NEUROSCIENCE

Neurologic assessment and management involve many branches of neuroscience. A neurologic diagnosis means identifying symptoms that characterize a particular disease and answering fundamental questions: What is the cause? Is it inflammatory, traumatic, genetic, psychological, or a combination? Which anatomic structures are involved? On what side of the neuroaxis (left or right) is the lesion located? As mentioned earlier, knowledge of the anatomy of the nervous system is often essential to diagnosing a neurologic problem, determining the cause, and localizing the lesion. The key for understanding the distribution and localization of deficits is knowledge of the neuroanatomic pathways in the nervous system, their cortical projections, sites of decussation, and interactions with other functional systems. Relating the signs and symptoms with the site of the lesion helps the clinician to arrive at a diagnosis and recommendation for treatment. Access to family history provides information about the onset, susceptibility, and severity of the deficit. The most important branches of neuroscience are listed in Table 1-1.

Table 1-1	
Branches of Neuroscience	

Branch	Domain
Neurology	Diagnosis and treatment of nervous system disorders
Neurosurgery	Surgery for removal of pathologic structures that impair functional organization of nervous system
Neuroanatomy	Structural framework of nervous system, consisting of nerve cells (neurons) and their tracts (fibers)
Neuroradiology	Imaging techniques for differentiating pathologic changes of central nervous system; radiation therapy for nervous system tumors is a subspecialty
Neuroembryology	Embryologic origins and development of nervous system
Neurophysiology	Chemical, electrical, and metabolic functions of nervous system
Neuropathology	Characteristics and origins of diseases and their effects on nervous system

Neurology

Neurology deals with diseases that disrupt the normal structural and physiologic properties of the nervous system. Neurologic conditions include the following: **vascular disorders** (thrombosis, embolism, hemorrhage); **neoplastic conditions** (benign or malignant tumor); **degenerative conditions** (amyotrophic lateral sclerosis, multiple sclerosis, Pick disease, Alzheimer disease); **motor disorders** (Parkinson disease and chorea); **deficiency disorders** (Wernicke-Korsakoff syndrome); **bacterial and viral infections** (meningitis, poliomyelitis, encephalitis); and **epileptic disorders** (Table 1-2). From clinical history, the neurologist derives crucial information about the disease process and uses the data obtained from the clinical examination of sensory and motor functions and laboratory testing to diagnose and determine the site, nature, and cause of the pathol-

ogy to recommend proper treatment. The neurologist, with a keen interest in human behavior, also uses information from the assessment of higher mental functions before making the final diagnosis (Table 1-3). The neurologist also employs data from disordered processes of communication and cognition to understand normal aspects of the neurolinguistic organization. For comprehensive assessment of higher mental functions (language, speech, memory, attention, and cognition), the neurologist depends on the speech-language-hearing pathologist.

Neurosurgery

Neurosurgery involves surgical intervention to treat a disease of the nervous system. Surgical access to the nervous system requires penetration of structures such as the skull, vertebral column, and meninges (brain and spinal cord

---

Table 1-2

Major Brain Diseases

Disorder	Description
Cerebrovascular accident (stroke)	Loss of sensory, motor, speech, and language functions caused by interruptions of blood supply to brain
Neoplasm	Abnormal or new formation of tissue (benign or malignant tumor), which may infiltrate, invade, and destroy normal structures
Demyelination	
Multiple sclerosis	Progressive autoimmune disease in which degeneration of axonal myelin in central nervous system affects nerve conduction Clinically characterized by symptoms such as weakness, incoordination, and speech disturbance, which often come and go
Degeneration	
Alzheimer disease	Progressive degenerative disease of brain Leading cause of dementia
Amyotrophic lateral sclerosis	Degenerative condition in which atrophy of motor neurons of spinal cord and cortex results in muscular weakness and spasticity
Motor disorders	
Huntington chorea	Progressive brain disease of dominant inheritance appearing in mid-30s Leads to dementia and chorea
Parkinson disease	Progressive disease of brain characterized by tremor, slowness of movement, and reduced muscular strength affecting motor speech
Cerebral palsy	Motor disorder with or without language and cognitive deficits in children Caused by damage to cerebrum before, during, or after birth
Deficiency disorders	Amnesia, confabulation, and psychosis caused by thiamine deficiency due to chronic alcoholism (Wernicke-Korsakoff syndrome)
Bacterial and viral infections	Inflammation of membranes covering spinal cord and cortical surface; also called meningitis
Epilepsy	Impairment of sensory, motor, cognitive, and affective functions caused by abnormal electrical activity in brain; also called seizures

Table 1-3

Common Areas Included in a Neurologic Assessment

Motor Examination	Sensory Examination	Mental Functions
Reflexes	Reflexes	Language
Superficial and tendon	Testing of sensory functions	Auditory comprehension (commands
Testing of motor functions	Pain and temperature	and yes/no questions)
Gait	Touch	Spontaneous speech (picture description
Muscle coordination	Nonlocalized touch	and conversation)
Involuntary movements	Two-point touch	Naming (common objects)
Muscle tone (resistance to	Kinesthetic sensation	Repetition (digits, words, and clauses)
passive limb manipulation)	Proprioceptive sensation	Reading (written commands)
Muscle strength	Sensation of vibration	Writing (dictation and picture description)
Cranial nerve examination	Stereognosis	Memory
Lens accommodation and pupil	Graphesthesia	Short term (recall of two objects in 4 min)
light reflex (CN II, CN III)	Cranial nerve examination	Long term (past presidents)
Eye movements (CN III, CN IV,	Smell (CN I)	Nonverbal tasks
CN VI)	Vision (CN II)	Copying (figures)
Facial movements	Visual acuity	Drawing (clock)
Jaw movement (CN V)	Visual fields	Calculation (multiplication tables and
Facial strength, expression,	Sensation from the face, mouth,	basic subtraction)
and articulation (CN VII)	nose, and eyes (CN V)	Abstraction (divergent/convergent
Resonance, phonation, and	Hearing and equilibrium (CN VIII)	thinking tasks)
speech (CN IX, CN X, CN XII)		
Head rotation & shoulder		
elevation (CN XI)		
Tongue movement (CN XII)		
Swallowing (CN IX, CN X)		

coverings). Neurosurgical intervention is used for common conditions such as removal of neoplastic (tumor) tissue, extraction of **blood clots** (hematoma), excision of **vascular aneurysms**, removal of **carotid arterial plaque**, ablation of functionally impaired "convulsing" tissues (epileptogenic scars), **placement of selective lesions** in the thalamus (thalamotomy) for Parkinson disease, placement of therapeutic brain stimulation electrodes in the mesothalamus (deep brain stimulation) for chronic pain and dyskinesia, and removal of **herniated disks** in the spine. Neurosurgery also involves intensive care management of patients neurologically ill from traumatic injury and other neurologic diseases. Pediatric neurosurgery has a special place in neurosurgery because of the high frequency of surgically amenable diseases that are diagnosed in infants and children.

Neuroanatomy

Neuroanatomy relates to the structural organization of the nervous system. It grossly and microscopically defines the structural elements of the nervous system, specifically neurons, fiber tracts, nerves, ventricular structures, vascular networks, and supporting glial and meningeal tissues.

Neuroradiology

Neuroradiology enables the diagnosis of cranial, spinal, and **peripheral nervous system** (PNS) abnormalities without intrusion into the cranial cavity and body tissues. It uses emission or transmission imaging to identify intact and pathologic structures of the nervous system. Some modern neuroradiologic techniques are **x-ray, angiography, computer tomography (CT), magnetic resonant imaging (MRI), single photon emission computed tomography (SPECT),** and **positron emission tomography (PET).** Advances in neuroradiology have not only revolutionized the study of the brain–behavior relationship but have also revealed the interaction between brain structures and behavioral (psychiatric) disorders. Therapeutic radiation is also used to treat various malignant body and brain tumors (with a γ-knife) and is often combined with drug treatment (chemotherapy) and tumor excision.

Neuroembryology

Neuroembryology deals with growth of the nervous system during the embryonic period of development extending from conception to 7 weeks, at which time all brain structures have anatomically emerged. **Teratology** is the study of fetal malformations and monstrosities, which have serious implications for the development of higher mental functions.

Neurophysiology

Neurophysiology focuses on the functional properties of the nervous system with respect to the structural, chemical, and electrical composition that is essential to living organisms.

Neuropathology

Neuropathology deals with the nature and cause of diseased tissue that structurally and functionally disrupts the nervous system.

PRINCIPLES GOVERNING FUNCTIONAL ORGANIZATION OF THE HUMAN BRAIN

Although the human brain has a complex anatomic organization, its functions are regulated by a set of simple principles. Taken together, these simple organizational principles account not only for complex anatomic details but also for all the processes underlying brain functions. Eight common regulating principles of the human brain are given in Table 1-4.

Interconnectivity in the Brain

All functionally specific primary sensory and motor regions in the **cerebrum** are connected through association and commissural fibers. The cortical association areas are directly connected to each other, whereas the primary cortical areas are indirectly connected through the cortical association areas. The homologous areas of the two hemispheres are connected through the **interhemispheric com-**

missural fibers. This integrated network allows constant interaction within each hemisphere and between the two hemispheres of the brain and explains how messages from multiple sources are rapidly integrated for an appropriate response to given stimuli.

Centrality of the Central Nervous System

The **central nervous system** (CNS) is responsible for integrating all incoming and outgoing information and for generating appropriate responses to the information received. The response can be volitional (internally generated), such as a spontaneous motor movement. Conversely, the response can be a reflex (environmentally elicited), such as withdrawal of a limb.

Because of the centrality of decision making and the all-encompassing response, no two parts in the peripheral body can directly communicate with each other, regardless of the distance between them. Even the simplest form of communication between two adjacent body parts, such as the thumb and palm (as exemplified in the basic reflexes), is mediated through the CNS. The outgoing motor response is always different from the incoming sensory information. A motor command in response to a sensory stimulus contains a directive that was refined and synthesized with additional informative stimuli from other sources of the neuraxis. The ability to analyze and synthesize multiple sources of information and to generate distinct responses exemplifies the centralized organization and function of the brain.

Hierarchy of Neuraxial Organization

The neuraxis of the CNS is hierarchically developed in complexity and organization of functions. Lower levels of organization perform inherent specific functions that are modified to varying degrees by the axial segments above. The spinal cord, the lowest level of organization, serves simple sensorimotor functions in the form of basic reflexes that are partly influenced by the upper axial levels. The complexity of information processing increases as the level of processing becomes more cephalic, or brain controlled. The cerebral cortex, the highest organizational level, is responsible for complex sensorimotor integration and higher mental functions (cognition, language, and speech). Functionally different neuronal structures also exist in the brainstem and **diencephalon**, the intermediate level of organization. These structures consist of autonomic, chemical, and visceral systems, all of which contribute to the regulation of consciousness, blood pressure, respiration, sleep, temperature, endocrine, and neurotransmitter interactions. Together these systems react to nonspecific stress and adverse bodily changes to maintain optimal homeostatic states. The intermediate level of organization, which may be considered the nonthinking part of the brain, is tightly integrated with the cerebral cortex, which serves the highest organization level of decision making.

Table 1-4
Organizational Principles of the Brain

Interconnectivity in brain
Centrality of central nervous system
Hierarchy of neuraxial organization
Laterality of brain organization
Structural and functional specialization
Topographical organization in cortical pathways
Plasticity in brain
Culturally neutral brain

Laterality of Brain Organization

The three most important aspects of brain organization are (1) bilateral anatomic symmetry between the two hemispheres, (2) unilateral functional differences, and (3) contralateral sensorimotor control of the nervous system.

Bilateral Anatomic Symmetry

Anatomically, the two cerebral hemispheres are essentially similar, with only minor differences. In terms of language dominance, there is a differential function of one region of the temporal lobe (**planum temporale**) between the two sides of the brain. Mostly, lesions on the left hemisphere affect language functions more than on the right side of the brain. Enlargement of the temporal planum on the left compared to the right is associated with the sidedness in function. Both hemispheres are connected through the **corpus callosum**, the largest of the commissural fibers.

Unilateral Functional Differences

Immediately after birth, the two cerebral hemispheres are functionally equipotential; each hemisphere has the functional capacity to develop all types of skills. However, after the first few years, each hemisphere acquires an advantage over the other for different specialized functions. Most people's left hemisphere becomes dominant for language, speech, and analytic processing irrespective of handedness; the right hemisphere dominates emotions, musical skills, metaphors, and humor. The right half of the brain is also involved with temporospatial attributes and regulating paralinguistic features, such as stress and intonation.

Contralateral Sensorimotor Control

A unique aspect of brain organization is that all sensory and motor fibers in the nervous system **decussate** (cross) the body's midline. The left motor cortex controls movements in the right half of the body; the sensory information from the left half of the body projects to the right sensory cortex (Fig. 1-1). Most sensory and motor fibers cross the midline in the caudal medulla of the brainstem. Fibers carrying pain and temperature cross the midline in the spinal cord. Some pathways, such as those for hearing, cross at numerous levels in the brainstem.

Functionally Specialized Networking

One striking aspect of cortical organization is that the neuronal systems are functionally specialized. Sensory and motor systems possess specialized nerve cells that are functionally specific, separable, and part of a selected network. Consequently, white matter in the brain is composed of many parallel pathways, each of which conducts different types of information. For example, sensory fibers carry sensations of pain, fine touch, and temperature; these fibers run parallel to one another and serve distinct functions that are determined by sensory receptor terminals in the peripheral body parts. The motor system also consists of several parallel but distinct pathways that transmit differentiated motor

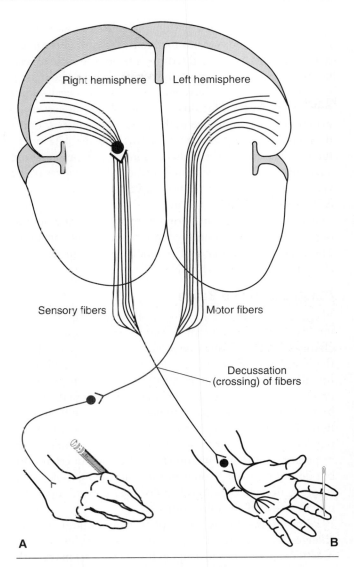

Figure 1-1 Contralateral brain organization. **A.** The descending motor fibers decussate before synapsing on the spinal motor neurons. **B.** The ascending sensory fibers also cross the midline before projecting to the contralateral somatosensory cortex.

information to different limbs. For example, one path mediates skilled hand movements from the cortical and subcortical structures to the upper spinal cord, whereas the second transmits postural adjustment messages throughout the spinal cord and brainstem for trunk and limb movements. A third pathway controls speech muscles in the face and neck through cranial nerves in the brainstem. The functional specialization of nerve cells refers to their increased adaptability, processing speed, and ability to make detailed analysis of selected signals.

Topographical Organization in Cortical Pathways

A remarkable feature of the somatosensory system is that the spatial arrangement of peripheral receptors in the body is discretely maintained within the information-carrying pathway and is projected to the brain. The spatial organization of neurons, tracts, and terminals reflects the spatial relationships of the body surface and functionally related muscle groups. Therefore, the cerebral cortex is organized with a **somatosensory homunculus.** For example, an orderly visual map is discretely projected to the visual cortex by way of the thalamus. This map is retained throughout the pathway to the visual cortex. There is also continuity of representation; adjacent visual fields are represented in adjacent areas of the visual cortex. A similar relationship exists between a delineated area in the auditory cortex and the frequency-specific cells in the cochlea. Furthermore, there is a topographical organization in the brain for sensory and motor functions. These topographic maps of functions help clinicians precisely locate lesions in the CNS.

Plasticity in the Brain

Plasticity refers to the brain's ability to reorganize and modify tissue functions and adapt to internal and external changes. The inherent plasticity of brain cells permits the integration of specific cortical areas to serve additional functions and to repair cortical circuitry in response to pathology, such as stroke. This adaptive property of the brain explains the reorganizational capacity of cellular functions. Regeneration of nerves (sprouting) occurs to varying degrees in the nervous system. However, inflammatory responses, scar tissue, and protein expression, interfere with but do not necessarily prevent the establishment of axonal reconnections in the CNS. The PNS has a greater opportunity to re-establish connections.

The brain's ability to adapt to external and internal changes has important implications for learning because functional plasticity and adaptability are greatest in the early years and gradually diminish with age; learning is better accomplished if one is given early experiences. Early exposure not only facilitates learning but also results in a finer and more efficient processing of information. Fine-tuning of the internal system is best illustrated by acquisition of a second language or musical knowledge in the early years.

Brain regions are genetically either committed or uncommitted to specific functions. For example, the brainstem possesses automatic control systems that are genetically acquired and cannot be modified. The functions involving the association of cortical areas are programmed through experience and are modifiable in the young. Developing cellular density, connectivity to target areas, and synaptic patterns plays an important role in the functional plasticity of cerebral tissue in early life. For the brain's functional reorganization, the **critical period** is another important concept; this is the period when an experience is most effective in influencing the brain's potential. It is best illustrated by the axonal connectivity to the visual cortex in the fetal period when the axons carrying visual input from both eyes have equal access to the visual cortex and equally compete for the available synaptic spaces. If for any reason,

axons from one eye are not functional during this developmentally critical period, they lose the claim for synaptic spaces in the visual cortex. This allows for the axonal fibers from the good eye to become dominant and take initiative for controlling the available synaptic space in the brain, suggesting that it is not the experience alone, but rather the timing of the experience that regulates the potential for functional plasticity.

Furthermore, the evidence involving the somatosensory representation in the cortex suggests that to a certain extent the tissue-function reorganization continues throughout adult life. If a digit is amputated, for example, the afferents to the cortex from this digit are lost, and the target cortical area receives no sensory inputs. However, with functional reorganization, the tissue in the affected sensory cortex has been found to respond to stimuli from the intact digits adjacent to the amputated digit (Kingsley 1999). Similar observations of a tissue functional reorganization have been made during cortical stimulation. Within hours of the resectioning of a motor nerve, researchers observed the brain area that earlier controlled the muscles innervated by the sectioned nerve now regulated a different group of muscles (Donohue and Sanes 1988).

Culturally Neutral Brain

Although the brain contains complex architectural organization, multiple interconnected pathways, and functionally independent specialized areas, its basic functioning is straightforward. Its operations are not governed by any personal characteristics of gender, color, or cultural variations. The brain's functioning is unaffected by normal variations in size, shape, or weight. Its power is judged by the efficiency with which it remembers, processes information, generates responses, attends to tasks, plans, programs, makes decisions, and projects information.

ORIENTATION TO BASIC TERMINOLOGY

A set of descriptive terms is used in neuroscience to indicate direction and position of structures with respect to their relative orientation within the brain. Special terminology is also used for visually delineating anatomic structures according to the various planes of brain sections.

Directional Brain Orientation

To understand the directional orientation of the human nervous system, it is important to consider first the brain of a mammal such as a dog, which because of its quadrupedal posture exemplifies a simpler axial organization. The CNS of the dog is organized in a straight (anteroposterior) line in the horizontal plane of the body. The term **rostral** refers to locations toward the nose; **caudal** refers to locations toward the tail; **dorsal** refers to locations toward the back, and **ventral** refers to locations toward the abdomen (Fig. 1-2).

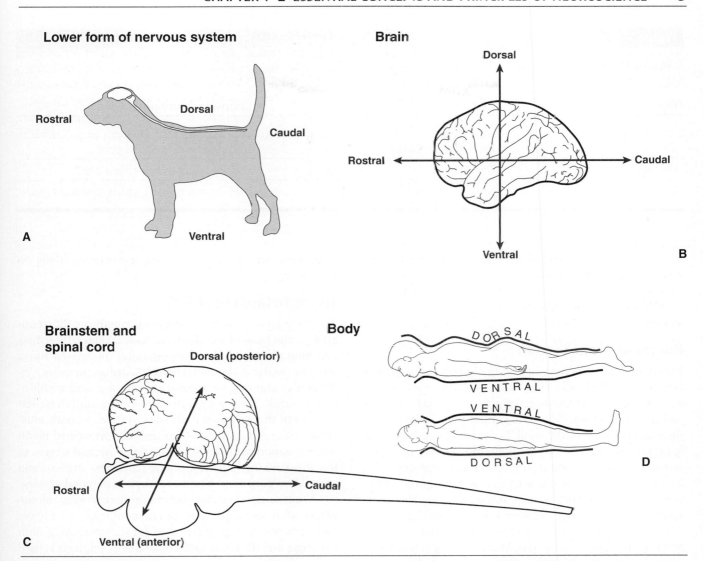

Figure 1-2 Nervous system axes and directional terms. **A.** The nervous system in lower primates develops along a straight line. **B.** The human nervous system is organized along horizontal and vertical axes because of the cephalic flexure at the junction of the cerebral hemisphere and midbrain. For the cerebral hemisphere and diencephalon, the directions of these terms change systematically. **C.** The directional terms used for the spinal cord and brainstem are similar to those employed for lower vertebrates. **D.** The directional terms on the human body surface.

This directional terminology is consistently used for referring to structures in the CNS; however, usage is slightly different in humans. During phylogenetic development, the longitudinal CNS system bends just above the brainstem. This cephalic flexure results in the spinal cord and brainstem developing vertically and the forebrain developing horizontally (Fig. 1-2). Therefore, in humans, the CNS (brain and spinal cord) is organized along two different axes: horizontal (brain) and vertical (spinal cord).

Because of this axial difference in structural orientation, the terms used for describing the positions of structures in the CNS vary (Table 1-5). For the forebrain above the cephalic flexure (bend), *rostral* refers to locations toward the nose and *caudal* refers to locations toward the back of the brain, whereas *dorsal* refers to the top of the brain and

ventral refers to the lower brain toward the jaw. The directions of these terms below the cephalic flexure (neuraxial bend) systematically change and are similar to the ones used for lower vertebrates. For the spinal cord and brainstem, *rostral* refers to locations toward the brain, *caudal* refers to the coccygeal end of the spinal cord, *dorsal* refers to locations toward the back of the body and *ventral* refers to locations toward the abdomen.

The PNS has two types of information-carrying fibers: **sensory (afferent)** and **motor (efferent)**. *Afferent fibers* carry sensory information from the body to the CNS. *Efferent fibers* carry motor impulses from the brain and spinal cord to the periphery of the body to contract muscles and activate gland secretion. **Decussation** refers to the crossing of incoming or outgoing fibers at the

Table 1-5		
Terms Indicating Direction		
Direction	Cerebrum	Brainstem and Spinal Cord
Rostral	Near front of head	Near or toward brain
Caudal	Back of brain or head	Coccygeal end of spinal cord
Dorsal	Top of brain	Back of brainstem or spinal cord
Ventral	Bottom of brain	Belly or anterior in quadrupeds and bipeds

midline (Fig. 1-1). **Proximal** and **distal** are defined by their relation to the CNS. Proximal refers to structures relatively close to a specific anatomic site of reference, whereas distal identifies the position of structures farther from the same anatomic site of reference.

Planes of Brain Section

Not all cortical structures are on the brain's surface. Some can be examined only after sectioning the brain, which may be cut into three primary planes: **sagittal, coronal,** and **horizontal** (Fig. 1-3). The sagittal plane, named after the sagittal suture in the skull, is a vertical cut that passes longitudinally and divides the brain into left and right portions. A sagittal section at the center separates the brain into two equal halves and is called the **midsagittal** cut. A coronal plane, a vertical section made perpendicular to the sagittal section, divides the brain into front and back parts. A horizontal plane, a cut perpendicular to both coronal and sagittal planes, divides the brain into upper and lower parts. A cross-section of the spinal cord at a right angle to its longitudinal axis divides the cord into upper and lower portions (Fig. 1-3; Table 1-6).

There are three other important orientation terms regarding brain planes: **transverse, lateral,** and **medial.** A transverse plane is a crosscut at a right angle to the longitudinal axis on a bend. Because of the curvature of the brainstem, this plane is diagonal to the horizontal (cross) plane (Fig. 1-3; Table 1-6). *Lateral* and *medial* derive their meanings from their context in a midsagittal section: *lateral* refers to structures away from a the midsagittal plane, whereas *medial* refers to a plane approaching the midsagittal plane.

Terms Related to Movement

Several technical terms are used to denote specific aspects of directional movement involving the muscular structures (Fig. 1-4). **Flexion** refers to the bending movement of a limb. **Extension** refers to the straightening movement of a limb. **Abduction** denotes a movement in which a limb is moved away from the central axis of the body. **Adduction** denotes a movement that brings a limb toward the central axis of the body. **Pronation** is the movement that turns the palm downward (or sleeping on the belly), and **supina-**

tion is the action that turns the palm upward (lying on the back).

Terms Related to Muscles

The three kinds of muscle fibers in the body are differentiated on the basis of histologic structure: **skeletal, cardiac,** and **smooth.** Skeletal muscles consist of striated fibers and are under volitional control. Cardiac muscles, although containing striated fibers, are not under voluntary control. They are controlled by the cardiovascular reflexes of the **autonomic nervous system.** Smooth muscles consist of nonstriated fibers and are considered involuntary. Smooth muscle is found in the internal organs of the digestive system, respiratory passages, urinary and genital tracts, urinary bladder, and walls of blood vessels.

Limb paralysis can involve one or more muscles: **monoplegia** refers to the paralysis of either an upper or a lower limb, whereas **hemiplegia** is used for the paralysis of both the upper and the lower limbs on one side. **Triplegia** is used to describe the paralysis of three limbs (both extremities on one side and one on the other side), and **quadriplegia** refers to a paralysis pattern involving all four limbs. **Paraplegia** refers to the paralysis of both lower limbs.

Terms Related to Anatomic Structures

The bony cavity of the skull restricts expansion of the cortical mantle containing nerve cells; consequently, the human cortex is highly convoluted, giving the brain a folded appearance (Fig. 2-3). The crest of every fold is called a **gyrus** (pl. gyri), or **convolution.** The groove or valley separating adjacent gyri is called the **sulcus** (pl. sulci), or **fissure** (in case of greater depth). **Opercular** refers to the margins of the cerebral convolutions serving as a cover. For example, the margins of the operculum of three lobes cover the **insular cortex** (see Fig. 2-13). A **commissure** is a band of fibers connecting part of the brain or spinal cord on one side with the same structures on the opposite side of the midline.

Somites are a series of mesodermal tissue blocks found on each side of the neural tube during the embryonic period (see Chapter 4). **Somatic structures** include most axial skeletal and associated muscles that are derived from the

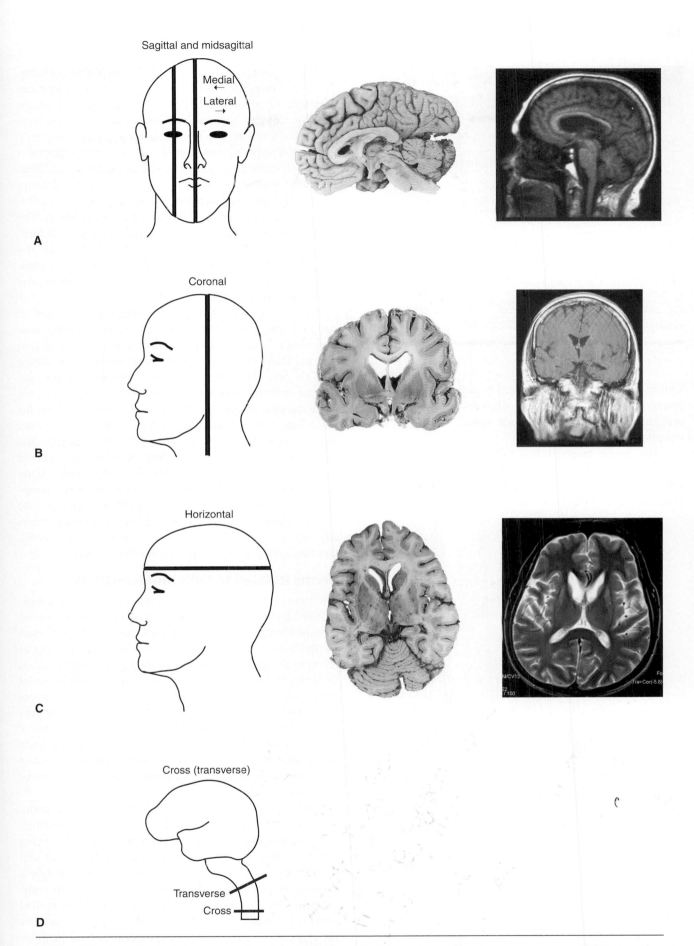

Figure 1-3 The planes of the human brain and spinal cord with corresponding brain sections and MRI images.

Table 1-6

Terms for Brain Sections

Section	Description
Coronal	Vertical section into front (rostral) and back (caudal)
Sagittal	Vertical division into left and right
Midsagittal	Vertical division into two equal parts
Horizontal	Cross-section division into upper and lower portions
Transverse	Diagonal to cross-plane at curving brainstem
Lateral	Structures away from midline
Medial	Structures toward midline

somite. **Viscera** refers to internal organs containing non-striated muscles, such as the digestive, respiratory, and urogenital organs; smooth glands; spleen; heart; and great vessels.

The prefix **inter-** denotes "between" and describes a structure common to both hemispheres. The *interhemispheric fissure,* for example, is a sulcus that divides the two hemispheres. Similarly, a fiber bundle that connects the

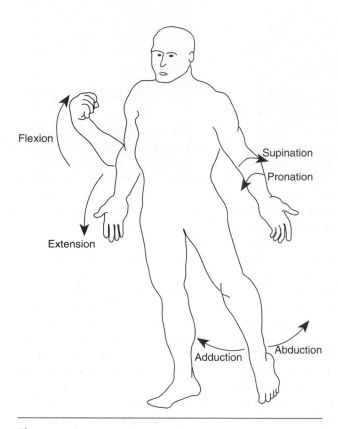

Figure 1-4 Body movements.

two hemispheres is called an **interhemispheric pathway.** The prefix **intra-** denotes "within"; consequently, an **intrahemispheric structure** is one that is located within the substance of that hemisphere. Fibers connecting two areas within the same hemisphere make up an **intrahemispheric pathway.** The prefix **ipsi-** denotes "same," and **ipsilateral** is used to describe lesions on one side of the brain that affect the same side of the body. Conversely, **contra-** denotes "opposite," and **contralateral** is used to describe involvement of the body on the side opposite a brain lesion. The prefix **pre-**, as in the word **presynaptic**, indicates "before" and is used to discuss the area on the proximal side of a synaptic cleft, the contact point between two cells; **postsynaptic** denotes the area distal to a synaptic cleft involving the second neuron.

A clinician should be familiar with the terms used to describe the temporal profile of neurologic symptoms. Neurologic symptoms can be classified as **transient** or **persistent.** Transient symptoms resolve completely; persistent ones do not. There are three types of persistent symptoms: symptoms that reach a maximum level of severity and do not change are called **static** or **stationary,** symptoms that reach a maximum severity and then begin to resolve are called **improving,** and symptoms that continue to worsen are called **progressive.** Terms referring to the rapidity of changes in the temporal profile are **acute, subacute,** and **chronic.** Acute symptoms evolve over minutes to hours. Subacute symptoms develop over days to weeks and fall between the acute and the chronic classifications. Subacute symptoms generally indicate the course of a disease of moderate severity. Chronic symptoms develop over months to years.

Terms Related to Cells and Functions

The brain consists of 10–15 billion nerve cells (**neurons,** grossly identified as **gray matter**) and their processes (axons, grossly identified as **white matter** and **dendrites**); two-thirds of the neurons are hidden within sulci. Gray matter refers to the gross appearance of the brain, which consists of nerve cells, supporting glia cells, and many unmyelinated fibers. Nerve cells are concentrated in the cerebral cortex as layers and in the subcortex as nuclei. The cells appear gray in the absence of myelin. White matter is made of nerve fibers that form tracts and carry information from one brain site to another. It is white because of the white appearance of the myelin lipid (fatlike) substance surrounding many of the axons.

The neuron is the basic building block in the brain, and it is responsible for generating, receiving, transmitting, and synthesizing electrical impulses as well as influencing other neurons or effector tissue. **Glial cells** protect and support the nerve cells. A typical neuron is bounded by a continuous plasma membrane and consists of a **cell body, dendrites,** and an **axon** (Fig. 1-5). The cell body, also called **soma** (pl. somata) or **perikaryon** (pl. perikarya), contains the cytoplasm with important organelles, such as the **mitochondria, ribosomes, rough endoplasmic reticulum,** and

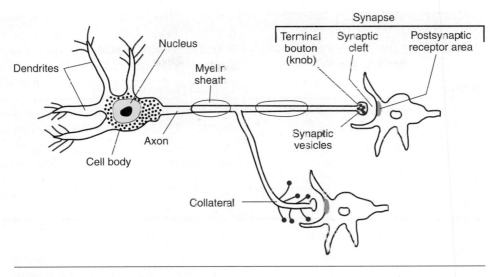

Figure 1-5 A typical nerve cell.

Golgi complex, needed for cellular metabolism. Also contained in the cytoplasm is a nucleus, which contains ladder-like micromolecules of DNA with the genetic blueprint and is responsible for vital cellular activities. Dendrites, highly specialized processes that look like trees, receive neural signals from other neurons through contacts (synapses).

The axon, arising from the cell body at an elevation called an **axon hillock**, transmits neural messages to other neurons through its synapses (contacts). **Synaptic terminals** (terminal boutons, knobs, or buttons) are the end portions of the axon and contain many vesicles that release neurotransmitters between the end of the axon and the surface of the next nerve cell. This narrow space is called the **synaptic cleft**. Once a neuron is adequately stimulated, a neural impulse travels along the axon, and the terminal boutons (knobs) release the neurotransmitters in the synaptic cleft to activate the receptor site of the next nerve cell. The **synapse** includes the boutons, synaptic cleft, and receptor site of the next nerve cell. A neuron that ends at the synapse is a **presynaptic nerve cell**. A neuron that receives an impulse from a presynaptic neuron is a **postsynaptic neuron**. Impulse movement in the axon can be **anterograde**, by which an impulse travels from the cell body to the axonal terminal, or **retrograde**, by which the flow is from the axonal terminals to the cell body.

Primary cells are responsible for generating the nerve impulses that underlie all sensorimotor and higher mental functions. Serving as supporting structures, glia cells ensure the survival of the primary cells by providing structural and metabolic support. Neurons are specialized for generating inhibitory or excitatory nerve action potentials and using the impulses to affect other cells. The nerve impulses also trigger the secretion of **neurotransmitters**, which are synthesized either in the cell bodies or in the synaptic terminals.

The most intriguing aspect of brain's cellular organization is the mechanism that guides the connectivity of axons to the predetermined target areas. The early developing axons are the pathfinding fibers, and their growth cones actively spot the target cell surfaces. Because not all of the synaptic connections survive, trophic factors must play an important role in the survival of neurons and their synapses. In general, an overabundance of neurons are produced during normal development and > 50% of neurons in some areas die a natural and programmed death during development (apoptosis); most of these cells die because of their inability to establish synaptic connections or because they develop weak connections.

Terminology of the Central and Peripheral Nervous Systems

A well-defined collection of nerve cells in the CNS is called a **nucleus** or **cell column**; a similar collection of nerve cells in the PNS is called a **ganglion** (Table 1-7). A sensory ganglion contains cell bodies of the sensory nerves; there are no synapses around cell bodies. A motor ganglion of the **autonomic nervous system** (ANS) contains cell bodies of fibers that supply the smooth muscles and glands.

Nerve fibers transmit information. A collection of nerve fibers that share a common origin is called a **tract** or **fasciculus** in the CNS. Another name for a bundle of connecting pathways is **brachium**, which is specifically used for the pathway connecting the **cerebellum** to the brainstem. **Stria** is used to denote a band of fibers that may differ in color and/or texture. **Colliculus** refers to a small prominence of nervous system tissue. A bundle of fibers in the PNS is called a **nerve** or **nerve trunk** (Table 1-7). Axial structures are differentiated from the appendicular structures. **Axial** refers to the central part of the body and is made up of the head and trunk. **Appendicular** relates to the limbs, which are attached to the axial structures.

Table 1-7

Terms Used for Describing the Neuronal Structures of the Nervous System

Central Nervous System	Peripheral Nervous System
Nucleus (pl. nuclei)—mass of neurons usually deep in brain; examples: caudate nucleus, lateral geniculate nucleus (body)	Ganglion (pl. ganglia)—collection of neurons; example: ganglion of trigeminal nerve or dorsal root
Tract—a bundle of parallel axons with a common point of origin and termination; example: corticospinal tract	Nerve—bundle of axons; example: facial nerve[a]
Fasciculus (pl. fasciculi, funiculi)—several tracts	

[a]The optic nerve is the only collection of axons in the central nervous system that is called a nerve.

GROSS STRUCTURES OF THE CENTRAL NERVOUS SYSTEM

The human nervous system is divided into the CNS and PNS. The CNS consists of the brain and the spinal cord. The brain consists of three major structures: cerebrum; brainstem (**midbrain, pons,** and **medulla**); and cerebellum (Fig. 1-6; Table 1-8). Each of these structures performs specific func-

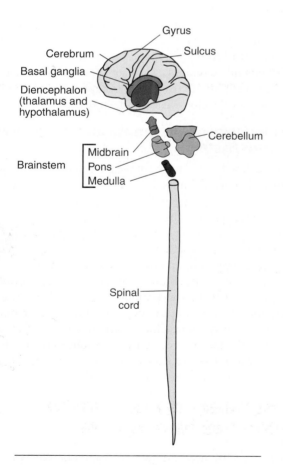

Figure 1-6 The major structures of the central nervous system.

tions. The cerebrum consists of two hemispheres separated by the interhemispheric fissure; each hemisphere contains the cerebral cortex, **basal ganglia,** and diencephalon (**thalamus** and **hypothalamus**).

The cerebral cortex refers to the 3- to 5-mm thick layer of neurons (gray matter) covering the entire surface of the cerebrum. The nerve cells of the cerebral cortex are arranged in horizontal layers. The basic three-layered pattern is called the **archicortex** (hippocampus, amygdala, and septum), the more complex three- to six-layered pattern is found in the highly evolved **mesocortex** (parahippocampal cortex and olfactory bulb), and the highly evolved six-layered pattern is found in the **neocortex** (most of the dorsal and lateral cerebral cortex). The three- to six-layered cortex is vital to short-term memory, emotion-related experiences, and emotional behavioral control. Representing the highest level of phylogenetic development, the six-layered cerebral cortex is essential for higher mental functions (Fig. 1-7). With 10–15 billion neurons, the cerebral cortex is a vital aspect of cortical thalamic circuits that enable all higher symbolic functions required of all vertebrates, and of special importance for humans, it controls language, thinking, memory, and attention.

The *basal ganglia* are the masses of gray matter in the depth of each cerebral hemisphere; the *basal ganglia* serve as an auxiliary motor system and play an important role in the regulation of motor activities by modifying the information received from the motor cortex and returning it to the motor cortex. Secondarily, they are also known to regulate symbolic functions (see Chapter 13).

The *thalamus* is a collection of subcortical nuclei; which are an essential part of the thalamus–cerebral cortex–thalamic circuit, the basic functional circuitry of the forebrain. Integrated closely with the cerebral hemispheres in sensorimotor functions, the thalamic nuclei control circuit activity by evaluating incoming sensory signals before directing them to the specific cortex. The *hypothalamus* is the central site of neuroendocrine production and the central structure for the control of various metabolic activities, such as water balance, sugar and fat metabolism, and body temperature.

Table 1-8

Functions of Brain Structures and the Spinal Cord

Brain Structure	Functions
☐ Cerebrum (cerebral hemispheres and cortex)	Serves higher mental functions (cognition, language, and memory) Regulates sensorimotor integration Relates perceptions with experiences
■ Basal ganglia (subcortical nuclei)	Regulate motor movements and muscle tone
■ Diencephalon	
Thalamus	Channels sensorimotor information to cortex Participates in cortex-mediated functions Regulates crude awareness of sensation
Hypothalamus	Regulates body temperature, food intake, water balance, hormonal secretions, emotional behavior, and sexual responses Controls the activities of autonomic nervous system
■ Midbrain	Mediates auditory and visual reflexes Regulates cortical arousal Houses cranial nerve nuclei
■ Cerebellum	Participates in the coordination of movements and regulation of equilibrium
■ Pons	Contains cranial nerve nuclei and sensory motor regulating fibers
■ Medulla	Contains cranial nerve nuclei Regulates respiration, phonation, heart beat, and blood pressure
☐ Spinal cord	Links body with central nervous system Regulates reflexes

The *brainstem* is composed of the midbrain, pons, and medulla. Besides linking the brainstem with the brain, the *midbrain* controls eye movements, pupil size, and auditory reflexes. The *pons* contains a center responsible for controlling the rhythm of respiration and also regulates facial movements and sensation. The *medulla* controls respiratory activity, heart rate, and blood pressure. In addition to serving specialized functions and controlling cranial nerves, the *midbrain, pons,* and *medulla* contain common sensorimotor fibers and the **reticular formation**, which regulates cortical arousal and attention. The *cerebellum* is dorsal to the brainstem and is attached to it but is not part of it. The *cerebellum* is important in the regulation of skilled movements. The *spinal cord* serves as the reflex-controlling center and contains fibers that run to and from the brain, connecting the brain with peripheral structures.

The PNS is formed by nerves that connect the brain and spinal cord with the peripheral structures. These include both sensory and motor nerves. Conveying pain, touch, and temperature information, the sensory fibers enter the spinal cord via the dorsal roots. The motor fibers that innervate muscles and glands exit through the ventral roots.

FUNCTIONAL CLASSIFICATION OF THE NERVOUS SYSTEM

The human nervous system processes information using two types of cells: **general** and **special**. General information originates from the surface of the body and is processed by

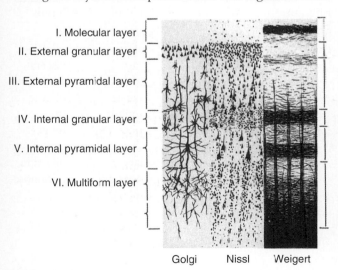

I. Molecular layer
II. External granular layer
III. External pyramidal layer
IV. Internal granular layer
V. Internal pyramidal layer
VI. Multiform layer

Golgi   Nissl   Weigert

Figure 1-7 The cellular layers of the neocortex, the most evolved type of cerebral cortex tissue.

general receptors. Special information is mediated by the receptors to specialized cells in the nervous system. Pain and temperature are examples of general information, whereas vision and audition are examples of special information. Each type (general and special) is involved with body structures that are either **somatic** or **visceral**. *Somatic* refers to striated skeletal muscles that are embryologically derived from somites. *Visceral* nonstriated muscles are concerned with vegetative tasks and relate to the internal vital body organs involved in the respiratory, vascular, and digestive systems. General and special information is divided into somatic and visceral subtypes, both of which include efferent (motor) and afferent (sensory) fibers. The only exception to this classification is the lack of a **special somatic efferent system**. The functional classification consists of seven components and is important for understanding the functioning of spinal and cranial nerves (Table 1-9).

CELLULAR ORGANIZATION (CYTOARCHITECTURE) AND BRODMANN AREAS

As noted, the cerebral neocortex consists of six cellular layers (laminae), which are classified by their neuronal density and architecture as seen under light microscopy: **molecular layer, external granular layer, external pyramidal layer, internal granular layer, internal pyramidal layer,** and **multiform layer** (Fig. 1-7; Table 1-10). Each layer func-

tions as a physiologic module, processing input and giving rise to axons. Some axons project to other cortical areas, and others form the descending tracts. The first three layers, with intercortical and intracortical connections, serve associational functions. The internal granular layer (granular cortex) participates in somatosensation; the fifth layer, with the pyramidal and large Betz cells, gives rise to the descending motor fibers.

Different cortical regions contain varied configurations (thickness) of the cellular layers, reflecting the specialized functions served by each brain area. Various **cyto-architectural** maps of the cellular architecture of the cortex have been constructed. The most frequently used cyto-architectural map in neurologic and neurolinguistic literature is that of Brodmann (1909). Brodmann's architectural map of the cerebral cortex divides the brain into approximately 50 regions and serves as a standard for referring to specific brain areas by a number (Fig. 1-8). For example, Brodmann area 4 is the primary motor cortex, which contains large pyramidal cells (Betz cells) in the leg and foot cortical areas. Sensory cortical areas have more densely packed granular cells and only a few pyramidal cells. Primary sensory areas include the somatosensory cortex in the postcentral gyrus (Brodmann areas 3, 1, 2), the primary visual cortex (Brodmann area 17), and the primary auditory cortex, or gyri of Heschl (Brodmann areas 41 and 42, in the superior temporal gyrus).

Tertiary areas of the temporal, parietal, and prefrontal cortex are called *association areas* of the brain. The association areas are concerned mostly with process-

Table 1-9

Functional Components of the Nervous System

General				Special			
Somatic		Visceral		Somatic		Visceral	
Efferent	Afferent	Efferent	Afferent	Efferent	Afferent	Efferent	Afferent
GSE	GSA	GVE	GVA	SSE	SSA	SVE	SVA
Activates muscles derived from somites, including skeletal, extra-ocular, and glossal (tongue) muscles	Mediates sensory inner-vation from somatic muscles, skin, ligaments, and joints	Projects to muscles of visceral organs, including pupillary constric-tion, gland secretion, and regulation of heart and tracheal muscles	Mediates sensory inner-vation from visceral organs, including larynx, pharynx, and abdomen	Does not exist	Mediates special sensations of vision from retina and of audition and equi-librium from inner ear	Projects to muscles of face, palate, mouth, pharynx, and larynx; does not include eye and tongue muscles	Mediates visceral sensations of taste from tongue and of olfaction from nose

Table 1-10

Six-layered Cerebral Gray Matter

Cellular Layer	Cellular Characteristics
Layer I: molecular	Terminal dendrites and axons from cortical neurons communicate with neighboring cortical areas
Layer II: external granular	Small granular interneurons receive inputs from other cortical regions
Layer III: external pyramidal	Small pyramidal neurons with projections to neighboring ipsilateral and contralateral cerebral cortex and basal ganglia
Layer IV: internal granular	Granular interneurons receive input from thalamus and other subcortical nuclei They form a thick layer in somatosensory, visual, auditory, and vestibular cortex
Layer V: internal pyramidal	Large pyramidal neurons (Betz cells of the primary motor cortex) that project to subcortical sites, such as brainstem, cerebellum, and spinal cord
Layer VI: multiform	Multiform layer with some neuronal projections to basal ganglia and remaining to superficial cellular layers within same cortical area

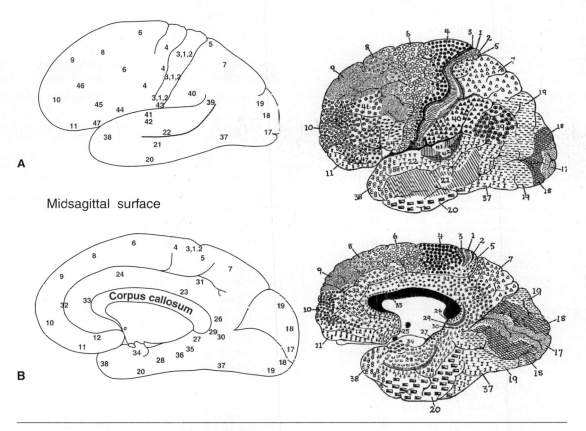

Figure 1-8 Cytoarchitectural map showing the Brodmann areas on the lateral (A) and medial (B) brain surfaces. Important areas include the following: *3, 1, 2,* primary sensory cortex; *4,* primary motor cortex; *5* and *7,* sensory association cortex; *6,* premotor cortex; *17,* primary visual cortex; *18* and *19,* visual association cortex; *22,* association language cortex (Wernicke area); *41,* primary auditory cortex; *42,* association auditory cortex; *44,* motor speech cortex (Broca area). See also Table 1-11.

ing of cross-modality input from other cortical areas and integrating and elaborating complex functions. Familiarity with the commonly used Brodmann areas is necessary for working in medical speech-language-hearing pathology (Table 1-11).

TECHNIQUES FOR SOLVING PROBLEMS WHEN LEARNING NEUROSCIENCE

Students in communicative disorders and disciplines related to human behavior need not feel overwhelmed by the technical terminology, abstract concepts, intricate connections, multiplicity of neuroanatomic structures, or amount of technical material to be learned. Progressively adding knowl-

edge in a methodical and persistent fashion is the best strategy for learning neuroscience. The following practical suggestions will simplify the technical terminology and the abstractness of the material presented. These suggestions will facilitate the learning process while making the time spent more enjoyable (Table 1-12).

Simplification of Technical Terminology

1. Learn the definitions and functions of each new technical term. Keep a list of new words in a notebook. If possible, use one word to define each term. The definition word should preferably portray an anatomic or physiologic function or description. Repeat that word mentally, write it several times, and pronounce it out loud, so that it becomes familiar. Electronic medical dictionaries provide the correct pronunciations of medical words.
2. Relate each technical word to its synonyms. For example *fissure* and *sulcus* refer to the same structure. The **superior cerebellar peduncle** and the **brachium conjunctivum** refer to the same cerebellar pathway, and the **cerebral aqueduct** and **sylvian aqueduct** refer to the canal connecting the third and fourth **ventricles** in the brain. **Iter** is also used as a synonym for the **cerebral aqueduct.**

Table 1-11

Important Brodmann Areas

Brodmann Area	Anatomic Location	Function
Frontal lobe		
4	Precentral gyrus	Primary motor cortex
6 and 8	Anterior to precentral gyrus	Premotor cortex
9–11	Prefrontal region	Cognitive association cortex
44, 45	Inferior frontal lobule	Frontal association language cortex; Broca area
Parietal lobe		
3, 1, 2	Postcentral gyrus	Primary sensory cortex
5, 7	Posterior to post-central gyrus	Somatosensory association cortex
39	Angular gyrus	Reading and writing
Temporal lobe		
22	Subtemporal and posterior temporal gyrus and planum temporale	Posterior association language cortex; Wernicke area
41, 42	Gyri of Heschl	Primary auditory cortex
Occipital lobe		
17	Calcarine cortex	Primary visual cortex
18, 19	Pericalcarine cortical area	Visual association cortex

Table 1-12

Strategies for Overcoming the Complexity of Neuroscience

Relate each structure to its definition and function.

Be familiar with the synonyms for each structure.

Relate each term with other functionally related terms.

Be familiar with the idiosyncratic patterns for coining technical terms based on the following:
- Visual appearance
- Researcher's name
- Anatomic projection
- Roots in Greek and Latin

Undertake a visual approach to neuroanatomy:
- Learn the shape, size, location, and function of each structure.
- Orient each structure in relation to its adjoining structures.

Apply clinical orientation to anatomic structures.

Find a functional context for neurologic concepts and structures.

Discover the meaning and purpose of each new concept by solving clinical problems.

Be familiar with the rules of lesion localization.

3. Relate each technical term to other functionally related terms. For example, **peduncle** refers to the fiber bundles connecting the cerebellum to the brainstem; thus, the superior, middle, and inferior cerebellar peduncles are functionally related anatomic structures.

4. Become familiar with the common principles of formulating medical terms.

   - Some neuroanatomic structures are named after their visual appearance: **lenticular** because of its lens shape; **colliculus** because of its hill like form; **corona radiata** because the sensory and motor fibers radiate in the form of a crown; **internal capsule** because of the capsulelike formation of the sensory and motor fibers deep in the brain between the diencephalon and basal ganglia; **amygdaloid nucleus** because of its almond shape; and **hippocampus** because of its seahorse shape in sagittal section.

   - Some terms are eponyms, coined from the names of researchers—for example, circle of Willis, Babinski reflex, Brodmann area, Huntington chorea, foramen of Monro, Sylvian fissure, fissure of Rolando, Parkinson disease, and area of Broca.

   - Names of pathways may be established according to sites of origin and termination. The **corticospinal tract**, for instance, originates in the motor cortex and terminates in the spinal cord. The **corticobulbar tract** originates in the cortex and terminates in the bulbar area (medulla and adjacent brainstem areas). The **reticulospinal system** extends from the reticular formation of the brainstem to its termination in the spinal cord. Although the names of fiber tracts primarily emphasize the points of origin and termination, they sometimes include unnamed brain structures along the entire length of the tract.

   - Most neurology terms are derived from Greek or Latin. Familiarity with roots and derivational morphemes can simplify learning. Some examples follow.
     - Ataxia: *a-* means "without," and the Greek root *taxis* means "order"; thus, *ataxia* is loss of motor coordination. (See Appendix B on the Point web site for common lexical roots.)
     - Chorea: the Greek root *choros* means "dance"; thus, *chorea* is a dancelike movement characterized by involuntary motor movements.
     - Lemniscus: the Greek root *lemniskos* means "a fillet or ribbon"; thus, *lemniscus* refers to a bundle of nerve fibers in the CNS.
     - Brachium: the Greek root *brachios* means "arm" (arm-like fiber bundle), as in **brachium conjunctivus**, the crossing fibers of the cerebellum.
     - Peduncle: the Latin root *pedunculus* means "foot," as in **cerebral peduncle**, the foot of the cerebrum for motor fibers descending through the midbrain.

   - Many medical terms derived from Greek or Latin roots have a combining form of the word that is different from its root form. For example, the combining form of the Greek root *skleros* (hard) is **scler-**, as in *sclerosis*; the combining form of Greek root *soma* (body) is **somat-**, as in *somatic*; the combining form of Greek root *stethos* (chest) is **stetho-**, as in *stethoscope* (see Appendix B on the Point web site for a list of such combining forms).

Visual Approach to Neuroscience

The human nervous system is complex, but it is organized logically. Most concepts can be understood and remembered after the learner has acquired the basics in neuroscience. Some concepts and facts, however, must be memorized and repeated until they become incorporated in a readily available bank of knowledge. Neuroanatomy is best learned by persistent repetition and visual orientation. Neuroanatomic structures are not abstract entities; they are real, occupy space, and serve specific functions. All brain structures are anatomically and physiologically integrated to form a whole entity with one purpose—preservation of the species. The visual learning of anatomic structures (with reference to shape, size, texture, function, and location in the nervous system and relationship to bordering structures) is the most successful tool. No other effective way has been found. Consequently, developing a visual memory by correlating written descriptions of cortical and subcortical structures with their anatomic illustrations, charts, and figures has been found to be invaluable. As a student learns more, he or she should become better equipped to solve clinical problems, a highly valued skill. Thus, some practical suggestions for learning the concepts and functions of neuroscience follow:

1. Take a visual approach to learning brain structures in the context of their locations. Each external and internal neuroanatomic structure is visually distinct. Visual familiarity with a structure as it appears in space facilitates learning neuroanatomy and reduces the fear of learning. For example, widely dispersed sensory and motor fibers are responsible in part for the bulging appearance of the pons; the four adjacent egg-shaped structures located dorsally in the midbrain are the **corpora quadrigemina** (four bodies), and the slit cleavage between two football-shaped thalami is the **third ventricle**. The fillet-shaped sensory fibers at the midbrain course through the **medial lemniscus** and the motor fibers, through the **pes pedunculi**, or **crus cerebri**.

2. Familiarity with adjacent structures and landmarks helps form a three-dimensional image that further facilitates learning. For example, it is easier to remember the location of various cortical and subcortical structures if they are visualized in relation to the **ventricular system**. Another important anatomic landmark is the shape of the sensorimotor fibers throughout the neuraxis (see Fig. 3-1).

Clinical Orientation to Neuroscience

There are two types of orientations involved in learning in neuroanatomy: anatomic and clinical. Structural neuroscience is learned from an anatomic orientation: in diagrams, the left brain structures are on the left side, and right brain structures are on the right. This is identical to the left and right of the clinician. In this orientation, the posteriorly (dorsal) located structures, like the colliculi (superior and inferior) and the cerebral aqueduct, are at the top of figures, whereas the anterior (ventral) structures, like the peduncle and pyramidal fibers, are located at the bottom of the figures.

The clinical orientation is opposite of the anatomic orientation, and it may generate some degree of confusion when it comes to reading MRI, CT, and PET studies. In clinical orientation, the patient lies supine on his or her back and the clinician looks at the patient from a pedal view, as if facing the patient's feet. This makes the patient's right and left, respectively, the physician's left and right (Fig. 1-9A); this reverse anatomic representation also applies to the brainstem and spinal cord anatomy (Fig. 1-9B). Clinical orientation not only facilitates reading radiological images (MRI, PET, and CT) but also enhances the ability of students in human behavior to use neuroradiologic studies in the management of neurologic patients.

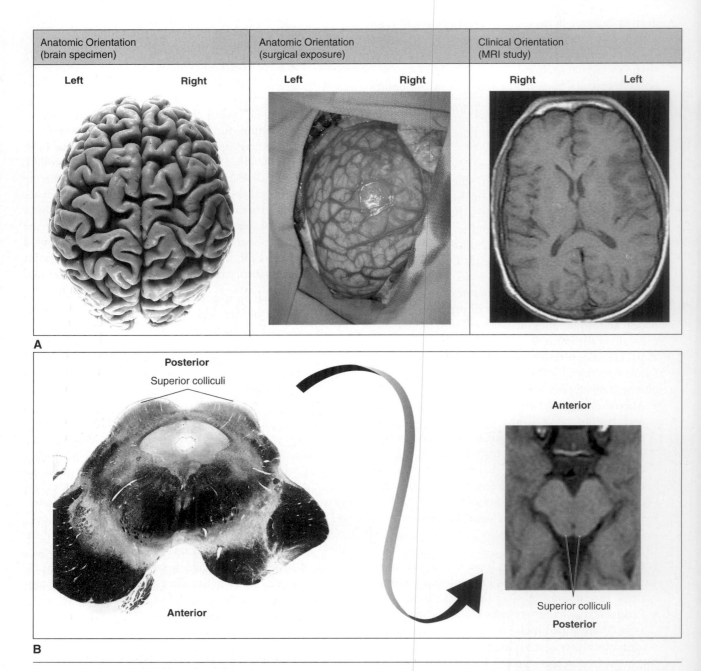

Figure 1-9 Reverse relationship between the anatomic and clinical orientations. A. Cerebral hemispheres. B. Midbrain.

Functional Context for Learning Neuroanatomy

Every structure in the nervous system has a purpose and is part of a functional system, with ascending and descending projections. Determine how each newly introduced structure fits into the broader organization of the brain. To what other structures is it functionally and/or anatomically related? For instance, the **medial lemniscus** in the brainstem conducts sensory information from the peripheral body parts to the thalamus, whereas the **lateral lemniscus** refers to fibers of the brainstem that conduct auditory impulses to the thalamus. The **superior colliculi** are concerned with visual reflexes, whereas the adjacent **inferior colliculi** are the auditory-relay structures in the midbrain.

Deductive Reasoning and Problem Solving

The most important aspect of training in neuroscience is to learn to localize a lesion in the nervous system using a multistep, clinical problem-solving approach (Box 1-2). The process of localizing a lesion involves finding the point of breakdown in the neural circuitry by examining both the spared and the disrupted functions. Basic knowledge of coexisting anatomic structures and understanding of the axonal pathways with respect to their origin, termination, and crossing (*decussation*) help determine how a patient with a particular lesion will exhibit a combination of symptoms on the body—ipsilateral or contralateral to the lesion site. For example, **oculomotor nerve** (cranial nerve III) palsy on the left side and hemiparesis on the right side of the body (**alternating ophthalmohemiplegia**) are most likely to result from a midbrain lesion in the left pes pedunculi (crus cerebri). A lesion affecting the oculomotor nerve before it emerges from the brainstem produces paralysis of the eye muscles on the same side (ipsilateral), but the paralysis of the limbs is contralateral because of the involvement of the corticospinal tract, which has not yet crossed in the medulla. Furthermore, loss of sensation (of pain and temperature) and paralysis in a single limb implies a lesion either in the spinal roots or nerves or in the brain. This is because these are the only two anatomic locations in which the sensory and motor fibers from the implicated limb are together. The bilateral presence of paralysis and sensory loss below a certain level on the trunk when there is normal function above suggests a spinal cord injury; a spinal disorder is likely to interrupt the fibers below the lesion while sparing those above. Reduced tone and reflexes are likely to result from a lesion in the PNS or one involving the lower (spinal or cranial) motor neurons. On the other hand, increased muscle tone and hyperactive reflexes are always associated with lesions involving the upper motor neurons in the forebrain or brainstem. Gradually expanding on such an analytical approach can make learning neuroanatomy and neurology enjoyable and invaluable.

Rules for Lesion Localization

Lesion localization is crucial to differential diagnosis in neurology and is perhaps the most challenging aspect of learning neuroscience. Most of the systems in the brain are considered to be line systems, vertically organized to connect the CNS to the peripheral body region. Each abnormal sign in a patient presumably reflects a breakdown at a point in the linear (ascending or descending) pathway. If the implicated linear fibers mediating sensory and motor information intersect, a lesion involving this single point impairs both sensory and motor functions. However, the intersection of fibers at two anatomic sites signifies two potential lesion sites. Localizing a lesion becomes complex in cases with multiple clinical symptoms that implicate numerous pathways and multiple points of intersection. Lesion localization in such patients requires a systematic analysis of symptoms, use of problem-solving skills, and in depth understanding of neuroanatomy; only neurologists may be able to complete the diagnosis.

Nevertheless, common neurologic symptoms follow a set of simple rules (Box 1-3), and some neurologic symptoms point to specific lesion sites (Table 1-13). The pathologic involvement of the sensorimotor cortex leads to impairment in the deliberate and voluntary control of movements. Basal ganglia lesions lead to increased muscle tone, resulting in stiff muscles and involuntary movements like tremors and chorea. Lesions in the cerebellum affect the ability to balance and are characterized by wide-based, unsteady (ataxic), clumsy, and inaccurate movements with a tendency to fall on the affected side. Additional symptoms associated with cerebellar pathology are tremors, and inaccurate (dysmetria) and irregular (asynergia) movements. These rules will become meaningful as students become more familiar with neuroanatomy and sensorimotor pathways. Common rules that assist in localizing a lesion are presented in Box 1-3.

BOX 1-2

Clinical Problem-Solving

Lesion localization, crucial for differential diagnosis, is the foundation for learning neurology. Perhaps the most challenging aspect of learning neuroscience is relating symptoms with their underlying lesion sites. The anatomic information that is vital to clinical problem solving is the knowledge of the neuraxial point of crossing for the sensorimotor fibers. The location of the crossing point helps determine if the symptoms of brain injuries will be present ipsilateral or contralateral to the lesion site.

Ten Rules That Assist in Localizing a Lesion

Rule 1: Symptoms Suggesting a Cortical Lesion

- **Presenting symptoms:** Contralateral hemiplegia; contralateral hemianesthesia of face, trunk, and upper extremity; and cortical sensory loss (failure to identify an object through touch or to identify a letter or word written on the surface of the skin) suggest a cortical lesion.
- **Dominant hemisphere:** In addition to the presenting symptoms, a dominant hemisphere lesion results in aphasia, apraxia, finger agnosia, and acalculia.
- **Nondominant hemisphere:** In addition to the presenting symptoms, an injury in the nondominant (right) hemisphere can also result in left-sided neglect or inattention, constructional and/or dressing deficits (apraxia), spatial and temporal disorientation, impaired prosody of speech, and impaired ability to recognize faces.

Rule 2: Symptoms Suggesting a Subcortical Lesion

- **Presenting symptoms:** Contralateral hemiplegia and diminution or loss of pain and temperature equally for the face, arms, and legs is associated with a subcortical (internal capsule) lesion. Emergence of involuntary movements suggests a basal ganglia lesion.

Rule 3: Symptoms Suggesting a Central Gray Spinal Lesion

- **Presenting symptoms:** Bilateral loss of pain and temperature sensation with a preserved sense of touch in the same limbs (usually the two upper limbs) implies a lesion (e.g., cavitation or syringomyelia) in the spinal central gray.

Rule 4: Symptoms Suggesting a Visual Pathway Lesion

- **Presenting symptoms:** Blindness in one eye suggests an optic nerve lesion anterior to the optic chiasm.
- **Presenting symptoms:** Bitemporal hemianopsia (the patient does not see things laterally in the visual fields) results from a lesion compressing or otherwise interrupting the crossing fibers from the nasal retina of each eye in the optic chiasm.
- **Presenting symptoms:** Homonymous hemianopsia is associated with a lesion in the optic tract fibers; this lesion can lie between the optic chiasm and the occipital lobe.
- **Presenting symptoms:** Visual agnosia, alexia (failure to comprehend written word), and homonymous hemianopsia, along with spared macular vision, are associated with a lesion of the primary visual cortex (area 17) and visual association cortex (areas 18 and 19).

Rule 5: Symptoms Suggesting a Complete Spinal Cord Lesion

- **Presenting symptoms:** Paralysis and sensory loss bilaterally below the level of the lesion with spared functions above indicates a complete spinal cord transsectional injury.

Rule 6: Symptoms Suggesting a Spinal Hemisection Lesion

- **Presenting symptoms:** Ipsilateral loss of position and vibratory sensation below the level of lesion, ipsilateral body paralysis, and contralateral loss of pain and temperature sensation indicate a spinal hemisection (Brown-Séquard syndrome).

Rule 7: Symptoms Suggesting a Peripheral or Central Lesion

- **Presenting symptoms:** Paralysis and sensory (pain and temperature) loss involving the same single limb suggest a lesion either in the peripheral nerve or in the cortex.

Rule 8: Symptoms Suggesting an Upper or Lower Motor Neuron Lesion

- **Presenting symptoms:** Increased reflexes and spastic tone in a symptomatic (sensorimotor) limb indicate an upper motor neuron lesion; reduced reflexes and weakness in the same symptomatic limb imply a peripheral or lower motor neuron lesion.

Rule 9: Symptoms Suggesting a Brainstem Lesion

- **Presenting symptoms:** Motor and sensory losses of the extremities associated with the cranial nerve (facial, ocular, lingual, trigeminal) imply a brainstem lesion.

BOX 1-3 *(Continued)*

- **Presenting symptoms:** An altered level of consciousness and cranial nerve impairments (facial paralysis, hearing impairment, nystagmus, dysarthria, dysphagia) on the same side (ipsilaterally) and hemianesthesia and paralysis of the body on the opposite side (alternating or crossed hemiplegia) imply a brainstem lesion.

Rule 10: Symptoms Suggesting a Disorder in Vascular System

- **Presenting symptoms:** Sudden development of contralateral paralysis of the lower face, arm, and upper extremity (more than the leg), with accompanying sensory loss, results from an occlusion of the middle cerebral artery that may be caused by either thrombosis or embolism. Additional symptoms may include the symptoms discussed under rule 1. (An abrupt onset of symptoms usually indicates vascular disease, whereas gradual progression of symptoms indicates a mass lesion.)
- **Presenting symptoms:** Toe, foot, and leg paralysis as well as sensory loss and mental impairments (distractibility, indecisiveness, and lack of spontaneity) are associated with ischemia owing to embolism or thrombosis in the anterior cerebral artery distribution.
- **Presenting symptoms:** Homonymous hemianopsia is associated with posterior cerebral artery involvement. Low pain threshold also is seen because of the thalamic involvement.

An understanding of the lesion-localizing rules facilitates the grasp of the rationale for using selected tasks and activities when examining a patient with left or right hemiplegia. For example, establishing a left cortical lesion in a patient with right hemiplegia requires that the patient be tested for aphasia (naming, verbal output, reading, and writing); the differential paralytic involvement of face, arm, and leg; right-sided cortical sensory loss; and homonymous hemianopsia. To determine a lesion in the nondominant hemisphere, testing should include the assessment of inattention to the left body space, left sensorimotor involvement, spatial orientation, constructional and/or dressing activities, and speech prosody and denial of disease. Determining a subcortical lesion requires that the patient be tested for contralateral hemiplegia and equal sensorimotor involvement of face, arm, and leg; dystonic postures; and reduced pain threshold. To confirm a brainstem lesion, one must test the patient for alternating hemiplegia, which is characterized by ipsilateral cranial nerve symptoms (left ear hearing loss, left tongue deviation, swallowing, and dysarthria) and crossed hemiplegia. Establishing a spinal cord lesion requires that the patient be examined for muscle tone, reflex quality, paralysis, and sensory loss. Both sensory and motor signs will be ipsilateral to the lesion at the segmental level of the damage.

Table 1-13

Important Lesion-Localizing Signs

Clinical Symptoms	Implicated Lesion Sites
Reduced deep tendon reflex (interrupted reflex path)	Impaired functioning of motor nuclei in brainstem or spinal cord
Muscle fasciculation (spontaneous muscle activation)	Motor nuclei dysfunctioning in brainstem or spinal cord
Muscle atrophy (waste of muscle fibers)	Loss of voluntary or reflexive muscle control subsequent to motor nuclei injuries in brainstem or spinal cord
Flaccid muscle tone (loss of natural muscle tension)	Injury to motor nuclei in the brainstem or spinal cord
Babinski sign (extension of great toe and abduction of other toes) plus hyperactive reflex (brisk reflex pattern)	Interruption in the descending motor corticospinal fibers
Decerebrate rigidity (increased extensor muscle tone)	Midbrain lesion

CLINICAL CONSIDERATIONS

PATIENT ONE

A 25-year-old speech language pathologist (SLP) on the first day of her medical placement received a case study with the following MRI study and a report identifying it as a glioblastoma involving the right frontal cortex. Because the lesion was clearly located on the left side of the image, the SLP thought the report localizing the tumor in the right hemisphere was in error.

Question: How can you explain the reason underlying this confusion in reading the MRI?

Discussion: The tumor is indeed in the right hemisphere. In clinical orientation, which is opposite of anatomic orientation, the clinician is looking from feet to head at a patient lying on his or her back. Consequently, the patient's right and left, respectively, are the examiner's left and right. This reversed clinical orientation applies to CT, PET, and MRI studies.

PATIENT TWO

On his first day of work at a hospital, a 28-year-old SLP met a neurologist who informally began discussing a 20-year-old patient she had seen that morning. The patient had no apparent cognitive or communicative problem but presented with a history of big appetite, excessive perspiration, irregular sleep–wake cycle, and altered sexual behavior, with no libido. The neurologist noted that this is a classical case of a lesion in the lower diencephalon.

Question: How can you explain these symptoms in relation to the lesion site?

Discussion: It is a hypothalamic syndrome. The hypothalamus, located below the thalamus, serves autonomic,

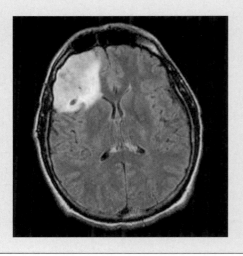

visceral, and endocrine functions, including sexual drive, appetite, sleep–wake cycle, and body heat production.

PATIENT THREE

A rookie SLP read the report of a patient with impaired speech, language, cognitive, and sensorimotor functions subsequent to a traumatic brain injury caused by an automobile accident. The neurologic report identified multiple sites with laceration and contusing tissues—most important, those involving Brodmann areas 4:3, 1, 2; 10, 11; and 38.

Question: What sensorimotor and behavioral symptoms are you likely to see in this patient?

Discussion: This patient is likely to exhibit impaired motor control (Brodmann area 4); altered somatic sensation (Brodmann areas 3, 1, and 2); cognitive disorders and personality changes (Brodmann areas 10 and 11); and aggression and agitation (Brodmann area 38) owing to involvement of the amygdala and surrounding region.

PATIENT FOUR

A beginning SLP went to a grand-round discussion, which focused on a patient who had profound aphasic symptoms disproportionate to the extent of the lesion displayed on a coronal MRI study. The SLP was asked what she could tell about this patient's language dysfunctions. The SLP said that she wanted to see a different view of the brain before commenting.

Question: Which view of the brain which would give the SLP a better clinical picture?

Discussion: Language is laterally located in the neocortex. This involves Brodmann areas 44 (expressive language cortex), 22 (receptive language cortex), and 39 and 40 (angular and supramarginal gyrus for reading and writing). The SLP needed to view the full extent of the lesion either on the leftmost parasagittal MRI slices or on a transverse view of the brain.

SUMMARY

Neuroscience and communicative disorders are two closely related disciplines. Basic understanding of neuroscience is essential for a comprehensive training in speech-language-hearing pathology. The rationale for training in neuroscience is that it provides a broad framework for diagnosing communication disorders and for providing effective remediation. Such background will also help students in communicative disorders and human behavior become creative partners in a team approach to managing a patient's clinical condition, nurturing good working relationships with colleagues in the medical and paramedical professions.

Although neuroscience is admittedly complex, there are ways to overcome its technical terminology. The basic neurologic concepts and technical tools that are prerequisite for learning neuroscience and are needed for solving clinical problems involving neurologically impaired patients have been presented. Familiarity with the rules of word formation and an approach that emphasizes persistent repetition, visual orientation, and deductive reasoning can make learning neuroscience easier. Visual familiarity with the graphic details given in Chapters 2 and 3 is necessary to develop the foundation for understanding the functional organization of the nervous system.

QUIZ QUESTIONS

1. Define the following technical terms: afferent, Brodmann area, cerebral cortex, cerebral plasticity, contralateral, decussation, efferent, interhemispheric, intrahemispheric, ipsilateral, somatic, visceral

2. Match each of the following numbered functional categories with its associated lettered statement.

   1. general somatic afferent (GSA)
   2. special somatic afferent (SSA)
   3. general visceral afferent (GVA)
   4. special visceral afferent (SVA)
   5. general somatic efferent (GSE)
   6. general visceral efferent (GVE)
   7. special visceral efferent (SVE)

   a. pain and temperature
   b. autonomic nervous system activity
   c. limb movement involving skeletal muscles
   d. audition
   e. organ content
   f. taste and smell
   g. articulation, phonation, facial expression, and swallowing

3. Define the following lexical roots (see Appendix C on the Point web site): kinesis, opsis, phagein, plege, prattein (praxis), presbys, taxis, tectum

4. Provide Brodmann area numbers for the following cortical regions.

   primary motor cortex
   primary somatosensory area
   primary visual cortex
   primary auditory cortex

5. Provide the directional terms for the structures above and below the neuroaxial bend.

   A. Above the neuraxial bend (the brain):
      _____ = toward the nose
      _____ = toward the top (vertex of the skull)
      _____ = toward the back
      _____ = toward the bottom (jaw)

   B. Below the neuraxial bend (the brainstem and spinal cord):
      _____ = toward the abdomen
      _____ = toward the nose (head)
      _____ = toward the back
      _____ = toward the spinal tail (coccyx)

6. Match each of the following numbered branches of neuroscience with its associated lettered definition.

   1. neurology
   2. neurosurgery
   3. neuroanatomy
   4. neuroradiology
   5. neuroembryology
   6. neurophysiology
   7. neuropathology

   a. nervous system and its diseases
   b. structure and anatomy of the CNS
   c. imaging techniques
   d. embryologic origin and development of the CNS
   e. chemical and physical processes of the CNS
   f. pathologic changes in the CNS
   g. surgical procedure involving the removal of pathologic tissue from the nervous system

7. Match each of the following numbered neurologic conditions with its associated lettered definition.

   1. Huntington disease
   2. cerebral palsy
   3. Parkinson disease
   4. Alzheimer disease
   5. stroke
   6. epilepsy
   7. multiple sclerosis

   a. a progressive degenerative disease of the aging brain associated with dementia
   b. a motor disorder caused by damage to the cerebrum before, during, or after birth
   c. an abnormality in the brain's electrical activity
   d. a progressive and hereditary disease of the brain leading to chorea and dementia
   e. a progressive CNS disease of sensorimotor dysfunctions that results from the degeneration of myelin
   f. a progressive disease of the brain characterized by involuntary tremor, reduced muscular strength, and slowed onset of voluntary movements
   g. a sudden loss of brain function caused by an interruption of the blood supply

TECHNICAL TERMS

abduction
adduction
afferent
anterograde
caudal
cerebral cortex
cerebral hemisphere

cerebrum
cognition
coronal
cytoarchitecture
decussation
dorsal
efferent

extension
flexion
ganglion
glial cell
interhemispheric
intrahemispheric
malignant
nerve cell
neuraxis

pronation
retrograde
rostral
sagittal
somatic
supination
teratology
ventral
visceral

Gross Anatomy of the Central Nervous System

LEARNING OBJECTIVES

After studying this chapter, students should be able to:

- Differentiate the central and peripheral nervous systems

- List structures in the central and peripheral nervous systems

- Describe the functions of the major structures of the central and peripheral nervous systems

- List principal embryonic divisions of the brain and gross anatomic structures related to each division

- Identify the gross anatomic structures of the brain, describe their locations, and explain their functions

- Identify the gross anatomic structures of the spinal cord and explain their functions

- Identify the internal structures of the cerebral cortex, midbrain, pons, medulla, and spinal cord and describe their functions

- Identify parts of the ventricular cavities

- Describe the meninges, their locations, and their functions

- Differentiate the various medullary fibers and describe their functions

- List the cranial nerves, cite their anatomic locations, and describe their major sensory and motor functions

- Discuss the anatomy and functions of the autonomic nervous system

- Appreciate the structural and functional connectivity of the brain structures

STRUCTURES OF CENTRAL AND PERIPHERAL NERVOUS SYSTEMS

The human nervous system can best be described as a cellular system specialized for rapid intercellular communication by means of the electrical and chemical energy distributed throughout the body, which it uses to respond to static or dynamic changes in the environment as they impinge on the body. With the endocrine system, it is able to reach target cells in all organs by long axons with multiple branches. Cellular communication along an axon involves rapid electrochemical changes in the cell membranes (action potential). The axonal branches terminate in close contact with the target cells, so the diffusion of the chemical messenger to the receptors of the target cell is rapid and localized.

Through rapid communication, complex integrative functions, and massive data storage, the network of neurons in the brain and spinal cord provides the mechanism of function for the nervous system. The nervous system has four categories of function: **sensor**, **effector**, **integrator**, and **regulator**. As the *sensor*, it receives all environmental and bodily generated changes, analyzes the information, and stores it. As the *effector*, it initiates and controls all body movements. As the *integrator*, it combines information received from all sources and modalities. As the *regulator*, it maintains the homeostatic state for the optimum control of peak body performance and repair.

Anatomically, the nervous system consists of two major parts: the **central nervous system** (CNS) and the **peripheral nervous system** (PNS). The CNS consists of the brain and spinal cord (Fig. 2-1A). The brain is responsible for initiating, controlling, and regulating all sensorimotor and cognitive (mental) functions that generate and regulate human behavior. The spinal cord is primarily a wired-cable structure in the CNS that transmits motor commands to various body parts, which interact with the environment. Also, the sensory information that is collected from the peripheral body parts and the environment is transmitted to the brain via the spinal cord. Some sensory input is processed locally in the spinal cord and regulates peripheral reflexive motor activity.

The CNS is protected by a bony shell. The brain is encased in a tough bony skull, and the spinal cord is similarly protected by the vertebral column, which consists of a series of bones and cartilaginous washerlike structures; the washers buffer body movements and weight bearing. The CNS is encased in three membranous coverings, known as the **meninges**. They may be visualized as three diapers, covering the CNS from the top of the brain to the tip of the spinal cord. Between the two inner diapers there is the **cerebrospinal fluid** (CSF), which serves both as a protective

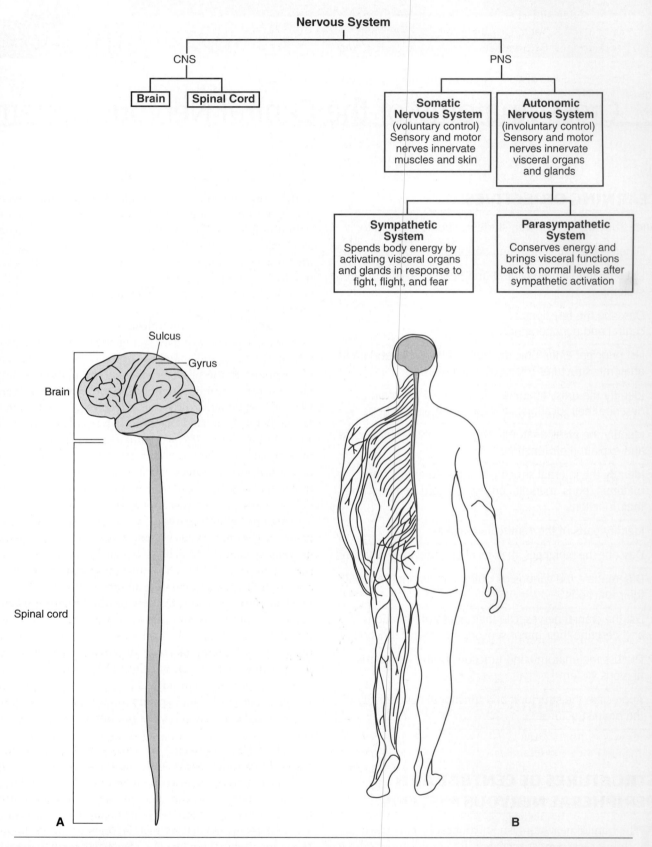

Figure 2-1 The human nervous system. **A.** The central nervous system (*CNS*) consists of the brain and spinal cord. **B.** The peripheral nervous system (*PNS*) consists of cranial nerves and spinal nerves, through which the CNS transmits commands to and receives information from the end organs.

mechanical buffer and as a chemical mediator for metabolic functions. The meninges also provide the supporting framework for the CNS vessels that carry blood to and from the heart.

The PNS consists of sensory and motor nerves that are connected to the spinal cord (**spinal nerves**) and the brainstem (**cranial nerves**). These nerves extend to the organs, muscles, joints, blood vessels, and skin surface, forming an extensive network of cables and fine wires throughout the body (Fig. 2-1B). The PNS consists of two major systems: the **somatic nervous system** and the **autonomic nervous system** (**ANS**). Each of these systems consists of two subsystems: sensory (**afferent**) and motor (**efferent**) fibers. The afferent fibers consist of nerves and cells that transmit sensory information to the CNS from receptors in the skin, muscles, and visceral organs. The efferent fibers transmit commands from the CNS to activate the muscles and glands located throughout the body.

The **somatic** afferents and efferents mediate the skeletal muscle reflexes. **Visceral sensory** inputs of the ANS communicate with **visceral motor** outputs to activate the visceral organ reflexes and glands. The ANS regulates the activity of organs, such as the salivary glands, heart, lung, blood vessels, stomach, intestines, kidneys, and bladder.

The ANS (also called the visceral, involuntary, autonomic, and vegetative system) is made up of two divisions: the **sympathetic nervous system** and the **parasympathetic nervous system**. **Sympathetic ganglia** (clusters of nerve cells) usually innervate many organs, whereas **parasympathetic ganglia** innervate a single organ. These systems produce opposite effects when innervating the same organ. For example, the *sympathetic system* spends energy (catabolic) and prepares for fight and flight. In so doing, it constricts the blood vessels of the skin, visceral organs, and bronchial passages, induces perspiration, dilates pupils, and mobilizes glucose. The *parasympathetic system* conserves energy (anabolic); dominant during relaxing or sleeping, it constricts the pupils and slows the heart rate. Together the *sympathetic* and *parasympathetic systems* monitor, regulate, and sustain optimum visceral functions essential to survival (see Chapter 16).

PRIMARY DIVISIONS OF THE BRAIN

Familiarity with the three major **vesicles** of the **embryonic brain** facilitates understanding the development of the human brain and its structures. The 4- to 5-week *embryonic brain* is well developed in terms of its structures. It has three **vesicles: prosencephalon** (forebrain), **mesencephalon** (midbrain), and **rhombencephalon** (hindbrain). These vesicles are demarcated by three brain **flexures: midbrain, pontine,** and **cervical** (Fig. 2-2). The midbrain flexure (also called the cephalic) demarcates the midbrain region in the brainstem. The cervical flexure is at the junction of the hindbrain and the spinal cord. An unequal development of

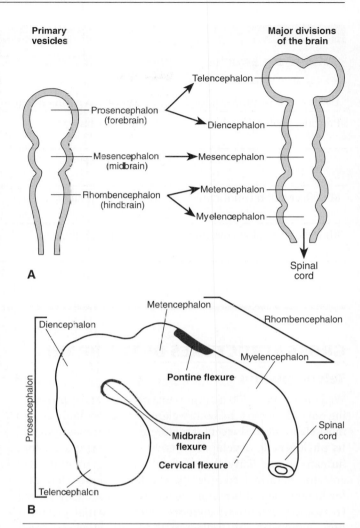

Figure 2-2 A. The three primary vesicles (*left*) in the embryonic brain from which the structures of the central nervous system are derived (*right*). **B.** Lateral view of the three flexures in the developing brain at end of embryonic week 5. These flexures divide the brain into the prosencephalon, mesencephalon, and rhombencephalon.

the hindbrain produces the pontine flexure, which causes the thinning of the hindbrain roof.

The *prosencephalon* develops into the **telencephalon** and **diencephalon**. The **cerebral hemispheres, limbic lobe,** and **basal ganglia** are the principal derivatives of the *telencephalon*, whereas the **thalamus** and **hypothalamus** are derived from the *diencephalon*. The midbrain structures are the developmental derivatives of the **mesencephalic vesicle**. The *rhombencephalon* further divides into **metencephalon** and **myelencephalon**. The *metencephalon* further develops into the **cerebellum** and **pons**; the *myelencephalon* becomes the **medulla oblongata** (Table 2-1). The brainstem, the upward extension of the spinal cord, vertically intersects the horizontal brain and includes, as a contiguous unit, the **midbrain** (mesencephalon), pons, and medulla (rhombencephalon).

Table 2-1

Adult Brain Structures Derived from Embryonic Vesicles

Embryonic Brain Vesicles	Major Divisions of the Brain	Gross Anatomic Structures
Prosencephalon (forebrain)	Telencephalon	Cerebral cortex, basal ganglia, and limbic system Lateral ventricles
	Diencephalon	Thalamus and hypothalamus Third ventricle
Mesencephalon (midbrain)	Mesencephalon	Midbrain structures Cerebral aqueduct
Rhombencephalon (hindbrain)	Metencephalon	Pons and cerebellum Fourth ventricle
	Myelencephalon	Medulla oblongata No ventricle

GROSS STRUCTURES OF THE BRAIN

Telencephalon

Weighing 1200–1400 g (approximately 3 lb) and representing only 2% of the total body weight, the human brain is the most elaborate and recent structure in the nervous system. Its phylogenetic development is especially significant for humans, particularly that of the frontal region. With its amazing neuronal complexity, the brain alone accounts for higher mental functions, such as language; cognition (reasoning, attention, memory, temporospatial orientation, judgment, and reflective thinking); emotion; consciousness; and imagination. These functions, however, are integrated by the combined activities of the *cerebral hemispheres* and *diencephalon*.

Cerebral Hemispheres

The **cerebrum** consists of the cerebral hemispheres, which make up the largest part of the brain (Fig. 2-3). Composed of a 3.5-mm thick layer of neurons, the *cerebral cortex* is the convoluted surface of the brain; it overlies the internal white matter and more deeply located basal ganglia. The convolutions form ridges and valleys (grooves): the cortical ridges are called **gyri**, and the grooves are called **fissures** or **sulci** (Fig. 2-3). The convolutions allow for the accommodation of a large cellular volume within a limited cranial space.

The cerebral hemispheres are separated along the midline by the **longitudinal fissure**, also called the **interhemispheric fissure**. The paired cerebral hemispheres are essentially mirror images, containing similar centers for processing sensory and motor functions. Each hemisphere controls the opposite side of the body (Fig. 1-1). In addition to basic sensorimotor functions, each hemisphere possesses specialized skills. For example, the left (dominant) hemisphere is superior in processing language, speech, calcula-

tion, and verbal memory, whereas the right (nondominant) hemisphere is better equipped to process and regulate pragmatic skills and visual and spatial concepts. Visual and spatial concepts refer to a series of cognitive processes that we use in recognizing visual objects, designing objects, orienting ourselves within the framework of time and space, and perceiving and expressing music and emotions.

Each cerebral hemisphere consists of five lobes: **frontal**, **parietal**, **occipital**, **temporal**, and **insular**. The first four, the primary lobes, are named after the overlying bones of the skull (Fig. 2-4). Considered a secondary lobe, the *insular lobe* (not a universally accepted nomenclature) is a small cortical island hidden in the depths of the lateral sulcus, covered by the overgrown opercular regions of the *frontal, parietal,* and *temporal* folds of cortex (Fig. 2-13). The primary lobes are divided by various sulci; the boundaries of these lobes, although well marked, are arbitrary, especially in the *temporal, parietal,* and *occipital* areas. The sulci and gyri markings of the brain are highly variable, particularly on the medial and basal surfaces of the brain. Consequently, maps of the hemispheric lobe boundaries serve as only rough frames of reference.

Cortical Surfaces

Dorsolateral Surface

Some sulci and gyri are always present in the human brain and therefore serve as important landmarks for describing the gross external topography and for dividing the hemisphere into lobes. Three major sulci are present on the dorsolateral surface of the brain: **central sulcus (fissure of Rolando)**, **lateral fissure (sylvian fissure)**, and **parieto-occipital sulcus** (Figs. 2-4 and 2-5). The *central sulcus* begins at the top of the brain, midway between the front and the back; extends along the dorsolateral surface in a downward and rostral (anterior) direction; and ends at the lateral fissure. The central sulcus is about 2 cm deep, a

Left hemisphere

Right hemisphere

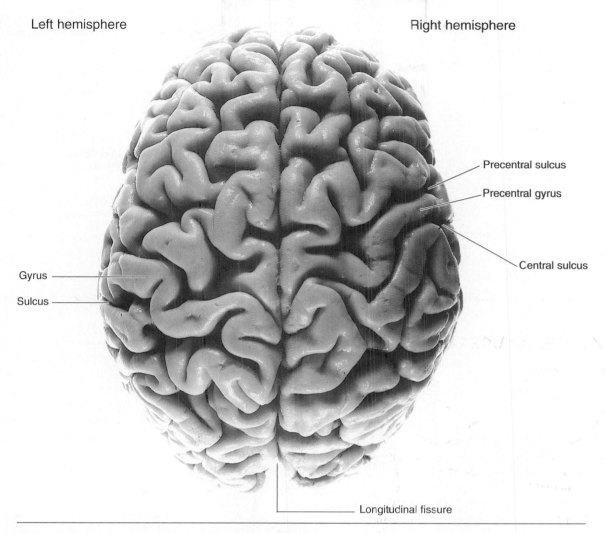

Precentral sulcus

Precentral gyrus

Central sulcus

Gyrus

Sulcus

Longitudinal fissure

Figure 2-3 Dorsal view of the human brain showing the cerebral hemispheres and their major sulci and gyri.

depth that marks the boundary between the frontal and the parietal lobes. It also separates the **primary motor cortex** from the **primary sensory cortex**. The *lateral fissure,* which is the most constant feature of the dorsolateral surface of the brain, begins rostrally below the frontal pole and extends posteriorly up toward the inferior parietal lobe. Anteriorly, the lateral fissure separates the frontal and temporal lobes; posteriorly, it extends partially between the parietal and the temporal lobes. The *parieto-occipital sulcus,* a deep and vertically oriented fissure on the lateral and medial surfaces of the cerebral cortex, separates the parietal lobe from the occipital lobe.

Frontal Lobe

The frontal lobe is rostral to the central sulcus and dorsal to the lateral fissure. As the largest lobe, it occupies about one-third of the hemisphere. It contains four important gyri: the vertical **precentral gyrus** and three horizontal gyri. The *precentral gyrus* lies rostral to the central sulcus; its ante-

rior boundary is marked by the **precentral sulcus**, which runs parallel to the central sulcus. The precentral gyrus, the site of the primary motor cortex (Brodmann area 4), contains the representation of the entire human body and regulates the fine and graded movements of the arms, legs, and face. (Note the disproportionate representation of various body parts in the homunculus, as presented in Figure 2-6.) Bioelectrical activity of nerve cells in this area is responsible for activating and controlling motor acts on the contralateral half of the body.

The area immediately rostral to the precentral sulcus is the **premotor cortex** (Brodmann area 6), which is involved with complex and skilled movements and regulates the responsiveness of the primary motor cortex. There are specific areas within the *premotor cortex* for controlling speech, hand, and finger movements and eye–head coordination.

The remaining anterior portion of the frontal lobe is the **prefrontal cortex** (Brodmann areas 10–12). As part of the cognitive brain and the biologic correlate of human

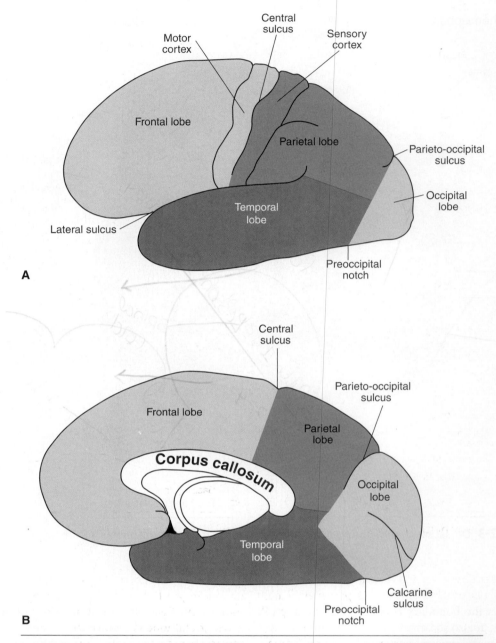

Figure 2-4 Lateral (A) and medial (B) views of the primary lobes of the cerebral hemisphere.

intelligence, it contributes to personality and the regulation of cognitive functions, such as reasoning, abstract thinking, self-monitoring, decision making, planning, and controlling executive decision and pragmatic behaviors.

Patients with a lesion of the lateral dorsal prefrontal region of the prefrontal cortex exhibit difficulty with planning, thinking, reasoning, and performing executive functions. Such patients appear normal but display difficulty in solving problems and planning the number and order of steps involved in task execution. Patients with orbital prefrontal region pathology are known to exhibit personality disorders, emotional disinhibition, and abnormal impulsive

social behaviors. A lesion of the medial prefrontal region affects the regulation of attention and motivation and the responsiveness to external cognitive stimuli. Such patients appear abulic, apathetic, and incognizant of their surroundings. Commonly seen in cases of traumatic brain injury, patients are usually apathetic, lazy, or confused. They are unaware of social expectations and the consequences of their actions and cannot regulate their behavior (Table 2-2).

This clinical symptomatology of the prefrontal lobe is best illustrated by the century-old case of an industrial worker named P. Gage. In an accident, a railway spike passed through his cheek and into the orbitofrontal region

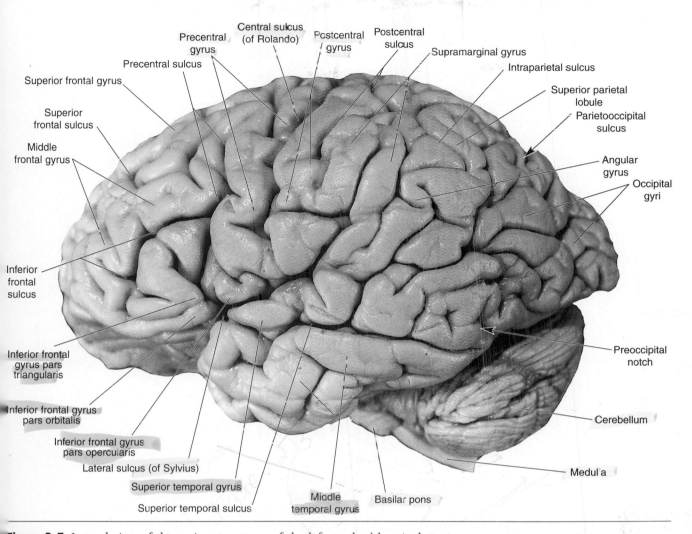

Figure 2-5 Lateral view of the major structures of the left cerebral hemisphere.

of the brain. He survived for many years with the spike protruding from his skull. However, his personality and social attitudes radically changed, and he became impulsive, rude, capricious, and erratic.

There are three large horizontal gyri in the frontal lobe: **superior** (first), **middle** (second), and **inferior** (third) **frontal gyri** (Fig. 2-5). The ascending rami of the lateral (sylvian) fissure intersect the inferior frontal gyrus and divide it into three sections: **pars opercularis**, **pars triangularis**, and **pars orbitalis**. The *opercular* and *triangular* portions of the *inferior frontal gyrus* in the dominant hemisphere constitute the **anterior language cortex**, or **Broca area** (Brodmann area 44). Broca area is important in spoken language. It is in front of the primary motor cortex area (Brodmann area 4), which controls jaw, lip, tongue, and vocal cord movement.

Parietal Lobe

The parietal lobe is between the frontal and the occipital lobes and above the temporal lobe. The central sulcus marks the anterior boundary of the parietal lobe. An arbitrary line from the ramus of the **parieto-occipital sulcus** extending to the **preoccipital notch** marks its posterior boundary (Figs. 2-4 and 2-5). The inferior boundary of the parietal lobe is represented by a line drawn from the posterior ramus of the lateral fissure to the middle of the line connecting the occipital notch to the parieto-occipital sulcus.

The parietal lobe is concerned with spatial orientation, cross-modality integration, memory, recognition and expression of emotions and prosodies, and cognition as well as the perceptual-interpretation and elaboration of somatic sensation. The **postcentral gyrus** (Brodmann areas 3, 1, 2) is the **primary sensory cortex**, in which all modalities of somatic sensation are received; these sensations are recognized as awareness in the parietal sensory association cortex, probably Brodmann areas 5 and 7 (Fig. 2-6B; see Fig. 1-8). The sensory representation of the entire body, like the motor representation in the precentral gyrus, is disproportionately perceived, beginning with the face and head in the lower third of the postcentral gyrus and the trunk, hands, arms, and legs in the upper portion of the gyrus.

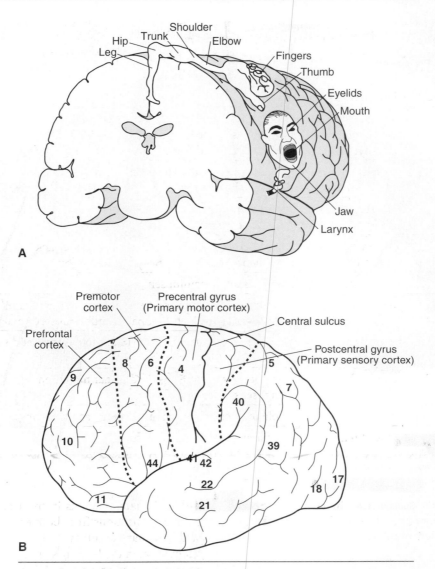

Figure 2-6 **A**. This distorted and disproportionate representation of the body parts is called the motor or sensory homunculus. The area allocated to each structure is based on its ability to participate in complex and/or skilled motor movements, not the mere size of the limbs. This representation is identical in both the precentral gyrus (motor cortex) and the postcentral gyrus (sensory cortex). **B**. The primary motor, premotor, prefrontal, and primary sensory cortices and central sulcus are depicted on the lateral surface of brain. *Numbers*, Brodmann areas.

The oblique **intraparietal sulcus** divides the remaining parietal lobe into the **superior** and the **inferior parietal lobules** (Fig. 2-5). The analysis and integration of sensory information in the *superior parietal lobule* contributes to complex perceptual experiences. Lesions in this parietal area result in contralateral sensory loss; complex perceptual disorders of constructional skills, spatial orientation, and memory deficit (Table 2-2). Lesions affecting the **angular** (Brodmann area 39) and **supramarginal** (Brodmann area 40) **gyri** in the *inferior parietal lobule* of the dominant hemisphere result in disorders of reading (alexia), writing (agraphia), calculation (acalculia), and language (aphasia). A pathology in the inferior parietal lobule of the nondominant hemisphere affects body schema and spatial attention and results in neglect of the contralateral half of the body.

Occipital Lobe

Only a small portion of the occipital lobe lies on the lateral surface (Figs. 2-4 and 2-5); it is more fully developed along the medial surface of the hemisphere. Containing the primary (Brodmann area 17) and secondary (Brodmann area 18) visual cortical areas, the anterior boundary of the

Table 2-2

Syndromes and Associated Neuroanatomic Localization of Lesions

Anatomic Structure	Associated Symptoms
Frontal lobe	Contralateral paralysis; impaired cognition (reasoning. self-monitoring, attention, abstraction, and problem solving); decreased spontaneity; impaired judgment; limited concentration; apathy; inappropriate or uninhibited social behavior; and expressive (Broca area) aphasia
Parietal lobe	Contralateral hemisensory loss, agnosia, inattention, constructional deficits, impaired tactile discrimination, contralateral hemianopsia, and aphasia (involvement of the left parietal lobe)
Occipital lobe	Blindness or scotoma in the opposite visual field, impaired recognition, visual agnosia, alexia, and impaired visual memories and recognition of color
Temporal lobe	Contralateral homonymous hemianopsia, receptive aphasia (Wernicke area in the left lobe), memory disturbance, epilepsy, and Klüver-Bucy syndrome (bilateral temporal lobes)
Thalamus	Impaired contralateral unpleasant or painful sensation
Hypothalamus	Impaired autonomic functions; disturbance in the regulation of temperature, salt, water metabolism, and the sleep–wake cycle; hormonal disorders; altered sexual functioning
Basal ganglia	Reduced (hypokinesia) movement, increased involuntary movement, and sustained abnormal posture
Brainstem	Altered consciousness, vertigo, nystagmus, impaired ocular movement, cranial nerve involvement, and crossed (alternating) sensorimotor deficits
Cerebellum	Reduced single or multiple limb coordination and synergy as well as impaired balance
Spinal cord	Reduced reflex as well as paralysis and sensory loss

occipital lobe is marked by an imaginary line extending from the **ramus** of the *parieto-occipital* sulcus to the *pre-occipital notch.*

Temporal Lobe

The temporal lobe, which serves audition, memory, language, and olfaction, is located ventral to the frontal and parietal lobes (Figs. 2-4 and 2-5). The *lateral fissure* and an arbitrary line extending from its posterior ramus toward the **occipital pole** mark the dorsal limit of the temporal lobe and separate it from the frontal and parietal lobes. The ventral continuation of the imaginary line connecting the parieto-occipital fissure to the preoccipital notch separates the temporal lobe from the occipital lobe.

The lateral surface of the temporal lobe contains three prominent gyri: **superior**; **middle**; and **inferior** (also called the first, second, and third) **temporal gyri**. The *superior temporal gyrus* and sulcus run parallel to the lateral fissure and posteriorly turn upward in the parietal lobe, where they are bordered on the parietal side by the *angular gyrus* (Brodmann area 39). The dorsal surface of the *superior temporal gyrus,* the area hidden by the opercular portions of the frontal, parietal, and temporal lobes, dips into the **insular cortex** and houses a few short, oblique convolutions, the **gyri of Heschl**. These gyri form the **primary auditory cortex** (Brodmann area 41), which is buried

within the lateral sulcus in front of the insular cortex. It receives projections from both ears. Thus, an involvement of the primary auditory cortex, may cause only a partial attenuation in the hearing sensitivity in both ears. The **language association cortex** (**Wernicke area**, or Brodmann area 22) lies in the posterior superior portion of the first temporal gyrus, the area surrounding the primary auditory cortex. This association cortex is concerned with the analysis and elaboration of speech sounds, comprehension of spoken language, and verbal memory and is committed to language in only the dominant hemisphere. The association cortex on the nondominant side of the brain is primarily concerned with the perception of nonverbal material, such as music and environmental sounds.

Ventral Surface

The ventral (inferior) surface of the brain displays structures of the frontal, temporal, and occipital lobes (Figs. 2-7 and 2-8); no parietal structure is visible. The two most visible structures are the orbital portion of the frontal lobe and the basal portion of the temporo-occipital lobes. The orbital-frontal region is known to serve emotions, personality, and inhibition. It also includes the olfactory region. Its pathologic involvement is associated with emotional disinhibition, detached personality, and behavioral disinhibition. The *interhemispheric fissure* extends to the

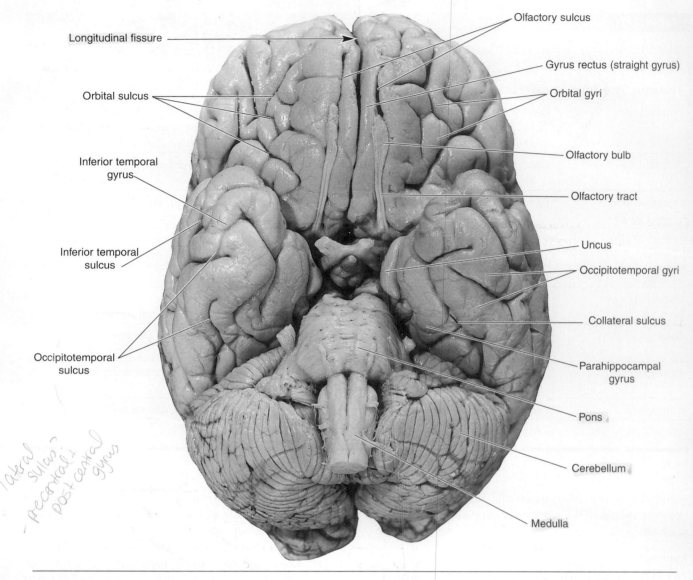

Figure 2-7 The ventral surface of the cerebral hemispheres with the pons, medulla, and cerebellum in place.

ventral surface separating the orbital portions of both frontal lobes. The **olfactory bulb** and **tract**, located in the **olfactory sulcus**, serve the sense of smell. The **gyrus rectus** is medial to the olfactory structures. The area lateral to the olfactory region is occupied by many small orbital gyri.

The posterior structures in the temporal and occipital lobes are the inferior temporal gyrus, **occipitotemporal gyrus**, **lingual gyrus**, **collateral sulcus**, **parahippocampal gyrus**, and **uncus**. The *inferior temporal gyrus* is on the lateral and ventral surfaces of the temporal lobe. *The hippocampus*, a structure identified with the encoding of short-term memory, is beneath the *parahippocampal gyrus* and can be seen after removal of this gyrus (Fig. 3-30). The *hippocampal gyrus* is posteriorly connected to the **cingulate gyrus** by a narrow isthmus beneath the splenium (posterior part) of the **corpus callosum** (Figs. 2-10 and 2-14). These structures (hippocampus, isthmus, and cingulate gyrus) are

components of the **limbic lobe**. The *collateral sulcus* marks the lateral limit of the parahippocampal and lingual gyri (Figs. 2-7 and 2-8).

Midsagittal Surface

Cortical structures on the medial surface of both hemispheres are best examined after the cerebral hemispheres are separated by sectioning the fibers of the corpus callosum (Figs. 2-9–2-11). Although portions of all four lobes are seen on the midsagittal surface, their sulci and gyri—except for the cingulate and parahippocampal gyri—do not present consistent lobar boundaries.

Frontal Lobe

A line drawn from the notch of the central sulcus to the cingulate sulcus marks the caudal boundary of the frontal lobe (Fig. 2-4). A portion of the frontal lobe on the medial

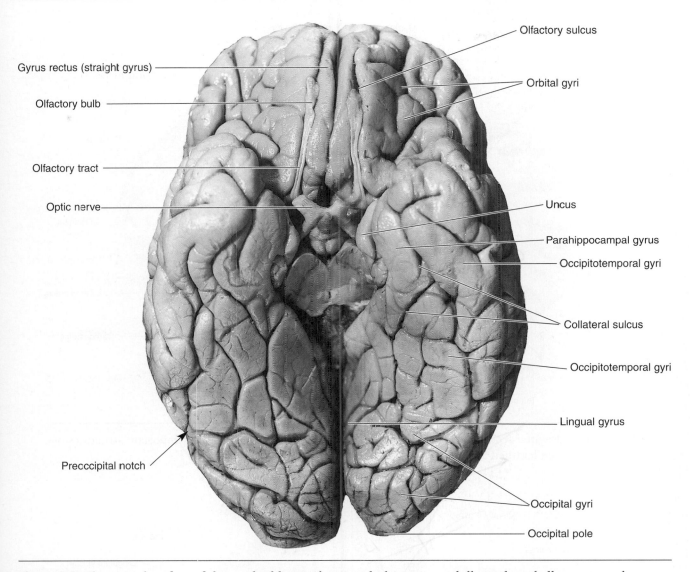

Olfactory sulcus

Gyrus rectus (straight gyrus)

Orbital gyri

Olfactory bulb

Olfactory tract

Optic nerve

Uncus

Parahippocampal gyrus

Occipitotemporal gyri

Collateral sulcus

Occipitotemporal gyri

Lingual gyrus

Precccipital notch

Occipital gyri

Occipital pole

Figure 2-8 The ventral surface of the cerebral hemispheres with the pons, medulla, and cerebellum removed.

surface is part of the superior frontal gyrus extending from the dorsolateral surface.

Parietal Lobe

Portions of the parietal lobe on the midsagittal surface extend from the superior parietal lobule of the lateral surface (Fig. 2-4). A line drawn from the notch of the central sulcus to the cingulate sulcus also demarcates the rostral boundary of the medial parietal lobe. The posterior boundary of the medial parietal lobe is marked by the *parieto-occipital sulcus* on the medial and the lateral surfaces. The precentral and postcentral gyri from the lateral surface continue midsagittally and constitute the **paracentral lobule**, an area notched by the central sulcus (Fig. 2-10).

Occipital Lobe

A larger portion of the occipital lobe is located on the medial surface than on the lateral surface. A line extending from the *parieto-occipital sulcus* to the *preoccipital notch* separates the occipital lobe from the parietal and the temporal lobes (Fig. 2-4). The occipital lobe has two important structures on the medial surface: **calcarine sulcus** and **lingual gyrus** (Fig. 2-10). The *calcarine sulcus* divides the **primary visual cortex** (Brodmann area 17) into the **upper** and **lower operculum**, which in turn are surrounded by the **secondary (association) visual cortex** (Brodmann areas 18 and 19). There are spatial patterns of representation in the primary visual cortex; the **upper calcarine operculum** receives information from the **lower quadrants** of the visual field, and the **lower calcarine operculum** receives visual impulses from the **upper quadrants** of the visual field. A destructive lesion in the primary visual cortex in one hemisphere causes blindness (homonomous hemianopsia) in the opposite visual field. A lesion in the *visual association area*, which participates in the recognition and appreciation of visual stimuli, results in visual agnosia, color agnosia,

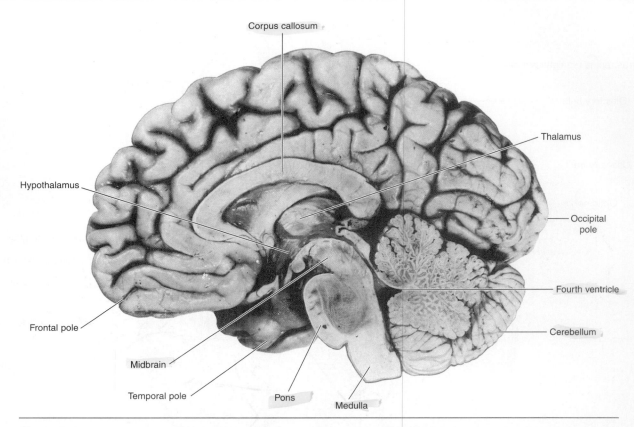

Figure 2-9 Midsagittal section of the brain with the brainstem structures in place. Important structures of the brainstem are identified in Figure 2-11.

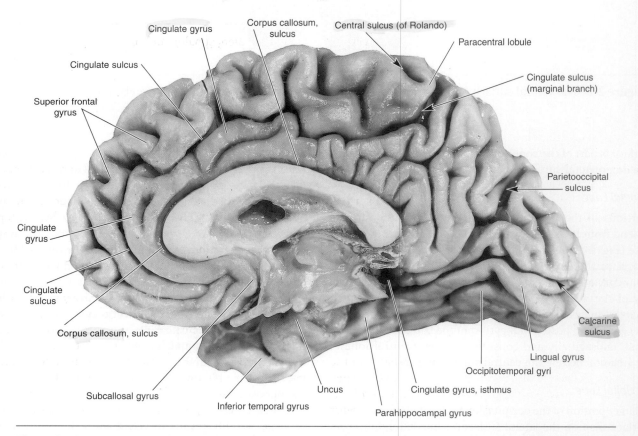

Figure 2-10 Midsagittal section of the right cerebral hemisphere with the brainstem and cerebellum removed.

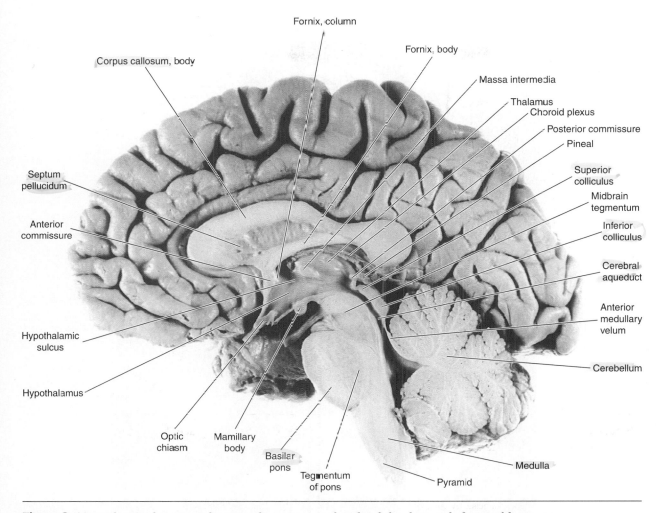

Figure 2-11 Midsagittal section showing the anatomic details of the diencephalon and brainstem.

alexia (inability to read), and impaired visual memories (Table 2-2).

The structure below the calcarine sulcus is the *lingual gyrus*. A bilateral involvement of the *primary visual cortices*—usually owing to an ischemic stroke involving the basilar artery, posterior cerebral arteries, or the calcarine arteries—results in **cortical blindness**. This is characterized by complete blindness, amnesia, and confusion, at least during the acute stage. A striking attribute of the syndrome is that, either because of parafoveal functioning or because of a natural recovery, patients are able to detect and localize light despite blindness. This processing of visual information is attributed to a subcortical integration of visual information.

Temporal Lobe

The medial temporal structures are contiguous with the ones that are visible on the ventral (basal) surface. They include the *uncus, parahippocampal gyrus, collateral sulcus, isthmus of cingulate gyrus,* and *occipitotemporal gyrus* (Fig. 2-10). The uncus and parahippocampal gyrus along with the **amygdaloid complex** form the **pyriform** (pear-shaped) **cortex.** The pyriform cortex includes the higher-order olfactory association cortex.

Additional Structures

Among other important structures on the midsagittal surface is the corpus callosum (Figs 2-9–2-12), the largest horizontal interhemispheric commissural fiber bundle. This massive, half moon–shaped myelinated fiber bundle interconnects most cortical areas of both hemispheres. Located in the floor of the *longitudinal (interhemispheric) fissure,* the myelinated fibers of the *corpus callosum* form the roof of the underlying *ventricular cavities.*

The *corpus callosum* consists of the following four parts, from its rostral to its caudal extent: **rostrum**, the most anterior portion; **genu**, the anterior bend; **body**, the large portion caudal to the genu; and **splenium**, the posterior region (Fig. 2-12). Memories, experiences, and actions of both hemispheres are shared and integrated by way of the corpus callosum.

A complete sectioning of the corpus callosum (**commissurotomy**) makes both hemispheres independent and incapable of communicating with each other or sharing

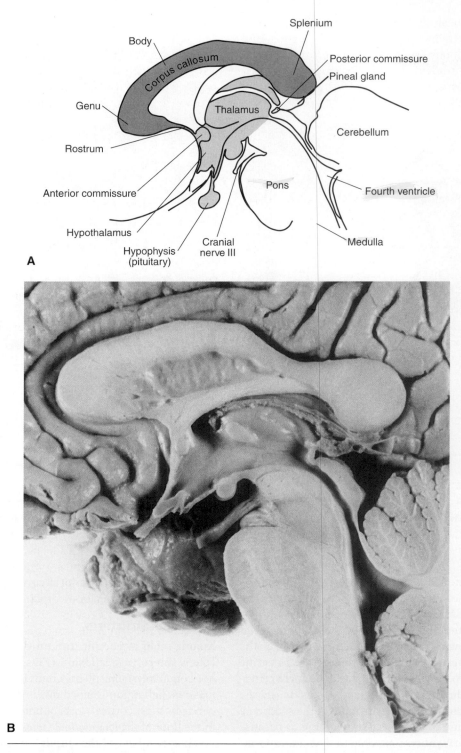

Figure 2-12 A. Midsagittal view showing the corpus callosum and its major parts. B. Midsagittal view of the brainstem, diencephalon, and corpus callosum.

information. Patients who had undergone commissurotomy for intractable seizures offered researchers a unique opportunity to map the independent neurolinguistic functions of each hemisphere, with no interference from the other half of the brain (Sperry 1977). That each hemisphere has exclusive skills and functions remains the outstanding neurolinguistic observation from that research. Findings revealed that the left hemisphere is dominant for analytic skills and receptive and expressive language (verbal expression). The right hemisphere seems to have merely adequate receptive language capacity but superior skills for facial recognition, music, temporal and spatial information, and paralinguistic functions (such as stress and intonation). Sperry extensively studied the functions of the commissural fibers in humans, receiving the 1981 Nobel Prize in physiology and medicine for this work.

Major structures dorsal to the callosal fibers are the **callosal sulcus**, the cingulate gyrus, and the **sulcus of the cingulate gyrus**. The *callosal sulcus* separates the corpus callosum from the overlying cingulate gyrus and surrounds the corpus callosum, curving ventrolaterally to become the **sulcus of the hippocampus**. The cingulate sulcus marks the inferior boundary of the *frontal lobe*. Running rostrocaudally, the cingulate sulcus turns dorsally to become its marginal branch (Fig. 2-10), which ascends and continues as the *postcentral sulcus* on the lateral surface. The cingulate gyrus, a part of the **limbic** or **visceral–emotional brain**, circles the corpus callosum and posteriorly curves ventrally to continue as the *parahippocampal gyrus* in the medial *temporal lobe* (Fig. 2-10).

Important structures ventral to the corpus callosum are the **septum pellucidum, fornix**, thalamus, hypothalamus and its sulcus, **massa intermedia (thalamic adhesion), anterior commissure, posterior commissure, mammillary body, hypophysis (pituitary gland), subcallosal gyrus, pineal body**, and **optic chiasm**. The *septum pellucidum*, consisting of a double paper-thin set of membranes, represents the medial walls of the anterior horns of the two lateral ventricles. At the base of the septum pellucidum (pl. septa pellucida), the medial cortex increases in thickness as the nucleus of the septum. This region, below the corpus callosum, is called the subcallosal gyrus (Fig. 2-14). Bidirectionally connecting the mamillary body of the *hypothalamus, septum*, and *hippocampus*, the *fornix* is important in regulating the *limbic brain* functions of emotions and memory. Forming the basic forebrain circuit, the *thalamus* is important in sensorimotor integration and speech-language-hearing functions. The hypothalamus, ventral to the thalamus, controls endocrine and autonomic functions. Specifically, it controls food and water intake, sexual behavior, and body temperature, important for preserving the survival capabilities of the organism. The boundary between the thalamus and the hypothalamus is identified by the *hypothalamic sulcus*, an indentation along the medial wall.

The *anterior commissure* connects the two *olfactory bulbs, amygdaloid complexes*, and the basal temporal pole cortices. The *posterior commissure* contains crossing fibers from the **pretectal nuclei**, the midbrain's visual reflex center. The *massa intermedia*, the interthalamic adhesion, located along the medial walls, connects the two thalami and is found in only 70–80% of humans.

The *mamillary body*, a *hypothalamic nucleus*, connects the anterior thalamus, septum, and hippocampus. The *hypophysis (pituitary gland)*, another hypothalamic structure and commonly called the master gland of the body, secretes hormones that regulate systems involved in sexual drive,

pain, emotional drive, temperature control, electrolyte control, and metabolism.

The *subcallosal gyrus*, also known as the paraolfactory area, may be considered part of the limbic lobe. The *pineal body* is a cone-shaped structure at the level of the posterior commissure. It secretes important neurotransmitters (**serotonin, melatonin**, and **norepinephrine**) that regulate the circadian rhythm and control the sexual reproduction cycles. The *optic chiasm* is the site at which optic fibers from the medial retina of each eye cross the midline, join the uncrossed fibers of the lateral retina, and continue to the opposite hemisphere.

Insular Lobe

The **insular cortex (isle of Reil)** is concealed within the depths of the lateral fissure by the overgrowth of the opercula of the frontal, parietal, and temporal lobes (Fig. 2-13). The structures of the insular cortex are exposed when these opercular tissues are removed or spread apart. Outlined by the **circular sulcus**, the insular cortex consists of short and long gyri, which run parallel to each other. The **limen insula** is the opening of the insula toward the lateral fissure. This structure is known for its nonelaboration of functions and undergoes little or no enlargement compared to the expansion of the surrounding cortex. Its anatomic location suggests that it is related to limbic and sensorimotor functions, including those of the intestine, and to vestibular and gustatory functions.

Limbic Lobe

The *limbic lobe*, one of the older parts of the brain, includes the mammalian brain structures that form a ring around the medial-most metabolic margins of the frontal, parietal, and temporal lobes (Fig. 2-14). The limbic lobe consists of the *cingulate gyrus, hippocampal formation, parahippocampal gyrus, uncus*, and *subcallosal gyrus*. All of these structures, through their connections with *diencephalic* and *brainstem nuclei*, provide the emotional drive to visceral and vegetative functions, which are fundamental to survival; these include instinctual reflexes and drives (fleeing, feeding, fighting, and mating behaviors); aggression; anxiety; and fear. The limbic circuit begins with hippocampal projections via the fornix to the hypothalamic mammillary bodies, which use the mammillothalamic tract for projecting to the cingulate gyrus by way of the anterior thalamic nuclei; the cingulate gyrus completes the circuit by projecting back to the parahippocampal gyrus (see Chapters 6 and 16).

The *fornix* is the principal *hippocampal output* to the *septum* and the *mamillary body* of the *hypothalamus*. The proximity of the hippocampal gyrus to the amygdala, uncus, and **olfactory system** emphasizes the importance of smell in visceral and emotional behaviors. The **Papez circuit** in the mammalian forebrain, which involves neuronal connections of the hypothalamus, limbic system, and thalamus, is considered the neurologic base of emotional expression (see Chapter 16). The limbic system also

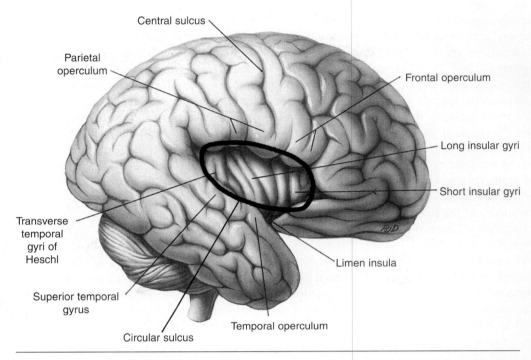

Figure 2-13 Lateral view of the right cerebral hemisphere with both banks of the lateral fissure separated to reveal the insular cortex and transverse gyrus of Heschl (*solid line*).

governs our values and decisions about perceptions and feelings, which regulate the intensity and strength of the emotional drive. Pathologic involvement of the Papez circuit produces profound deficits in emotional behavior.

Basal Ganglia

Formed by a series of complex circuits, the basal ganglia involve cortical output processing, which impinges on the thalamocortical-thalamic circuits by slowing or inhibiting the activity of other loops and the motor cortex. Basal ganglia are believed to regulate motor functions and muscle tone; however, recently these structures are also found to participate in processes that regulate drives, action execution, and cognitive functions. Basal ganglia structures, best seen on horizontal or coronal sections of the brain, consist of five nuclear masses: **caudate nucleus**, **putamen**, **globus pallidus**, **claustrum**, and **amygdaloid nucleus** (Figs. 2-15–2-17). Various anatomic terms are used for grouping the

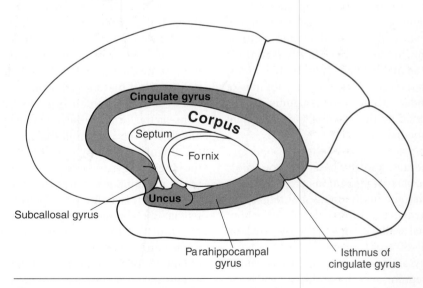

Figure 2-14 Midsagittal view. *Shaded area*, limbic structures, including the cingulate gyrus, parahippocampal gyrus, and uncus.

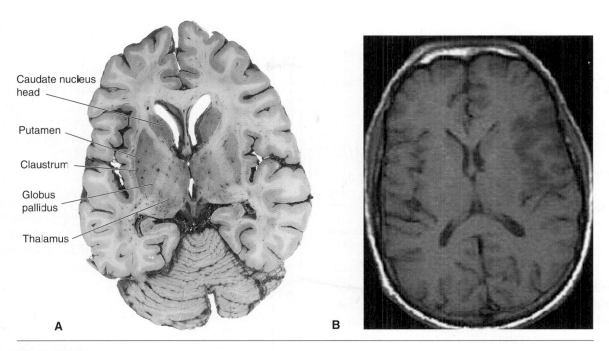

Figure 2-15 Horizontal section (A) and the corresponding MRI (B) showing the subcortical basal ganglia structures in relation to the internal capsule and its parts.

basal ganglia nuclei (Table 2-3). The caudate nucleus and putamen, as a histologically identical group of nuclei, constitute the **neostriatum** or **striatum**. The **lenticular nucleus**, which is also called the **pallidum**, includes the putamen and globus pallidus.

Damage to the basal ganglia circuitry by physical injury or by the loss of neurotransmitters results in disinhibition and the release of inappropriate behavioral patterns as seen in patients with Parkinson disease, Huntington disease, Tourette syndrome, and Sydenham chorea. Basal ganglia

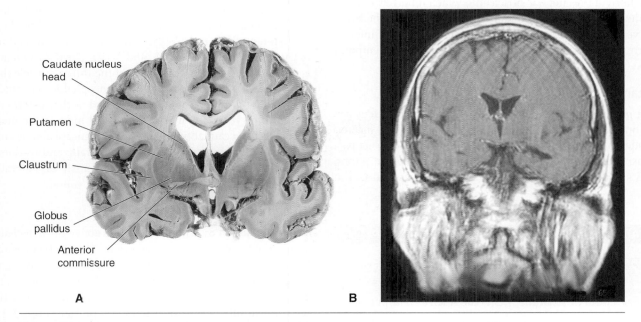

Figure 2-16 Rostral surface of a coronal section of the brain (A) and the corresponding MRI (B) showing the basal ganglia nuclei and other subcortical structures in relation to the internal capsule.

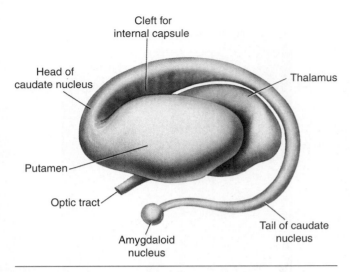

Cleft for
internal capsule

Head of
caudate nucleus

Thalamus

Putamen

Optic tract

Amygdaloid
nucleus

Tail of caudate
nucleus

Figure 2-17 General anatomy of an isolated striatum. Rostrally, the caudate nucleus merges with the putamen. The tail of the caudate nucleus travels in the floor of the lateral ventricle and ends in the amygdaloid nucleus. Fibers of the internal capsule pass through the cleft between the putamen and the thalamus.

lesions do not cause paralysis or paresis. Rather, they produce involuntary movements, such as the tremor, chorea, ticks, and ballism (Table 1-2).

Caudate Nucleus

The *caudate nucleus* is a large C-shaped structure. It has a massive pear-shaped head and a long curved tail. Rostrally, the head of the caudate forms the lateral wall of the anterior horn of the lateral ventricle into which it bulges. The tail of the caudate extends caudally (posteriorly) from the head, curves around the **ventricular trigone** to enter the inferior horn, and ends at the level of the *amygdala* in the temporal lobe (Figs. 2-17 and 3-30).

Putamen

The *putamen,* a half moon–shaped basal ganglia nucleus lies within the subcortical white core of the brain. It is located caudal-lateral to the *caudate* and lateral to the *globus pallidus*. Lateral to the putamen is the **external capsule**, a long and slender fiber bundle. Other structures lateral to the

putamen are the *claustrum* and **extreme capsule**, underlying the *insular cortex* (Figs. 2-15 and 2-16).

Globus Pallidus

The wedge-shaped *globus pallidus* is medial to the *putamen* (Fig. 2-15). It consists of medial and lateral components. The globus pallidus is bordered by the optic tract fibers and *amygdala* ventrally and by the **internal capsule** medially (Fig. 2-16).

Claustrum

The *claustrum* is a slender mass of gray matter buried in the white matter between the *insular cortex* and the lateral margin of the *lenticular nucleus* (Figs. 2-15 and 2-16). It is connected with sensory cortical areas and contributes to visceral functions and sensory integration.

Amygdaloid Nucleus

The *amygdaloid nucleus* is a small round nucleus that lies in the rostral-medial temporal lobe at the end of the temporal horn and is contiguous to the tail end of the *caudate nucleus* (Fig. 2-17). Although anatomically included in the basal ganglia, the amygdaloid nucleus is related functionally to the limbic system.

The **substantia nigra**, **red nucleus**, and **subthalamic nucleus** are additional important subcortical nuclei that participate in motor activity (Figs 2-19 and 2-24). Although functionally related, these are not true *basal ganglia* structures. The structural and functional details of these structures are discussed in Chapter 13.

Diencephalon

The diencephalon includes the subcortical nuclear masses that form the central core of the brain. The *thalamus* and *hypothalamus* are the two major substructures of the diencephalon and can be seen on sagittal and coronal sections of the brain (Figs. 2-11, 2-18, and 2-19). The diencephalon is divided in half by a vertical slit of the third ventricle that demarcates the medial limit of the diencephalon. The **interventricular foramen**, bilaterally located at the rostral end of the third ventricle, marks the rostral limit of the diencephalon. The caudal boundary of the diencephalon is contiguous with the rostral end of the midbrain, and its dorsal boundary is delineated by the lateral ventricles. Laterally, the diencephalon extends to the *internal capsule*.

Thalamus

The *thalamus,* an oval nuclear mass, is above the *hypothalamus* in the floor of the lateral ventricle. The interventricular foramen and the posterior commissure, respectively, mark the anterior and posterior limits of the thalamus (Fig. 2-11). The third ventricle delineates the medial border, and the *internal capsule* delineates the lateral border (Figs. 2-15, 2-18, and 2-19). Both *thalami* are bridged by a loose fibrous tissue, the *massa intermedia* (thalamic adhesion), that crosses the midline through the *third ventricle* (Fig. 2-11).

Table 2-3	
Terms for the Basal Ganglia Structures	
Neostriatum or striatum	Caudate nucleus and putamen
Lenticular nucleus	Putamen and globus pallidus
Pallidum	Globus pallidus

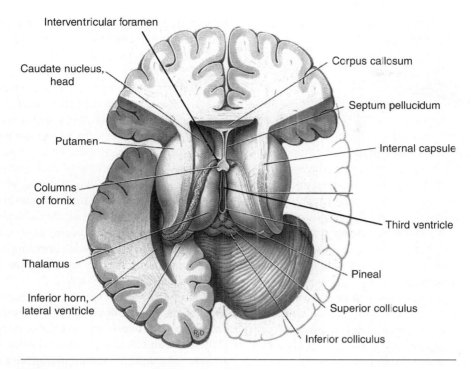

Figure 2-18 A horizontally dissected brain showing the general locations of the thalamus, striatum (caudate and putamen), internal capsule, and cavity of the lateral ventricle.

The thalamus is made up of numerous small specific and nonspecific nuclei, each serving definite functions and projecting to different parts of the brain. A major function of the thalamus is to relay sensorimotor information to the cortex. Research evidence from patients with thalamic infarcts and thalamotomy (surgically induced lesion of the thalamus for treatment of intractable pain and motor disorders) suggests that the thalamus also contributes to cortically mediated speech and language functions. Vascular or neoplastic thalamic lesions produce impaired contralateral

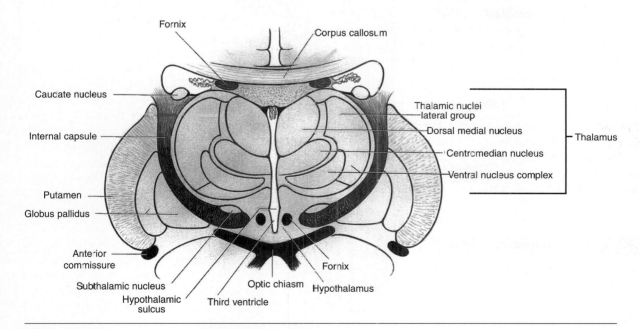

Figure 2-19 Coronal section through the diencephalon showing the thalamus and hypothalamus in relation to the third ventricle. Additional structures are the internal capsule, striatum, corpus callosum, and fornix.

somatic sensation, a burning sensation of pain, and a low threshold of pain (Table 2-2). The anatomy and function of the thalamus are discussed in Chapter 6.

Hypothalamus

The *hypothalamic sulcus* separates the *hypothalamus* from the dorsally located *thalamus* (Fig. 2-19). The **optic chiasm** and *anterior commissure* mark the anterior limit, and the *mamillary body* marks the caudal limit of the hypothalamus (Fig. 2-11). Consisting of many nuclei, the hypothalamus communicates with the brain, brainstem, and spinal cord by neural and hormonal efferents. The hypothalamus uses overlapping neuronal circuitry to serve four primary functions: autonomic, endocrinic, regulatory, and drive and emotion. With efferent projections to the brainstem and spinal cord, it controls the autonomic nervous system. By releasing various hormones directly into the blood system, it regulates all endocrinic functions of the body. Major regulatory functions of the hypothalamus include maintaining body temperature, blood volume, food and water intake, body mass, reproduction, and the regulation of circadian rhythms. With projections to the limbic system, the hypothalamus contributes to drives and emotions.

The structures and functions of the hypothalamus are discussed in Chapter 16. Hypothalamic pathology results in impaired control of body temperature regulation, food and water intake, salt metabolism, sleep–wake cycles, and endocrine functions (Table 2-2).

Brainstem

The *brainstem* is a short extension of the brain that connects the diencephalon to the *spinal cord* (Figs. 2-20–2-22). It consists of the midbrain, pons, and medulla oblongata, but it does not include the cerebellum. Integrating and coordinating both centrally and peripherally acquired information, the brainstem monitors all brain outputs. It possesses automatic control systems that are genetically acquired. This is opposite of the cortical functions, which are programmed through daily experience and learning. Brainstem syndrome includes impaired ocular control, altered consciousness, and sensorimotor deficit of the opposite half of the body (Table 2-2).

The entire ventral surface of the brainstem can be seen in Figure 2-20. The dorsal and lateral surfaces are exposed only after the overlying cerebellar tissues are removed (Figs. 2-21 and 2-22). The ventral surface of the midbrain consists of a midline **peduncular groove** and a **pes pedunculi** (crus cerebri) on each side. Caudal to the peduncular groove and *pes pedunculi* is the large protruding body of the pons. Caudally attached to the *pons* is the *medulla,*

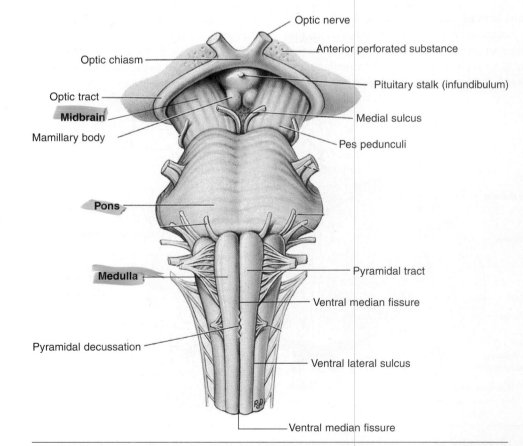

Figure 2-20 The ventral brainstem showing the locations of the midbrain, pons, and medulla as well as several cranial nerve rootlets.

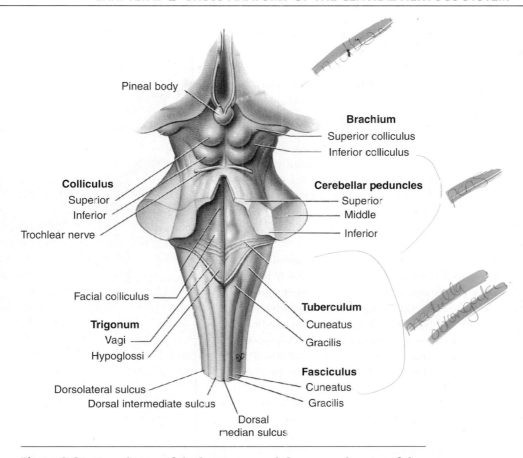

Pineal body

Brachium
Superior colliculus
Inferior colliculus

Colliculus
Superior
Inferior
Trochlear nerve

Cerebellar peduncles
Superior
Middle
Inferior

Facial colliculus

Tuberculum
Cuneatus
Gracilis

Trigonum
Vagi
Hypoglossi

Fasciculus
Cuneatus
Gracilis

Dorsolateral sulcus
Dorsal intermediate sulcus

Dorsal median sulcus

Figure 2-21 Dorsal view of the brainstem and the exposed cavity of the fourth ventricle with the overlying cerebellum removed.

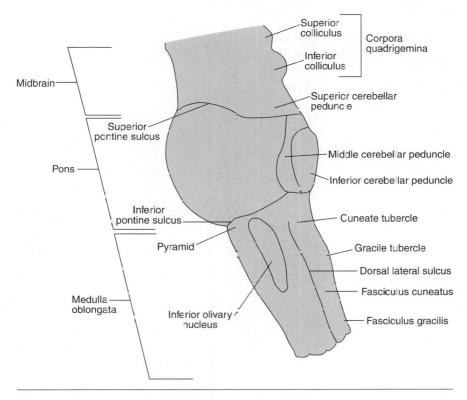

Midbrain

Superior colliculus
Inferior colliculus
Corpora quadrigemina

Superior pontine sulcus

Superior cerebellar peduncle

Pons

Middle cerebellar peduncle
Inferior cerebellar peduncle

Inferior pontine sulcus

Cuneate tubercle

Pyramid

Gracile tubercle

Dorsal lateral sulcus

Medulla oblongata

Fasciculus cuneatus

Inferior olivary nucleus

Fasciculus gracilis

Figure 2-22 Lateral view of the brainstem showing the relation of the midbrain, pons, and medulla to the cerebellar peduncles.

the cone-shaped caudal portion of the brainstem, which becomes contiguous with the spinal cord at the level of the **foramen magnum** (Fig. 2-31).

The superior surface of the brainstem is seen after the cerebellum is removed (Fig. 2-21). The structures on brainstem's dorsal surface are the **corpora quadrigemina** (**superior** and **inferior colliculi**), the floor of the **fourth ventricle**, and three **cerebellar peduncles**. The fourth ventricle floor contains many cranial nerve nuclei. The **cuneate tubercle**, **fasciculus gracilis**, and **fasciculus cuneatus** are the most evident structures of the dorsal medulla. These structures mediate fine discriminative touch from the body (see Chapter 7). Figure 2-22 provides a lateral view of the entire brainstem and its gross anatomic structures.

Internally, the brainstem consists of **cranial nerve nuclei**, **longitudinal fiber tracts**, and the **reticular formation**. The *reticular formation* collectively represents groups of diffusely located specialized nerve cells that are entangled in a network of fibers, which are interconnected with parallel- and serial-running neuronal circuits. Composing most of the brainstem, the divergent circuitry of the reticular formation is functionally wired to nuclei in the thalamus and spinal cord (Fig. 2-23). By virtue of their central locations, the reticular neuronal circuits inhibit, facilitate, modify, and regulate all cortical functions. The reticular formation integrates all sensorimotor stimuli with internally generated thoughts, emotions, and cognition. It is also responsible for maintaining the homeostatic state of the brain, which is essential for regulating visceral, sensorimotor, and neuroendocrine activities, including blood pressure and movement.

The complex multisynaptic ascending projections of the reticular formation to the brain, thalamus, hypothalamus, and basal ganglia form the **reticular activating system** (**RAS**), which has a controlling influence on the levels of cortical arousal and consciousness. A lesion of the RAS can produce altered states of arousal, such as drowsiness, stupor, or prolonged unconsciousness (comatose). The level of alertness is correlated with the electroencephalic activity of the brain. While the neocortex (cerebral hemispheres) is sleeping, the specialized nuclei of the brainstem turn on the body's metabolic repair systems; after the body repair is completed and energy replenished, the reticular formation clock turns and reawakens the brain.

Besides alertness, two functions of the reticular formation that are closely related to communicative disorders are the regulation of **respiration** and **swallowing**. The **pontine pneumotaxic center** not only refines the respiration but also regulates the depth and rhythm of the **medullary respiratory center**, which regulates the basic inspiration and expiration rhythm, which in turn is controlled by the carbon dioxide level in the blood. Damage to the respiratory centers in the medulla and pons can be life-threatening. The reticular formation regulates swallowing by integrating the sensorimotor functions of the **trigeminal nerve** (**cranial nerve [CN] V**), **facial nerve** (**CN VII**), **glossopharyngeal**

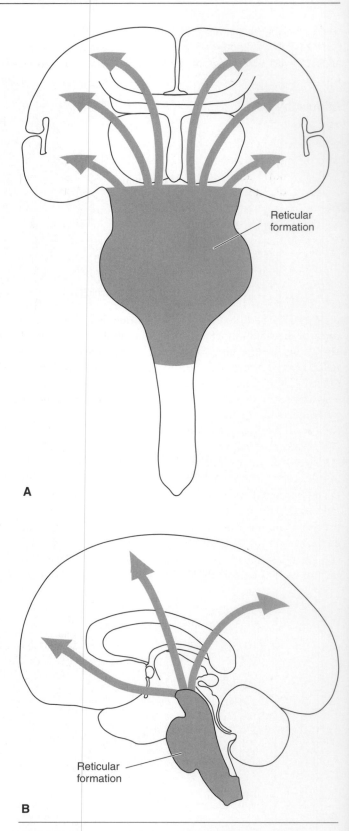

A

B

Figure 2-23 Frontal (A) and lateral (B) views of the brainstem reticular formation.

Reticular formation

Reticular formation

nerve (CN IX), **vagus nerve** (CN X), and **hypoglossal nerve** (CN XII). See Chapter 16 for a detailed discussion of the anatomy and physiology of the reticular formation and its functions.

Midbrain

The *midbrain* is a link between the *cerebral hemispheres* and peripheral and cranial sensory input systems. It contains all incoming sensory and outgoing motor fibers and important reticular and cranial nerve nuclei. It is also responsible for generating neurotransmitters vital to *telencephalic, diencephalic, brainstem,* and *spinal cord* functions.

Ventrally, the midbrain has an **interpeduncular fossa,** which is divided by a longitudinal indentation (peduncular groove). The elevation on each side is formed by the *pes pedunculi tracts* of pyramidal motor fibers (Fig. 2-20). Dorsally, the midbrain has four rounded elevations (corpora quadrigemina), which are located just beneath the overlapping *pineal gland* of the thalamus and form the roof (**tectum**) of the midbrain (Fig. 2-21). The upper two rounded elevations are the *superior colliculi,* which participate in reflex control of eye movements, visual reflexes, and coordination of vestibular-generated head and eye movements. The lower two rounded elevations are the *inferior colliculi,* which mediate the transmission of auditory impulses from the ear to the thalamus and auditory cortex. The inferior colliculi also mediate reflexes triggered by auditory stimuli.

Lateral to the *corpora quadrigemina* are swellings of the two **brachia** (sing. brachium). Fibers of the **brachium of the superior colliculus** connect the superior colliculi with the visual relay nucleus of the thalamus, and fibers of the **brachium of the inferior colliculus** connect the inferior colliculi with the auditory relay nucleus of the thalamus.

Internally, the midbrain contains many important nuclei and bundles of sensory and motor fibers (Fig. 2-24). There are three subdivisions in the midbrain: **tectum** (roof), **tegmentum,** and **basis pedunculi**. The *tectum* is located dorsal to the cerebral aqueduct, a small tubular connection between the third and the fourth ventricles. The *tectum* has an important role in the survival of the organism because it provides the organism with a three-dimensional orientation map. This map guides eye movements and head and body turning in response to bright light and directional sounds. The tectum also mediates visual reflexes, such as pupil constriction and lens accommodation. The *tegmentum,* the central part of the midbrain, contains numerous scattered nuclei, such as the *red nucleus, cranial nerve nuclei,* and *reticular central gray region.* The *basis pedunculi* is ventral to the tegmentum; it consists of the pes pedunculi (crus cerebri), a group of cortical pyramidal tract fibers, which terminate in the brainstem, spinal cord, and the *substantia nigra. The* substantia nigra contains a group of nuclei that produce dopamine, an inhibitory neurotransmitter; a degenerative lesion involving these cells leads to Parkinson disease (Box 2-1).

Pons

The *pons,* a metencephalic structure, is separated from the midbrain by the **superior pontine sulcus** and from the medulla by the **inferior pontine sulcus** (Fig. 2-22). The ventral pontine surface is convex both longitudinally and horizontally, whereas dorsally the pontine structures are hidden by the overlying cerebellum. The pons contains all descending motor fibers and ascending sensory fibers; numerous cranial nuclei; the reticular formation; and transverse fibers that form the **middle cerebellar peduncle,** which attaches the cerebellum to the brainstem. The rhomboid fourth ventricle is dorsal to the pons and is visible after removal of the overlying cerebellum. The ventricular floor is broad in the middle and narrows toward its

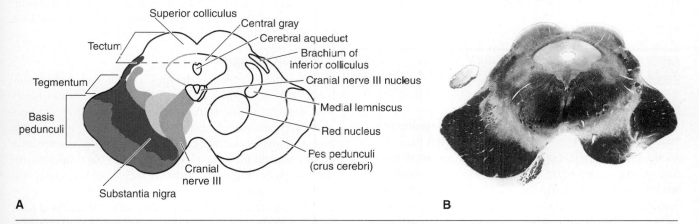

A **B**

Figure 2-24 **A.** Transverse section of the rostral midbrain at the level of the superior colliculus showing the internal anatomy of the midbrain. The tectum, containing the superior and inferior colliculi, is dorsal to the cerebral aqueduct. The tegmentum contains the sensorimotor nuclei, many passing tracts, and the reticular formation. The pedunculi region contains the motor fibers of the corticospinal and corticobulbar systems. **B.** The corresponding transverse section of the midbrain.

(Continued)

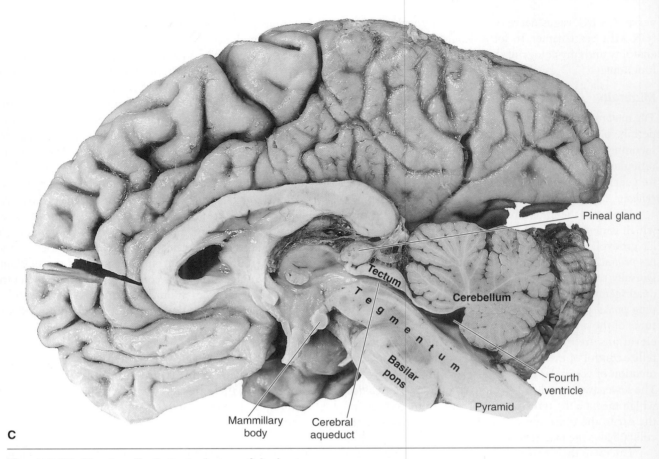

C

Figure 2-24 *(Continued)* C. Sagittal view of the brainstem.

caudal end. The floor is divided in half by the dorsal median sulcus, and it contains important cranial nerve nuclei (Fig. 2-21). Along the medial eminence of the ventricular floor is a small round protrusion, the **facial colliculus**, formed by the facial nerve (CN VII) fibers.

Internally, the pons consists of two parts: the **pontine tegmentum** and the **basis pontis**, which is also called the

base of the pons (Fig. 2-25). The *tegmentum* of the pons contains ascending and descending fibers and numerous diffusely scattered pontine reticular nuclei. The fibers of the **medial lemniscus** are responsible for mediating fine discriminative touch. The *basis pontis* contains the cortical descending fiber tracts, pontine nuclei, and pontocerebellar fibers. The base of the pons also contains descending corticospinal fibers, which form the medullary pyramids in the medulla and continue in the spinal cord.

Medulla Oblongata

The *medulla oblongata* is the most caudal part of the brainstem (Fig. 2-20 and 2-22). It contains all the motor fibers that descend to the spinal cord and all the sensory fibers that carry sensory information from the body to the more rostral brain areas. Major surface structures of the medulla are the **ventral median sulcus**, **pyramidal tract**, **inferior olivary nucleus**, and **dorsal tubercula** (gracile fasciculus and cuneate fasciculus).

The ventral median fissure divides the medulla in half. Parallel to the ventral median fissure is the **ventrolateral sulcus**. Between both these sulci is the pyramidal tract, which carries motor information from the motor cortex to the spinal cord for activation of skeletal muscles. The descending fibers of the pyramidal pathway decussate at the level of the caudal medulla. After the motor fibers cross

---

BOX 2-1

Parkinson Disease

Associated with the deficiency of a neurotransmitter, Parkinson disease results from the degeneration of dopaminergic neurons in the substantia nigra of the midbrain. This condition, usually involving the body bilaterally, generally afflicts the elderly and is characterized by rhythmic tremors, rigidity of movement, stooped posture, mask-like expressionless face, slowness of movements, and unintelligible speech because of dysarthria; cognitive symptoms may emerge in the late stages of the disease.

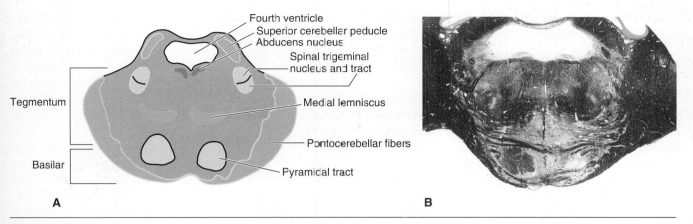

Figure 2-25 **A**. Transverse section of the mid-pons showing its internal anatomy, which consists of the tegmentum and basilar pons. The tegmentum of the pons contains diffusely scattered sensorimotor nuclei of cranial nerves, the core of the reticular formation, and multiple ascending and descending fibers. The basilar pons largely contains pyramidal fibers of the corticobulbar and corticospinal systems. **B**. Corresponding transverse section of the pons.

the midline, they form the **lateral corticospinal tract**, a motor pathway of the spinal cord.

The **dorsal median sulcus** divides the dorsal surface of the medulla in half; the caudal floor of the fourth ventricle forms a **trigonum**, which contains the **hypoglossal** and **vagus nuclear complexes** (Fig. 2-21). Located between the **dorsolateral sulcus** and the dorsal median sulcus are two sensory pathways, the gracile fasciculus and cuneate fasciculus, that carry fine discriminatory sensory information from the body to the medulla and then to the thalamus. On the lateral medullary surface is an oval protrusion produced by the underlying enlarged **inferior olivary nucleus**. Fibers from the inferior olivary nucleus project to the cerebellum by way of the inferior cerebellar peduncle.

Internally, the medulla consists of two parts: the tegmentum and **pyramid** (Fig. 2-26). The tegmental area contains several nuclei, the reticular formation, medial lemniscus fibers, and fibers projecting to the cerebellum. Numerous cranial nerve nuclei are anchored and interconnected through the reticular bed that extends up and down the brainstem tegmentum. Some nuclei of the medullary reticular formation form three vital reflex centers. The **cardiac center** regulates the rate and strength of heartbeat. The **vasomotor center** monitors and alters the diameter of the blood vessels. The **respiratory center**, in conjunction with the pontine pneumotaxic center, controls the rhythm and rate of breathing. Consequently, injuries to the medulla that implicate those centers may

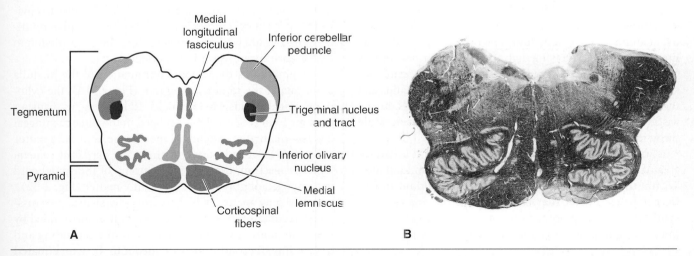

Figure 2-26 **A**. Transverse section of the medulla showing the internal anatomic regions of the tegmentum and pyramid. The tegmentum contains sensorimotor nuclei, the reticular formation, and passing fibers; the pyramidal region contains pyramidal motor fibers. **B**. Corresponding transverse section of the medulla.

be fatal. The pyramid contains the descending motor fibers that are ventral in the medulla and cross the midline in the caudal medulla.

Cerebellum

The cerebellum is dorsal to the *pons* and *medulla* (Figs. 2-9, 2-11, and 2-12). It is separated from the cerebral hemispheres above by a **meningeal layer** of **dura mater** and from the brainstem by the fourth ventricle.

It contributes to the maintenance of equilibrium and coordination of motor activity by modifying cortical motor functions, but it does not initiate motor activity. Through direct and indirect projections to the motor cortex, basal ganglia, and spinal cord, the cerebellum coordinates and modifies the tone, speed, and range of muscular excursions in the execution of motor functions. For example, it adjusts the strength needed to lift, for example, 10 lb versus 200 lb and ensures smooth movement. The cerebellar projections to the vestibular system make crucial contributions to equilibrium-maintaining mechanisms. A lesion in the cerebellum leads to mild weakness, tremor, paucity of movement, ataxia (muscular incoordination), and impaired equilibrium.

The cerebellum has a highly distinctive appearance; its surface consists of a large number of transverse thin sulci formed by narrow rows of tightly packed gyri called **folia**. The wedge-shaped cerebellum is divided into the cerebellar hemispheres (Fig. 2-27). The structures in the midline portion of the cerebellum are grouped into the **vermis** (Fig. 2-28). Each cerebellar hemisphere is divided into three lobes: **anterior**, **posterior**, and **flocculonodular** (Fig. 2-28). The portion of the cerebellum rostral to the primary fissure is the anterior lobe. The posterior lobe lies between the primary fissure and the posterolateral fissure. The flocculonodular lobe, the oldest part of the cerebellum, is on the inferior surface; it consists of the **nodulus** and the paired **flocculi** which are two vermal structures (Fig. 2-29).

A midsagittal section of the *vermis* reveals its central structures and provides a better view of the overall internal anatomy of the cerebellum. The nodulus portion of the flocculonodular lobe is medial; the remaining part of this older lobe, the paired flocculi, is ventrolateral on the inferior surface of the cerebellum (Fig. 2-29). Both the flocculus and the nodulus are involved in coordinating movements during vestibular system activation, such as falling to the side while throwing a ball.

Structurally, the cerebellar lobes consist of a surface area of gray matter and a medullary core of white matter. Within the core of the white matter are important intrinsic cerebellar nuclei that participate in the analysis and synthesis of sensorimotor information and project motor-modulating impulses to all motor control centers.

Cerebellar Peduncles

The *cerebellum* is connected to the *brainstem* through three fiber bundles called the **superior (brachium conjunctivum)**, middle **(brachium pontis)**, and **inferior (restiform body) cerebellar peduncles**. The lateral inferior surface of the cerebellum reveals the connections of the peduncles to the brainstem (Figs. 2-29 and 2-30). The superior peduncle is stem shaped. Ventrally, the middle and inferior peduncles appear as a bulging, thick semicircular collar attached to the pontine ventrolateral brainstem.

Input to the Cerebellum

The *cerebellum* receives its input information from two sources. Afferents from the motor cortex by way of the pontine nuclei enter through fibers of the *middle cerebellar peduncle*. Fibers of the *inferior cerebellar peduncle* transmit proprioceptive afferent information from the trunk and limbs and the vestibular information to the cerebellum (Fig. 2-30). The cerebellar cortex near the midline (vermis), which receives all the input, plays an important role in the integration of vestibular data with the ongoing movement mechanism.

Output from the Cerebellum

After analysis and synthesis of the received sensorimotor information, the cerebellum projects its corrective feedback predominantly to the opposite motor cortex, reticular formation, and spinal cord primarily through the *superior cerebellar peduncle* (Fig. 2-30).

Spinal Cord
Anatomic Structure

The *spinal cord* is the transmission link between the brain and the body. As a bidirectional pathway, it transmits motor impulses from the brain to the visceral organs and muscles and carries sensory information—such as pain, touch, temperature, and proprioception—from the body to the brain. Sensory input that requires an immediate response may not reach the level of awareness. Instead, the spinal cord locally integrates such information via collaterals, thereby generating its own reflex ad an immediate response to environmental changes. Even the reflexes that involve multiple synapses are well under way before the transmission to the cerebrum can result in experience.

Beginning as the caudal continuation of the medulla oblongata at the **foramen magnum** (Fig. 2.31*A*), the cylindrical spinal cord is 42–45 cm (16–18 in.) long; its diameter is about 1 cm (Fig. 2-31*B*). Wrapped in the three meningeal layers—**pia mater**, **arachnoid membrane**, and **dura mater** (Fig. 2-32)—it is housed in the bony *vertebral column*. On cross-section, the internal anatomy of the spinal cord is composed of gray matter and white matter (Fig. 2-32).

The gray matter, which is butterfly-shaped in cross-section, contains all spinal nerve cells. It is surrounded by the white matter, which is made up of the ascending and descending fibers arbitrarily divided into three **myelinated funiculi** (fasciculi): dorsal, lateral, and ventral. The gray matter consists of two **dorsal horns** and two **ventral horns**. The *dorsal horns* contain the nerve cells that receive sensory

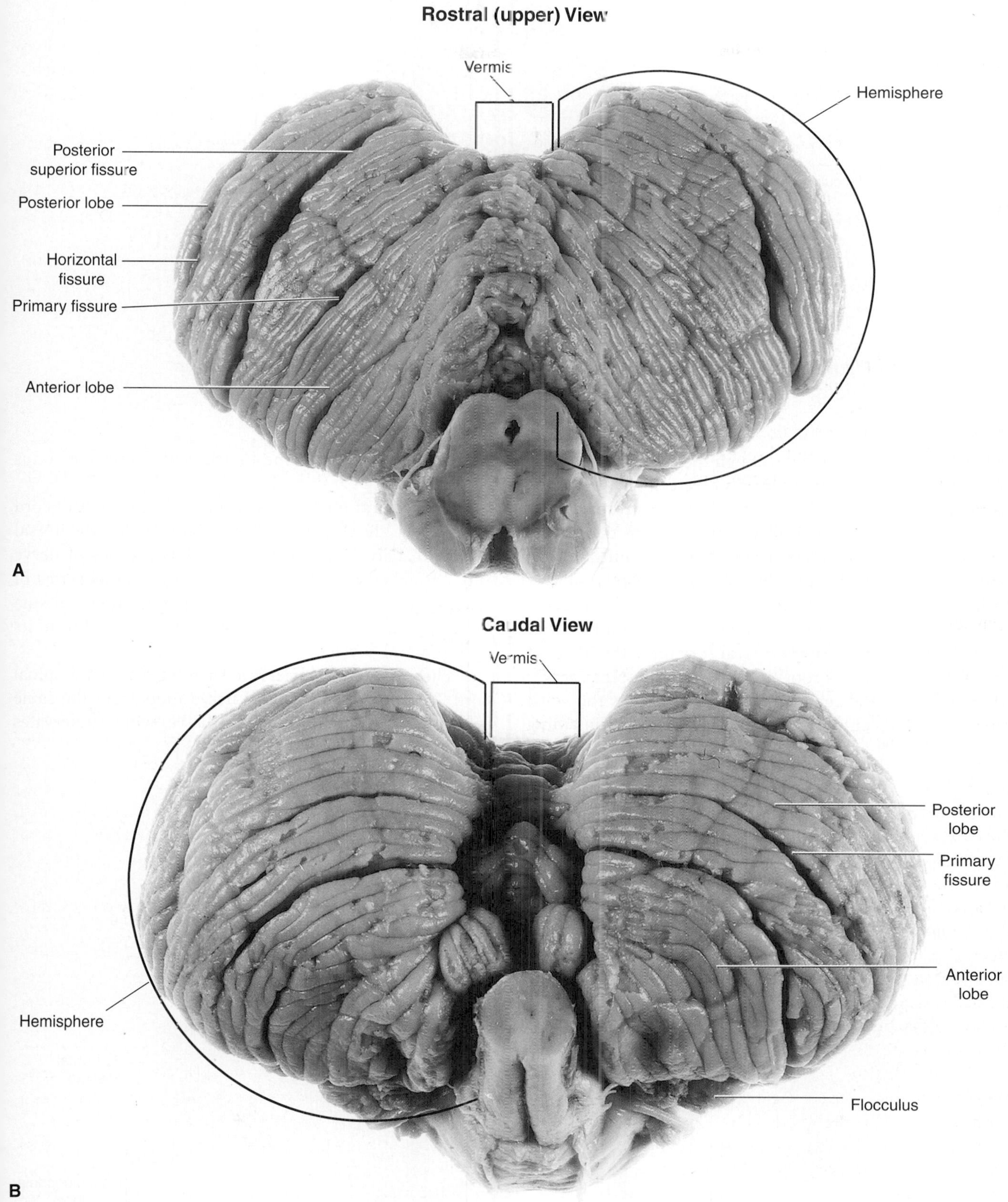

Rostral (upper) View

Vermis

Hemisphere

Posterior superior fissure

Posterior lobe

Horizontal fissure

Primary fissure

Anterior lobe

A

Caudal View

Vermis

Posterior lobe

Primary fissure

Anterior lobe

Hemisphere

Flocculus

B

Figure 2-27 Rostral (A) and caudal (B) views of the cerebellum revealing the cerebellar hemispheres, primary lobes, vermis, and fissures.

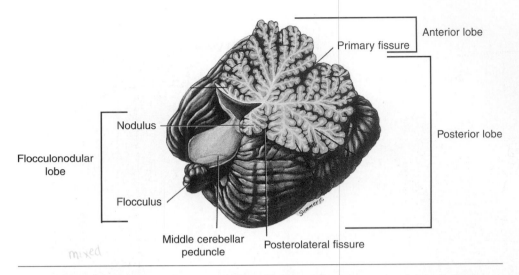

Figure 2-28 Sagittal view of the cerebellum showing the structures of the cerebellar vermis.

information from the body through the **dorsal root fibers**. The *ventral horns* contain motor nerve cells whose axons leave the cord through the anterior roots to activate visceral and skeletal muscles and glands. In addition, the ventral horns contain many interneurons that communicate with each other and the **lower motor neurons** (**LMNs**) of synergistic motor units and agonistic and antagonistic muscles, producing coordinated movements of limbs. After exiting through the **intervertebral foramina**, the fibers of the dorsal and ventral roots join to form the spinal nerves (Fig. 2-32). In the center of the spinal cord is the small opening of the **central canal**, an invisible duct containing

CSF that extends from the fourth ventricle to the conus medullaris.

The **ventral median fissure** divides the ventral cord into halves; the **dorsal median sulcus** divides the dorsal cord into halves. The spinal cord has a series of nerve roots attached to it (Fig. 2-32). A continuous series of dorsal rootlets enters the cord on its posterolateral surface. Similarly, a series of rootlets exits the cord from its anterolateral surface.

There is one spinal nerve at each segment of the spinal cord. The dorsal and ventral nerve roots from the same side join to form the *peripheral nerve*, which innervates

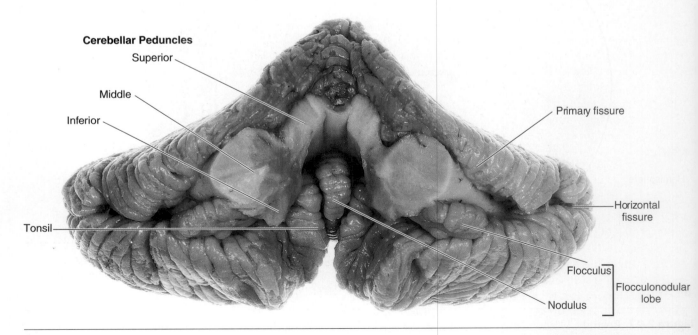

Figure 2-29 Inferior surface of the cerebellum with the brainstem removed to expose the three cerebellar peduncles and vermal structures.

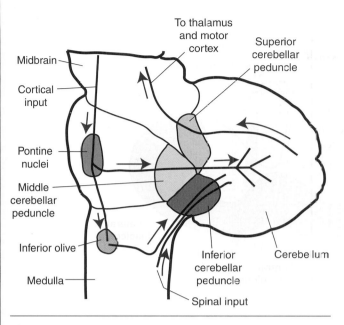

Figure 2-30 A lateral view of the brainstem and a mid-sagittal section of the cerebellum showing the three connecting cerebellar peduncles.

that side of the body (Fig. 2-32). The cell bodies of the dorsal root fibers form the **dorsal root ganglion**, which is proximal to the site at which the dorsal root fibers join the **ventral root fibers** to form a spinal nerve. The region of the spinal cord that gives rise to the fibers making up a spinal nerve is called a spinal cord segment. Without the rootlet fibers, the spinal cord would show no signs of its segmental nature; rather it would appear as a continuous column of gray and white matter.

There are 31 segments in the spinal cord and 31 spinal nerves on each side (Fig. 2-33). These segments are grouped into five divisions of the spinal cord: **cervical** ($n = 8$), **thoracic** ($n = 12$), **lumbar** ($n = 5$), **sacral** ($n = 5$), and **coccygeal** ($n = 1$). The segmental sensorimotor organization of the spinal cord is reflected by the peripheral overlapping of sensory and motor innervations for body parts and areas. The area of the body innervated by the neurons in a single dorsal root ganglion or a single dorsal root is termed a **dermatome**. The entire body is divided into numerous dermatomes. The muscles or parts of muscles innervated by all the axons exiting the cord via single ventral root is called a **myotome**. Familiarity with a dermatome–myotome chart and the corresponding spinal segments can aid in making clinical diagnoses of sensorimotor disorders (Fig. 2-34; Table 2-4).

In earthworms and fish, the body area (dermatome) related to each spinal segment is not only equal in width to the spinal cord but is also parallel to the spinal segment. The segmental organization of spinal innervation did not change during phylogenetic development. What has changed is the level of the innervated area that used to be parallel to the cord. In humans, before approximately fetal

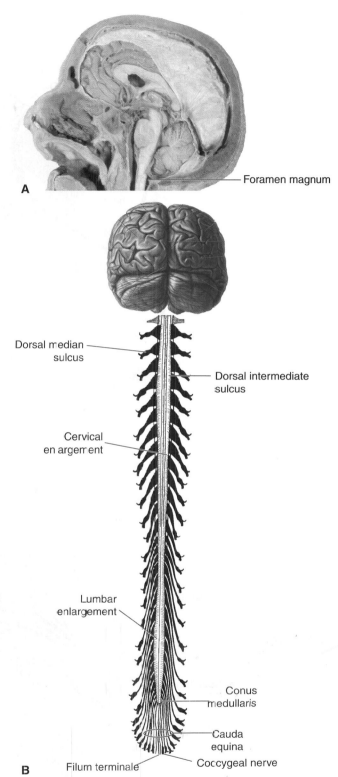

Figure 2-31 A. Sagittal view of the foramen magnum. B. Posterior view of the spinal cord with a series of dorsal root ganglia and spinal nerves.

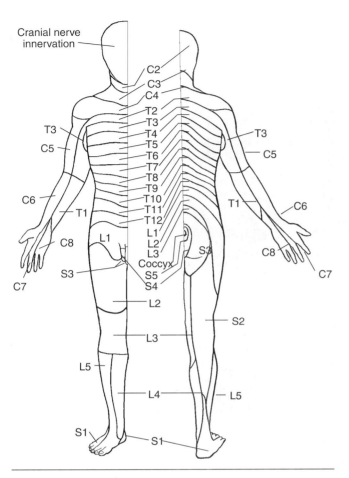

Figure 2-34 The dermatomes and their innervation by the spinal nerves.

Networking of Spinal Nerves

The 31 pairs of spinal nerves, named after the regions from which they arise, are formed by the merging of the dorsal (sensory) and ventral (motor) roots of the spinal cord. After traveling a centimeter, each nerve divides into two rami: **dorsal** and **ventral**. Each ramus, like a spinal nerve, contains both sensory and motor fibers. Thus a lesion of a ramus or spinal nerve results in paralysis and loss of sensation (pain and touch) for a specific limb. The dorsal rami serve the sensorimotor functions of the posterior trunk (skin and dorsal back muscles). The ventral rami, which contain a greater number of fibers, innervate a larger area of the body. Other than those originating from T1–T12, ventral rami do not go directly to body structures. Rather they form a **plexus** near the cervical and lumbar enlargements of the spinal cord by merging with the adjacent ventral rami (Fig. 2-35). There are four major plexuses: **cervical**, **brachial**, **lumbar**, and **sacral** (Table 2-5). Peripheral nerves, containing fibers from several adjacent spinal roots, ensure a substantial overlap in the sensorimotor innervations to the skin and muscles.

The *cervical plexus*, formed primarily by the projections from C1 to C4, supplies the muscles and skin of the head, neck, and part of the shoulders and the diaphragm. Its pathology results in cervical pain and respiratory palsy. The *brachial plexus*, with efferents from C5 to C8, provides the nerve supply for the shoulders and upper limbs. Its pathologic involvement is characterized by sensory loss and/or weakness in the arm and reflex loss. The *lumbar plexus*, with efferents from L1 to L4, supplies the abdominal

---

Table 2-4

Spinal Roots and Their Distribution (Myotome and Dermatome) Landmarks

Roots	Myotomal Activity	Dermatomal Distribution
C5	Shoulder abduction	Shoulder, lateral
C5–C6	Forearm flexion	Biceps
C6	Elbow supination/pronation	Thumb
C7	Finger extension; forearm extension at elbow	Third finger
C8–T1	Digital abduction and adduction (Check patient's ability to move fingers apart and together against resistance)	Finger, ring
T4		Nipple
T10	Umbilical contraction	Umbilicus
L2–L4	Knee extension, hip flexion, and adduction	Anterior-medial thigh and medial leg below the knee
L5	Ankle and great toe dorsiflexion (Check patient's ability to walk on heels)	Foot, dorsal
S1	Ankle plantar flexion (Check patient's ability to walk on tiptoes)	Sole of foot, lateral

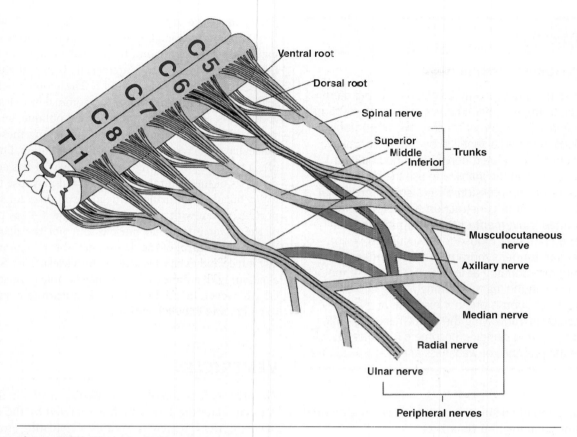

Figure 2-35 The spinal plexuses.

wall, external genitals, and part of the lower limbs (thigh, leg, and foot). Inability to extend the leg and loss of sensation from the genitals and lower limbs are associated with the involvement of the lumbar plexus. The *sacral plexus,* with spinal efferents from L4 to S4, supplies the buttocks, perineum, and lower limbs. Foot-drop and pain extending down from the buttocks to the leg indicates involvement of the sacral plexus.

Neuritis marks the common pathologic condition involving peripheral (spinal or cranial) nerves; it is marked

Table 2-5			

Nerve Plexus and Motor Functions

Plexus and Origin	Nerves	Served Body Areas	Clinical Characteristics
Cervical (C1–C5)	Phrenic	Diaphragm; muscles of shoulder and neck	Respiratory paralysis
Brachial (C5–C8, T1)	Radial	Triceps and extensors of arm	Wrist-drop and inability to extend hand at wrist
	Median	Flexors of forearm	Inability to pick up objects; failure to abduct thumb and index finger; neuropathy associated with carpal tunnel syndrome
	Ulnar	Wrist muscles	Inability to spread fingers
Lumbar (T12, L1–L4)	Femoral	Lower abdomen, buttocks, and anterior thigh	Inability to extend leg and flex hip
Sacral (L4–L5, S1–S4)	Sciatic	Lower trunk and posterior surface of thigh and leg	Inability to the extend hip and flex knee
	Peroneal	Foot and lateral leg	Foot-drop and inability to dorsiflex foot

by inflammation of one more nerves from either structural irritation or inflammation (Box 2-2).

Spinal Regulation of Muscles for Respiration

Understanding the spinal control of the muscles of respiration is an important aspect of training for students in communicative disorders (Table 2-6). In addition to being vital for survival, respiration entails a patterned cycle of inhalation and exhalation, which also regulates our speaking. The contraction of the **diaphragm** and **external intercostal muscles** increases the intrathoracic volume, triggering the process of inspiration. An increase in intra-abdominal pressure by the **abdominal muscles** and rib depression by **internal intercostal muscles** initiates exhalation. The motor nuclei from the anterior horns of the C3–C5 segments (predominantly from C4) form the phrenic nerve, which innervates the diaphragm, the primary muscle of inspiration. The efferents to the intercostals (internal and external) exit from segments T1–T12. The motor nuclei from segments T6–T12 innervate the abdominal muscles (rectus abdominus, internal oblique, external oblique, and transversus abdominus). Spinal lesions involving these motor nuclei have different implications for respiration. For example, a patient with a spinal lesion above C4 has complete paralysis of the respiratory muscles and may lose the ability to breathe, requiring artificial respiration for life support. A patient with a spinal injury below C4 has paralysis of the lower intercostal muscles but not the diaphragm. With basic control of the diaphragm, this patient may quietly inhale and exhale because of muscle elasticity. Similarly, a patient with a thoracic lesion may be able to breathe quietly; however, he or she may have to learn to compensate to cough and exhale forcefully.

VENTRICLES

The primary function of the ventricular cavities in the brain is to circulate the CSF, which is secreted by the **choroid plexus** in the **ventricular cavities**. Circulating around the CNS, the CSF forms a spongy cushion to protect the brain and spinal cord from excessive accelerating and decelerating head movements.

There are four interconnected ventricles within the brain (Figs. 2-36 and 2-37): two lateral ventricles (one in each hemisphere; the first and second ventricles), the third ventricle, and the fourth ventricle. Both lateral ventricles are connected by way of the interventricular foramen to the midline third ventricle. The third ventricle is connected to the fourth ventricle in the brainstem through the *cerebral aqueduct*. The inner wall of these interconnected ventricular cavities is lined with a layer of **ependymal cells**; these

Table 2-6		
Spinal Control of the Muscles of Respiration		
Spinal Roots	Muscles	Functions
C3–C5	Diaphragm	Contracts to increase thoracic diameter for inspiration
T1–T12	External intercostals	Contract to raise ribs for inspiration
T1–T12	Internal intercostals	Assist in rib depression for forced expiration

T6–T12	Abdominal muscles
	  Rectus abdominus
	  Internal oblique
	  External oblique
	  Transversus abdominus
		Increase intrathoracic pressure for forced expiration

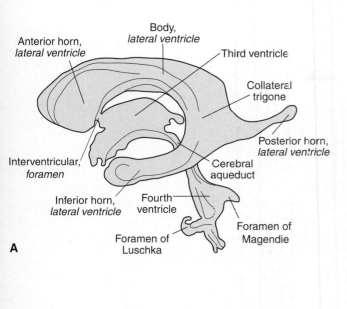

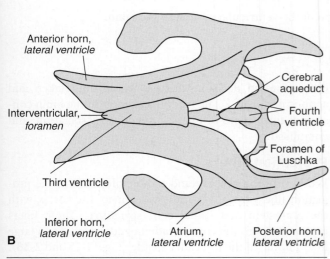

Figure 2-36 Lateral (A) and dorsal (B) views of the entire ventricular system in the brain.

glial cells, in part, prevent diffusion of substances from the CSF into the brain. A common pathologic condition associated with CSF circulation is **hydrocephalus** (Box 2-3).

Lateral Ventricles

The lateral ventricles are C-shaped structures that form an arch (Fig. 2-36). Each lateral ventricle consists of the central part, or body, and three extensions: **anterior**, **posterior** (occipital), and **inferior** (temporal) **horns**. The roof of the body of the lateral ventricle is formed by the fibers of the corpus callosum. The superior surface of the thalamus constitutes the floor of the lateral ventricle. The body of the lateral ventricle extends from the interventricular foramen (of Monro) to an imprecisely defined point near the splenium of the corpus callosum. The arch-shaped body of the lateral ventricle enlarges near the **collateral trigone area**, the broader portion in the posterior floor of the

lateral ventricle. At this point, the ventricular body diverges into the posterior and inferior horns. The anterior horn refers to the extension of the lateral ventricle in the frontal lobe rostral to the interventricular foramen. The membranous thin part of the *septum pellucidum* forms the medial wall of the anterior ventricular horns (Figs. 2-11 and 2-16). The posterior horn, shaped like an elongated slender finger, is the caudal extension of the ventricle from the trigone area into the occipital lobe. The inferior horn is the curved inferior extension of the lateral ventricle from the trigone area into the temporal lobe. Some important anatomic structures in the floor of the inferior horn are the *hippocampus, amygdala,* tail of the *caudate nucleus,* and crus (leg) of the *fornix.*

Third Ventricle

The third ventricle is a narrow vertical space between the two thalami and is rostrally connected to the lateral ventricles through the foramen of Monro (Fig. 2-36). The hypothalamic nuclei form the floor of the third ventricle (Fig. 2-19). Caudally in the midbrain, the cavity of the third ventricle narrows to become the *cerebral aqueduct,* which connects the third ventricle with the fourth ventricle of the brainstem (Fig. 2-11).

The cerebral aqueduct is ventral to the corpora quadrigemina in the midbrain and is surrounded by the central gray matter (Fig. 2-24). The cerebral aqueduct is an important reference point for the transition between the dorsal and the ventral midbrain areas. The area dorsal to the cerebral aqueduct, the tectum, includes the corpora quadrigemina in addition to the tectal nuclei. The midbrain region ventral to the cerebral aqueduct is the tegmentum, which contains important structures, such as the red nucleus and reticular formation nuclei. Clinically, it is important to note that the cerebral aqueduct undergoes a 90° bend downward, corresponding to the cephalic flexure at this point.

Fourth Ventricle

The tegmentum of the pons and medulla constitute the triangular floor of the fourth ventricle; the cerebellum forms its roof. The rhomboid floor of the fourth ventricle can be completely seen after removal of the cerebellum (Figs. 2-9 and 2-21). Beneath the floor of the ventricle are the nuclei of CN V–CN XII. At the widest portion of the fourth ventricle, there are three openings: two lateral apertures (**foramina of Luschka**) and one medial aperture (**foramen of Magendie**) (Fig. 2-36). Through these three openings, the CSF gains access to the subarachnoid space surrounding the CNS (see Chapter 18).

MEDULLARY CENTERS IN THE BRAIN

Besides containing the cellular gray matter and ventricular cavities, each cerebral hemisphere includes a large volume

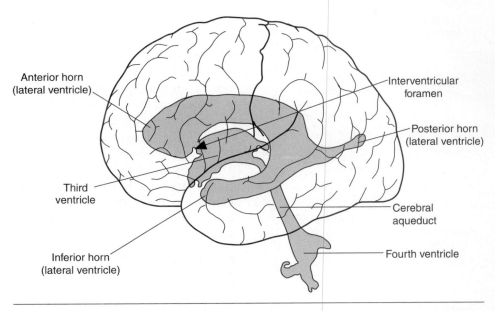

Figure 2-37 Lateral view showing the relation of the ventricular system to the brain.

of white matter (fibers). The myelinated fibers form the medullary center of the brain and account for all **inter-hemispheric** (between hemispheres) and **intrahemispheric** (within a hemisphere) axonal connections. The comprehensive and well-organized connectivity through these fibers within and between both cerebral hemispheres accounts for the efficiency with which external information is quickly analyzed, synthesized, and transferred from one modality to another and adequate responses are formulated and executed promptly with the left, right, or both limbs. These interconnecting fibers keep all brain areas informed of

data processed, decisions made, activities undertaken, and actions performed. The medullary center in the brain consists of three types of fibers: **projection**, **association**, and **commissural**.

Projection Fibers

While carrying sensory and motor information, the projection fibers travel vertically to connect the cortex with the brainstem and spinal cord structures. These fibers project through the **corona radiata** and coalesce as a large fiber bundle in the **internal capsule** (Figs. 2-15 and 2-38). The internal capsule, a subcortical band of fibers, contains all ascending (projecting to the cerebral cortex) and descending (projecting downward from the telencephalon) fibers as they pass between the basal ganglia and the thalamus. Appearing as a left-facing V-shaped structure, the internal capsule can be seen on a coronal or horizontal section; it consists of an **anterior limb**, **genu**, and **posterior limb** (Figs. 2-15, 2-16, and 2-38). The anterior limb contains corticothalamic and thalamocortical fibers, which connect the thalamic nuclei with the frontal cortex and limbic cingulate gyrus. Also located here are the corticopontine fibers that mediate frontal projections. The genu of the internal capsule is the site for the corticobulbar fibers that descend to innervate the cranial nerve nuclei and play an important role in motor speech processes. The posterior limb is much larger and is known to contain the corticospinal fibers that project to the spinal motor neurons.

The motor fibers of the corticospinal (pyramidal) tract primarily originate from the precentral gyrus and descend through the corona radiata, internal capsule between the basal ganglia and the thalamus, and pes pedunculi in the

BOX 2-3

Hydrocephalus

Hydrocephalus is a pathologic condition associated with impaired CSF circulation. It is characterized in children by dilated ventricles, prominent forehead, brain atrophy, convulsion, and mental deficiency. The adult skull does not increase in size; instead, only the ventricles enlarge at the expense of the surrounding cortical tissues. This condition is caused by an obstruction in the flow of CSF from its sites of production (in the lateral ventricle) to its site of reabsorption into the bloodstream, the superior sagittal sinus, a structure of the dural meninges between the cerebral hemispheres.

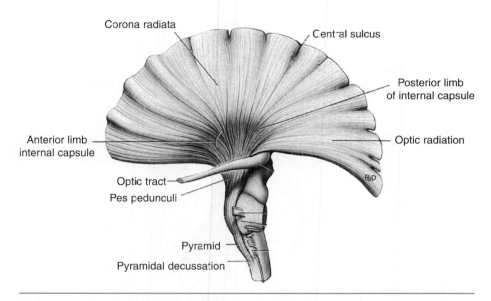

Corona radiata

Central sulcus

Posterior limb
of internal capsule

Anterior limb
internal capsule

Optic radiation

Optic tract

Pes pedunculi

Pyramid

Pyramidal decussation

Figure 2-38 Continuity of the longitudinally arranged projection fibers from the cortex through the corona radiata, internal capsule, and midbrain pedunculi to the pyramids in the medulla.

midbrain (Fig. 2-38). They form the pyramid in the medulla before crossing the midline and entering the spinal cord. The **sensory projection fibers** collect cutaneous and proprioceptive sensation from the skin and joints and project to the CNS. These sensory fibers enter the spinal cord, ascend through the brainstem and internal capsule, then fan out through the corona radiata and project to the primary sensory cortex in the parietal lobe.

Motor projection fibers include **corticospinal** and **corticobulbar fibers**. Corticospinal fibers originate from the motor cortex and terminate in the spinal cord. Corticobulbar fibers originate from the motor cortex and terminate in the brainstem (the bulbar area). Interruption of the projection fibers results in sensorimotor syndromes.

Association Fibers

Association fibers, the most numerous of the three types of fibers, are confined within the hemisphere. Some of the association fibers are short and connect adjacent gyri, whereas some are long and connect distant cortical areas. Functionally, they share the same goal, which is to provide efficient bidirectional channels for communication among cortical areas within each hemisphere. They are also important in refined and integrated behavioral responses. Lesions involving these pathways result in disconnections between two areas within a hemisphere. Selective involvement of one or more of these pathways may result in a peculiar symptom complex, such as the disconnection syndrome.

Short association fibers are U-shaped arcuate fibers that bend sharply around a sulcus and connect two adjacent gyri. The important **long association fiber bundles** are the following: **superior longitudinal fasciculus, cingulum, inferior longitudinal fasciculus,** and **uncinate fasciculus**. The general location of these pathways can be best seen on a coronal section of the brain (Fig. 2-39).

The *superior longitudinal fasciculus,* also known as the **arcuate fasciculus,** lies anteroposterior above the insular cortex. This associational fasciculus connects the frontal lobe with the occipital lobe. Many of its fibers diverge from the parietal lobe, curve around as the **arcuate fasciculus,** and project to the temporal lobe (Fig. 2-40). This fasciculus is an important communication link among the frontal, parietal, occipital, and temporal lobes. The curved arcuate fibers of the fasciculus are known to connect the classical Wernicke area (posterior language cortex) in the temporal lobe with Broca area (anterior language cortex) in the frontal lobe. This pathway is significant in the normal acquisition of language functions, auditory–verbal (repetition) memory, and propositional communication.

The *inferior longitudinal fasciculus* is a well-defined compressed bundle of fibers beneath the sylvian fissure and the insular cortex. It connects the temporal and occipital lobes. Its fibers travel anteroposteriorly from the occipital to the temporal lobe. Traveling parallel to the inferior longitudinal fasciculus are the short fibers of the uncinate fasciculus (Fig. 2-40A); some anatomists consider it to be an extension of the inferior occipitofrontal fasciculus. These fibers connect the orbital frontal gyri with the rostral region in the temporal lobe.

The *cingulum,* a C-shaped association fiber bundle, is beneath the cingulate gyrus, which lies above the corpus callosum. The cingulum is an association fiber bundle of

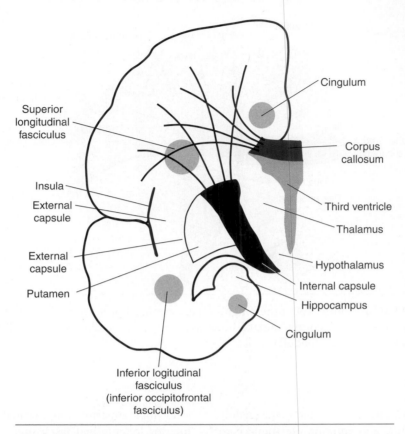

Figure 2-39 Coronal section showing the intrahemispheric location of the major associational pathways.

the limbic lobe connecting the medial, frontal, and parietal cortices with the temporal cortex. Its fibers originate in the subcallosal area beneath the genu of the corpus callosum, circle around the corpus callosum within the cingulate gyrus, and terminate in the parahippocampal gyrus of the medial temporal lobe (Fig. 2-40*B*).

Commissural Fibers

Commissural fibers in the brain run horizontally and connect the corresponding cortical areas in both cerebral hemispheres. Most neocortical commissural fibers are included in the *corpus callosum*, and the remainder of the fibers constitute the *anterior commissure*. The corpus callosum, the largest commissural bundle of fibers, is a thick plate of 300–400 million fibers (Figs. 2-15, 2-16, and 2-41). The fibers of the corpus callosum connect the corresponding cortical areas in both hemispheres, except for the primary centers for motor, sensory, auditory, and visual functions. The primary centers in both hemispheres are connected to each other only through the association cortical areas, which in turn are interconnected through the callosal fibers.

The corpus callosum contains four parts: rostrum, genu, body, and splenium (Figs. 2-12 and 2-41). The fibers in the *genu* and *rostrum* of the corpus callosum interconnect the anterior and orbital regions of the frontal lobes. The

fibers from the posterior frontal lobes and the parietal lobes pass through the body of the corpus callosum. The fibers forming the *splenium* originate from the occipital and temporal lobes. Because the corpus callosum is shorter than the hemispheres from front to back, its fiber radiations extend anteriorly and posteriorly to the frontal and occipital poles.

The fibers of the corpus callosum allow each hemisphere to access the memory traces, experiences, and unique learning abilities of the contralateral hemisphere. This close interaction underlying normal behavior is best illustrated by the studies conducted on patients who had undergone **commissurotomy**, described earlier in this chapter, which produces the so-called split brain. Surgical sectioning of the callosal fibers, undertaken as a medical treatment for epilepsy, renders the cerebral hemispheres functionally independent. As noted, this research provided insight into the neurolinguistic functions of the hemispheres.

The smaller **anterior commissure**, a second commissural bundle, contains crossing fibers other than the neocortical ones (Figs. 2-11 and 2-16). It is rostral to the thalamus. Originating from the ventral temporal lobe cortices, the anterior commissure interconnects two amygdaloid complexes and both olfactory systems.

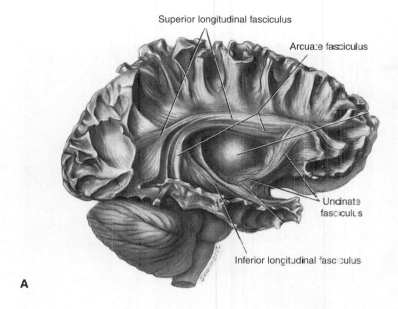

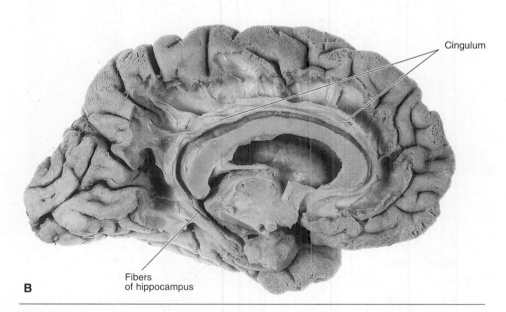

Figure 2-40 A. Lateral view of the long intrahemispheric association fibers. B. Dissection showing the medial aspect of the left hemisphere to reveal the cingulum and fibers of hippocampus.

MENINGES OF THE BRAIN

The soft and gelatinous nature of the CNS makes the brain and spinal cord susceptible to traumatic injuries. The structures that provide the basic protections to the CNS include the three **meningeal** layers, the cushioning CSF, the bony wall of the skull, and the vertebral column. The meninges consist of three concentric fibrous tissue membranes that encase the CNS: dura mater, arachnoid membrane, and pia mater (Fig. 2-42; Table 2-7). A pathologic condition associated with membranes of the CNS is viral or bacterial meningitis, which is associated with meningeal inflammation (Box 2-4).

Dura Mater

The dura mater, the gray outermost membrane, consists of dense, fibrous connective tissue and provides the maximum meningeal protection to the CNS. It is thick and tough in comparison with the pia and arachnoid. The dura is attached to the inner surface of the skull and overlies the

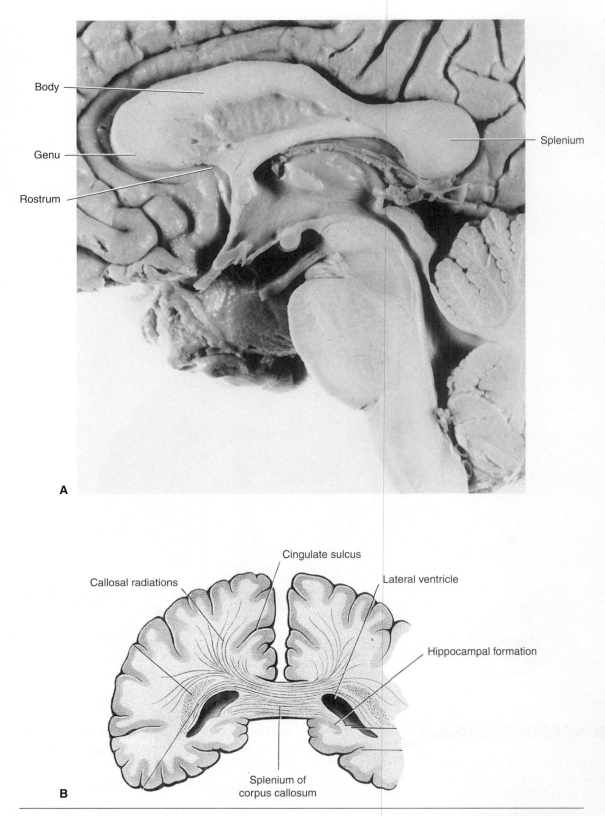

Figure 2-41 **A.** Midsagittal view of the corpus callosum. **B.** Coronal view showing the course of the corpus callosal fibers.

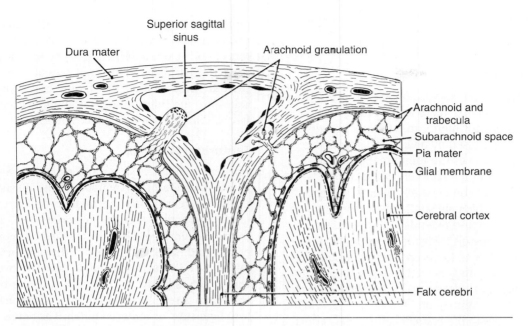

Figure 2-42 The three meninges in relation to the surfaces of the brain, subarachnoid space, and sagittal sinus. Also shown are the arachnoid villi (granulations) that drain the cerebrospinal fluid in the sagittal sinus.

underlying arachnoid. There are two potential (not real) spaces around the cranial dura: **epidural** and **subdural spaces**. The epidural refers to the space between the dura mater and the bone. The subdural is the space between the dura mater and the arachnoid. Dura mater consists of two fibrous layers: external **periosteal** and internal **meningeal**. The two layers are attached to each other, except where they separate to form sinuses that carry the blood from veins and absorb the circulated CSF (Fig. 2-43). The outer periosteal layer of the dura mater is attached to the inner surface of the cranium, and its meningeal layer

forms various **septa** (**dural extensions**), which form two lateral compartments for the cerebral hemispheres and one posterior compartment for the cerebellum (Fig. 2-44).

Falx Cerebri

The *falx cerebri*, a dural extension, is named for its sickle shape and is the largest dural reflection. It extends longitudinally in the interhemispheric fissure and forms a vertical partition in the cranial cavity between the cerebral hemispheres (Fig. 2-44). Anteriorly, this dural reflection is attached to the **crista galli** of the **ethmoid bone** in the inner

Table 2-7	
Cerebral versus Spinal Meninges	

Cerebral Meninges	Spinal Meninges
Dura	
Adheres to inner skull; composed of two fused (periosteal and meningeal) layers that split to form sinuses	Composed of only meningeal layer; separates from vertebrae by epidural (potential) space
Arachnoid	
Attaches to dura in living condition (no subdural space); subarachnoid space with several cisterns	Attaches to dura in living condition (no subdural space); subarachnoid space with sacral cistern
Pia	
Adheres to surface of brain, with extension within depth of sulci; follows vessels as they pierce cerebral cortex	Adheres to surface of cord; specializations in form of denticulate ligaments and filum terminale that attach to dural sac

BOX 2-4

Meningitis

Meningitis, a pathologic condition of the CNS, can cause serious injury to the brain and has implications for higher mental function disorders. It is caused by a viral or bacterial infection and involves the inflammation of the membranes of the brain and spinal cord. The bacterial infection generally affects the leptomeninges, which are subdural membranes. The inflammation also extends to the nerve roots and blood vessels penetrating the meninges, causing the neck to become stiff; any stretching of the nerves triggers intense pain. The infection generally starts elsewhere in the body, such as the sinuses or throat, and travels through via the bloodstream to the brain. It can severely affect the cognitive functions and result in speech and language disorders. Bacterial meningitis carries serious risks, such as permanent brain damage and death. Group B streptococcus (in newborns), pneumococcus, *Haemophilus influenzae* type B, and meningococcus are common bacteria associated with meningitis. Viral meningitis is not likely to have serious consequences, and it clears up on its own within a few weeks.

cranium; posteriorly, it extends to the **internal occipital protuberance** and the **tentorium cerebelli**, another dural reflection. At the dorsal edge of the interhemispheric fissure, the falx cerebri forms the cavity for the **superior sagittal sinus**. Within this fissure and above the corpus callosum, the **inferior sagittal sinus** is located along the free inferior margin of the falx cerebri.

Tentorium Cerebelli

The *tentorium cerebelli*, a dural extension, arises from the petrous portion of the temporal bone. Its attachments to the falx cerebri along the midline pull it up, creating a tentlike structure over the posterior fossa, which houses the cerebellum (Fig. 2-44). Its margins are between the cerebellum and the basal surface of the temporal and occipital lobes, so that the occipital lobes lie over it and the cerebellum is below it. Anteriorly, the free borders of the tentorium cerebelli constitute the opening named the **tentorial incisure**, or **tentorial notch**. The brainstem descends through the tentorial notch toward the foramen magnum. The space above the tentorium, the **supratentorial space**, contains the cerebral cortex. The space below the tentorium, the **infratentorial space**, contains the cerebellum and brainstem (Fig. 2-45).

Falx Cerebelli

The falx cerebelli is a small triangular vertical extension from the tentorium cerebelli that separates the cerebellar hemispheres (Figs. 2-44 and 2-45).

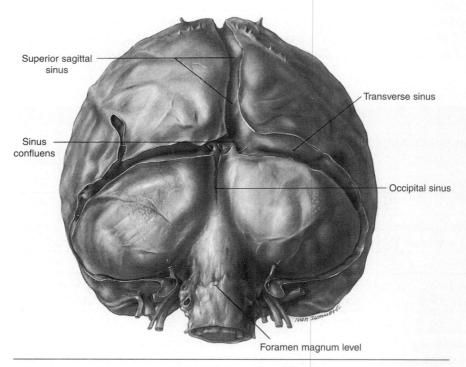

Figure 2-43 The dura surrounding the brain. The periosteal layer of the dura mater has been removed to expose the prominent dural sinuses.

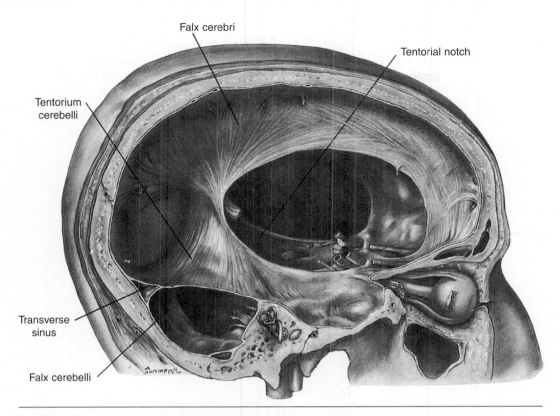

Figure 2-44 Midsagittal section revealing the dural extensions (falx cerebri, falx cerebelli, and tentorium cerebelli).

Arachnoid Membrane

The arachnoid membrane is a thin, nonvascular membrane between the internal pia mater and the external dura mater. It does not adhere to the cortical surface like the pia mater (Figs. 2-42 and 2-46) but bridges the cortical surface and the pia mater. The space between the pia and the arachnoid is traversed by the **arachnoid trabeculae**, which consist of fibrous and elastic connective tissue. Located between the arachnoid and the pia mater, the **subarachnoid space**, which envelops the CNS, is filled with CSF.

The arachnoid membrane is separated from the dura mater by the potential subdural space. However, the arachnoid pushes through the dura to form flower-shaped **arachnoid granulations** (villi) near the vertex of the brain

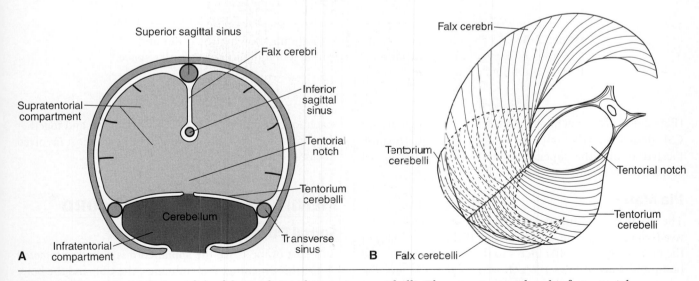

Figure 2-45 **A.** Coronal view of the falx cerebri and tentorium cerebelli. The supratentorial and infratentorial compartments are also shown. **B.** Locations of the three dural extensions.

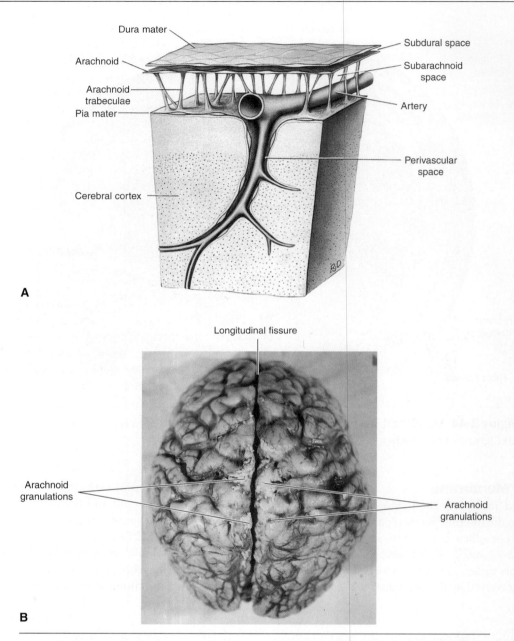

Figure 2-46 A. The meningeal structures of the brain showing the order and locations of the meninges in relation to the subarachnoid and perivascular space. B. The arachnoid granulations.

(Fig. 2-46). The arachnoid granulations, through which CSF drains into the vascular system, are predominantly located around the superior sagittal sinus on the dorsal surface of the brain.

Pia Mater

The pia mater, a thin, transparent, collagenous (connective tissue) membrane, is closely attached to the surface of the brain (Fig. 2-42). It adheres to the entire surface of the brain and thus follows the contours of the gyri and the sulci (Fig. 2-46). The pia mater also surrounds the blood vessels and forms the **perivascular space**. Both the pia and

arachnoid membranes are relatively delicate, and together they are called the **leptomeninges**; they are most involved in cases of meningitis.

MENINGES OF THE SPINAL CORD

Spinal Dura Mater

As a part of the CNS, the spinal cord is equally protected by the three meningeal membranes, the CSF, and the bony vertebral column (Figs. 2-32 and 2-47). However, the spinal dura mater is a single-layer meningeal membrane; it lacks

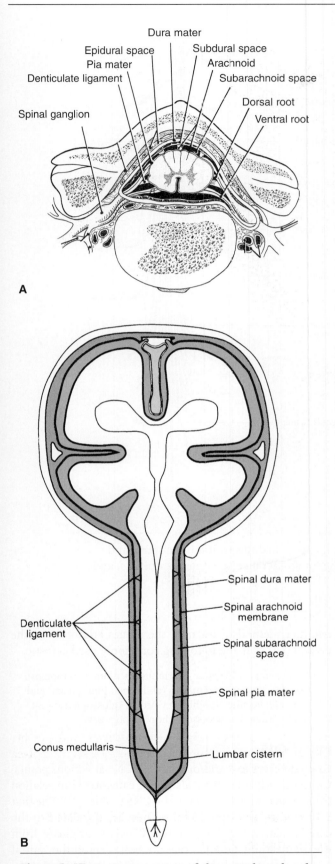

the cranial pericsteal layer (Table 2-7). The spinal dura looks like a loose tube pierced by the spinal nerve roots. It is rostrally attached to the foramen magnum, the opening in the occipital bone through which the spinal cord passes. The spinal dura is separated from the wall of spinal canal by an extradural space and extends in a sac formation to the S2 vertebral level, at which point it merges with the filum terminale to form the coccygeal ligament, a thin fibrous cord. The spinal dura is surrounded by an actual epidural space, which is normally obliterated (Fig. 2-47). Anesthetic agents are injected to the epidural space for anesthetizing the lower body by blocking nerve transmission of pain.

Spinal Arachnoid Membrane

The arachnoid covering for the spinal cord begins at the *foramen magnum* and extends to the cauda equina. The subarachnoid space around the cord is filled with CSF. The arachnoid also invests the tubular projections of the spinal nerve roots from the cord to their foramina of exit. At the lumbar level of the spinal column, with the diminished cord size, the subarachnoid space extends into the **lumbar cistern**. With no cord structure present, the lumbar level serves as the best site for the **lumbar puncture** (spinal tap). Anesthesiologists use this sac to administer anesthetics, producing spinal anesthesia. Removal of CSF (spinal tap) for chemical examination is done at the level below L1 or L2; the dura and arachnoid are punctured, allowing the clinician access to the subarachnoid space (Fig. 2-48).

Spinal Pia Mater

The pia, the innermost protective layer, surrounds and tightly adheres to the spinal cord. The fibers of the dorsal and ventral spinal roots pierce the pia membrane. The cord suspended within the dural tube is not free; it is attached to the surrounding dura mater by a series of **denticulate ligaments** on both sides. These fibrous ligaments originate from the pia mater at the lateral surface of the spinal cord between both roots and connect to the inner dura. Below the termination of the cord at the conus medullaris, the pia mater continues with the filum terminale and eventually merges with the dura at the sacral level.

CRANIAL NERVES

The PNS consists of **spinal** and **cranial nerves**. The efferent fibers of the spinal nerves innervate skeletal muscles and the visceral organs, whereas the afferent fibers transmit sensory information from the skin and visceral organs to the CNS. The cranial nerves originate from the brainstem and innervate the muscles of the head, neck, face, larynx, tongue, pharynx, and glands. The cranial nerves are essential for speech, resonance, and phonation. In

Figure 2-47 A. Cross-section of the spinal cord and its meningeal coverings. B. The relationship of the meningeal membranes to the brain and spinal cord.

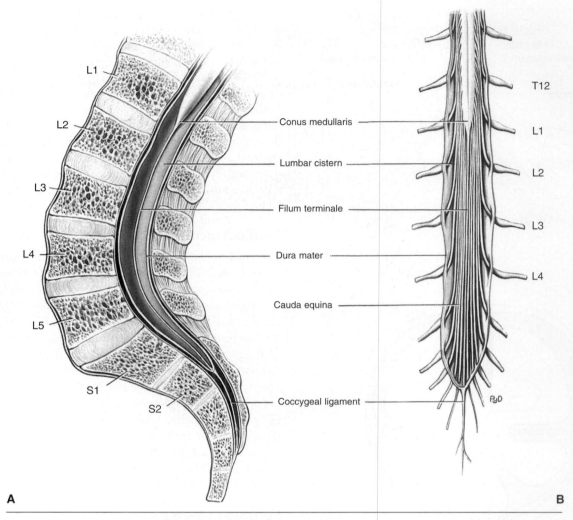

Figure 2-48 **A.** Sagittal view of the caudal spinal cord, conus medullaris, lumbar cistern, and lumbosacral vertebral column. **B.** Posterior view of the lumbosacral cord, conus medullaris, and lumbar cistern.

addition, they serve the special senses—vision, audition, smell, and taste. Of the 12 pairs of cranial nerves, some mediate either sensory or motor functions, and others serve both (Table 2-8).

Nomenclature

Cranial nerves are both numbered and named. The Roman numerals (CN I–CN XII) indicate the sequence in which the cranial nerves exit and/or enter the brain. The names contain information describing some or all the functional characteristics of the nerves (Table 2-8). A series of acronyms can be used to facilitate learning the names of the cranial nerves:

OOO = olfactory, optic, oculomotor
TTA = trochlear, trigeminal, abducens
FAG = facial, acoustic (vestibulocochlear),
    glossopharyngeal
VAH = vagus, accessory, hypoglossal

Another method of learning the names and order of the cranial nerves is the following commonly used acrostic:

On (olfactory) old (optic) Olympus' (oculomotor) topmost (trochlear) top (trigeminal), **a** (abducens) Finn (facial) and (acoustic; vestibulocochlear) German (glossopharyngeal) viewed (vagus) **a** (accessory) hop (hypoglossal).

Functions

Cranial nerves exit and/or enter the CNS at various points. Consequently, they have also been categorized in relation to their anatomic location in the CNS (Table 2-9). The first 2 (olfactory and optic) cranial nerves are related to the cerebral cortex; the remaining 10 nerves originate from the brainstem. Cranial nerves are best seen on the ventral or lateral surface of the brainstem (Figs. 2-49–2-51).

The **olfactory nerve** (**CN I**), a sensory nerve, is responsible for the perception of smell. It originates from the receptor cells in the mucosa of the nasal cavity and synapses

Table 2-8

Cranial Nerves and Their Functions

Number	Name	Major Motor Function	Major Sensory Function
I	Olfactory		Smell: sends information from nasal mucosa to olfactory bulb
II	Optic		Vision: sends messages from retina to visual cortex (vision) and superior colliculus (reflexes)
III	Oculomotor	Eye movement; regulation of pupil; accommodation of lens for near vision; upper lid elevation	
IV	Trochlear	Eye movement	
V	Trigeminal	Mastication	Sensation: face, orbit, and oral structures
VI	Abducens	Eye movement	
VII	Facial	Facial expression; secretion of saliva and tears	Taste: anterior two-thirds of tongue
VIII	Acoustic; vestibulocochlear		Equilibrium and audition
IX	Glossopharyngeal	Swallowing	Taste: posterior third of tongue; visceral sensation from oral pharynx
X	Vagus	Phonation and swallowing	Sensation: thoracic and abdominal organs
XI	Accessory	Head movement and shoulder elevation	
XII	Hypoglossal	Tongue movement	

Table 2-9

Anatomic Classification of the Cranial Nerves

Location	Cranial Nerves
Prosencephalon (forebrain)	
Telencephalon	I (olfactory)
Diencephalon	II (optic)
Mesencephalon (midbrain)	III (oculomotor)
	IV (trochlear)
Rhombencephalon (hindbrain)	
Metencephalon (pons)	V (trigeminal)
	VI (abducens)
	VII (facial)
	VIII (acoustic; vestibulocochlear)
Myelencephalon (medulla oblongata)	IX (glossopharyngeal)
	X (vagus)
	XI (spinal accessory)
	XII (hypoglossal)

in the olfactory bulbs on the orbital surface of the frontal lobe. The axons from the bulb travel in the olfactory tract and terminate in the olfactory area (pyriform cortex) of the basal medial temporal lobe (Figs. 2-7 and 2-8). An interruption of olfactory fibers produces anosmia, a condition of impaired sense of smell.

The **optic nerve (CN II)** is a brain tract concerned with visual sensation. Optic nerves originate from the retina (a part of the brain) in both eyes and unite at the optic chiasm at the base of the brain. The crossed and uncrossed optic fibers continue in the optic tract and, via the thalamus, project information from each eye to the visual cortex in the occipital lobes. Owing to the direct projections to the thalamus, it is considered a diencephalic (forebrain) nerve (Figs. 2-7 and 2-8). Injury to any part of the visual pathway results in a selective visual field loss (scotoma).

The **oculomotor nerve (CN III)**, a motor nerve, controls four of the six muscles responsible for moving the eyeball. It emerges from the ventral surface of the midbrain medial to the pes pedunculi and enters the interpeduncular fossa. Complete interruption of the oculomotor nerve results in ptosis of the eyelid, dilation of the pupil, and an abducted (laterally deviated) position of the eye. This eye

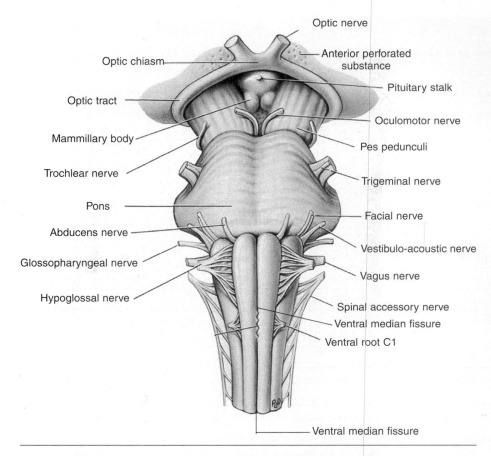

Figure 2-49 Ventral view showing the cranial nerves exiting from the midbrain, pons, and medulla.

deviation is produced by unopposed action of the lateral rectus muscle, which is supplied by abducens, (**CN VI**). The oculomotor nerve also innervates the **levator palpebrae**, which raises the upper eyelid. Interruption of the nerve to this muscle causes ptosis through the loss of this function.

The **trochlear nerve** (**CN IV**), a motor nerve, controls one of the muscles responsible for eye movement. The trochlear nerve exits from the brainstem below the inferior colliculus. It is the only motor nerve to exit the brainstem from the dorsal surface. A trochlear lesion or injury is associated with impaired downward gaze.

The **trigeminal nerve** (**CN V**) and the next three nerves (CN VI–CN VIII) originate from the tegmentum of the pons. The trigeminal is a functionally mixed nerve with both sensory and motor functions. Primarily, it is a sensory nerve for the face, head, and oral structures and a motor nerve for jaw movements. It is a large nerve in the pons, and its sensory and motor roots leave the brainstem from the ventrolateral surface of the pons. Loss of trigeminal function is associated with facial sensory loss and paralysis of the jaw.

The **abducens nerve** (**CN VI**), a motor nerve, controls the lateral rectus muscle, which turns the eyeball away from the nose. Fibers of the abducens nerve originate from the tegmentum of the pons and emerge ventrally from the junction of the pons and the medulla oblongata. Inter-

ruption of this nerve results in partial ocular paralysis with a medially fixed eye.

The **facial nerve** (**CN VII**) is primarily a motor nerve, but it also has some sensory functions. As the name implies, this nerve controls all muscles of facial expression. It also serves the sense of taste from the anterior two-thirds of the tongue. Fibers of this nerve exit from the ventrolateral surface of the pons at its border with the medulla. A facial nerve lesion results in facial paralysis and loss of taste sensation. It may also interfere with production of tears and saliva.

The **vestibulocochlear**, or **acoustic**, **nerve** (**CN VIII**) is a sensory nerve with, as its name implies, two divisions: **vestibular** and **acoustic**. The vestibular division is concerned with the position of the head in space; the acoustic portion is concerned with hearing. This is a large nerve, and its fibers enter the brainstem at the ventrolateral surface of the pons at its junction with the medulla. Its rootlets are lateral to the roots of the facial nerve, and its location is the landmark of the pontomedullary junction. Interruption of the vestibulocochlear nerve is associated with impaired hearing and equilibrium disorders.

The **glossopharyngeal nerve** (**CN IX**) originates from the medulla oblongata. It serves both sensory and motor functions. Its motor function is to contribute to swallow-

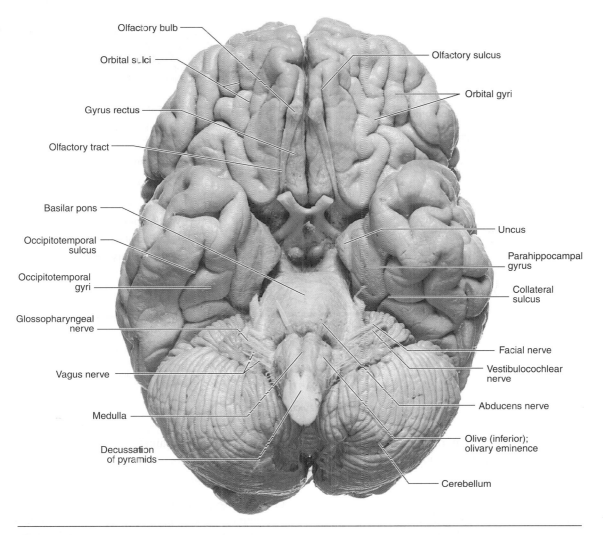

Figure 2-50 Ventral view of the cerebral hemispheres, brainstem, and cerebellum with exposed cranial nerves.

ing, and its sensory function is to process the sensation of touch and taste from the posterior third of the tongue and of the oral pharynx. Its nuclei are in the medulla, and its fibers leave the medulla just below the acoustic nerve from the lateral surface. A glossopharyngeal lesion results in the loss of taste sensation from the posterior third of the tongue and mild dysphagia (swallowing disorder). It may also cause loss of the gag reflex.

The **vagus nerve (CN X)**, the largest cranial nerve, has a wide distribution of its fibers. Its fibers leave the brainstem from the lateral medulla just below the point of exit for the glossopharyngeal nerve. Although the vagus is primarily a sensory nerve, it has a motor component, which activates the muscles of the pharynx, larynx, and soft palate. Vagus nerve pathology results in decreased sensation from and activation of visceral organs and paralysis of the larynx and pharynx.

The **spinal accessory nerve (CN XI)**, a motor nerve, innervates muscles for controlling head movement. The

spinal roots exit from the four cervical segments and contribute to the innervation of neck and shoulder muscles. A spinal accessory nerve injury causes restricted neck movement and weakness of the shoulder.

The **hypoglossal nerve (CN XII)** is a motor nerve, innervating the muscles of tongue. The nucleus is in the medulla, and its fibers exit the medulla just lateral to the pyramid (formed by axons of the corticospinal tract). The branches of this nerve innervate all intrinsic and some extrinsic muscles of the tongue. A pathologic condition of the hypoglossal nerve results in paralysis of half of the tongue.

AUTONOMIC NERVOUS SYSTEM

The autonomic nervous system (ANS), an autonomous and self-monitoring system, is regulated by the hypothalamus in the CNS. The ANS consists of sensory and motor

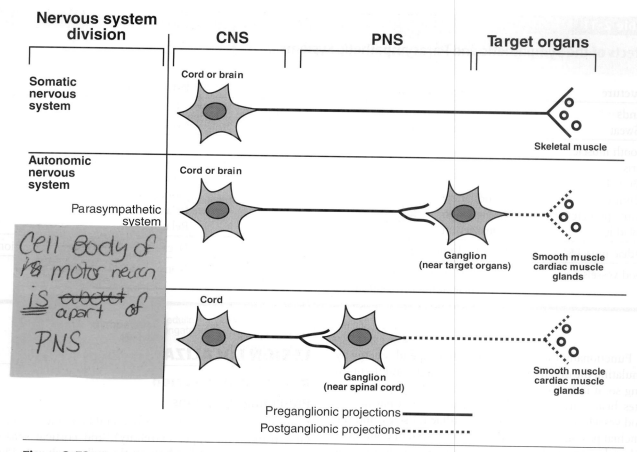

Figure 2-52 Comparison between the somatic and the autonomic nervous systems. *CNS*, central nervous system; *PNS*, peripheral nervous system.

[handwritten note: Cell Body of ~~its~~ motor neuron is ~~about~~ apart of PNS]

- The left cerebral cortex contains sites for language (aphasia).
- The right (nondominant) hemisphere regulates visuospatial orientation, emotional and prosodic function, attention, and sensorimotor control for the left half of the body.

Additional Information

See Chapter 7 for somatic sensation, Chapters 11–14 for the physiology of motor systems, Chapter 17 for the vascular system, and Chapter 19 for neurolinguistic properties of the brain and higher mental functions.

Rule 2: Subcortical Lesion

Presenting Symptoms

Contralateral hemiplegia and diminution or loss of pain and temperature equally for the face, arms, and legs are associated with a subcortical (internal capsule) lesion. Emergence of involuntary movements suggests a basal ganglia lesion.

Rationale

- All of the descending motor fibers and ascending sensory fibers pass through the internal capsule. Thus any involvement of the internal capsule is likely to produce equal sensorimotor deficits for the contralateral face, arm, and leg.
- Involuntary movements, such as tremor, athetosis, and chorea imply basal ganglia involvement.

Additional Information

See Chapters 7 and 11–14 for a discussion of the physiology of sensory and motor systems.

CLINICAL CONSIDERATIONS

PATIENT ONE

A 52-year-old man was taken to a neurologist because for over 2 months he had been exhibiting progressively greater amounts of confusion about time. He had also been experiencing difficulty organizing his thoughts and making decisions. Lately, he had begun speaking a little incoherently with fewer structures and words. The attending neurologist noticed the following signs:

- Time-related confusion
- Mild right-sided hemiparesis (face, arm, and leg)

- Right hemianopsia
- Increased deep tendon reflexes and Babinski sign
- Altered personality (the patient appeared reclusive and unconcerned)
- Expressive aphasia (disfluent verbal output consisting of a few words and phrases)
- Good auditory comprehension

The physician suspected a brain tumor (neoplastic growth) because of the progressive nature of the deficit. MRI studies revealed a left cortical neoplastic mass bordering the frontoparietotemporal region. The patient was referred for biopsy; surgical removal of the tumor, if possible; and then radiation treatment, if needed.

Question: How can you relate these clinical signs to the structures involved?

Discussion: The involvement of the frontoparietotemporal tissue accounts for all of the reported symptoms:

- Time-related confusion is characteristic of parietal involvement.
- Expressive aphasia reflects the involvement of the anterior language area, and the altered personality results from the involvement of the prefrontal projections.
- Right-sided paralysis and a positive Babinski sign indicates involvement of the motor and surrounding cortex.

PATIENT TWO

The family of a 75-year-old man with poor bladder control took him to the family physician, who noted that the patient's failure to control the sphincters had resulted in impaired urinary retention and fecal incontinence. The physician suspected an interruption of the sacral spinal nerves. MRI studies revealed a tumor involving the cauda equina region of the spinal cord.

Question: How can you relate these symptoms to the structures involved?

Discussion: The spinal nerves from the sacral region (S3–S5) innervate the bladder and anal sphincters (Fig. 2-34). Interruption of these nerves affects bowel and bladder function; incontinence issues are common after lower spinal cord injuries.

PATIENT THREE

A 30-year-old man who had a history of being social, detail oriented, and focused had gradually changed, becoming depressed, indifferent, and socially detached. For the past 2–3 months, he did not want to work and spent time sitting, staring, and procrastinating. He was seen by a neurologist who noted the following:

- Indifferent attitude and little desire to do anything
- Easy distractibility

- Socially inappropriate use of language
- Impaired sense of smell
- Nose picking in public
- Paucity of verbalization

A brain MRI study revealed a tumor in the anterior cranial fossa bilaterally affecting the frontal lobes.

Question: Can you relate these symptoms to the associated region of the brain?

Discussion: This bilaterally located tumor had affected the inferior frontal cortex.

- The inferior frontal cortex (Brodmann areas 10–12) deals with personality and regulates executive–cognitive functions, such as reasoning, abstract thinking, self-monitoring, decision making, planning, and pragmatic behaviors.
- The reported behavioral deficits (altered personality, profanity, inactivity, and inappropriate behavior) implicate the orbitofrontal region.
- The tumor had also compressed the olfactory bulb and its tract, which accounts for the loss of the sensation of smell.

PATIENT FOUR

A husband and wife speech language pathologist (SLP) team participated in a cognitive experiment in which they were examined with functional brain MRI studies. Both were horrified to see that one had a structure bridging the space in the third ventricle, but the other did not. Each attributed this as the cause of the other's weird personality and psychosomatic discomforts.

Question: Can you identify the structure that crosses through the third ventricle to connect both thalami?

Discussion: Massa intermedia, also called interthalamic adhesion, is present in only 70–80% of the human brains; it, however, is not related to any known neurologic (linguistic or cognitive) deficit.

PATIENT FIVE

A 60-year-old woman developed severe dysarthria after undergoing carotid endarterectomy. This is a surgical procedure used to clean the atherosclerotic plaque from the right internal carotid artery, a major artery that supplies blood to the brain. The surgeon assured the patient that the symptoms would resolve soon and she could expect a full recovery. The consulting SLP noted the woman exhibited the following:

- Paresis involving the right half of the face
- Paralysis of the right half of the tongue
- Unintelligible speech owing to slurred speech
- Slow articulatory movements
- Distorted consonants and vowel prolongation

- Aphonia, diplophonia, and breathiness
- Difficulty with swallowing
- Good auditory comprehension and no signs of aphasia

Question: Can you discuss the cranial nerves that were affected in this patient?

Discussion: The observed symptoms indicate that three cranial nerves were affected:

- Facial cranial nucleus/nerve: related to the paralysis of the right face and contributed to dysarthria
- Hypoglossal nerve: involved with the paralysis of the tongue and contributed to dysarthria
- Vagus nerve: contributed to the vocal cord paralysis and to the aphonia, diplophonia, and breathiness
- All three nerves: contributed to the articulatory precision causing the speech to be unintelligible

PATIENT SIX

A 55-year-old man, who initially complained of a constant headache, had gradually developed poor balance and lacked concentration. He was seen by a neurologist who noted the following:

- Difficulty walking, with small shuffled steps
- Slow thinking and inattentiveness, which caused loss of immediate memory
- No signs of motor weakness or sensory loss
- Bladder incontinence

The brain MRI study revealed two large lateral ventricles, a wide third ventricle, and a normal size fourth ventricle.

Question: Can you identify the foramen that was blocked in this case?

- Foramen of Magendie
- Foramen of Luschka
- Interventricular foramen
- Cerebral aqueduct
- Foramina of Magendie and Luschka

Discussion: The lateral ventricles are connected to the third ventricles through the interventricular foramina of Monro. The CSF from the third ventricle drains into the fourth ventricle through the cerebral aqueduct. A block involving the cerebral aqueduct in the midbrain region had resulted in an obstructive type of hydrocephalus.

PATIENT SEVEN

A 75-year-old right-handed man, who was diagnosed with stroke and aphasia, was seen by a SLP, who noted the following:

- Fluently spoken and well-articulated speech
- Speech consisting a meaningless strings of words

- Poor repetitions
- Impaired comprehension for both spoken and written language
- Moderate anomia
- Optimistic attitude

The MRI study revealed a large ischemic stroke in the left inferior parietal lobule involving Brodmann areas 22, 39, and 40.

Question: Can you identify the type of aphasia and the lesion site?

- Transcortical aphasia related to a lesion in the pars triangularis region
- Conduction aphasia related to a postcentral gyrus lesion
- Wernicke aphasia related to a lesion affecting the posterosuperior temporal, angular, and supramarginal gyri
- Visual agnosia related to a lesion in the anterior temporal gyrus
- Anomic aphasia related to a prefrontal lesion

Discussion: This neurolinguistic symptomatology (fluently spoken, asemantic verbal output with anomia and impaired comprehension) indicates Wernicke aphasia. This type of aphasia is associated with damage to the posterosuperior temporal region and the inferior parietal lobule in the dominant hemisphere, which, in this case, includes the left supramarginal and angular gyri.

SUMMARY

The human nervous system, which consists of the CNS (brain and spinal cord) and PNS (spinal and cranial nerves), is the generator of the electrical and chemical energy that controls body parts and their functions. The brain is responsible for initiating, controlling, and regulating all sensorimotor and cognitive (mental) functions. The spinal cord mediates sensory and motor commands, both somatic and visceral, to and from body parts that interact with the environment. The bony shell of the skull; the vertebral column; and the dural, arachnoid, and pial layers of the meninges protect the CNS. CSF in the subarachnoid space also helps protect the brain and spinal cord by serving as a mechanical buffer. Embryologically, the brain is derived from three vesicles: prosencephalon, mesencephalon, and rhombencephalon. The cerebral hemispheres, basal ganglia, limbic lobe, thalamus, hypothalamus, and lateral and third ventricles are derived from the prosencephalon. The mesencephalon develops into the midbrain and cerebral aqueduct, whereas the rhombencephalon gives rise to the pons, cerebellum, medulla oblongata, and fourth ventricle. Each of these structures serves a specific sensorimotor or regulating function. The PNS, which includes spinal and cranial nerves, extends to organs, muscles, joints, blood vessels, and skin surfaces, forming an extensive network of cables and fine wires throughout the body. The PNS consists of the somatic and autonomic nervous systems. The somatic motor and sensory nerves innervate skeletal muscles, whereas the autonomic sensory and motor nerves innervate the visceral organs and glands. Cranial nerves regulate the sensory and motor functions of the face and head.

QUIZ QUESTIONS

1. Define the following terms: basal ganglia, brainstem, dermatome, foramen magnum, hippocampus, hypothalamus, limbic lobe, meninges, septum pellucidum, tectum, tegmentum, thalamus

2. Match each of the following numbered structures with its associated lettered vesicle.
   1. pes pedunculi
   2. limbic system
   3. fourth ventricle
   4. basal ganglia
   5. thalamus
   6. substantia nigra
   7. medulla
   8. pons

   a. telencephalon
   b. diencephalon
   c. mesencephalon
   d. metencephalon
   e. myelencephalon

3. Match each of the following numbered structures to its associated lettered state.
   1. supramarginal gyrus
   2. angular gyrus
   3. calcarine sulcus
   4. olfactory sulcus
   5. uncus
   6. parahippocampal gyrus
   7. third frontal convolution
   8. superior temporal gyrus
   9. superior frontal sulcus
   10. postcentral gyrus

   a. frontal
   b. parietal
   c. temporal
   d. occipital

4. Match each of the following numbered structures to its associated lettered cortical surface.
   1. central sulcus
   2. lateral sulcus
   3. supramarginal gyrus
   4. angular gyrus
   5. calcarine sulcus
   6. olfactory sulcus
   7. parahippocampal gyrus
   8. collateral sulcus

   a. dorsal-lateral
   b. ventral
   c. mid-sagittal

   9. orbital frontal cortex
   10. olfactory nerve
   11. cingulate gyrus
   12. corpus callosum

5. Which ventricular spaces are found in the forebrain? In the diencephalon?

6. List the number of spinal nerves that exit from the following regions of the spinal cord:
   cervical
   thoracic
   lumbar
   sacral

7. List the cranial nerves by name and in the order they exit the brainstem.

8. Match each of the following numbered pathologies to its associated lettered statement.
   1. lesion in area of 17 on the left side
   2. destruction of area 41 on the left side
   3. destruction of area 22 on the left side
   4. damage to the white matter of the prefrontal lobe
   5. cutting the corpus callosum

   a. Wernicke aphasia
   b. right hemianopsia
   c. loss of executive function
   d. auditory imperceptibility
   e. separation of hemispheres

TECHNICAL TERMS

afferent
arachnoid trabeculae
basal ganglia
brainstem
cauda equina
choroid plexus
conus medullaris
corpora quadrigemina
denticulate ligaments
dermatome
efferent
filum terminale
foramen magnum
fornix
hippocampus

homeostasis
hypothalamus
insula
limbic lobe
meninges
parasympathetic
peduncle
septum pellucidum
subarachnoid space
subdural space
sympathetic
tectum
tegmentum
thalamus

Internal Anatomy of the Central Nervous System

LEARNING OBJECTIVES

After studying this chapter, students should be able to:

- Identify the shapes of corticospinal fibers at different neuraxial levels

- Recognize the ventricular cavity at various neuroaxial levels

- Recognize major internal anatomic structures of the spinal cord and describe their functions

- Recognize important internal anatomic structures of the medulla and explain their functions

- Recognize important internal anatomic structures of the pons and describe their functions

- Identify important internal anatomic structures of the midbrain and discuss their functions

- Recognize important internal anatomic structures of the forebrain (diencephalon, basal ganglia, and limbic structures) and describe their functions

- Follow the continuation of major anatomic structures and relate them in each sequential section of the brain

The gross anatomic (cortical, subcortical, meninges, ventricles, and medullary centers) structures were discussed in relation to their functions and locations in Chapter 2. The next step is to use specific and easily identified anatomic structures as signposts for developing an orientation to the internal anatomy of the brain in relation to the surrounding structures. Exposure to the internal brain structures often is neglected in teaching neuroscience to students of communicative disorders and human behavior. Learning internal brain anatomy is the most significant part of training in neuroscience, and this knowledge is essential for solving clinical problems and reading brain images. Internal anatomy is best learned by repeated exposure to the serial sections of the spinal cord, brainstem, and forebrain. In this chapter, the spinal cord, brainstem, and diencephalon are examined via stained sections, and the forebrain is studied on unstained sections.

Nuclear structures and fiber tracts related to various functional systems exist side by side at each level of the nervous system. Because disease processes in the brain rarely strike only one anatomic structure or pathway, there is a tendency for a series of related and unrelated clinical symptoms to emerge after a brain injury. A thorough knowledge of the internal brain structures, including their shape, size, location, and proximity, makes it easier to understand their functional significance. In addition, the proximity of nuclear structures and fiber tracts explains multiple symptoms that may develop from a single lesion site.

ANATOMIC ORIENTATION LANDMARKS

Two distinct anatomic landmarks used for visual orientation to the internal anatomy of the brain are the shapes of the descending **corticospinal fibers** and the **ventricular cavity** (Fig. 3-1). Both are present throughout the brain, although their shape and size vary as one progresses caudally from the rostral forebrain (telencephalon) to the caudal brainstem. Consequently, familiarity with the progressively changing shapes and sizes of these structures is essential for identifying the various brain levels that they represent.

Shapes of Corticospinal Fibers

Immediately after their origin in the sensorimotor cortex, the corticospinal fibers fan down through the **corona radiata** (see Fig. 2-38) to enter the wedge-shaped **internal capsule** at the *diencephalic level* (Fig. 3-1*A*; see Figs. 2-15 and 2-16). Along the ventral surface of the midbrain, they form the **pes pedunculi** (crus cerebri), a bilaterally compact fillet-shaped mass of fibers on a cross-sectional view (Fig. 3-1*B*; see Fig. 2-24). The fibers of the corticospinal tract later disperse among the scattered pontine nuclei and appear as many irregular round masses scattered throughout the basal pons (Fig. 3-1*C*; see Fig. 2-25). The corticospinal tract fibers recombine when entering the medulla and form a **pyramid**, which is best viewed in gross and microscopic cross section of the caudal brainstem (Fig. 3-1*D*; see Fig. 2-26). The term *pyramid* gave origin to the term *pyramidal tract*, which is synonymous with *corticospinal tract*. Pyramidal fibers cross the midline at the

Motor Fibers and Ventricle Shapes

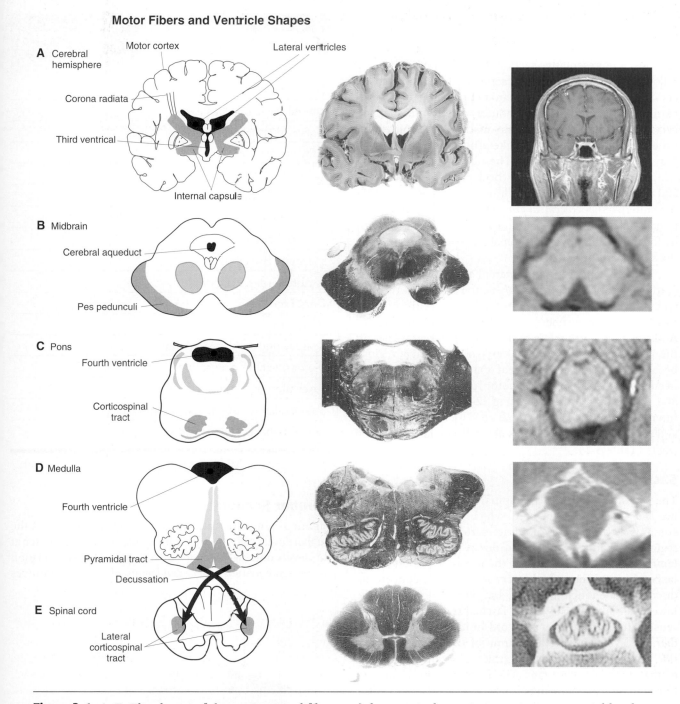

A Cerebral hemisphere
Motor cortex
Lateral ventricles
Corona radiata
Third ventrical
Internal capsule

B Midbrain
Cerebral aqueduct
Pes pedunculi

C Pons
Fourth ventricle
Corticospinal tract

D Medulla
Fourth ventricle
Pyramidal tract
Decussation

E Spinal cord
Lateral corticospinal tract

Figure 3-1 A–E. The shapes of the corticospinal fibers and the ventricular cavity at various neuroaxial levels.

caudal medulla; after crossing, they enter the **lateral funiculus** of the spinal cord and are known as the **lateral corticospinal tract** (Fig. 3-1E).

Shape of the Ventricular Cavity

The **lateral** and **third ventricles** together are butterfly-shaped in a cross-section of the rostral brain (Fig. 3-1A; see Fig. 2-16). The wings represent the two lateral ventricles and the body; the narrow slit in the middle marks the third ventricle. The **cerebral aqueduct** of Sylvius is the

small tube-shaped midbrain canal (Fig. 3-1B; see Fig. 2-24) that connects the **third** and **fourth ventricles**. The fourth ventricle overlies the pons (Fig. 3-1D; see Fig. 2-9); it tapers to end in the rostral medulla (Fig. 3-1E).

Important internal anatomic landmarks of central nervous system (CNS) have been serially examined. The spinal cord is examined in cross section. The midbrain, pons, and medulla are reviewed in transverse section. The **forebrain structures** (cerebral cortex, diencephalon, and basal ganglia) are studied in both coronal and horizontal sections.

SPINAL CORD IN CROSS-SECTIONS

The internal anatomy of the spinal cord is studied in four sections; a representative section is taken from each of the following anatomic divisions: **sacral**, **lumbar**, **thoracic**, and **cervical**. The basic internal anatomic pattern of the spinal cord remains the same throughout its extent from sacral to cervical regions. The **central gray matter** of the cord, made up of cell bodies, is shaped like a butterfly and appears gray in freshly cut sections. The outer part of the cord, which looks like the rim of a wheel, consists of ascending and descending fiber tracts (**white matter**) and surrounds the butterfly-shaped *central gray*. The fiber tracts form functionally related longitudinal funiculi, which are demarcated by longitudinal grooves and spinal nerve attachments along the surface of the spinal cord.

The only change in the internal anatomy of the spinal cord is the ratio of *white* to *gray matter* at each of the four spinal levels. That ratio gradually increases, from sacral to cervical, as new fibers are added to the afferent tracts. Additional changes relate to the shape of the gray matter; the spinal cord enlarges in the cervical and lumbar regions because of the relatively great extent of nerve supply needed for the sensory and motor functions of the upper and lower extremities (see Fig. 2-33). The important internal structures of the spinal cord include the sensory and motor nuclei and various ascending and descending tracts (Table 3-1).

Sacral Section

The *sacral structures* of the spinal cord are seen in Figure 3-2. This level of the cord, which is small in diameter, contains a thin mantle of white matter and a larger gray region with bulky **ventral** and **dorsal horns**. The **dorsal lemniscal column** consists of the ascending fibers of the **fasciculus gracilis**, which carry information concerning discriminative touch, pressure, and limb position from the lower half of the body. The fasciculus gracilis contains sensory fibers that enter the cord from the *sacral* to *mid-thoracic level*. The lateral column of the white matter at this level contains the lateral corticospinal tract and fibers of the anterolateral system. The *lateral corticospinal tract* transmits motor commands from the motor cortex via the **lower motor neurons** to the muscles. The **anterolateral system** consists of the **anterior** and **lateral spinothalamic tracts**, which mediate sensations of diffuse touch, pain, and temperature.

The large *ventral horns* are the sites of motor nuclei. The *dorsal horns* contain the sensory nuclei, which include the **substantia gelatinosa** and **nucleus proprius** (see Chapter 7); these nuclei are present throughout the spinal cord and receive input predominantly from spinal sensory nerves. Other sensory spinal cells include the **nucleus dorsalis of Clark**. Many dorsal horn cells give rise to fibers of the *spinocerebellar* (unconscious proprioception) and *anterolateral system* (pain and temperature).

Table 3-1

Anatomic Structures of the Spinal Cord

Dorsal median sulcus
Ventral median sulcus
Dorsal intermediate sulcus
Gray matter
   Dorsal horns
   Ventral horns
White matter
   Dorsal fasciculus
   Lateral fasciculus
   Anterior fasciculus
Dorsal root
Ventral root
Sensory nuclei in gray column
Motor nuclei in gray column
Fasciculus gracilis and cuneatus
Spinothalamic (lateral and anterior) tracts
Spinocerebellar (dorsal and ventral) tracts

Lumbar Section

Figure 3-3 demonstrates the anatomic appearance of the *lumbar level* (at L4) of the spinal cord. The gray matter at this level contains larger *dorsal* and *ventral horns* in relation to the white matter. The *dorsal lemniscal* column continues

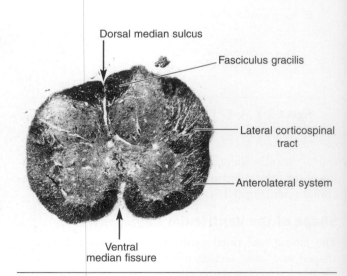

Figure 3-2 Cross-section of the spinal cord at the sacral level.

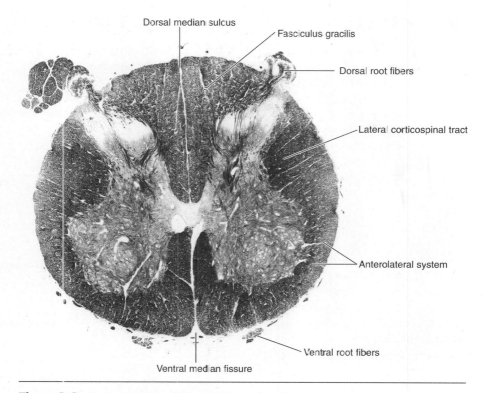

Figure 3-3 Cross-section of the spinal cord at the L4 level.

to exclusively represent fibers of the *fasciculus gracilis*, which is located lateral to the *dorsal median sulcus*. This level also contains the *lateral corticospinal tract* and the *anterolateral system*, consisting of the *spinothalamic* and *spinocerebellar tracts*. (The *spinocerebellar tract* is not identified in Fig. 3-3.) The dorsal horns contain the sensory nuclei, and the ventral

horns contain the motor nuclei. Also present in this cross section are the *dorsal* and *ventral root fibers*.

Thoracic Section

The anatomic characteristics of the *thoracic* region (T4) of the spinal cord are shown in Figure 3-4. This spinal cord

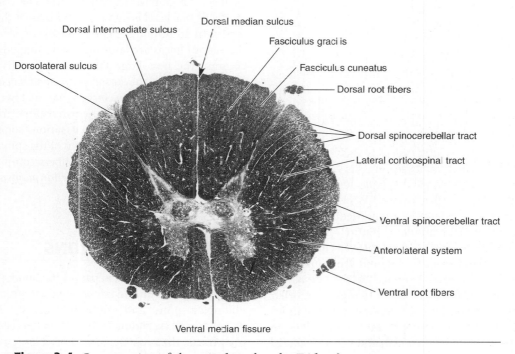

Figure 3-4 Cross-section of the spinal cord at the T4 level.

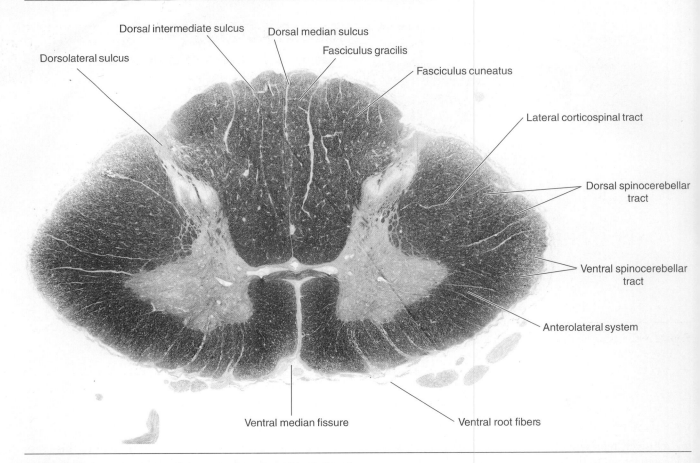

Figure 3-5 Cross-section of the spinal cord at the C7 level.

level is characterized by the reduced size of the gray matter and the enlarged share of white matter. Compared the previously discussed sections, the *dorsal* and *ventral horns* are smaller and tapered. The *dorsal lemniscal column* at this level is larger because of additional sensory fibers from the higher body levels. The additional sensory fibers form the **fasciculus cuneatus**, which ascend lateral to the *fasciculus gracilis* in the dorsal columns of the spinal cord. The fasciculus cuneatus fibers carry the sensations of fine discriminative touch, pressure, and limb position from the upper body; its fibers enter the spinal cord at the midthoracic through cervical levels. With emergence of the fasciculus cuneatus, the *dorsal intermediate sulcus* is visible as it separates the medially located fasciculus gracilis from the laterally located fibers of the fasciculus cuneatus. The *lateral corticospinal tract* is larger than at lower levels, although it retains the same relative lateral location. Mediating sensations of diffuse touch, pain, and temperature, the fibers of the *spinothalamic tracts (anterolateral system)* continue to occupy the same general space throughout the spinal cord.

Appearing along the lateral surface are the **dorsal** and **ventral spinocerebellar tracts**. Fibers of the spinocerebellar tracts mediate unconscious proprioception from the limbs to the cerebellum. Unconscious proprioception plays an important role in the acquisition and maintenance of skilled motor activities.

Cervical Section

Figure 3-5 displays the anatomic characteristics of the *cervical* (C7) region of the spinal cord. The volume of white matter at this level is much greater than at the lower spinal levels. In addition, the *dorsal horns* are slender, whereas the *ventral horns* are large and wing shaped. In the dorsal column, the now-large *fasciculi* of *gracilis* and *cuneatus* are demarcated by the *dorsal intermediate sulcus*. The *corticospinal tract* is relatively larger than at lower levels. This configuration of the lateral corticospinal tract marks the level below the **pyramidal decussation** (soon to take place rostral to this level at the junction of the spinal cord and the medulla). The lateral column of fibers continues to contain the *spinothalamic* and *spinocerebellar pathways*.

BRAINSTEM IN TRANSVERSE SECTIONS

The brainstem, as the axial part of the brain, protrudes from the base of the brain and consists of three structures: medulla oblongata, pons, and midbrain (see Fig. 2-22). Besides containing all ascending (sensory) and descending (motor) fiber tracts, the brainstem includes a large group of nuclei that relate to the sensorimotor functions of the cranial

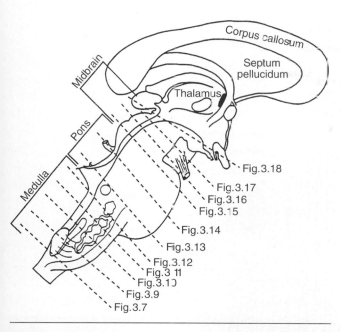

Figure 3-6 Location of the transverse sections of the brainstem shown in the specified figures.

Table 3-2

Anatomic Structures of the Medulla

Caudal (low) medulla
  Pyramid
  Decussation of pyramidal fibers
  Lateral corticospinal tract
  Fasciculus gracilis and cuneatus
  Nucleus gracilis and cuneatus
  Spinal trigeminal nucleus and tract

Middle medulla
  Nucleus gracilis and cuneatus
  Fasciculus gracilis and cuneatus
  Inferior cerebellar peduncle (restiform body)
  Sensory decussation
    Internal arcuate fibers
    Medial lemniscus
  Principal inferior olivary nucleus
  Pyramid
  Spinal trigeminal nucleus and tract

Rostral (high) medulla
  Principal inferior olivary nucleus
  Inferior cerebellar peduncle
  Cochlear nucleus
  Vestibular nucleus
  Medial lemniscus
  Pyramid
  Spinal trigeminal nucleus and tract

nerves, serve various vital visceral (cardiac and respiratory) functions, and mediate the special senses and reflexive functions. The transverse sections of the brainstem discussed here are indicated in Figure 3-6.

Medulla Oblongata

The *medulla oblongata,* the most caudal portion of the brainstem, begins above the rootlets of the first cervical spinal nerve and gradually increases in size until rostrally it merges with the pons. Important structures in the medulla are the *corticospinal fibers* (pyramidal tract), *pyramidal decussation* (crossing of motor fibers), dorsal lemniscal column (*fasciculus gracilis* and *fasciculus cuneatus*), sensory decussation, medial lemniscus, inferior cerebellar peduncle, principal (inferior) olivary nucleus, reticular formation, and many cranial nerve nuclei (Table 3-2).

Caudal Medulla

The transverse section in Figure 3-7 is the most caudal view of the brainstem, where the medulla merges with the spinal cord at the foramen magnum (see Fig. 2-31A). Four important structures in the dorsal medulla are the *nucleus gracilis, fasciculus gracilis, nucleus cuneatus,* and *fasciculus cuneatus.*

The ascending fibers of the fasciculus gracilis synapse on the cells of the nucleus gracilis, and those of the fasciculus cuneatus synapse on the cells of the nucleus cuneatus. In the center of this medullary section is the crossing of the pyramidal fibers. After the crossing, the descending pyramidal fibers move to a lateral position in the spinal column and form the *lateral corticospinal tract* (Fig. 3-5). This crossing of the *corticospinal fibers* accounts for the motor cortex of one side of the brain controlling the opposite

side of the body. Lateral to the fasciculus cuneatus is the massive formation of the **spinal trigeminal nucleus** and the **spinal trigeminal tract.**

The *spinal trigeminal tract* consists of fibers of the *trigeminal (CN V) nerve,* which mediates pain and temperature from the face. Fibers of this tract enter the brainstem, descend ipsilaterally in the medulla, and terminate in the *spinal trigeminal nucleus.* Secondary fibers from the spinal trigeminal nucleus cross the midline and ascend to the thalamus, from which impulses are relayed to the sensory cortex (see Chapter 7).

Medial to the trigeminal tract and nucleus are diffusely located cellular and fibrous components of the *reticular formation,* which extend throughout the brainstem. The reticular formation integrates complex behaviors and regulates cortical arousal (see Fig. 2-23). The *reticular formation* integrates all sensorimotor stimuli with internally generated thoughts, emotions, and cognition. It is also responsible for maintaining the homeostatic state of the brain, which is essential for regulating visceral (cardiovascular), sensorimotor (respiration), and neuroendocrine activities such as blood pressure and movement.

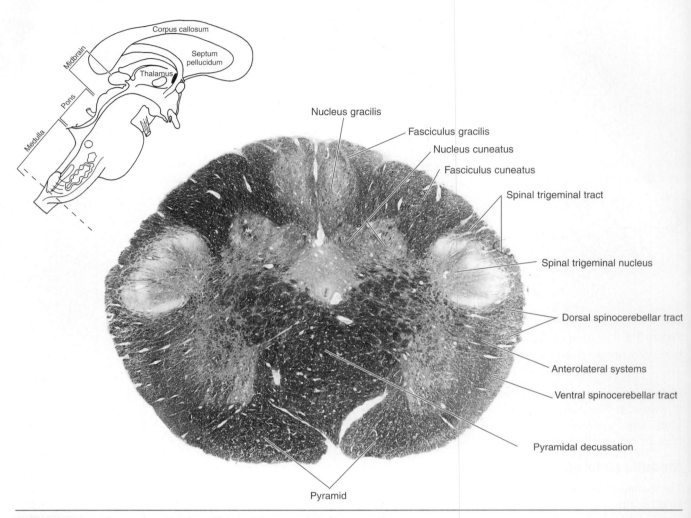

Figure 3-7 Transverse section of the medulla through the pyramidal decussation.

A discussion of the events related to the crossing of sensory fibers is important for an orientation to the course of the *dorsal column fibers* and their level of crossing (Fig. 3-8). The *fasciculi of gracilis* and *cuneatus* are the first-order sensory fibers; their sensory neurons are in the spinal *dorsal root ganglion.* Fibers of these two fasciculi enter the spinal cord and ascend on the same side in the *dorsal lemniscal column* and synapse on their respective nuclei in the medulla. These nuclei project secondary fibers across the midline as the **internal arcuate fibers**, which form the **medial lemniscus** and travel upward to relay information related to fine discriminative touch (deep touch, two-point touch, stereognosis, and proprioception) to the thalamus. The thalamocortical projections transmit the sensory information to the **primary sensory cortex** (Brodmann areas 3, 1, 2). Thus it becomes clear why three different terms (*dorsal lemniscal column, internal arcuate fibers,* and *medial lemniscus*) relate to fibers that mediate the same sensory information received from the *fasciculi of gracilis* and *cuneatus,* which transmit sensation from the lower and the upper body, respectively.

Caudal (Lower) Third of the Medulla

The transverse section in Figure 3-9 provides a better view of the *internal arcuate fibers* that arise from the *gracilis* and *cuneatus nuclei* and cross the midline. The gracile and cuneate nuclei attain their largest size at this level. The internal arcuate fibers from those nuclei cross the midline to form the medial lemniscus and then travel rostrally to the thalamus. At the medullary level, this *decussation* thus allows for the transmission of tactile and discriminative sensation from one side of the body to the opposite half of the brain. The *pyramids* in the ventromedial medulla appear as a compact *bundle* of fibers just rostral to the level at which they decussate. The decussations of the sensory internal arcuate fibers and motor *pyramidal fibers* are two landmarks of the caudal medulla.

The core of the *reticular formation* in the central third of the medulla is continuous with the lower levels. It is a net-like arrangement of cell bodies and interwoven projections that interact with virtually all sensorimotor systems and regulate brain functioning (see Fig. 2-23). The *central gray matter* is the *midbrain reticular–limbic area,* which regulates somatic and visceral functions. Beneath the central gray

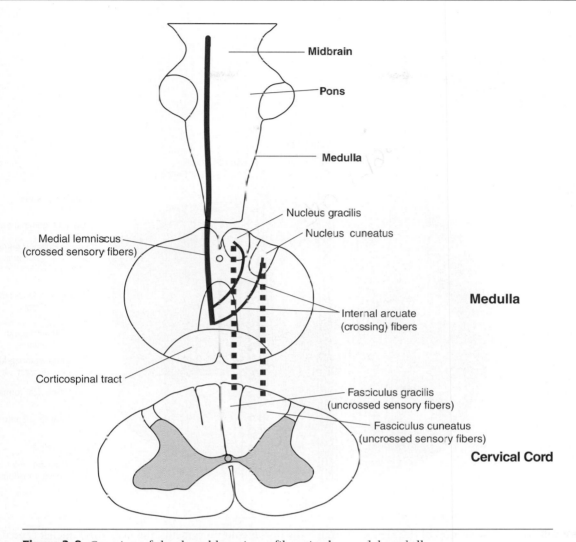

Figure 3-8 Crossing of the dorsal lemniscus fibers in the caudal medulla.

is the nucleus of the **hypoglossal nerve** (CN XII). It controls all intrinsic and most extrinsic tongue muscles and is an important nerve for speech production and swallowing.

The structure below the *hypoglossal nucleus* is the **medial longitudinal fasciculus**; this fiber bundle receives visual and vestibular projections and is located longitudinally from the cervical cord to the brainstem. It interconnects the motor nuclei of four cranial nerves (oculomotor [CN III], trochlear [CN IV], abducens [CN VI], and spinal accessory [CN XI]) and regulates head–eye coordination. The principal (inferior) olivary nucleus, also seen in this area, relays spinal and brainstem afferents to the cerebellum. Some of the previously described structures also appear in this section of the brainstem.

Middle Third of the Medulla

Figure 3-10 presents structures of the middle third of the medulla. The rostral portion of the *hypoglossal nucleus* is larger here than the lower third of the medulla. Located above the pyramidal tract, the *principal (inferior) olivary*

nucleus occupies a major portion of the lower half of the medulla. The principal olivary nucleus, a wrinkled and saggy structure, is an important relay center for motor and proprioceptive information to the cerebellum. This nucleus receives input related to pain, touch, and position of the limbs from the spinal cord (**spino-olivary**) and reticular formation (**reticulo-olivary**). The **olivocerebellar fibers** cross the midline and project to the opposite cerebellar hemisphere through the *inferior cerebellar peduncle* (**restiform body**). The inferior cerebellar peduncle appears along the lateral dorsal surface of the upper half of the medulla. Furthermore, it is the most caudal of the three peduncles that connect the brainstem to the cerebellum (see Figs. 2-29 and 2-30).

The **cranial nerve nuclei**, which are related to the **glossopharyngeal** (CN IX) and **vagus** (CN X) **nerves**, are found in the region between the *inferior cerebellar peduncle* and the *reticular formation*. One of the important nuclei at this level is the **nucleus ambiguus**, the motor nucleus of the glossopharyngeal (CN IX) and vagus (CN X) nerves; it supplies muscles of the soft palate, pharynx, larynx, and

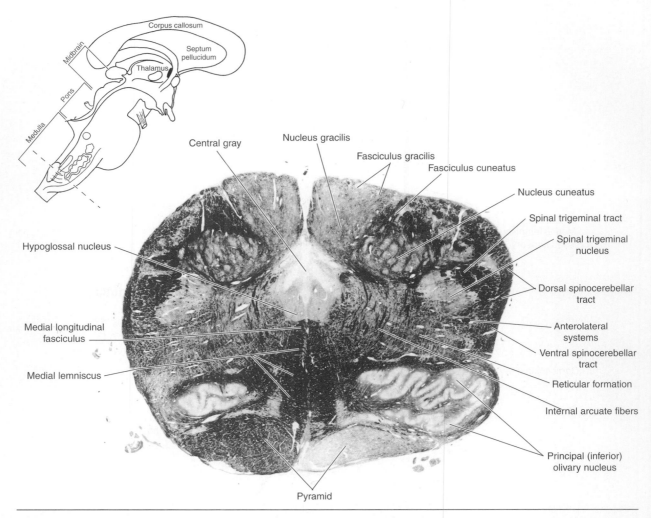

Figure 3-9   Transverse section of the medulla through the dorsal column (gracilis and cuneatus) nuclei, caudal portions of hypoglossal nucleus, caudal end of inferior olivary nucleus, and middle portions of the sensory decussation.

upper esophagus and controls swallowing and phonation. The nuclei of the reticular formation are scattered and occupy a larger core area in the center of the medulla.

Rostral Third of the Medulla

In the transverse section through the rostral third of the medulla shown in Figure 3-11, the *inferior cerebellar peduncle* and *principal (inferior) olivary nucleus* are larger than they are at the level shown in Figure 3-10. Among the newly appearing structures are the **cochlear complex** and glossopharyngeal (CN IX) nerve. The *cochlear (CN IX) nuclear complex,* located above the restiform body in the dorsolateral medulla, receives projections from the inner ear. The *glossopharyngeal nerve* mediates taste and contributes to swallowing.

The compact **pyramidal motor fibers** are in the ventral medulla. The *principal (inferior) olivary nucleus* is present in its fully developed form. The *medial lemniscus* (mediating fine and discriminative touch) and the *medial longitudinal fasciculus* (interconnecting the motor nuclei of the ocular cranial nerves with vestibular input) are present along the

midline in the medulla dorsal to the *pyramids*. The *spinal trigeminal nucleus* and its tract can also be seen in this section. The *reticular formation* occupies a large core in the middle third of the medulla, spanning the area dorsal to the principal (inferior) olivary nucleus.

Pons

The major pontine structures are the corticospinal fibers interspersed with diffused **pontine nuclei**, the crown-shaped cavity of the fourth ventricle, the massive **middle cerebellar peduncle (brachium pontis)**, the medial lemniscus, the **crossing pontocerebellar fibers**, the **trigeminal nuclear complex**, the spinal trigeminal nucleus and tract, the **superior cerebellar peduncle (brachium conjunctivum)**, remnants of the inferior cerebellar peduncle, and many cranial nerve structures (Table 3-3).

Lower Pons

The transitional anatomic structures between the medulla and pons are presented in Figure 3-12. The enlarged *fourth*

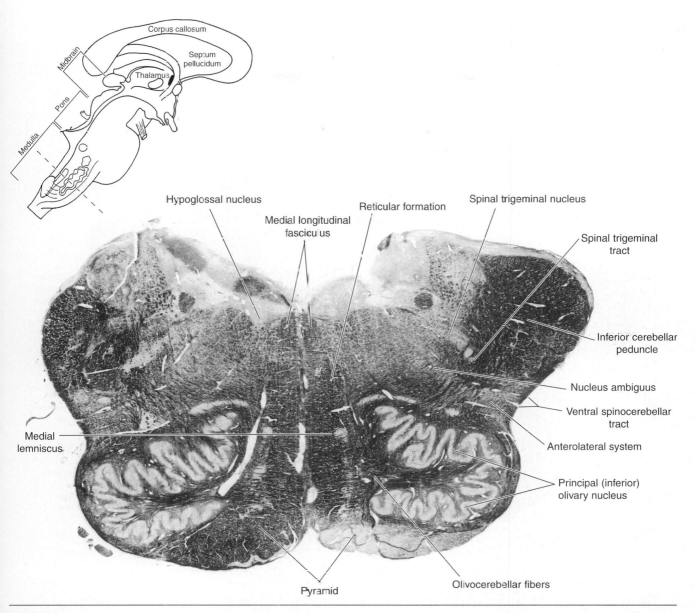

Figure 3-10 Transverse section of the medulla through the rostral portions of the hypoglossal nucleus and middle portions of the principal (inferior) olivary nucleus.

ventricle and diffuse pontine nuclei represent the pons, whereas the *pyramid* characterizes the medulla. The *superior cerebellar peduncle* forms part of the lateral roof of the fourth ventricle. The convex **anterior medullary velum**, in the dorsal area of this section, forms the roof of the fourth ventricle. The ventral teardrop-shaped pyramid does not hug the ventromedial area here, as it does in the lower medullary levels.

The **vestibular nuclear complex** appears beneath the floor of the *fourth ventricle*. The *cochlear nucleus*, seen in Figure 3-11, is no longer present. The *vestibular complex* receives projections from the semicircular canals in the inner ear and plays a role in equilibrium and head–eye coordination (see Chapter 10).

The fibers of the **vestibular branch** of the **vestibulocochlear nerve** exit laterally from the pontomedullary junction along the ventral surface of the *middle* and *inferior cerebellar peduncles*. The structures beneath the vestibular complex are the *spinal trigeminal tract* and *spinal trigeminal nucleus*.

The *spinal tract* fibers of the *trigeminal nerve* descend ipsilaterally to synapse in the *trigeminal nucleus*, which relays somatosensory sensation from the face through its fiber tracts. After crossing, the trigeminal spinal tract fibers join the *medial lemniscus* to terminate in the thalamus. The nucleus of the **facial nerve** (CN VII) is present in the pontine tegmentum. The facial (CN VII) nerve innervates the muscles of facial expression and controls smiling, frowning,

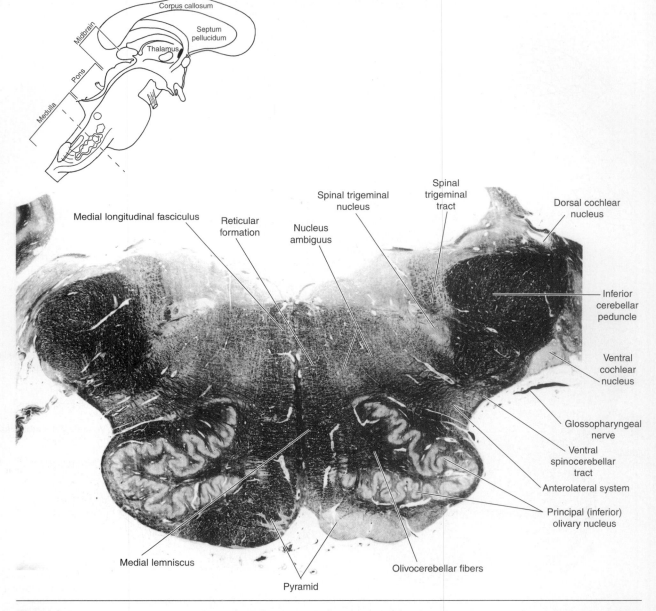

Figure 3-11 Transverse section of the medulla through the dorsal and ventral cochlear nuclei and the root of the glossopharyngeal nerve.

Table 3-3

Anatomic Structures of the Pons

Lower pons
- Full-size crown-shaped fourth ventricle
- Diffuse pyramidal fibers piercing basal pons
- Remnants of inferior cerebellar peduncle
- Facial nucleus and nerve
- Middle cerebellar peduncle (brachium pontis)
- Medial lemniscus (marking upper limit of basal pons)
- Anterior medullary velum
- Spinal trigeminal nucleus and tract
- Superior cerebellar peduncle (brachium conjunctivum)

Middle pons
- Middle cerebellar peduncle
- Trigeminal nuclear complex
- Pontine nuclei
- Superior cerebellar peduncle
- Fourth ventricle cavity
- Anterior medullary velum
- Medial lemniscus
- Diffuse corticospinal fibers

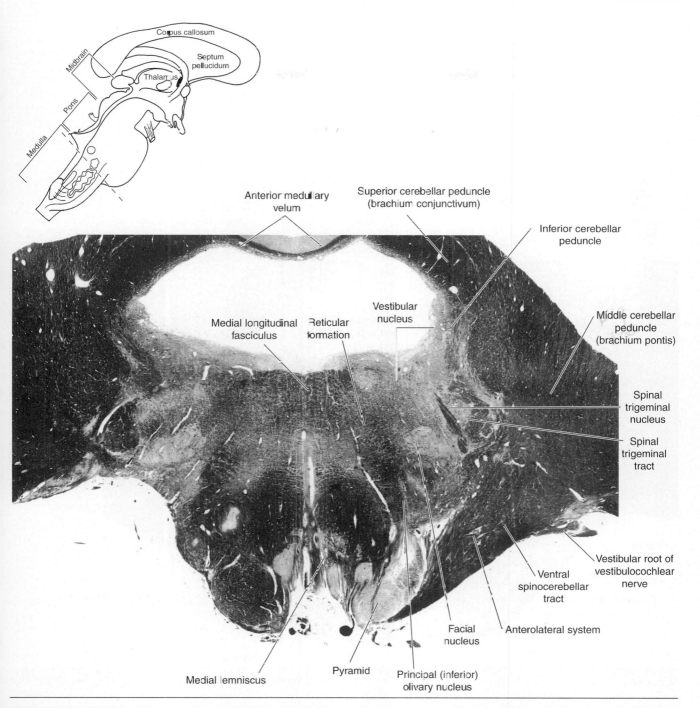

Figure 3-12 Transverse section of the pontomedullary junction through the rostral pole of the inferior olivary nucleus and facial nucleus.

and laughing as well as assists in speaking. Fibers of the facial (CN VII) nerve exit laterally from the pontomedullary junction (see Figs. 2-49–2-51).

The massive body of the *middle cerebellar peduncle*, by far the largest of the cerebellar peduncles, is located laterally in this section. Its fibers connect the pons with the cerebellum and mediate information from the motor cortex to the cerebellum. The fibers located medial to the middle cerebellar peduncle belong to the *inferior cerebellar peduncle*, which mediates vestibular and spinal afferents to the cerebellum. The crescent-shaped fibers of the *superior cerebellar peduncle* emerge dorsally and form the dorsolateral roof of the *fourth ventricle*.

Middle Pons

The transverse section of the middle pons shown in Figure 3-13 is at the level of the *trigeminal* (CN V) nerve (the principal sensory nerve for the face) as it exits laterally

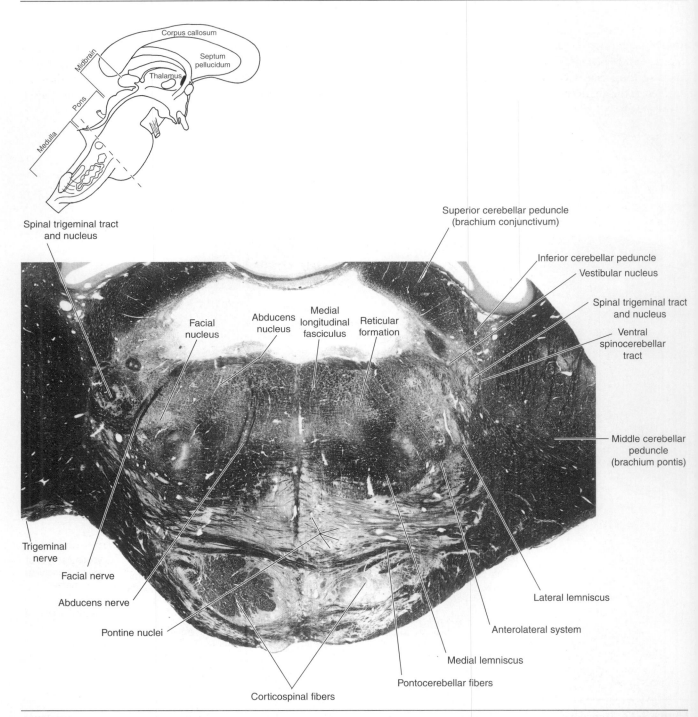

Figure 3-13 Transverse section of the pons through the rostral pole of the facial nucleus and internal genu of the facial nerve.

through the *middle cerebellar peduncle*. The most characteristic features of the pons are the interspersed **corticospinal–corticopontine fibers** and the crown-shaped lumen of the *fourth ventricle*. Fibers of all three *cerebellar peduncles* are present laterally in this section, although the *inferior cerebellar* and *superior cerebellar peduncles* are relatively small.

Scattered pontine nuclei receive massive input from the ipsilateral primary motor and sensory cortices and project the **pontocerebellar fibers** to the cerebellum; these fibers

cross the midline before entering the cerebellum via the *middle cerebellar peduncle*. These fibers mediate information from the opposite primary motor, sensory, and visual cortices and are concerned with limb movement during skilled acts. Laterally, the crescent-shaped *superior cerebellar peduncle* provides cerebellar feedback to the primary motor cortex via the **red nucleus**. Located ventrolaterally are fibers of the **lateral lemniscus**, which carry auditory information from both ears to the cortex (see Chapter 9).

This pontine section also demonstrates spatial relationships among the *facial nucleus, facial nerve, abducens nucleus,* and *abducens nerve.* The internal genu refers to fibers of the facial (CN VII) nerve as they curve over the nucleus of the abducens (CN VI) nerve just below the floor of the *fourth ventricle* (see Figs. 15-3 and 15-4).

Pons–Midbrain Junction

The section shown in Figure 3-14 is located at the transition between the rostral pons and the midbrain. This transition is marked by a reduction in the size of the *fourth ventricle.* The ventricular floor is formed by the enlarged *central gray of the reticular formation,* which contains important somatic and visceral nuclei. Located dorsally in this section is the **trochlear nerve root,** which is one of three cranial nerves (the other two are **oculomotor** [CN III] and **abducens** [CN VI]) responsible for innervating the eye and is the only motor nerve that exits dorsally. The *medial longitudinal fasciculus* is buried within the central gray substance of the reticular formation. The massive cerebellum is dorsal to the ventricular cavity.

Ventral to the *central gray* of the *reticular formation* are fibers of the *superior cerebellar peduncle,* which occupy the outer third of the tegmentum and decussate at a higher level in the midbrain. These fibers originate in the deep cerebellar nuclei and provide feedback to the opposite thalamic

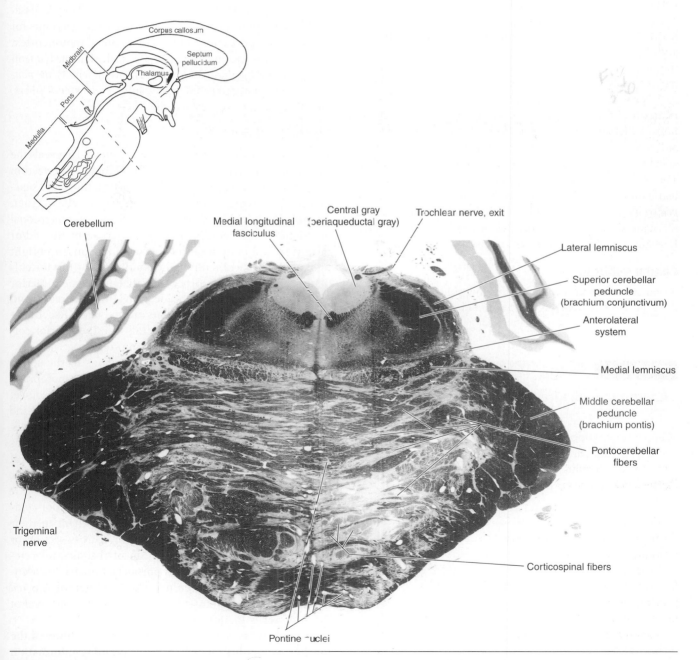

Figure 3-14 Transverse section of the rostral pons through the exits of the trochlear and trigeminal nerves.

and cortical centers. Lateral to the fibers of the superior cerebellar peduncle are the *lateral lemniscus* fibers, which relay information from both ears to the primary auditory cortex in the temporal lobe. The ventral region in this section contains diffuse pontine nuclei and a massive amount of crossing pontocerebellar fibers that make up the large *middle cerebellar peduncles;* also seen here are the scattered corticospinal tract fibers on each side of the midline. Located laterally is the root of the *trigeminal nerve* (CN V).

Midbrain

The midbrain consists of the **tectum**, **tegmentum**, and **basis pedunculi** (see Fig. 2-24). The tectum consists of the **corpora quadrigemina**, which refers to four egg-shaped structures (see Figs. 2-21 and 2-22). The upper two bodies of the corpora quadrigemina are the **superior colliculi**, and the lower two bodies are the **inferior colliculi**. Below the **midbrain tectal structure** is the **cerebral aqueduct**, a narrow canal that connects the third and fourth ventricles.

The *tegmentum* is an elongated mass of nuclei and white matter in the center of the brainstem that includes decussation of the *superior cerebellar peduncle, reticular formation,* and *red nucleus.* The *tectum* and tegmentum are distinguishable by their locations with respect to the *cerebral aqueduct.* The tectum is dorsal to the cerebral aqueduct, whereas the tegmentum is beneath the cerebral aqueduct. The *basis pedunculi* is ventral, and it includes the *substantia nigra* and the wing-shaped fibers of the pes pedunculi (crus cerebri). Important midbrain structures are given in Table 3-4.

Caudal Midbrain

A transverse section through the low midbrain and high pons is presented in Figure 3-15. The two round struc-

---

Table 3-4

Anatomic Structures of the Midbrain

Caudal (low) midbrain
    Cerebral aqueduct
    Inferior colliculus
    Superior cerebellar peduncle and decussation
    Medial lemniscus

Rostral (high) midbrain
    Pes pedunculi (crus cerebri)
    Substantia nigra
    Red nucleus
    Superior colliculus
    Central gray
    Cerebral aqueduct
    Oculomotor nucleus and nerve
    Medial lemniscus

---

tures located dorsally are the *inferior colliculi.* The inferior colliculus is a relay center in the transmission of information from the ears to the auditory cortex; it also regulates auditory reflexes. The fibers of the *lateral lemniscus* that carry auditory information are visible as they merge with the inferior colliculus. Rostrally, the *fourth ventricle* communicates with the *cerebral aqueduct,* which is a frequent site of obstruction in congenital hydrocephalus because of its small lumen. The *central gray* region and reticular formation are located around the cerebral aqueduct and mediate affective behavior.

Originating from the deep *dentate cerebellar nucleus* are the fibers of the *superior cerebellar peduncle;* these fibers course ventromedially below the aqueduct to cross the midline before going to the thalamus and cortex. This decussation of the superior cerebellar peduncle fibers accounts for the cerebellar projections to the contralateral motor cortex. Also present is the emerging *pes pedunculi.* The *medial lemniscus, medial longitudinal fasciculus, lateral lemniscus, pontine nuclei, pontocerebellar fibers,* and *corticospinal fibers,* identified earlier, are also seen in this section.

Rostral Midbrain

The slightly oblique section shown in Figure 3-16 reveals the anatomic characteristics of the high midbrain. The tectum consists of two dorsally located round structures, the *superior colliculi,* which also serve as the visual reflex center. The tectum provides the organism with a three-dimensional orientation map according to which eye movements and/or head turn and body rotations occur in response to bright lights (superior colliculus) and loud noises (inferior colliculus). Besides the cortex and thalamus, the superior colliculus also receives light locations from the retina and is where the spatial retinal points are activated. Ascending auditory signals also send collaterals into the inferior colliculus for similar spatial orientation processing.

Tectobulbar and tectospinal projections to the spinal cord and brainstem motor nuclei result in the appropriate turning of the eyes, head, and body toward the sound source. These startle reflexes are quite rapid, occurring before the cerebral cortex becomes aware of them. The *superior colliculus* and the adjacent **pretectal area** mediate reflexes involving intrinsic eye muscles; they also regulate pupil constriction (light reflex) and lens accommodation for near vision (see Chapter 8).

The *superior colliculi* look similar to the *inferior colliculi,* but can be differentiated by relating them to their co-occurring structures. When seen on a cross-section or transverse section, the decussation of the *superior cerebellar peduncle* fibers is the important landmark for identifying the inferior colliculus. The presence of the *red nucleus* and the substantia nigra characterizes the level of the superior colliculus.

Lateral to the *superior colliculus* is the **brachium of the inferior colliculus**, which carries auditory information from the *inferior colliculus* to the **medial geniculate body**,

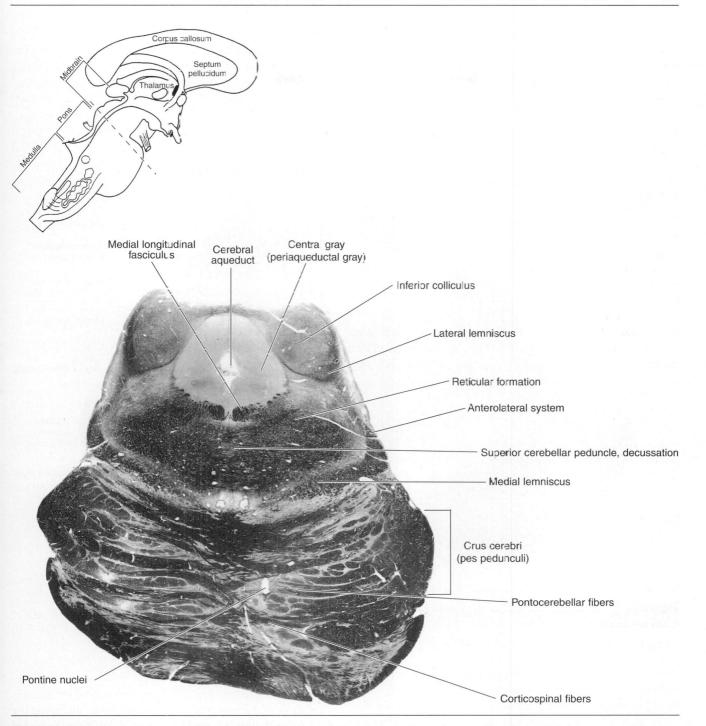

Figure 3-15 Transverse section of the pons–midbrain junction through the inferior colliculus, caudal portions of the decussation of the superior cerebellar peduncle, and rostral parts of the basilar pons.

the thalamic relay nucleus for audition to the brain. The round nucleus in the midbrain tegmentum is the *red nucleus,* which has two important functions. First, it receives the cerebellar projections through the crossed *superior cerebellar peduncle* fibers and sends cerebellar feedback to the thalamus. Second, it transmits descending motor information to the spinal and cranial motor nuclei and regulates muscle tone.

Below the *red nucleus* is the *substantia nigra,* which is important in the extrapyramidal circuitry. Cells of the substantia nigra have been identified as the producers of **dopamine,** an inhibitory basal ganglia neurotransmitter; the nigrostriatal fibers project dopamine from the substantia nigra to the **caudate nucleus** of the **neostriatum.** The degeneration of the substantia nigra's dopamine-producing cells is associated with **Parkinson disease,** a

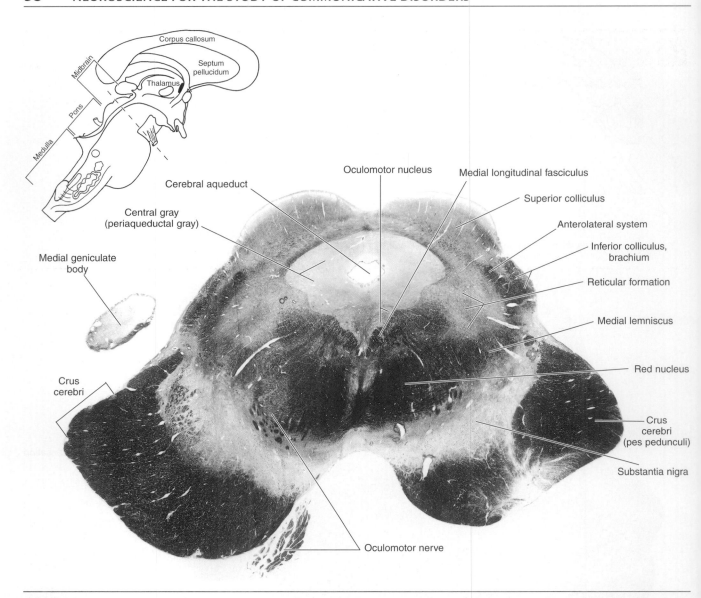

Figure 3-16 Transverse section of the midbrain through the superior colliculus, caudal parts of the oculomotor nucleus, and red nucleus.

slowly progressive degenerative condition characterized by resting tremor, expressionless face, muscular rigidity, flexed posture, and moderate to severe motor speech difficulty (Box 3-1; see Chapter 13).

Ventrally located in this section are the wing-shaped fibers of the *pes pedunculi* (crus cerebri), which indicate the midbrain location of the corticospinal and **corticobulbar fibers**. In the floor of the *central gray* is the *oculomotor nerve nucleus,* one of the three cranial nerves responsible for eye movements. Fibers of the *oculomotor nerve* exit in the interpeduncular fossa (see Fig. 2-50). The *medial longitudinal fasciculus* is below the oculomotor nucleus and is an important fiber bundle, interconnecting three cranial nerves (*oculomotor* [CN III], *trochlear* [CN IV], and *abducens* [CN VI]) with the vestibular system. It is also important in coordinated eye movements.

High Rostral Midbrain

A transverse section through the rostral midbrain contains structures that are not present at lower levels, including the **posterior thalamus, optic tract,** and **Edinger-Westphal nucleus** (Fig. 3-17; see Fig. 15-10). The Edinger-Westphal nucleus is the visceral nucleus of the *oculomotor nerve,* which mediates pupillary constriction and lens accommodation reflexes. The posterior thalamus includes **pulvinar, lateral geniculate,** and medial geniculate bodies (see Chapter 6). The lateral geniculate body is the thalamic relay center for vision. The medial geniculate body is the thalamic relay for audition. The oculomotor nerve runs along the medial border of the midbrain next to the medial border of the large red nucleus (see Fig. 2-24). The *substantia nigra* sits in the hammock of the pes pedunculi just beneath the red nucleus. The large red nucleus located

BOX 3-1

Parkinson Disease

Parkinson disease is associated with the degeneration of dopaminergic neurons in the pars compacta region of the substantia nigra. Discovery of this underlying neurotransmitter deficiency led to a pharmacologic method of treating the disease; levodopa, a precursor of dopamine, has the ability to pass through the **blood–brain barrier.** Although promising when first introduced; this drug is known to lose its effectiveness in the later stages of the disease.

The lack of adequate treatment for progressive Parkinson disease provided an incentive for surgical intervention involving the neural circuitry of the basal ganglia. The procedure, known as stereotaxic neurosurgery and introduced in 1947, involved placing stereotactic lesions in the pallidum or its efferent pathways or in the ventrolateral thalamic nucleus. More recent surgical treatment focuses on deep-brain stimulation of the subthalamic nucleus using a permanently implanted depth electrode.

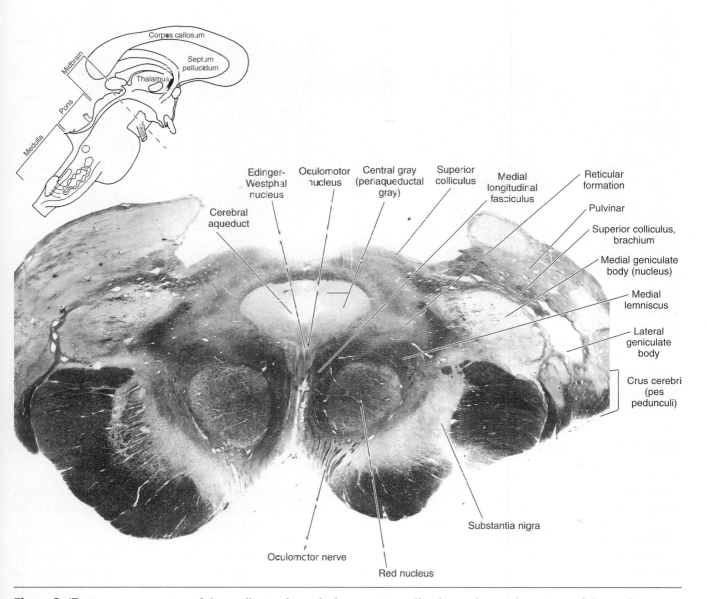

Figure 3-17 Transverse section of the midbrain through the superior colliculus and rostral portions of the oculomotor nucleus.

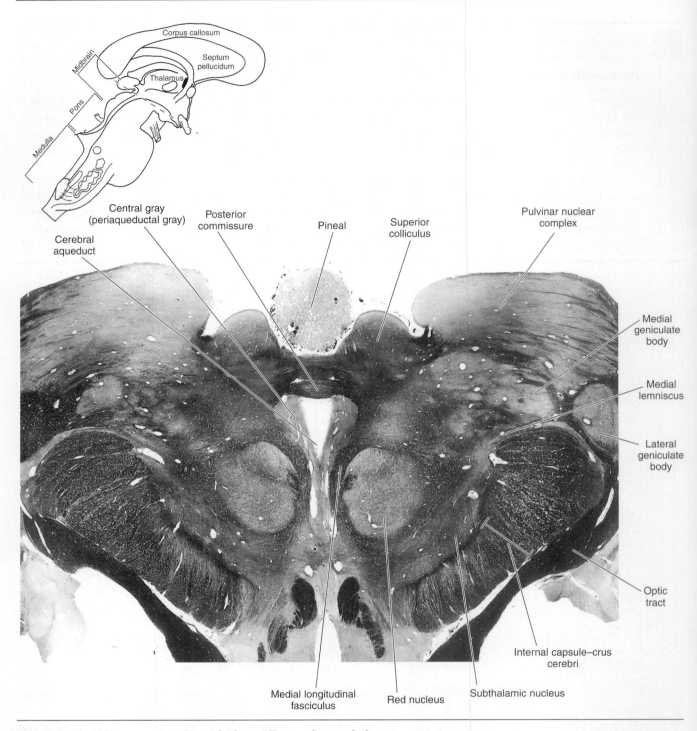

Figure 3-18 Oblique section through the midbrain–diencephalon junction.

between the central gray and the large *pes pedunculi* identifies this level of the midbrain.

Midbrain–Diencephalon Junction

The oblique section in Figure 3-18 is located in a transitional area, revealing structures from both the midbrain and the diencephalon. The important structures are the **posterior commissure** with the overlying **pineal gland** in the dorsal midline, neposterior part of the **pulvinar nucleus**, the rostral end of the *red nucleus* flanked laterally by the *medial*

lemniscus, and the large diagonal internal capsule–pes pedunculi. Fibers of the *internal capsule*, which were identified as the *pes pedunculi* below this level, are hugged by the optic tract that runs along its ventrolateral border. The **subthalamic nucleus** is sandwiched between the *internal capsule* and the red nucleus, the area that was occupied by the *substantia nigra* at the caudal midbrain levels. Both the subthalamic nucleus and substantia nigra are major contributors to movement, and their dysfunction is associated with movement disorders.

The *pineal gland,* an endocrine organ, is located dorsally and is important in the body's diurnal rhythm. Inhibition of its secretion has also been associated with the onset of puberty. The *posterior commissure* is considered to connect the two *superior colliculi.* The posterior thalamus includes the *pulvinar, lateral,* and *medial geniculate bodies.* The lateral geniculate body is the thalamic relay center for vision. The medial geniculate body is the thalamic relay center for audition. The pulvinar—the most caudal part of the thalamus—is reciprocally connected with the parietotemporal association cortex. It also has been associated with speech and language functions (see Chapter 6).

The *subthalamic nucleus,* which is mediodorsal to the *crus cerebri,* is an important extrapyramidal structure; its pathology results in **hemiballism**, a neurologic condition characterized by violent and flinging movements. Ventrally situated in the section is the optic tract.

FOREBRAIN IN CORONAL SECTIONS

Learning the forebrain anatomy entails orientation to the subcortical structures: **basal ganglia (caudate nucleus, putamen, globus pallidus,** and functionally related sub-thalamic nucleus), **diencephalon (thalamus** and **hypothalamus), ventricular cavity (lateral** and **third ventricles),** and **limbic structures (amygdala, fornix, hippocampal formation,** and **cingulate gyrus)** Other important structures are the **corpus callosum, optic chiasm, insular cortex** (isle of Reil), **septum pellucidum, anterior commissure, cingulate gyrus, internal capsule, external capsule, extreme capsule,** and **claustrum** (Table 3-5).

These structures are in fixed positions with respect to each other; a review of their relative locations on a horizontal section facilitates the orientation to them on subsequent coronal serial sections of the brain (Figs. 3-19 and 3-20).

Located rostrally in a horizontal section of the brain are the **frontal lobes** on each side of the midline *corpus callosum* (genu) (Fig. 3-19). The fibers of the corpus callosum connect the homologous cortical areas in both hemispheres by corticocortical fibers. The *septum pellucidum* is in the midline extending from the ventral surface of the corpus callosum and ending along the anterior limits of the thalamus. On each side of the septum pellucidum are the **anterior horns** of the *lateral ventricle.* The septal nuclei are located at the base of the anterior ventricular horns. With connections to the limbic (hippocampal formation and

---

Table 3-5

Anatomic Structures of the Basal Ganglia and Diencephalon at Different Levels

Posterior thalamus	
Pineal gland	Lateral geniculate body
Corpus callosum, splenium	Medial geniculate body
Pulvinar of thalamus	Internal capsule merging in crus cerebri/pes pedunculi
Cerebral aqueduct	
Midthalamus	
Corpus callosum, body	Third ventricle
Fornix	Hypothalamus
Subthalamic nucleus	Diminishing globus pallidus and putamen
Lateral ventricle	
Anterior thalamus	
Anterior commissure	Internal capsule, genu
Caudate	Corpus callosum, body
Putamen	External capsule
Globus pallidus	Extreme capsule
Third ventricle	Septum pellucidum
Hypothalamus	Claustrum
Anterior limb of internal capsule	
Corpus callosum, body	Septum pellucidum
Head of the caudate nucleus	Internal capsule, anterior limb
Putamen	External capsule
Attachment of the caudate and putamen	Claustrum
Lateral ventricle, anterior horn	Extreme capsule

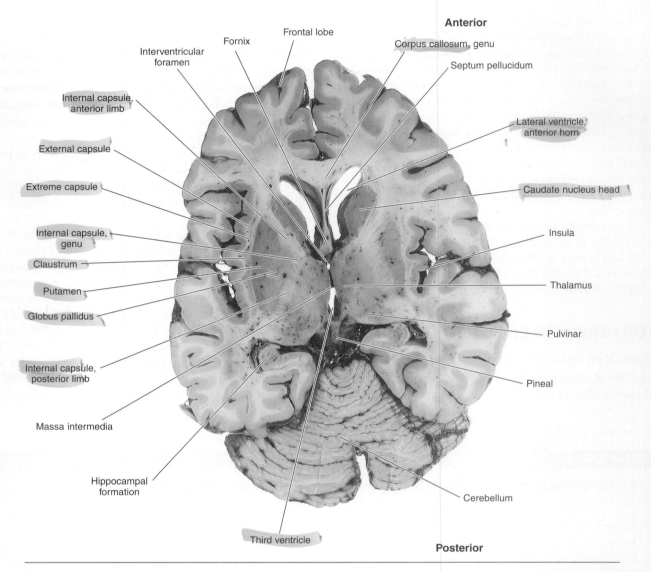

Figure 3-19 Dorsal view of a horizontal section through the interventricular foramina, third ventricle, and pulvinar.

amygdala), hypothalamic (mammillary) structures, and **hippocampus**, the septal nuclei are known to play a role in autonomic (reproductive) behaviors and memory regulation. The *third ventricle* is in the midline between two the thalami. Each lateral ventricle communicates with the midline third ventricle through the **interventricular foramina of Monro.** The interventricular foramen is located at the junction of the septum and thalamus on each side of the midline.

The two large nuclear masses projecting into the *lateral ventricles* are the heads of the *caudate nuclei,* which are important contributors to motor functions. Caudal to the caudate nuclei are the two thalami on each side of the *third ventricle.* The junctional area between the caudate and the thalamus is indented by the **genu** of *internal capsule,* which connects the **anterior limb** to **posterior limb**. The anterior limb is associated predominantly with cortical motor projections, and the poste-

rior limb is associated with the ascending (sensory) cortical projections.

The bend of the *internal capsule* is produced in part by the **lenticular nucleus** (putamen and **globus pallidus**). These two nuclei contribute to motor control and, in conjunction with the *caudate nucleus,* constitute the basal ganglia. Just lateral to the *putamen* is the *claustrum,* a thin, wavy line of cells that possesses two-way projections predominantly with the sensory cortical areas of the brain. The **insular cortex**, concerned with visceral functions, overlies the claustrum and lenticular nucleus.

The caudal end of the third ventricle is identified by the **posterior commissure** and the **pineal gland** in the midline. This level is the transitional area between the posterior thalamus and the midbrain. More caudally, the cerebellum is in the midline between the occipital lobes. The cerebellum overlies the *fourth ventricle* and is attached to the brainstem by the *cerebellar peduncles.*

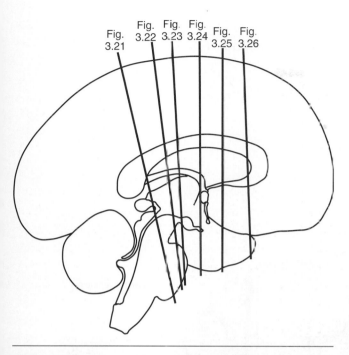

Figure 3-20 Midsagittal view identifying the locations of the coronal brain sections shown in the indicated figures.

Coronal Section Through the Posterior Thalamus

The coronal brain section shown in Figure 3-21 clearly shows the distinction between white and gray matter with sulci and gyri markings. The large fissure in the middle separating the hemispheres is the interhemispheric **longitudinal fissure**. The body of the *corpus callosum* forms the roof of the *lateral ventricles*. The **splenium** of the corpus callosum connects both *occipital lobes*.

The large cavities in this section are the bodies of the *lateral ventricles*; the small cavities in the temporal lobe are the **inferior horns** of the lateral ventricles. In the floor of the lateral ventricle is the fornix, a bundle of fibers that serves as a two-way connection between the hypothalamic structures (mammillary body) and hippocampus. Forming the medial wall of the inferior horn of the lateral ventricles is the **hippocampal formation**, which is thought to serve memory functions by consolidating new information.

The thalamic nucleus in this section is the *pulvinar*, the most posterior nucleus of the thalamus, which is connected reciprocally to the parietal association cortex and participates in language functions. Ventral to the pulvinar are the *geniculate* (medial and lateral) *bodies*, which serve as thalamic relay centers. The medial geniculate body mediates auditory information from the ears to the primary auditory cortices in the **gyrus of Heschl** (Brodmann area 41). The lateral geniculate body transmits visual information from homonymous halves of the retinas to the primary visual cortex in the occipital lobe (Brodmann area 17).

Dorsal to the inferior horn and lateral to the thalamus is the posterior limb of the *internal capsule*, which contains the ascending (sensory) and descending (motor) fibers. In the middle of this section the following brainstem structures can be seen: *cerebral aqueduct, decussation of the superior cerebellar peduncle, basal pons,* and the *pretectal structure.* The *pretectal area* regulates visual reflexes (see Chapters 8 and 15).

Coronal Section Through the Midthalamus

The section of the brain shown in Figure 3-22 retains most of the previously identified structures at the posterior thalamic level and a few newly visible structures. Emerging bilaterally from the walls of the *lateral ventricle* is the larger body of the *caudate nucleus*. The caudate nucleus, with its long tail, is a C-shaped structure in sagittal views of the brain (see Fig. 2-17): it can be seen in many sequential coronal sections of the brain. The caudate is an important nucleus, contributing to motor activity; it may have a role in cognitive processing. Its pathologic involvement of this structure is associated with Huntington chorea, a neurodegenerative disease characterized by dysarthria, chorea, and dementia. This genetically transmitted condition is characterized by dominant inheritance with complete penetrance and onset in the third decade of life. The mutation, a repeat of the Huntington gene (HD) locus, has been mapped to chromosome 4p (Box 3-2).

Forming the floor of the lateral ventricles in this section are the large gray masses of the thalamus. Both thalami are connected through the **massa intermedia**, a thalamic loose fibrous tissue. In the midline between the two lateral ventricles, is the septum pellucidum. Through the base of the septum courses the *fornix*, an important C-shaped limbic structure that connects the mamillary bodies of the *hypothalamus* to the *hippocampus* and *septum* and is involved in autonomic functions. Located lateral to the *internal capsule*, the *lenticular nucleus* consists of the *globus pallidus* and *putamen*. The globus pallidus and putamen are parts of the basal ganglia and are important in regulating motor functions and muscle tone.

The *external capsule* is a thin band of fibers lateral to the *lenticular nucleus*. Lateral to the *external capsule* is the *claustrum*, a thin layer of gray matter. The thin bundle of fibers lateral to the claustrum is the *extreme capsule*. The most lateral structure in this section is the *insular cortex*. The vertical slit in the center is the *third ventricle*, formed by the medial walls of each thalamus. In the center of the section, the remaining brainstem structures include the *crus cerebri* (pes pedunculi), *basilar pons, red nucleus,* and *substantia nigra*.

Coronal Section Through the Anterior Thalamus

The general orientation of the forebrain anatomy in a coronal section through the anterior thalamus is similar to that of the previous section, although the one shown in Figure 3-23

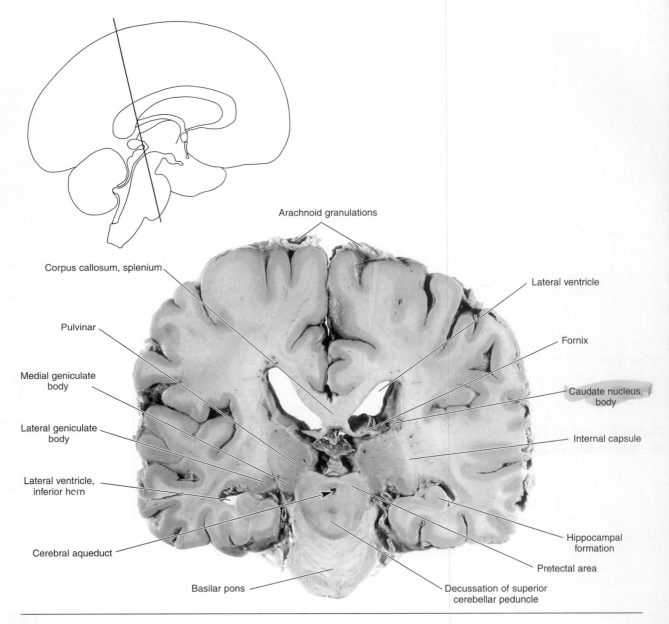

Figure 3-21 Caudal surface of a coronal section through the posterior thalamus.

is more rostral at the anterior thalamic nucleus level. The rough, saggy, and worm-shaped structure in the lateral ventricles is the **choroid plexus**, which secretes **cerebrospinal fluid (CSF)**. Forming the floor of the lateral ventricle is the **anterior nucleus**, the most rostral nucleus of the thalamus. This nucleus receives afferents from the **mamillary bodies** of the hypothalamus and projects to the cingulate gyrus of the **limbic lobe**. Along the lateral wall of the *lateral ventricles* is the *caudate nucleus,* a C-shaped structure. This section of the forebrain is unique because it simultaneously reveals the dorsal component (body of the caudate nucleus in the lateral ventricle) and ventral component (tail of the *caudate nucleus* in the lateral wall of the temporal horn).

Medial to the *internal capsule* is the biconvex-shaped *subthalamic nucleus,* which receives afferents from the lateral segment of the *globus pallidus* and projects to both of the pal-

lidal segments and to the pars reticulata region of the **substantia nigra**. Subthalamic pathology results in hemiballism.

Coronal Section Through the Anterior Commissure

A coronal section of the forebrain through the *anterior commissure* and the *internal capsule genu,* marks the anterior limit of the thalamus (Fig. 3-24). The head of the *caudate nucleus* emerges in the ventricular cavity as a larger structure than at the more caudal levels. There is a clear view of the anterior commissure and its crossing. The anterior commissure is a small forebrain fiber bundle that contains bidirectional olfactory fibers and connects the temporal cortices. At this level, the internal capsule fibers, which are somewhat diminished, suggest the beginning of its *anterior limb.*

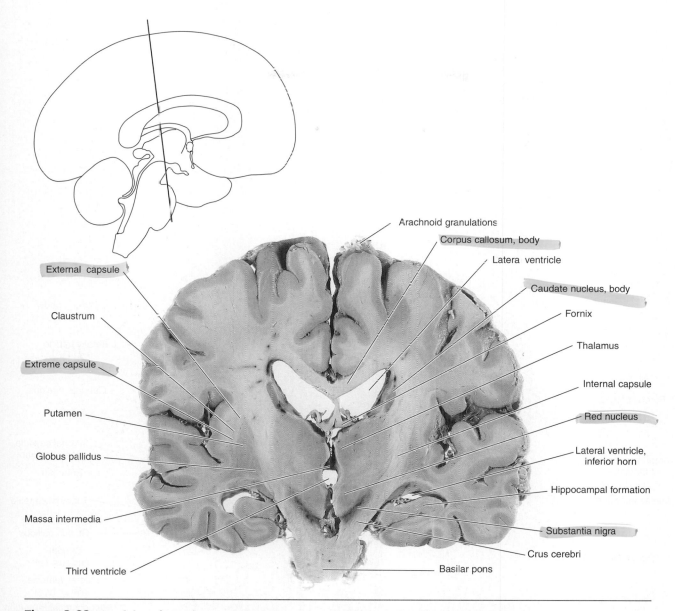

External capsule

Claustrum

Extreme capsule

Putamen

Globus pallidus

Massa intermedia

Third ventricle

Arachnoid granulations

Corpus callosum, body

Latera ventricle

Caudate nucleus, body

Fornix

Thalamus

Internal capsule

Red nucleus

Lateral ventricle, inferior horn

Hippocampal formation

Substantia nigra

Crus cerebri

Basilar pons

Figure 3-22 Caudal surface of a coronal section through the medial thalamus and massa intermedia.

The *septum*, which anteriorly separates the *lateral ventricles*, is centrally located in the section. All *hippocampal* projections terminate in the *septum verum nuclei*, which are part of the limbic system. Forming the lateral walls of the third ventricle below the level of the *anterior commissure* is the *hypothalamus*. Two important structures of the hypothalamus, not seen in this section, are the *mammillary body* and *pituitary gland*. Hypothalamic nuclei produce neurosecretions that are important in controlling water balance, sugar and fat metabolism, body temperature, and hormone production. The hypothalamus is also the regulator of the autonomic (sympathetic and parasympathetic) nervous system.

The **amygdaloid nucleus** is seen here at the level at which the tail of the *caudate nucleus* terminates (see Fig. 2-17). The *amygdala*, a massive round structure in the medial temporal lobe, is generally responsible for activating

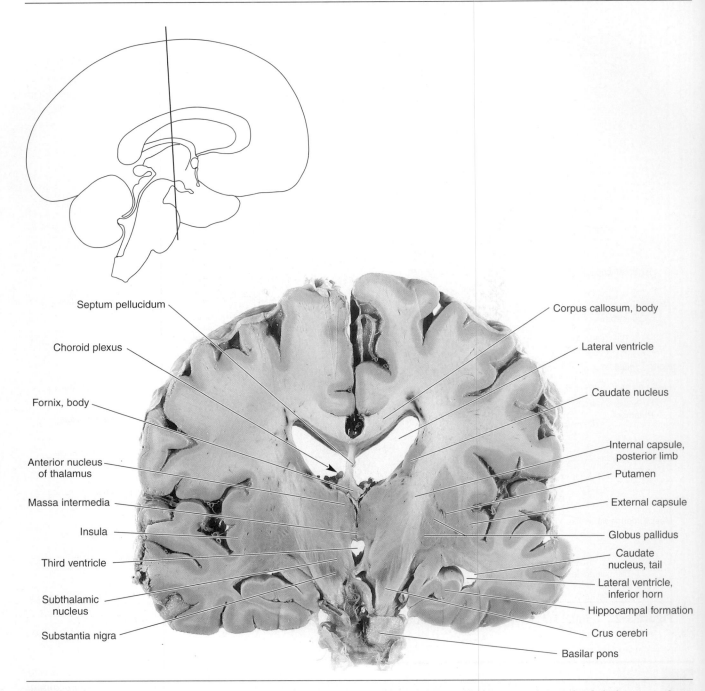

Septum pellucidum

Choroid plexus

Fornix, body

Anterior nucleus
of thalamus

Massa intermedia

Insula

Third ventricle

Subthalamic
nucleus

Substantia nigra

Corpus callosum, body

Lateral ventricle

Caudate nucleus

Internal capsule,
posterior limb

Putamen

External capsule

Globus pallidus

Caudate
nucleus, tail

Lateral ventricle,
inferior horn

Hippocampal formation

Crus cerebri

Basilar pons

Figure 3-23 Rostral surface of a coronal section through the rostral thalamus, massa intermedia, and subthalamic nucleus.

emotional behavior. Pathology of this structure has been known to lead to aggression and other abnormal behavior, such as hypersexuality; surgical removal in animals has caused aggressive animals to become docile and hyposexual.

The following previously identified structures are also present in this section and are unchanged in basic configuration: *corpus callosum, septum pellucidum, fornix, caudate nucleus, putamen, globus pallidus, internal capsule, external capsule, claustrum, extreme capsule,* and *insular cortex.*

Coronal Section Through the Anterior Limb of the Internal Capsule and Caudate Head

A coronal section of the forebrain at the rostral region of the basal ganglia reveals the large head of the *caudate nucleus,* the *anterior horn* of the *lateral ventricles,* and the *anterior limb* of the *internal capsule* (Fig. 3-25). At this level of the brain, the thalamus and *globus pallidus* are no longer present (Fig. 3-19). The massive caudate nucleus head forms the ventrolateral wall of the lateral ventricle at the level of

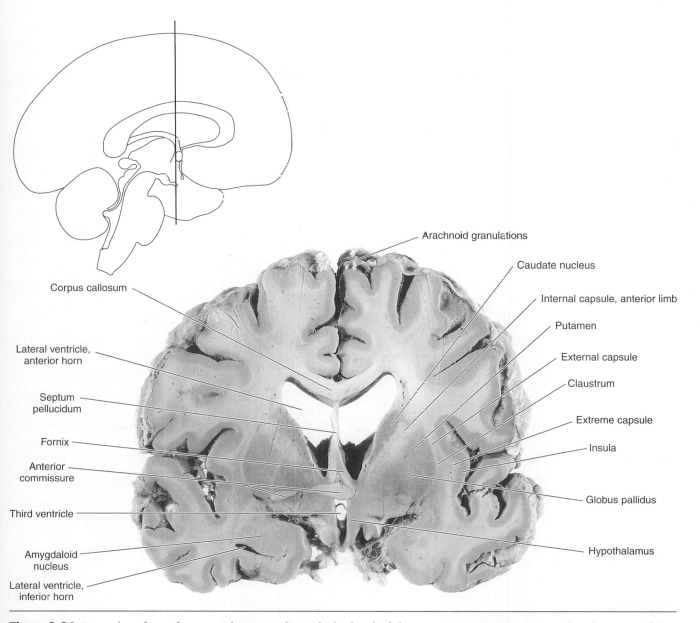

Corpus callosum

Arachnoid granulations

Caudate nucleus

Internal capsule, anterior limb

Putamen

External capsule

Claustrum

Extreme capsule

Insula

Globus pallidus

Hypothalamus

Lateral ventricle, anterior horn

Septum pellucidum

Fornix

Anterior commissure

Third ventricle

Amygdaloid nucleus

Lateral ventricle, inferior horn

Figure 3-24 Rostral surface of a coronal section through the level of the anterior commissure rostral to the genu of the internal capsule.

the anterior horn. Laterally, the ventral component of the caudate nucleus merges with the *putamen* to form the **corpus striatum**.

The portion of the *internal capsule* at this level is the *anterior limb,* which courses between the bodies of the caudate and *putamen*. In the middle, forming the medial ventricular wall, is the *septum pellucidum,* which is attached to the medial basal forebrain area. The *cingulate gyrus,* a limbic structure involved with emotional drive and anxiety, is dorsal to the body of the corpus callosum. The **cingulum,** a bundle of mediofrontal parietal cingulate association fibers, is beneath the cingulate gyrus. Also visible is the *septum pellucidum* with its underlying nucleus, a limbic structure related to visceral functions, reward, and gratification.

The cortical regions rostral to this level undergo only a few changes. The *ventricular cavity* rostrally ends at the *genu* of the *corpus callosum* (see Fig. 2-12). Anterior to the corpus callosum is the massive accumulation of white matter that consists of *callosal radiations* and *corona radiata*. These changes can be seen in Figure 3-26.

Coronal Section Through the Anterior Horn

A coronal section of the forebrain at the *genu* of the *corpus callosum* reveals the end of the *lateral ventricle* (anterior horn) and the *rostral striatum* (caudate head and putamen) (Fig. 3-26). Other previously identified rostral structures seen here include the *septum, internal* and *external capsules, claustrum, cingulate gyrus,* and *cingulum*.

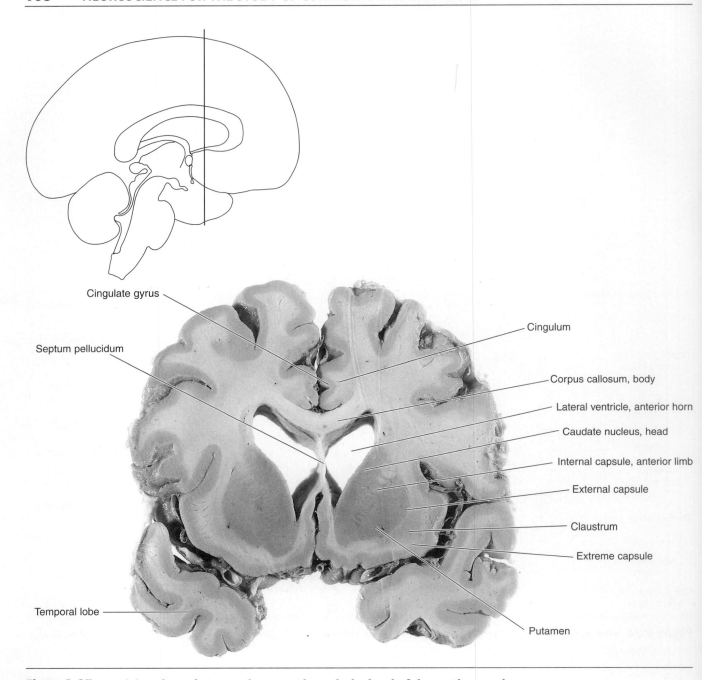

Cingulate gyrus

Septum pellucidum

Temporal lobe

Cingulum

Corpus callosum, body

Lateral ventricle, anterior horn

Caudate nucleus, head

Internal capsule, anterior limb

External capsule

Claustrum

Extreme capsule

Putamen

Figure 3-25   Caudal surface of a coronal section through the head of the caudate nucleus.

FOREBRAIN IN HORIZONTAL SECTIONS

A review of the forebrain anatomy on horizontal sections contributes to the visual orientation of the internal anatomy of the brain and helps consolidate previous learning. In Figures 3-27 to 3-30, the human brain has been dissected horizontally to provide a three-dimensional view of the *corpus callosum, ventricular cavity, thalamus,* and *basal ganglia* structures.

In Figure 3-27, a 1-cm-thick layer of the cerebral cortex has been removed to expose the underlying brain structures. The residual indentation of the interhemispheric longitudinal fissure is evident in the middle, including the *central sulcus;* other sulci and gyri are seen in the periphery of this section. Each hemisphere contains a **semiovale center,** a massive accumulation of white matter that contains the blended **association, commissural,** and **projection fibers** above the *internal capsule* level. The sensorimotor fibers form the *corona radiata,* in which the descending motor fibers fan down toward the internal capsule and the ascending sensory fibers fan out to reach the cerebral cortex. (See Fig. 2-38.)

The removal of an additional 1–2 cm of cortical substance, which includes the *cingulate gyrus* and *cingulum,* exposes the dorsal surface of the *corpus callosum* (Fig. 3-28). Starting rostrally in this section are the *genu, body,* and *splenium* of the corpus callosum. The densely packed radiating fibers of the corpus callosum connect the hemispheres. The

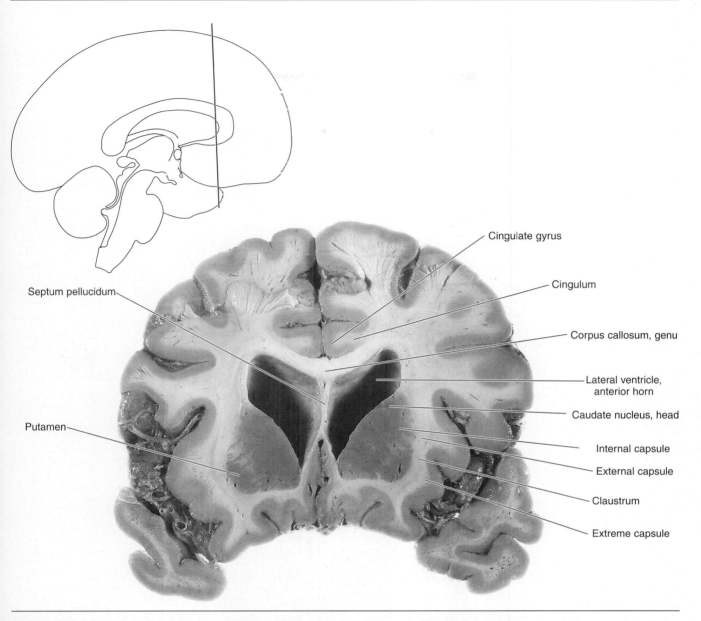

Figure 3-26 Caudal surface of a coronal section just caudal to the genu of the corpus callosum and the rostral end of the anterior horns.

body of the corpus callosum and its lateral radiations form the roof of the *lateral ventricles.*

Further removal of the *corpus callosum* and its radiating cortical fibers reveals the large underlying subcortical structures and *lateral ventricles* (Fig. 3-29). Laterally located are the fibers constituting the *corona radiata*, the condensed projection fibers before they enter the *internal capsule.* The spaces on both sides of the corpus callosum mark the cavities of the lateral ventricles. The two prominent structures in the floor of the ventricles are the *caudate nucleus* and the *thalamus.*

The massive balloon-shaped structure located rostrally and laterally in the ventricular cavity is the head of the *caudate nucleus*; its C-shaped tail is buried within the adjoining white matter. The head of the caudate nucleus forms the lateral anterior wall of the *lateral ventricles.* The

thalamus, the largest diencephalic structure, is located posteriorly in the floor of the ventricular cavity. Removal of *parietal* and *occipital* tissues has also exposed the caudal portion of the lateral ventricles, particularly the posterior horns in the **occipital lobe regions**. The remaining *genu, body,* and *splenium* portions of the *corpus callosum* are identified easily above the lateral ventricles. Also present is the point at which the tail of the caudate nucleus enters the temporal lobe.

Further removal of the overlying white **medullary substance**, *caudate nucleus,* and thalamus by sectioning rostral to the *genu* of the *corpus callosum* exposes the cavity of the *lateral ventricles* and the surrounding subcortical structures (Fig. 3-30). The exposed inner temporal lobe contains the slender temporal horns of the lateral ventricles. The hippo-

(text continues on page 113)

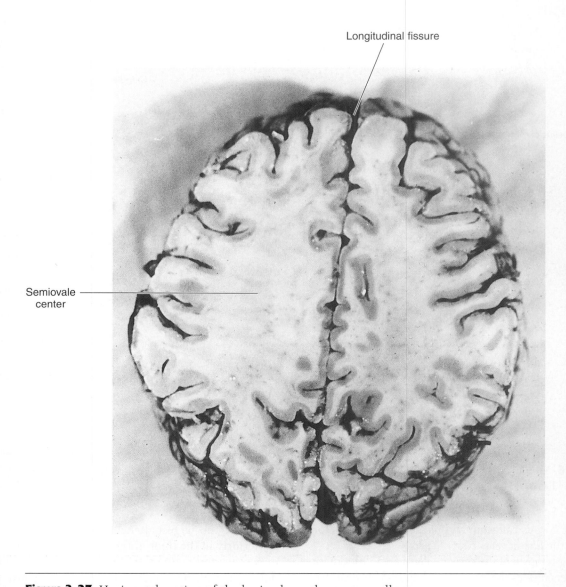

Longitudinal fissure

Semiovale center

Figure 3-27 Horizontal section of the brain above the corpus callosum.

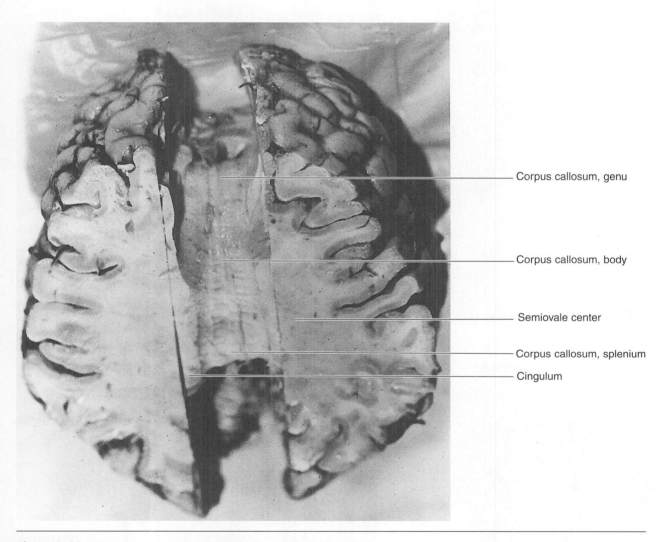

Corpus callosum, genu

Corpus callosum, body

Semiovale center

Corpus callosum, splenium

Cingulum

Figure 3-28 Horizontal section exposing the corpus callosum.

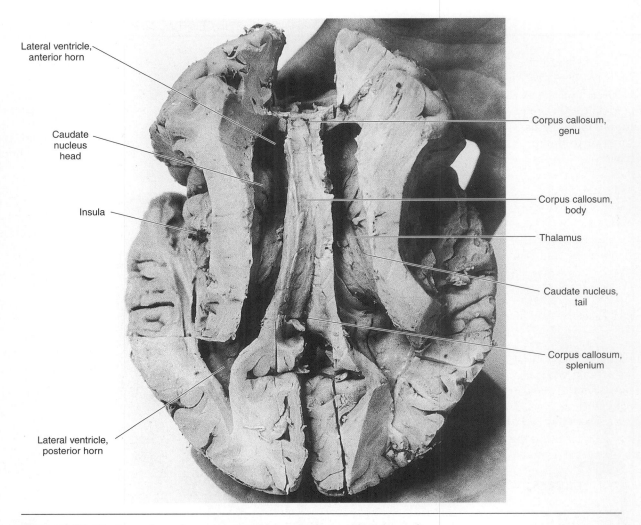

Lateral ventricle, anterior horn

Caudate nucleus head

Insula

Lateral ventricle, posterior horn

Corpus callosum, genu

Corpus callosum, body

Thalamus

Caudate nucleus, tail

Corpus callosum, splenium

Figure 3-29 Horizontal section exposing the ventricles and basal ganglia.

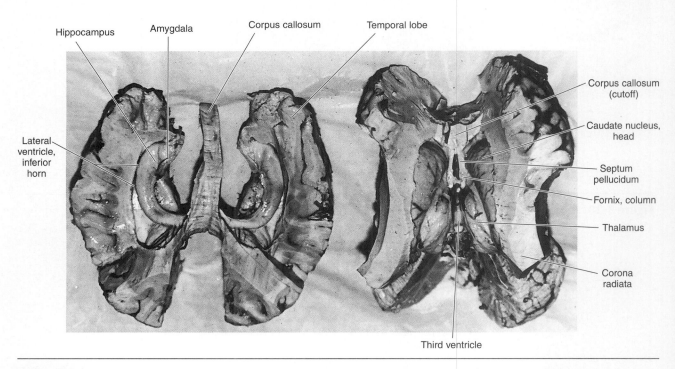

Hippocampus

Amygdala

Corpus callosum

Temporal lobe

Lateral ventricle, inferior horn

Corpus callosum (cutoff)

Caudate nucleus, head

Septum pellucidum

Fornix, column

Thalamus

Corona radiata

Third ventricle

Figure 3-30 Horizontal section in which sectioning of the corpus callosum from the adjacent cortical structure exposes the hippocampus, ventricular cavity, and basal ganglia structure.

campus, amygdala, and **uncus** are located medially in the *inferior horn*. The *hippocampus* forms the medial wall of the *temporal horns*. It receives direct projections from the fornix and indirect projections from the *cingulum* via the **parahippocampal gyrus**.

Anterior to the tip of the *hippocampus* is the *amygdaloid nucleus*, an important limbic structure with a protruding cortical component called the *uncus*. With a complete removal of the *callosal fibers*, the floor of the *lateral ventricles* becomes fully visible. The *septum* is seen rostrally, separating the *anterior horns* of the lateral ventricles. The structure at the base of the *septum* is the **fornix column**. Also present are the head of the caudate nucleus, the medial dorsal *thalamus*, and the *third ventricle*.

SUMMARY

Knowledge of the internal brain anatomy is the most important part of training in neuroscience and is essential for solving clinical problems. It is learned best by repeated study of the internal structures on serial sections of the spinal cord, brainstem, and forebrain and by relating the structures to their functions. Visual orientation to the structures and functional knowledge of the internal anatomy are essential because the form the basis for the overall understanding of brain structures and their relation to clinical symptoms.

QUIZ QUESTIONS

1. Define the following terms: cerebral aqueduct, inferior colliculus, lateral geniculate body, medial geniculate body, medial longitudinal fasciculus, pyramidal decussation, red nucleus, substantia nigra, subthalamic nucleus, superior colliculus

2. Identify three landmark structures of the internal medulla and define their functions.

3. What ventricular cavity is located dorsal to the pons?

4. Identify three landmarks of the internal pons and define their functions.

5. What differentiates the tectal and tegmental regions in the midbrain?

6. Name three major internal structures of the midbrain and define their functions.

7. List five structures that are present on a coronal section of the forebrain cut at the caudate head level and define their functions.

8. Explain why a hemorrhage in the right caudal medulla involving the corticospinal fibers will cause a left hemiplegia?

TECHNICAL TERMS

amygdaloid nucleus
anterior medullary velum
caudate nucleus
central gray
cerebral aqueduct
choroid plexus
cingulate gyrus
collateral trigone
corona radiata
fornix
hippocampus
    (hippocampal formation)
hypothalamus
inferior cerebellar peduncle
    (restiform body)
inferior colliculus
insula (isle of Reil)
internal arcuate fibers
lateral geniculate body
lateral lemniscus
medial geniculate body

medial lemniscus
medial longitudinal
    fasciculus
middle cerebellar peduncle
    (brachium pontis)
pineal
principal (inferior) olivary
    nucleus
pyramidal decussation
red nucleus
reticular formation
semiovale center
spinocerebellar tract
substantia nigra
subthalamic nucleus
superior cerebellar
    peduncle (brachium
    conjunctivum)
superior colliculus
thalamus

Development of the Central Nervous System*

LEARNING OBJECTIVES

After studying this chapter, students should be able to:

- Define embryologic terms

- Describe the developmental processes of sperm and ovum from single cells to the adult form

- Discuss the differences between oogenesis and spermatogenesis

- Explain how the mother's lifestyle is so vital for normal embryologic development

- Explain human development during the first 3 weeks

- Discuss the ways in which the central and peripheral nervous systems form

- Describe the major brain structures that are derived from the three primary brain vesicles

- Construct a flow diagram of human development from the zygote to the three germ layers and their derivatives

- Discuss the critical periods of susceptibility to teratogenesis for the central nervous system and for other related organ systems

- Describe the common cerebrospinal malformations

HUMAN CHROMOSOMES, GENES, AND CELL DIVISION

Abnormalities in Chromosome Number

Human somatic cells are **diploid**, or contain $2n$ chromosomes—that is, 46 chromosomes: 44 autosomes and 2 sex chromosomes (either 46, XY for the male, or 46, XX for the female as per international code). The **haploid** normal **gamete**, or sex cell, contains n chromosomes—that is 23 chromosomes: either 23, Y or 23, X. It is only the male gamete that has either an X or a Y chromosome. (The division of the primary **spermatocyte** into four spermatids—two 23, X and two 23, Y—is discussed later in this chapter.) The term **euploid** refers to any exact multiple of n chromosomes, such as **triploid** (23×3) or

tetraploid (23×4). **Aneuploid** is the term used for any chromosome number that is not euploid (e.g., when an extra chromosome is present, as in trisomy of chromosomes 13, 18, or 21 or when one chromosome is missing, as in monosomy). Such abnormalities in chromosome number originate during **gametogenesis**. Some of these abnormalities are listed in Table 4-1.

The diploid human **genome** is made up of 6–7 billion base pairs of deoxyribonucleic acid (**DNA**) arranged linearly on the autosomal and sex chromosomes. Molecularly defined, a **gene** is the sequence of chromosomal DNA required for a functional product—a polypeptide or ribonucleic acid (**RNA**) molecule—to be produced. The human genome consists of 31,778 known genes and gene predictions that encode a similar number of proteins. The total number of human genes is still in question and is subject to change as research continues (Lander et al. 2001).

Except for the small mitochondrial chromosome, each chromosome is made up of a single continuous DNA double helix, or DNA molecule. DNA molecules have been estimated to range in size from about 50 million base pairs for the smallest (chromosome 21) to 250 million base pairs for the largest (chromosome 1). The DNA molecule appears along with **histones** (chromosomal proteins) and other proteins. The combined DNA and protein complex is called the **chromatin**.

Cell division is indispensable for living organisms. Whereas embryonic cells and some adult cells divide by **mitosis** (equal division), sex cells, or **gametes**, form by a special type of cell division called **meiosis**. Meiosis is the reduction division that occurs during gametogenesis. In meiosis, the chromosome number is reduced to half the usual number, ensuring the constancy of chromosome number from generation to generation. Maternal and paternal chromosomes are independently assorted and crossed over, which shuffles the genes and recombines genetic material, creating a unique genome.

Mitosis has four phases: **prophase**, **metaphase**, **anaphase**, and **telophase**. During prophase, the chromosomes appear within the nucleus and double longitudinally (fold in half), forming two **chromatids** united at a **centromere** (Fig. 4-1). During **prometaphase**, the nuclear envelope breaks down and kinetochore fibers form. The chromo-

Table 4-1

Trisomies of the Autosomal and Sex Chromosomes

Condition	Incidence	Characteristics
Autosomal chromosomes		
Trisomy 13[a]	1/25,000 births	Mental retardation; severe central nervous system malformations; bilateral cleft lip and/or palate; polydactyly; malformed ears
Trisomy 18[a]	1/8,000 births	Mental retardation; growth retardation; low-set, malformed ears
Trisomy 21 (Down syndrome)	1/800 births	Mental retardation; flat nasal bridge; upward or slant to palpebral fissures; protruding tongue; simian crease (a single transverse palmar crease)
Sex chromosomes		
45, X (Turner syndrome); monosomy	1/8,000 births	Short neck; gonadal dysgenesis (faulty development); puffiness and swelling of feet
47, XXX	1/960 female births	15–25% are mentally retarded
47, XXY (Klinefelter syndrome)	1/1,080 male births	Small testes; disproportionately longer lower limbs; impaired intelligence; 40% of males with abnormally developed mammary glands
47, XYY	1/1,080 male births	Tall; exhibit aggressive behavior

[a]Rarely survive beyond 6 months after birth.
Data from Moore and Persaud (2003).

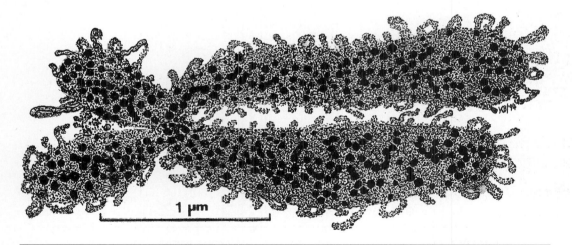

Figure 4-1 An unsectioned human chromosome 12 from a dividing cell as seen by electron micrography. The chromosome is divided in half along its length (into two chromatids) except at the centromere. This chromosome contains about 4 cm of DNA double helix per chromatid. Some of the looping and coiling that allows all the DNA to be contained in a chromosome 3 μm long is visible (40,200×).

somes then arrange themselves on the equatorial plate, or metaphase plate. The chromosomes move apart during anaphase and reach the spindle poles during telophase. The division of the cytoplasm takes place and leads to the formation of two sibling cells. The increase in cell numbers and, consequently, the growth of tissue, leads to development and maturation. Details of mitosis are readily available in human biology textbooks.

EARLY HUMAN DEVELOPMENT

Even though human development is a continuous process, its origin is found in gametogenesis, or the formation of the male and female gametes, the spermatozoa and the ova, respectively. With the union of a spermatozoon and an ovum (secondary oocyte), fertilization is complete. The large cell that results is called a **zygote**. The zygote undergoes repeated divisions, giving rise to the multicellular human form.

Gametogenesis

The formation of **germ cells** called gametes (**spermatozoa** and **ova**) involves the halving of chromosomes (i.e., haploid cells are created from diploid cells) and an alteration in cell shape. The reduction of chromosome number, from 46, XY for males and 46, XX for females to 23, Y (spermatozoa) or 23, X (ovum and spermatozoa), occurs during a unique process of cell division called meiosis (Figs. 4-2 and 4-3). Remember that in mitosis, the new cells remain diploid.

During gametogenesis, two meiotic divisions occur, one after the other. During the first meiotic division, the homologous chromosomes (one from each parent) in the primary spermatocyte or oocyte pair during prophase (Fig. 4-2A). They separate during anaphase, with each chromosome going to one of the poles of the cell (Fig. 4-2E). Therefore, at the end of this process, each of the two resulting cells (the secondary spermatocyte or oocyte) contains half of the original number of chromosomes (Fig. 4-2G). This

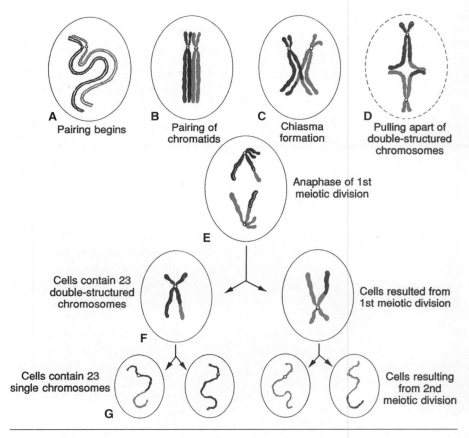

A Pairing begins

B Pairing of chromatids

C Chiasma formation

D Pulling apart of double-structured chromosomes

Anaphase of 1st meiotic division

E

Cells contain 23 double-structured chromosomes

Cells resulted from 1st meiotic division

F

Cells contain 23 single chromosomes

Cells resulting from 2nd meiotic division

G

Figure 4-2 First and second meiotic divisions with crossover. **A.** Homologous chromosomes approach each other. **B.** The homologous chromosomes pair, and each member of the pair consists of two chromatids. **C.** The intimately paired homologous chromosomes interchange chromatid fragments (crossover). Note the chiasma. **D.** The double-structured chromosomes pull apart. **E.** Anaphase of the first meiotic division. **F and G.** During the second meiotic division, the double-structured chromosomes split at the centromere. At the completion of division, the chromosomes in each of the four daughter cells are different from each other.

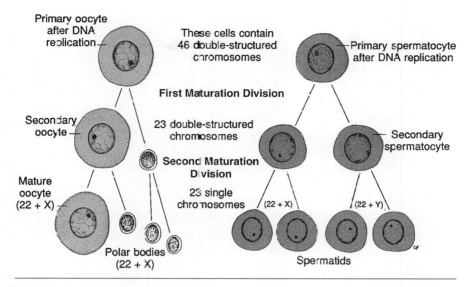

Figure 4-3 Reduction in the number of chromosomes during the maturation divisions. A. Female germ cell. B. Male germ cell.

disjunction of homologous chromosomes enables the separation of the **allelic genes** during meiosis. Without an interphase (break in the process of cell division), the second meiotic division follows. Each chromosome, consisting of two **chromatids**, divides; the chromatids are drawn to opposite poles of the cell during division (Fig. 4-2F and G). The haploid number of chromosomes in the resulting daughter cells is maintained. Meiosis ensures that the number of chromosomes in the next generation remains the same and that chromosomes are recombined to create a mix of genetic material from each parent.

Nondisjunction is one cause of abnormal gametes that are able to develop into a fetus. The resulting newborns tend to display congenital malformations. During gametogenesis, each primary spermatocyte gives rise to four spermatozoa. However, each primary oocyte develops into only one mature ovum and three nonfunctional polar **bodies**, which soon degenerate.

In the human male, spermatogonia lie dormant in the testes from the fetal period through puberty. **Spermatogenesis** begins at puberty and continues through life. In males, the BMP8B gene (bone morphogenetic protein 8b or osteogenic protein 2), the DAZ1 gene (deleted in azoospermia 1), and paternal effect genes influence gametogenesis. In the human female, however, oogenesis begins before birth. All oogonia, possibly as many as 2 million, develop into primary oocytes before birth and are retained as primordial follicles. These begin the first meiotic division before birth. However, prophase is not complete until after puberty, at which time no more than 40,000 primary oocytes can be seen. Of these, it is estimated that only about 400 become secondary oocytes and are expelled one at a time on a monthly cycle (Moore and Persaud 2003). Thus the entire reproductive period of a human female can be considered to last only about 400

months, or 33 years, from about age 12 to about age 45. A small number of the expelled ova never reach the status of secondary oocytes.

Fertilization and the First Week of Development

Once spermatozoa and the secondary oocyte are united, human development begins. Only one spermatozoon can gain entry through the thick zona pellucida surrounding the secondary oocyte. Binding of spermatozoon to zona pellucida is brought about by the proteins zona pellucida 3 (ZP3), the zona pellucida–binding protein sp56, zona receptor kinase (ZRK), and galactosyl transferase. At the time of contact between the two gametes, the secondary oocyte completes the second meiotic division and becomes a mature ovum. Its nucleus becomes the female pronucleus. The head of the spermatozoon forms the male pronucleus. With the fusion of these pronuclei, a **zygote** is formed.

Within 24 hr of ovulation, fertilization is complete, the diploid number of chromosomes is restored, and sex and species variation are determined. The zygote then begins to divide slowly by mitotic division. Mitosis-promoting factor (MPF), cyclins, and cdc-25 phosphatase participate in the cleavage. The new cells, called **blastomeres**, gradually become smaller because they remain confined within the zona pellucida. After the 2-, 3-, and 4-cell stages, the ball of 12–16 blastomeres (embryonic cells) is called a **morula** (Fig. 4-4).

This stage, about 3 days after fertilization, occurs when the morula enters the uterus. The morula develops a central cavity—the **blastocyst cavity**—that gets larger as more uterine fluid gains access to it. Cells are now clustered into an outer ringlike cell mass (**trophoblast**) and a group of cell clusters, or the inner cell mass (**embryoblast**) (Fig. 4-5). The blastocyst formation plays

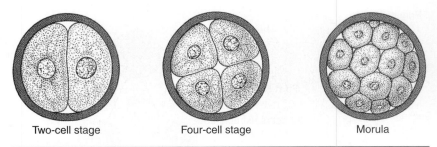

Two-cell stage   Four-cell stage   Morula

Figure 4-4 Development of the zygote from the two-cell stage to the late morula stage. The two-cell stage is reached approximately 30 hr after fertilization; the four-cell stage, at approximately 40 hr; the 12- and 16-cell stages, at approximately 3 days; and the late morula stage, at approximately 4 days.

a role in the adhesion molecules, including cadherin. The blastocyst remains free in the uterine cavity for about 2 days, during which time the zona pellucida gradually degenerates, allowing the blastocyst to grow in all directions. About 6 days after fertilization, the blastocyst attaches to the **uterine endometrium** at the embryonic pole, most frequently on the upper part of the posterior fundic wall near the midsagittal plane. The 1st week of human development begins with fertilization and ends with the blastocyst superficially implanted in the uterine lining (endometrium).

Second Week of Development

In week 2, the blastocyst becomes completely implanted, and the **bilaminar embryo** develops. Other structures that develop during this period are the **cytotrophoblast** and **syncytiotrophoblast** (both differentiated from the trophoblast), **amniotic cavity**, **amnion**, **chorion**, **primary** and **secondary yolk sacs**, **connecting stalk**, **chorionic cavity** or **extra-embryonic coelom**, **extra-embryonic mesoderm**, and the two components of the bilaminar embryo (the epi-

blast and the **hypoblast**). Another important structure that emerges during this time is the prechordal plate, a thickened cranial region of the hypoblast and epiblast combined that is the site of the future mouth (Fig. 4-6).

Third Week of Development

The 3rd week of gestation generally coincides with the week after the first missed menstrual period—that is, the 5th week after the onset of the last normal menstrual period. The embryo becomes **trilaminar**; the three germ layers are **ectoderm**, **mesoderm**, and **endoderm** (Fig. 4-7). A caudal midline thickening on the dorsal embryonic disc forms. Through this **primitive streak**, epiblastic cells move between the epiblast and the hypoblast, ultimately giving rise to the mesoderm and the endoderm. The rest of the epiblastic cells become ectoderm.

The notochord is the first skeletal structure that develops, and it is retained in the adult intervertebral discs as the **nucleus pulposus** (Fig. 4-8). Mesodermal masses arrange themselves segmentally into paired **somites**, which give rise to muscles and other tissues (Fig. 4-9). The **allantois**

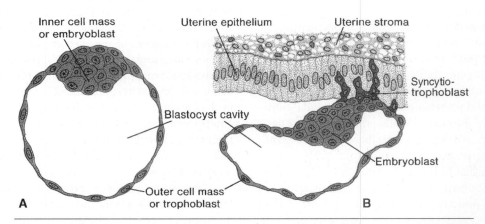

Figure 4-5 **A.** A section through a human blastocyst recovered from the uterine cavity at approximately 4.5 days. **B.** A section of a blastocyst at day 9 of development. The human blastocyst likely begins to penetrate the uterine mucosa by day 5 or 6.

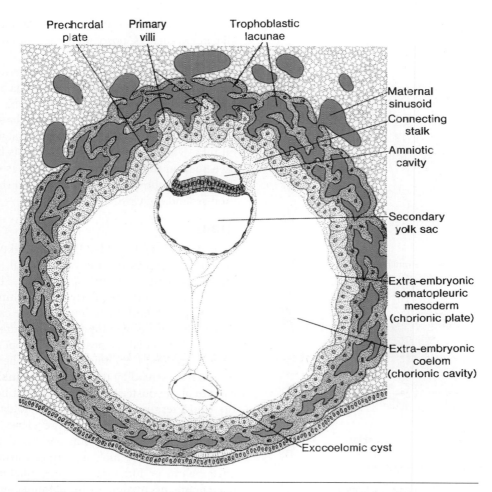

Figure 4-6 A 13-day-old human blastocyst is completely embedded in the endometrium. The dark region between the amniotic cavity and the secondary yolk sac is the bilaminar germ disc.

appears, and the **neural plate**, the forerunner of the nervous system, develops. The **neural crest** separates as the **neural tube** closes and gives rise to numerous components of the peripheral nervous system (PNS). Any disturbance in the development of the neural plate results in severe abnormalities of the nervous system. The intra-embryonic coelom, the primitive placenta, and the cardiovascular system—including the plasma and blood cells—also develop in week 3. Of the 8 weeks of embryonic development, week 3 can be considered the most significant because of the definitive beginnings of numerous structures.

THE CENTRAL NERVOUS SYSTEM

Development of the brain and spinal cord begins early in week 3 of gestation under the inductive influence of the notochord and the paraxial mesoderm adjacent to it. Neurulation is one of several important processes that begin during the trilaminar stage of human development and is complete by the end of week 4. The entire trilaminar stage is completed in week 3.

The 2-week-old embryo is essentially in the form of a bilaminar embryonic disc (Fig. 4-6); the two layers are the epiblast and hypoblast. The primitive streak forms under the influence of **Nodal, Goosecoid, Lim-1,** and hepatocyte nuclear factor 1 (**hnf-1**). The notochord forms under the expression of the **sonic hedgehog gene**.

As the embryo enters week 3, epiblastic cells give rise to endoderm and mesoderm through the region of the primitive streak. The remaining epiblastic cells are now called ectodermal cells. The hypoblast moves to form the secondary yolk sac. Thus in the 3rd week of gestation the three primary germ layers (ectoderm, mesoderm, and endoderm) are established. Anterior to the primitive streak, the ectodermal cells in the dorsal midline of the embryonic disc thicken to become the neuroectodermal layer, the forerunner of the entire CNS and PNS.

Neural Plate, Neural Tube, and Neural Crest

The neuroectoderm overlying the midline notochord thickens to form the neural plate, cranial to the primitive knot. The neural plate later extends caudally with the receding

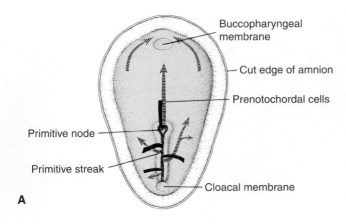

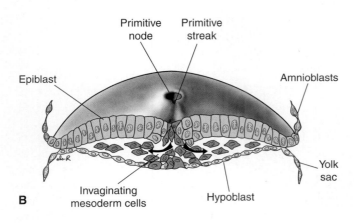

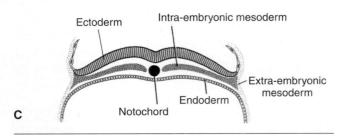

Figure 4-7 **A.** The germ disc of a 16-day-old embryo from the dorsal aspect indicating the movement of the surface epiblastic cells (*solid lines*) through the primitive streak and the subsequent cellular migration between the hypoblast and the epiblast (*broken lines*). **B.** A cross-section through the cranial primitive streak showing the invaginating epiblastic cells. **C.** Cross-section of the three primary germ layers: ectoderm, mesoderm, and endoderm.

primitive streak. On day 18, the neural plate invaginates along the midline to form a neural groove flanked by neural folds on either side (Fig. 4-8). At this time, some neuroectodermal cells on the crest of each neural fold are identifiable. These cells first fuse and later split to lie on the right and left sides of the neural tube when it closes on approximately day 22. The neural tube develops into the brain and the spinal cord, and the segmentally arranged

neural crest tissue develops into the **cranial** and **spinal ganglia**, **nerve sheaths**, **postganglionic autonomic nerves**, and other structures (Figs. 4-8, 4-9, and 4-13). The neural tube soon separates from the adjacent ectoderm and differentiates into a **posterior (dorsal) alar lamina** or **alar plate** and an **anterior (ventral) basal lamina** or **basal plate**. These two regions are separated by a groove, the **sulcus limitans**, midway on the inner surface of the lateral walls of the neural tube. The gap over the neural tube is bridged dorsally by ectoderm that will become skin. Mesoderm will later develop into the bony cranial vault and the vertebral column around the CNS.

Brain

Early in week 4 (days 22–23), the rostral two-thirds of the neural tube represents the future brain, and the caudal third represents the future spinal cord. The fusion of the neural folds occurs irregularly. The resulting neural tube is at first open at both the cranial and the caudal ends (Fig. 4-10). The rostral opening (anterior neuropore) closes on day 25. The caudal, or posterior, neuropore closes 2 days later. In the brain, the final closure of the anterior neuropore is represented by the **lamina terminalis**; a sign of the closure of the posterior neuropore must be sought within the filum terminale. As the neural folds fuse dorsocranially and the rostral neuropore closes, three primary brain **vesicles** form. The brain proper develops from the following vesicles, which are formed during week 4: **prosencephalon**, or forebrain; **mesencephalon**, or midbrain; and **rhombencephalon**, or hindbrain (Figs. 4-11–4-13). A week later, the prosencephalon develops into two secondary vesicles, the **telencephalon** and the **diencephalon**. Likewise, the rhombencephalon develops into the **metencephalon** and **myelencephalon**. The mesencephalon does not divide. The brain is now represented by five secondary brain vesicles, each with its own wall of neuroectoderm that gives rise to motor, sensory, association, and **preganglionic autonomic neurons**, **glia**, and **ependyma**. Cavities in each vesicle differentiate into brain ventricles (Table 4-2).

Three **brain flexures**, or bends, develop with the rapid growth and folding of the brain. The **midbrain** and **cervical flexures** develop ventrally in the midbrain region and at the junction of the hindbrain and spinal cord. The **pontine flexure** develops dorsally between these two flexures, thinning the roof of the hindbrain.

Prosencephalon (Forebrain)

The forebrain develops into two subdivisions: **telencephalon** and **diencephalon**.

Telencephalon

Early in week 4, a pair of lateral outgrowths from the forebrain appears. These optic vesicles are the primordia for retinas and **optic nerves** (Fig. 4-11). Soon another pair of diverticula, the telencephalic vesicles, appears dorsal and rostral to the optic vesicles. These grow into cerebral

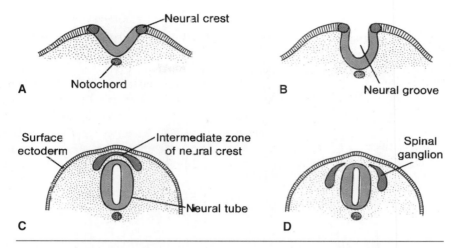

Figure 4-8 Transverse sections through successively older embryos showing the formation of the neural crest (A), neural groove (B), and neural tube (C). The cells of the neural crest, initially forming an intermediate zone between the neural tube and the surface ectoderm, develop into the spinal and cranial sensory ganglia (D) and other structures.

hemispheres, each with a **lateral ventricle**. The median connection between the cerebral vesicles develops into the lamina terminalis, the site of closure of the **rostral neuropore**. The cerebral vesicles give rise to three main structures: **olfactory lobe**, **corpus striatum** (**caudate nucleus and lentiform nucleus**), and **cerebral cortex**. The timeline for the maturation of the cortical areas, tracts, and myelination is known (Table 4-3).

The olfactory lobe consists of the **olfactory bulb**, **olfactory tract**, **anterior perforated substance**, and certain other olfactory structures collectively known as the **pyri-**form lobe. The olfactory parts of the brain constitute the rhinencephalon (see Chapter 15). An accessory olfactory (vomeronasal) system complex develops in the human embryo but degenerates in the fetal stage (Bhatnagar and Smith 2001).

The entire forebrain is considered to be an alar lamina derivative. The cerebral cortex in early development consists of three concentric zones: a germinal zone surrounding the lateral ventricles; an intermediate zone, which becomes the white matter; and an outer cortical zone, which develops into the six-layered isocortex. The olfactory cortex, the hippocampal formation, and the dentate gyrus constitute the allocortex, because these do not have six layers.

The cerebral hemispheres are smooth (lissencephalic) up to about 20 weeks of gestation. By week 24, various sulci and gyri gradually appear. At birth, all topographical features of the adult brain are present. The various lobes (**frontal, parietal, occipital, temporal,** and **insula**) become clearly identifiable during the third trimester. Commissures connecting the right and left hemispheres develop. The principal ones are the **anterior commissure, commissure of the fornix, corpus callosum, habenular commissure,** and **posterior commissure**. The latter two develop in relation to the **pineal body**.

Diencephalon

The caudal forebrain develops into the diencephalon. Its cavity is the **third ventricle**, to which small contributions are added from the telencephalic cavities. The **epithalamus, thalamus, metathalamus, hypothalamus,** and **subthalamus** develop in the lateral walls of the third ventricle. The epithalamus differentiates into the pineal body, **habenular trigone, stria medullaris, tenia thalami,** and posterior

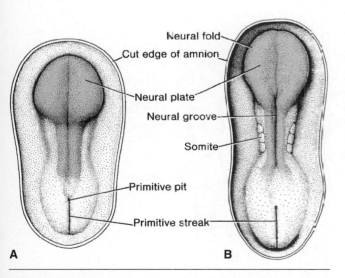

Figure 4-9 A. Dorsal view of a late presomite embryo (~ 18 days). The amnion has been removed, and the neural plate is clearly visible. **B.** Dorsal view at ~ 20 days. Note the somites, neural groove, and neural folds.

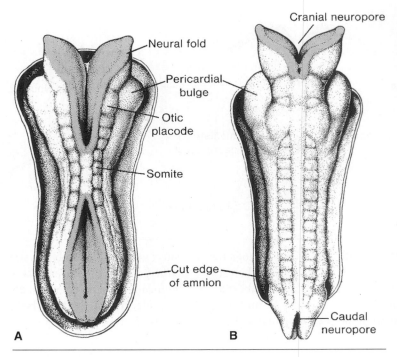

Figure 4-10 **A.** Dorsal view of a human embryo at approximately day 22. Seven distinct somites are visible on each side of the neural tube. **B.** Dorsal view of a human embryo at approximately day 23. The central canal is in communication with the amniotic cavity through the open cranial and caudal neuropores.

commissure. The posterior commissure separates the diencephalon from the mesencephalon. The thalamus is a large structure. Its rapid development reduces the third ventricle to a narrow cavity. In about 70% of humans the two thalami fuse, forming the **massa intermedia**. The **medial** and **lateral geniculate bodies** constitute the metathalamus.

The hypothalamus develops into the inferior lateral wall and floor of the third ventricle. The optic chiasm, infundibulum, tuber cinereum, mamillary bodies, and neurohypophysis are grossly identifiable hypothalamic structures. The subthalamus is small and lies between the thalamus and the tegmentum.

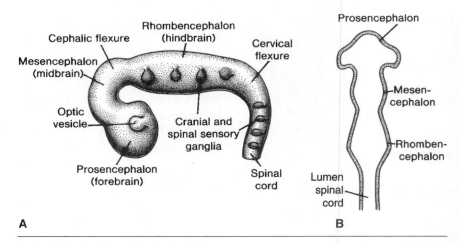

Figure 4-11 **A.** Lateral view of the brain vesicles and part of the spinal cord in a 4-week-old embryo. Note the sensory ganglia formed by the neural crest on each side of the rhombencephalon and spinal cord. **B.** Lumina of the three brain vesicles and spinal cord.

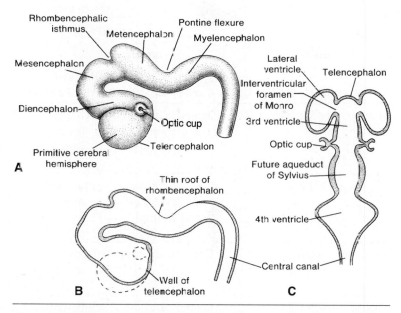

Figure 4-12 Brain vesicles at the beginning of week 6. A. Lateral view of the brain vesicles. B. Midline section through the brain vesicles and spinal cord. Note the thin roof of the rhombencephalon. C. The lumina of the spinal cord and brain vesicles.

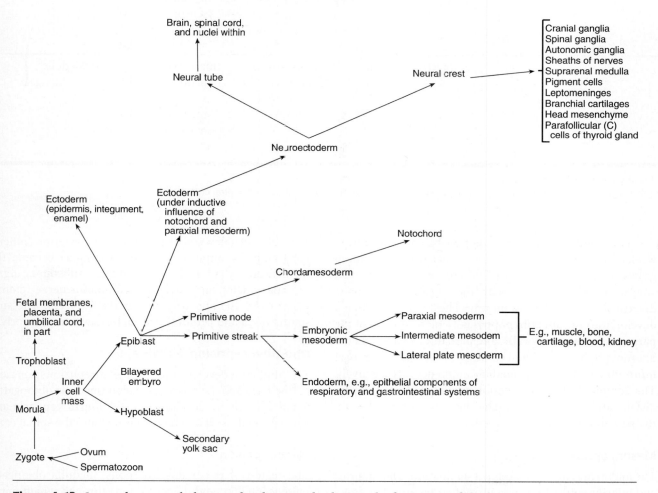

Figure 4-13 Stages during early human development leading to the formation of the brain and spinal cord.

Table 4-2

Development of the Human Brain[a]

Week 3	Week 4	Week 5	Cavity	Weeks 6–12: Alar Lamina	Basal Lamina
Neural tube	Prosencephalon[c]	Telencephalon	Lateral ventricles and choroid plexus; rostral third ventricle	Cerebral hemispheres, cortex, and corpus striatum	None
		Diencephalon	Caudal part of the third ventricle and choroid plexus	Thalamus, hypothalamus, and epithalamus, including pineal body	None
	Mesencephalon	Mesencephalon	Cerebral aqueduct	Tectum: superior and inferior colliculi	Cerebral peduncles and tegmentum
	Rhombencephalon	Isthmus rhombencephali	Rostral part of fourth ventricle	Superior cerebellar peduncles	None
		Metencephalon	Middle part of fourth ventricle	Cerebellum, middle cerebellar peduncles, and sensory nuclei of cranial nerves V and VIII (in part)	Pons
		Myelencephalon	Posterior part of fourth ventricle and choroid plexus	Inferior cerebellar peduncles and sensory relay nuclei of cranial nerves VII, IX, and X (in part)	Medulla oblongata

[a]See also Figures 4-11 and 4-12.
[c]"Many embryologists consider that the prosencephalon is formed of alar laminae alone" (Hamilton et al. 1972).

The **pituitary gland**, or **hypophysis**, develops during weeks 4 and 5 of gestation. An ectodermal diverticulum grows dorsally from the roof of the mouth cavity and comes into close contact with the ventral diencephalic diverticulum, the infundibulum. These two diverticula develop into the **adenohypophysis** (which consists of the **pars distalis**, **pars tuberalis**, and **pars intermedia**) and the **neurohypophysis** (which consists of the **pars nervosa**, **infundibular stem**, and **median eminence**), respectively. The commonly known anterior lobe is made of the pars distalis and pars tuberalis. The posterior lobe makes up the pars intermedia and pars nervosa.

Mesencephalon (Midbrain)

The midbrain is the least modified subdivision. The **superior** and **inferior colliculi** form in its roof, or **tectum**. The supe-

rior colliculi relay visual impulses. The inferior colliculi relay auditory impulses. The basal laminae become the **tegmentum**, which includes **red nuclei**, **substantia nigra**, **reticular nuclei**, and nuclei of **oculomotor nerve** (cranial nerve [CN] III) and **trochlear nerve** (CN IV). The substantia nigra and **cerebral peduncles** develop anteriorly.

Rhombencephalon (Hindbrain)

The hindbrain develops into the metencephalon (pons and cerebellum) and the myelencephalon (**medulla oblongata**), whereas its cavity develops into the **fourth ventricle** and **central canal**, both of which continue into the spinal cord.

Metencephalon

The region of the brainstem (pons, medulla oblongata, mesencephalon, and diencephalon) through which nerve

Table 4-3

Gradients of Maturation for Cortical Areas and Myelination of Tracts

Period	Maturation for Cortical Areas and Myelination
8th week of gestation to birth	Cerebral cortex is established from deeper layers toward surface Neuroepithelial cells in ventricular zone, which cease to divide, are postmitotic; these are guided by glial cells toward cortex
4th month to 2–3 years after birth	Process of myelination is related to functional maturation of neuronal interconnections Myelination starts at soma and proceeds distally Tracts concerned with tasks necessary for life are myelinated first In spinal cord: myelination starts in cervical region and proceeds caudally Anterior root motor fibers are myelinated first; then posterior root sensory fibers Ascending spinal tracts start myelination in the fetal 6th month, followed by descending tracts Pyramidal tract fibers are fully myelinated about 2 years after birth
6th fetal month to before birth	Myelination of cranial nerves takes place (optic nerve myelinated before birth) Nuclear groups develop in their own time, but not simultaneously
Newborn to adult	Synaptic density per neuron at time of birth begins to decline gradually By puberty, number of synapses are drastically reduced Formation of new synapses is closely related to learning

Data from Brodal (2004).

fibers connect the cerebellar and cerebral cortices with the spinal cord develops in the anterior region of the metencephalon as the pons. The tegmental part of the pons is derived from the basal laminae. The pons receives contributions from the alar laminae of the myelencephalon.

The cerebellum is derived from the dorsal alar laminae of the metencephalon, which comes together as the rhombic lips. The cranial region of each rhombic lip thickens, forming the cerebellar rudiment, which later fuses with its opposite. The extraventricular portion, which does not project into the fourth ventricle, becomes larger. By the end of the 4th month, it develops a small midline vermis, the lateral lobes, and the surface fissures. Development of secondary fissures gives rise to the characteristic folia of the cerebellum.

Myelencephalon

The medulla oblongata develops from the most caudal brain region, the myelencephalon. It is continuous with the brainstem superiorly and the spinal cord inferiorly. Here, the **sulcus limitans** divides the alar lamina and the basal lamina in such a manner that the alar region lies lateral to the basal lamina. The bilaminar roof plate in the region of the fourth ventricle consists of an outer thin layer of pia mater and an inner layer of ependymal cells. Together these two layers constitute the tela choroidea, which projects into the fourth ventricle (and into other ventricles in a similar manner) as the choroid plexus. Two

lateral apertures (**foramina of Luschka**) and a median aperture (**foramen of Magendie**) connect the fourth ventricle and the entire ventricular system, including the spinal central canal, with the cerebellomedullary cistern.

Spinal Cord

As the neural tube begins to close, its walls thicken and stratify. Three layers—an **inner ependymal**, a **middle mantle**, and an **external marginal**—differentiate. As the layers develop by proliferation of neuroblasts, they give rise to alar and basal laminae; roof and floor plates; and a sulcus limitans, which separates the alar from the basal regions. With the formation of the anterior median fissure, the central canal is greatly reduced in size. The large neuroblasts near the central canal rapidly divide and form neurons and neuroglia. The mantle layer develops into gray matter, and the marginal layer becomes the white matter of the spinal cord.

CLINICAL CONCERNS

Abnormal Development of the Central Nervous System

The brain and spinal cord, with the exception of the cerebellum, reach the full complement of neurons by week 25 of gestation. After this point and well into the postnatal years, glial cells develop and multiply, various neuronal

Table 4-4

Teratogenic Sensitivity of Some Developing Human Organ Systems

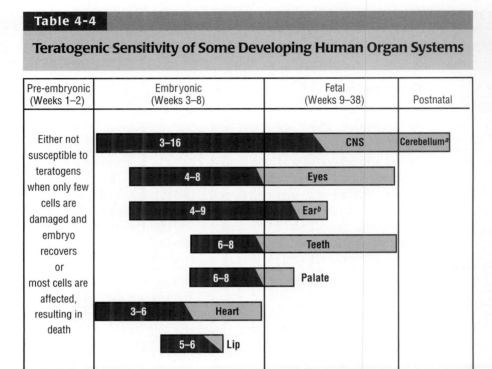

Pre-embryonic (Weeks 1–2)	Embryonic (Weeks 3–8)	Fetal (Weeks 9–38)	Postnatal
Either not susceptible to teratogens when only few cells are damaged and embryo recovers or most cells are affected, resulting in death	3–16	CNS	Cerebellum[a]
	4–8	Eyes	
	4–9	Ear[b]	
	6–8	Teeth	
	6–8	Palate	
	3–6 Heart		
	5–6 Lip		

[a]DNA synthesis has been reported to occur in the cerebellar granular layer during first few years of life; antiviral therapy in infants may cause extensive damage to the developing cerebellar neurons (Langman et al. 1972). Other brain regions in infants are also known to continue mitotic division of neurons postnatally.
[b]Week 16.
CNS, central nervous system; *dark red,* major congenital defect; *light red,* minor defect or functional malformation.

processes develop, and **synaptogenesis** occurs. Glial cells proliferate from midgestation to the end of the 2nd year of life and beyond. **Myelinogenesis** begins at the end of the first trimester (month 3 of gestation) and extends to age 4. In **embryogenesis**, the timing of an insult is more detrimental than the nature of the insult in causing cerebrospinal malformations; hence **teratogenesis** is time-specific but insult-nonspecific phenomenon (Table 4-4). Of patients with cerebrospinal disorders admitted to hospitals, some 90% relate to neural tube closure, notably spina bifida cystica and anencephaly. Table 4-5 summarizes the critical periods and relative vulnerability of the neural regions to insult leading to specific defects.

Anencephaly

Defective fusion of the neural tube results in **anencephaly**, in which the cranial vault is congenitally absent. Cerebral hemispheres are either missing or reduced and attached to the base of the skull. This abnormality has an incidence of 1/1,000 deliveries and occurs more commonly in females. Indications of the defects include absence of the optic nerves, although the eyes appear normal, and exposure or herniation of cerebral tissue (Fig. 4-14). Folic acid with a

multivitamin preparation taken by the mother even before conception has been used to prevent such a defect. Anencephaly is incompatible with extrauterine existence; survival in many cases lasts between 3 and 48 hr after birth.

Cranium Bifidum

Cranium bifidum is a condition in which bone fusion is prevented in the posterior midline of the skull. As a result, the brain or spinal cord protrudes through the opening.

Spina Bifida

When a defect similar to cranium bifidum occurs in the vertebral column, it is called **spina bifida**. Spina bifida can be classified into several subtypes, based on severity and tissue involvement. In **spina bifida cystica**, the posterior vertebral arches fail to fuse, and meninges herniate but neural tissues do not; lumbar or lumbosacral defects are common. In **spina bifida occulta**, the skin of the back is epithelialized and always shows a surface marking in the form of a dimple, a dermal sinus, or a hairy region. Several skin, spinal cord, and bone deformities of this kind can be

Table 4-5

Critical Periods of Development of the Human Central Nervous System

Gestational Age (days)	Developmental Stage	Malformation
14	Bilaminar germ disc	Not vulnerable; either all cells are damaged, resulting in death, or only a few cells are affected and may recover fully
18	Neural plate and neural groove	Anterior midline defects
22	Optic vesicles	Hydrocephalus
25	Rostral neuropore (anterior neuropore) closes	Anencephaly (after 23 days), exencephaly, and microcephaly
27	Caudal neuropore (posterior neuropore) closes	Cranium bifidum, spina bifida cystica, and spina bifida occulta (after 26 days)
32	Cerebellar primordium	Microcephaly (30–130 days)
33–35	Five cerebral vesicles, choroid plexuses, and dorsal root ganglia	Vulnerable
56	Differentiation of cerebral cortex, meninges, ventricular foramina, and cerebrospinal fluid circulation	Vulnerable
70–100	Corpus callosum	Vulnerable
140–175	Neuronal proliferation in the central nervous system (except cerebellum) fully completed	Defects of cellular circuitry and myelin
175 days to 4 years of life	Neuronal migration, glia, and myelin formation and synaptic connections	Vulnerable

revealed through radiograms. These defects are extremely common.

Hydrocephalus

Hydrocephalus is characterized by an enlarged head, a prominent forehead, brain atrophy, mental deficiency, and convulsions. Cerebral ventricles enlarge because of excessive production of cerebrospinal fluid and/or obstruction of the cerebrospinal fluid drainage pathways. Hydrocephalus is caused by the obstruction of cerebrospinal fluid circulation. The ventricles are enlarged and the cerebral mantle is thin. Neurologic findings are abnormal.

Microcephaly

Microcephaly is an uncommon condition in which the brain and **calvaria** (skull cap) and the face are small. Because the brain is underdeveloped, infants with this condition are mentally retarded. Environmental disturbances, genetic abnormalities, and ionizing radiation during the critical period of CNS development have been implicated as the primary causes of the defect.

Other less common abnormalities of the nervous system are craniorachischisis, encephalocele, meningocele, cyclopia, and agenesis of the cortex, corpus callosum, and cerebellum.

Developmental Disabilities

Commonly known developmental disabilities are **mental retardation**, **Down syndrome**, **fragile X syndrome**, **Williams syndrome**, childhood **autism**, and **attention deficit hyperactivity disorder (ADHD)**. The origins of some of these disabilities have been identified, but the causes of other such conditions remain unknown.

Mental Retardation

Mental retardation is a disability characterized by significant limitations both in intellectual functioning and in adaptive behaviors (Luckasson, American Association on Mental Retardation 2002). This disability originates before age 16 and affects one's ability to conceptualize age-appropriate cognitive skills and social functioning. Its causes can include idiopathic factors and genetic conditions. The genetic causes include chromosomal abnormalities (e.g., Down syndrome)

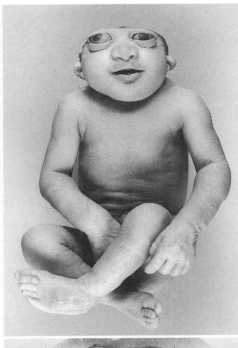

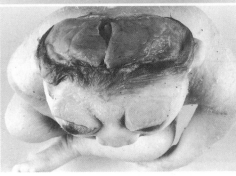

Figure 4-14 Newborn female with anencephaly. **A.** Front view showing the large eyes and absence of the cranial vault. **B.** Dorsal view showing the exposed, poorly formed brain.

or gene mutations. The most common preventable cause of mental retardation is maternal alcohol abuse. Gestational weeks 3–16 is the period of greatest sensitivity for fetal brain damage (Table 4-5). Cell depletion in the cerebral cortex results in severe mental retardation and social/communicative disorders.

Down Syndrome

Marked by a range of cognitive abnormalities, Down syndrome results from a translocation of chromosome 21. The affected individual has three copies of this chromosome; this condition is also known as trisomy 21. Its clinical findings include mental retardation, retarded growth, flat face with short nose, low-set ears, thickened tongue, broad hands and feet, and stubby fingers (Table 4-1).

Fragile X Syndrome

Fragile X syndrome is one of the most common causes of mental retardation. Affected individuals have a fragile site near the end of the long arm of the X chromosome, which looks almost as if it were a detached segment. Special culture conditions are required for demonstration. It has a frequency of 1/1,500 male births and may account for the excess of males in the mentally retarded population.

Williams Syndrome

Williams syndrome, another genetic cause of mental retardation, is characterized by distinct facial features, a small nose, and a high level of empathy (overly friendly). Most subjects develop a sensorineural hearing loss by the age 30. Additional symptoms are high anxiety, attention deficit disorder, and phobia to loud sounds. This is a contiguous gene deletion syndrome.

Childhood Autism

Autism is a mental disorder of unknown cause characterized by abnormal development of brain circuitry that is essential for integrating social interaction and communicative skills. Affected individuals have limited interests and keep busy by being involved with only a few selected items. Their disability is life long and affects their capacity to deal with social-emotional-communicative skills and their linguistic interaction with people. Early intervention using controlled social and linguistic stimulation has been found to make significant improvement in the functional skills of these patients.

Attention Deficit Hyperactivity Disorder

ADHD, one of the most common developmental disabilities, has serious implications for cognitive development, social interaction, and educational performance. The origins of ADHD are mostly unknown. The condition is characterized by persistent inattention, chronic hyperactivity, and impulsivity. Early diagnosis of children with ADHD is important because it saves them, along with parents and teachers, from frustration, anger, and anxiety. It also helps in providing them with systematic treatment to promote their cognitive and linguistic functions.

Peripheral Nervous System
Normal Development

The **PNS** is composed of cranial and spinal ganglia and nerves and the ganglia and nerves of the **autonomic nervous system** (ANS). The **suprarenal gland medulla**, which is derived from the postganglionic sympathetic neurons, also falls in this category. Of the 12 pairs of cranial nerves, 4—oculomotor (CN III), facial (CN VII), glossopharyngeal (CN IX), and vagus (CN X)—belong to the cranial parasympathetic system. Likewise, the S2, S3, and S4 spinal nerves form the components of the sacral parasympathetic system.

The PNS as a whole is derived from the neural tube because the motor nuclei for all cranial and spinal nerves, along with all preganglionic neurons for the autonomic nervous system, are derived from the neural tube. Both are within the brain and the spinal cord. Therefore, **axons** of all such neurons, even though they collectively form peripheral nerves, are derived from the CNS. The spiral or dorsal root ganglia, sensory ganglia of the cranial nerves, all autonomic ganglia, and postganglionic autonomic neurons are derived from the neural crest in a similar manner from tissue that separated from the closing neural tube. The suprarenal medulla, the **mucosal** and **submucosal enteric ganglia**, the **capsular cells** that enclose the sensory nerve bodies, and the myelin-producing **Schwann cells** also develop from the neural crest. Some cranial ganglia—glossopharyngeal (CN IX) and vagus (CN X)—and the first-order olfactory and accessory olfactory (vomeronasal) neurons arise not from the neural tube but from the surface ectoderm—that is, they have a placodal origin.

Variations and abnormalities in the muscles are fairly common. In such cases, the nerves to the affected muscles develop abnormally. Sternocleidomastoid muscle fibrosis, absence of the head of the pectoralis major muscle, and appearance of the sternalis muscle are examples of muscle abnormalities that cause the abnormal development of nerves.

Abnormal Development

Abnormal development of the PNS cannot ordinarily be distinguished from the developing central nervous structures. Anencephalic fetuses lack optic nerves, but the eyes, although large, appear normal. Another example of such a disorder is congenital **aganglionic megacolon (Hirschsprung disease)**. In this condition, the colon is greatly dilated because of lack of muscular tone and contractile activity of the bowel segment, which causes fecal retention. This is because the postganglionic parasympathetic neurons are congenitally decreased in the myenteric plexus, which is located in the distal segment of the large intestine. The innervation of the muscle layers is defective even when ganglionic neurons are present. Only the rectum and sigmoid colon are generally involved, but occasionally more proximal parts of the colon are affected.

SUMMARY

There are 46 human somatic chromosomes. The current estimate of the number of human genes is 31,778. Human sex cells divide by meiosis. Growth occurs through mitosis. Human development begins with the union of a spermatozoon and with a secondary oocyte. During week 1 of development, a zygote forms and divides into blastomeres that pass through the 2-, 3-, and 4-cell stages. In the 12- to 16-cell stages, on about day 6, the morula becomes the blastocyst and attaches to the endometrium. During week 2, trophoblast differentiation and formation of the amnion and chorion, the two yolk sacs, and the two germ layers (epiblast and hypoblast layers) occur. In week 3, the mesoderm and endoderm form from the epiblast through the primitive streak, and the ectoderm differentiates. Somites and the neural tube develop at this time. The five brain vesicles appear early in week 4 and gradually differentiate into corresponding brain structures and ventricles. Sulci and gyri appear in approximately week 24. Abnormal development of the central nervous system causes deficits such as anencephaly, cranium bifidum, spina bifida, hydrocephaly, and microcephaly. The peripheral nervous system is derived from a specialized portion of the neural tube, the neural crest. The nervous system continues to develop for many years after birth.

*This chapter is written by K.P. Bhatnagar, PhD, University of Louisville School of Medicine, Louisville, KY.

QUIZ QUESTIONS

1. Define the following terms: chromosomes, disjunction, embryo, gametogenesis, meiosis, mitosis, neural crest, neural plate, nondisjunction, teratogenesis

2. What is the normal number of human somatic chromosomes?

3. True or false? Normally developing humans have 46 somatic chromosomes.

4. True or false? There are 24 types of human chromosomes; 22 autosomes, and one X and one Y chromosome.

5. True or false? The neural plate is the forerunner of the nervous system.

6. True or false? The neural tube develops into the brain and the spinal cord.

7. True or false? The CNS is most susceptible to major congenital defects during weeks 3–16 of development.

8. Match the following numbered disorders with their associated lettered statements.

1. anencephaly	a. failure of the brain to form two hemispheres
2. holoprosencephaly	
3. lissencephaly	b. developmental failure of the gyri/sulci formation
4. microcephaly	c. miniature brain and small skull cap with normal face size
	d. congenital absence of the cranial vault with missing or reduced forebrain

TECHNICAL TERMS

abembryonic (or vegetal) pole

allantois

allelic gene

amnion

anaphase

aneuploid

anlagen (primordium)

attention deficit hyperactive disorder (ADHD)

basal lamina

bilaminar embryo

blast

blastocyst

blastomere

chorion

chromosomes

cleavage

coelom

Klinefelter syndrome

lamina terminalis (lamina terminalis hypothalami)

maturation

meiosis

mental retardation

mesoderm

metaphase

mitosis

monosomy

morula

myelination

neural crest

neural plate

neural tube

nondisjunction

notochord

nucleus pulposus

conceptus

connecting stalk

cytotrophoblast

diploid

disjunction

Down syndrome

ectoderm

embryoblast

embryonic (or animal) pole

endoderm

epiblast

euploid

extra-embryonic

fragile-X syndrome

gametes

gametogenesis

gene

genome

haploid

hypoblast

oogonia

polar bodies

prechordal plate

primitive streak

primordium (anlagen)

prophase

somite

spermatogonia

syncytiotrophoblast

telophase

trilaminar embryo

trisomy

trophoblast

Turner syndrome

vesicle (brain)

Williams syndrome

yolk sac (primary)

yolk sac (secondary)

zygote

Basic Physiology of Nerve Cells

LEARNING OBJECTIVES

After studying this chapter, students should be able to:

- Explain the parts of a typical nerve cell and describe their functions

- Discuss the common types of nerve and glial cells

- Describe the functions of nerve and glial cells

- Explain the electrical and chemical properties of nerve cells

- Describe the mechanism of impulse generation and its conduction

- Explain nerve cell responses to injuries in the nervous system

- Explain differential regenerative processes between the central and peripheral nervous systems

- Discuss the functions of common neurotransmitters

The **nerve cell** is the basic functional unit in the CNS. Each nerve cell participates in activities that are vital to the life of the cell and organ. Each cell uses identical mechanisms to synthesize protein, thereby using and transforming energy. More than 15 billion nerve cells in the human brain generate nerve impulses and are the main means of communication within the nervous system and between the nervous system and body parts. The CNS consists of two primary types of cells: nerve cells (**neurons**) and **neuroglial cells** (or simply **glia**). These cells form the structure of the nervous system that is responsible for functional behavior. Through excitatory and inhibitory nerve impulses, nerve cells serve all sensorimotor activities and higher mental functions, including attention, problem solving, memory, thinking, reasoning, calculation, and language. Neuroglial cells support and protect nerve cells, proliferate, and participate in tissue repair in response to brain injury and disease.

NEURON

A nerve cell primarily consists of three elements: **cell body** (soma), **dendrites**, and **axon** (Fig. 5-1A). Cells receive impulses primarily via the dendrites and secondarily through the soma and the initial segment of the axons. Cells conduct nerve impulses through their axonal fibers. The axons travel various distances and **synapse** on the receptive ends of other nerve cells, muscles, and target organs. Whether the effect is excitatory or inhibitory on the target cell depends on the identity of the neurotransmitter released by the neuron. Nerve cells are highly specialized in responding to excitatory and inhibitory neurotransmitters. Factors that add to the operational complexity of nerve cells are the various ways in which the cell bodies are interconnected and respond to electrochemical signals.

Nerve Cell Structure

Cell Body

The cell body of a neuron consists of two major components a **nucleus** and **cytoplasm**. The nucleus and cytoplasm work closely together to maintain the viability of the organ. Cytoplasm consists of protein molecules and an aqueous substance enclosed within the cell membrane. The cytoplasmic material of the cell contains many **microscopic organelles** (Fig. 5-1B), which include **mitochondria**, **ribosomes**, **lysosomes**, **rough** and **smooth endoplasmic reticulum** (**ER**), and the **Golgi apparatus**. The primary function of these organelles and associated structures is to metabolize protein essential for the maintenance and growth of the cell body and its processes and to add to the viability of the cell and organ. Nerve cells have a high metabolic activity that depends on the availability of glucose. Cells also manufacture their own proteins, which can be transported throughout the cell via a network of cylindrical **microtubules**. Transport can occur both from the cell body to axons and dendrites and from the processes back to the cell body.

The nucleus contains deoxyribonucleic acid (**DNA**), micromolecules with genetic information that determines the characteristics of specific cell types. The transformation and replication of DNA through cell division make up the mechanism for genetic inheritance (see Chapter 4). Visible within the nucleus is the **nucleolus**, which is the site of the

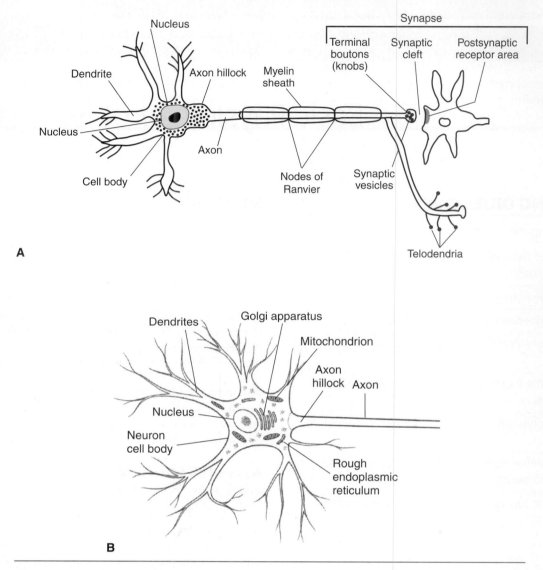

Figure 5-1 **A.** A nerve cell and its major parts: body, dendrites, and axon. **B.** Soma organelles, the most important of which are neurofibrils, mitochondria, Nissl bodies, and Golgi apparatus.

assembly of ribosomes and contains RNA. The ribosomes are transported out of the nucleus into the cytoplasm, where they play a key role in protein synthesis. Proteins destined to be free in the cytoplasm are synthesized by free ribosomes, whereas all other proteins (membrane bound or within organelles) are synthesized by ribosomes attached to the rough ER. Further processing of proteins occurs in the smooth ER and Golgi apparatus. Mitochondria, scattered throughout the cell body, contain enzymes involved with cellular metabolic energy. Lysosomes contain the enzymes that participate in intracellular digestion.

The cytoskeleton consists of three components: **microtubules**, **neurofilaments**, and **microfilaments**. These components of the cytoskeleton act together to provide a dynamic scaffolding, giving neurons their characteristic shape and acting as roadways for the transport of proteins and small organelles throughout the cell. Microtubules, neurofilaments, and microfilaments are all long strands of proteins. Microtubules are the largest of the three, and microfilaments are the smallest.

Dendritic and Axonal Processes

Dendrites and axons are cytoplasmic extensions that extend from the cell body and mediate impulses. Dendrites are afferent (receptive), transmitting information to the cell body from other cells via synaptic sites. They tend to be short and have many branches. The branching dendrites sometimes have small spines that add to their arborization (sub-branching); this increases the surface available for synapses with other nerve cells.

The term **nerve fiber** refers to an axon and its covering myelin sheath. Nerves are composed of many nerve fibers. Axons are efferent structures that transmit information away from the cell body to other neurons or target organs. Axons do not produce their own protein and thus depend on the cytoplasmic substance of the cell body for survival. Axons originate from a cone-shaped region of the cell, the **axon hillock** (initial segment) and extend longer distances than do dendrites. On their way to a terminal destination, axons give off collaterals that communicate with many intervening nerve cells along the way. Axons terminate by branching into smaller multiple fibers that include synaptic terminals at their ends. Within the synaptic terminals are synaptic vesicles that contain a variety of neurotransmitters, the chemical communication molecules that are released on stimulation of the cell.

Myelin Sheath

The speed of nerve conduction is determined by the diameter of the nerve and its myelin sheath. **Myelin** is a multilayered lipid material that insulates and protects the nerve fiber. An important function of this insulation is to prevent the escape of electrical energy during impulse transmission, which affects the speed of nerve impulses. **Oligodendroglial cells** produce the myelin sheath in the CNS. The myelin sheath is formed in small segments that are interrupted by intervals called the **nodes of Ranvier.** The segment of myelin between two nodes is the **internode.** In a longitudinal section, the nerve fiber looks like a string of sausages (Fig. 5-1A).

Electrical impulses jump from one node of Ranvier to the next (**saltatory conduction**), which facilitates rapid nerve fiber conduction of up to 120 m/sec (typical rate = 10 m/sec). The myelin formation process begins during the fetal period and continues to cortical maturity and beyond to adulthood. The growth rate and time span for myelin formation (myelogenesis) are directly related to sensorimotor and cognitive development (Lecours 1975; Lenneberg 1967; Yakovlev and Lecours 1967). The incomplete or impaired maturation process of myelination has definite implications for the development of sensorimotor functions, learning, and speech-language-cognitive skills. Damaged myelin in the CNS impairs nerve impulse conduction, a deficit found in **multiple sclerosis.**

In the peripheral nervous system (PNS), the myelin sheath is produced by the **Schwann cells,** which are located along the axons. One characteristic of myelin formation in the PNS is that each Schwann cell is associated with only one axon, whereas an oligodendroglial cell contributes to the myelination of a group of adjacent axons in the CNS.

Synapse

The synapse is the connection point between neurons. It includes three parts: **presynaptic terminal, synaptic cleft,** and **postsynaptic cell.** Structurally, the presynaptic terminal may be a clearly defined bouton, or it may occur merely where there is close opposition of the membrane of two cells. The synaptic terminals contain vesicles filled with neurotransmitters that mediate communication between

cells. The membrane of the postsynaptic cell contains receptor proteins for the neurotransmitter molecules. The synaptic cleft is the space between the presynaptic terminal and the postsynaptic cell.

Nerve impulses do not actually cross the synapse. Communication at the synapse occurs through a neurotransmitter released from the terminals. The presynaptic cell is stimulated to release its neurotransmitter by a nerve impulse that travels down the axon. Electrical impulse transmission through the axon causes the vesicles at the axon terminals to release stored neurotransmitters into the cleft area. Activation of the postsynaptic receptors can lead to myriad effects, such as depolarizing the postsynaptic membrane, hyperpolarizing the postsynaptic membrane, and activating various second messenger pathways depending on the neurotransmitter and receptor type involved in the synapse. If a depolarization of the postsynaptic membrane is sufficiently large to cause the membrane potential to reach threshold, the cell will fire an action potential that will move up the dendrite to the cell body. (For details, see "Nerve Impulse" later in this chapter.) Axons usually synapse with dendrites (**axodendritic synapse**) but may synapse with axons (**axoaxonic synapse**) or directly on cell bodies (**axosomatic synapse**).

Nerve Cell Types

The ability of a cell to process specialized information depends not only on how it is connected with other cells but also on its shape, size, and structural configuration. Accordingly, this structural diversity serves as the basis for nerve cell classification. Nerve cells are classified according to the number of receptive processes coming out of their bodies and by the length of their axons. Both dendritic and axonal processes add to a cell's ability to respond differentially to various types of sensorimotor information.

Based on the number of processes arising from the cell body, nerve cells are either **multipolar, bipolar,** or **unipolar** (Fig. 5-2). Multipolar cells have many dendrites and one axon. Differing in size and shape, the cells make numerous synaptic contacts with other cells. Most multipolar cells are in the CNS. Spinal interneurons and cerebellar **Purkinje cells** are the best examples of the multipolar type. Bipolar cells have two processes (dendrite and axon), one extending from each pole of the body. These are found in retina and inner ear. Unipolar cells are T-shaped, with one process extending from the body. It divides into an axon and dendrite away from the cell body. Cells in the spinal dorsal roots, for example, are unipolar.

An alternative classification of neurons is based on axon length. **Golgi type I** cells have a long axon, ranging from inches to feet; many form the sensory or motor tracts connecting cells across long distances. **Golgi type II** cells, such as the interneurons that connect with other adjacent cells, have a short axonal process.

Neuronal Circuits

The CNS contains billions of cells that are organized into specific patterns of neuronal pools. Each pool or circuit

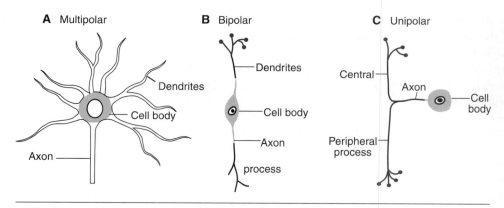

Figure 5-2 A–C. Types of nerve cells based on their processes.

processes information differently, and each is concerned with the facilitation and inhibition of information. The common neuronal circuits are networks used for divergent and convergent processing, lateral inhibition, and reverberating information feedback (Fig. 5-3). A **divergent circuit** amplifies an impulse when an impulse from a single presynaptic cell activates several postsynaptic cells. A **convergent circuit** has two patterns of connections. In the first neuronal circuit of convergence, the postsynaptic neuron receives impulses from several diverged fibers of the same presynaptic nerve cell. In the second pattern, impulses from different nerve cells converge on one postsynaptic nerve cell.

In **lateral inhibition**, the signal or cellular message is sharpened by inhibiting the adjacent nerve cells. The **reverberating circuit** is a self-propagating system between cells that, if activated, can discharge the signal continuously until its operation is blocked by an external source. In the reverberating circuitry, neurons are arranged in a chain formation. The incoming impulse activates the first nerve cell, which activates the second cell, which stimulates the third, and so on. Branches from the second, third, and fourth cells send impulses back to activate the previous nerve cell, forming a closed neuronal loop.

Neuroglial Cells

The function of neuroglia glia cells is to support and protect the nerve cells (Table 5-1). Glial cells are in the gray and white matter of the brain, and there are 40–50 times as many glial cells as nerve cells. However, the glial cells are small and do not participate in the generation and transmission of nerve impulses. There are four types of glial cells in the CNS: **astrocytes, oligodendroglia, ependymal cells,** and **microglia** (Fig. 5-4). Glial cells of the PNS are **Schwann cells** and **satellite cells**. Schwann cells may be capable of acting as **fibroblasts** (connective tissue).

Located predominantly in the white matter, the **astrocytes** function as connective tissue and provide skeletal support for the brain cells and their processes. In the gray matter, the astrocytes protect the brain by forming **external** and **internal limiting membranes**. By contacting capillary surfaces with their end feet and by forming tight junctions,

astrocytes contribute to the **blood–brain barrier** (the selective **permeability** of capillaries and arteries that restricts the movement of harmful substances from the blood to the brain; see Chapter 17). *Astrocytes* also regulate the extracellular concentration of ions and in some instances can degrade released neurotransmitters. After an injury to the brain, astroglial cells are important in recovery. In cerebral vascular accidents, the astrocytes and microglial cells proliferate and migrate to the lesion site. *Microglia* phagocytose (engulf and digest) cellular debris, leaving a cavity. In the case of a large lesion, astrocytes seal the cavity, which is called a **cyst**. In the case of a limited-size lesion, astrocytes fill the space with a glial scar; this process is called **replacement gliosis**.

Oligodendroglia cells form and maintain the myelin sheath in the CNS. Each of the processes that radiate from the oligodendrocyte contributes to forming myelin. Thus each oligodendrocyte may supply myelin for 25 or more axons. The sheath of myelin insulates the axons and speeds up impulse conduction. The myelin that covers PNS fibers is formed by Schwann cells, which are derived from the neural crest.

Ependymal cells primarily form the inner surface of the **ventricles**. In conjunction with the astrocytes, the ependymal cells form the internal limiting membrane. The **choroid plexus**, which secretes cerebrospinal fluid (CSF) and is in the ventricular cavity, consists of vascular pia surrounded by an epithelial layer of *ependymal* cells. *Microglial* cells do not perform day-to-day functions in the nervous system but are called on during injury. These cells are the scavengers of the CNS. In response to injury, the microglia proliferate and migrate to the injury site. Once at the site, the *microglia* transform into macrophages that phagocytose dead tissue debris and pathogens.

CENTRAL AND PERIPHERAL NERVOUS SYSTEMS

The two important cytologic differences between the CNS and the PNS are different myelin-forming cells and the

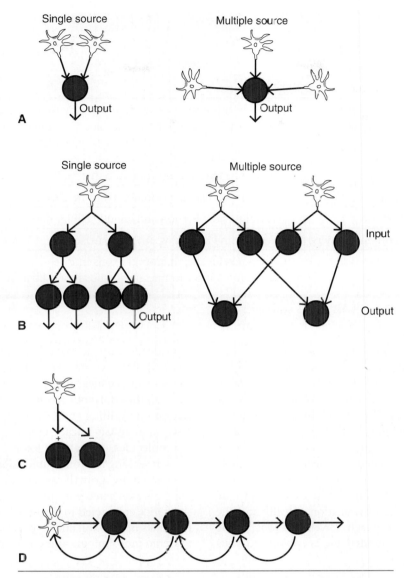

Figure 5-3 Common types of neuronal circuits. **A.** Convergent circuit. **B.** Divergent circuit. **C.** Lateral inhibition. **D.** Reverberating circuit.

presence in the PNS of **endoneurium**, a fibrous connective tissue covering for axons. Schwann cells myelinate the fibers in a jelly-roll manner—that is, the myelin consists of layers of Schwann cell membranes. One Schwann cell forms myelin exclusively for one internode of a peripheral nerve fiber, whereas one oligodendrocyte myelinates many axons in the CNS. Myelin formation by these two types of cells is otherwise similar.

The composition of nerve fibers differs between the CNS and PNS. Peripheral nerve fiber bundles are held together by connective tissues, such as the collagen fibers of the fibroblasts and other cells that form the **endoneurial membrane** (Fig. 5-5). This is a fragile covering that surrounds each peripheral nerve individually. This fibrous connective tissue (endoneurial membrane) is not known to exist in the CNS and may be related to the lack of regenerative growth in the CNS.

NEURONAL PRUNING AND SYNAPSE ESTABLISHMENT IN THE BRAIN

The human brain's ability to serve cognitive-linguistic-speech functions relates to its unique neuronal growth pattern during its embryonic period, which reflects a balanced development between the cellular density and the establishment of patterned axonal connections. This cellular growth involves an extensive proliferation and migration of cells that is regulated either by cyclic proteins or by trophic (nutritional) factors. The potentially full complement of nerve cells in the human brain is typically reached by the 25th gestational week and is virtually over by the time of birth.

Embryogenesis (establishment of the anatomic configuration) is known to produce an overabundance of neurons in the brain; most of these cells are active throughout

Table 5-1

Neuroglia and Their Functions

Glia Cells	Locations	Functions
Astrocytes	CNS (gray and white matter)	Provide supporting network in brain by forming a complete lining around external surface of brain and blood vessels in CNS
		Contribute to blood–brain barrier by regulating transmission of substances across blood vessels
		Form scars around dead brain tissue
Oligodendrocytes	CNS	Form myelin sheaths around axons in CNS
Microglia	CNS	Travel to site of lesion and engulf cellular debris before removing it
Ependymal cells	Ventricular cavity	Form lining around ventricular surface
Schwann cells	PNS	Form myelin sheath around axons in PNS
		Constitute fibrous connective tissue around fibers in PNS

CNS, central nervous system; *PNS*, peripheral nervous system.

the life of the individual, but some do not survive. Postembryonic and postfetal neuronal (neuroblast and glioblast) growth involves a cellular reduction and rapid synaptic growth, which causes a 350% increase in the brain size within the first 2 years of life. As an active process, programmed cellular death (apoptosis) involves approximately 50% of the original cells and applies to the neurons that are either incorrectly connected or are unable to develop synaptic connections to the target areas.

During the development of the brain, there are specific mechanisms that guide the organization of cells and the ways they are connected through traveling axons in the brain. Once a neuron has migrated and is established in its final destination, it extends an axon with **growth cones** (path finders) containing sensory or motor inclination. These growth cones guide the axonal paths by finding ways through the enormous tissue density to connect with target neurons by sniffing and/or navigating through the biologic environment. Chemical factors, such as cell adhesive guiding molecules, that attract axons also regulate the axonal growth seeking neuronal targets. Axonal target seeking also is affected by **growth-associated protein 43 (GAP-43)**, which is associated with repair of the CNS.

Once connected to the target neurons, the presynaptic terminals of the axon and its postsynaptic (receptive) region undergo morphologic and chemical changes that are regu-

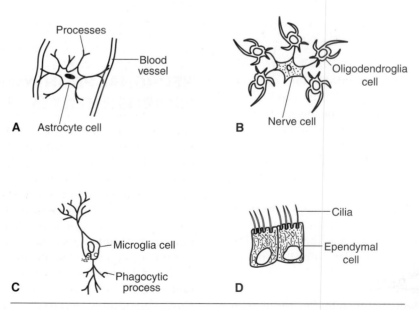

Figure 5-4 Glia cells. A. Astrocyte. B. Oligodendroglia. C. Microglia. D. Ependyma.

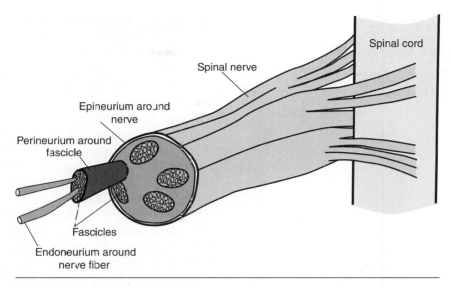

Figure 5-5 Peripheral nerve components.

lated by physiologic compatibility of both sides of the synapse. Only synaptic connections that meet the criterion of biochemical compatibility involving both ends survive. This results in the retention of only a few synapses out of many competing connections. This networking stabilization is the basis for the formation of mature axonal pathways, which are functionally reinforced by experience on each repeated activation.

Repeated activation influences the brain's organization and contributes to its astonishing capacity for serving a variety of human cognitive behaviors and allocating functions to different regions. Some of these mechanisms are retention of particular connections through use and function, removal of redundant and incompatible connections, and reduction of additional neurons through the process of programmed cell death during the critical period of the first 5 years of age (Box 5-1). Cerebral plasticity and the brain's ability to re-establish functional communication are most visible in the early years of life; however, cerebral plasticity remains somewhat functional into adult life.

Knowledge of the physiologic processes involved in nervous system development and the identification of growth factors that can interrupt programmed cell death have allowed researchers to evaluate the natural restitution seen in some brain-damaged patients. Research is under way to find methods of stopping, or slowing the rate of, cellular death in the brains of stroke patients by administering nerve growth proteins and incorporating the brain's own trophic factors.

NERVE IMPULSE

Nerve cells communicate with one another through impulses that represent all neuronal activity. Nerve impulses have a chemical component that underlies the electric potential of the cells (Fig. 5-6). The excitability of nerve cells depends on the ion channels in the neuronal membrane. An action potential results from charged particles (ions) moving through the cell membranes. Nerve impulses activate the release of a neurotransmitter in a presynaptic neuron. The transmitter often causes the adjacent postsynaptic receptors to open an ion channel (either directly or indirectly through second messengers). By selectively open-

BOX 5-1

Neuronal Pruning and Establishment of Synapses

Cellular growth during the embryonic and fetal periods involves an overabundance of cells. However, not all the cells live to function. The only those cells to survive and become operative are those that are connected optimally and assigned functions. However, a widespread neuronal loss involving > 50% of the cells occurs during normal development. This programmed attrition of neurons largely involves neurons that are either not connected, are weakly connected, or have redundant connections. Thus the programmed death of neurons and the establishment of synapses are essential for the cortical maturation needed for regulating higher mental functions. Attenuated synapse development and altered or reduced programmed cellular death may have implications for learning disorders and developmentally impaired cognitive and linguistic functions.

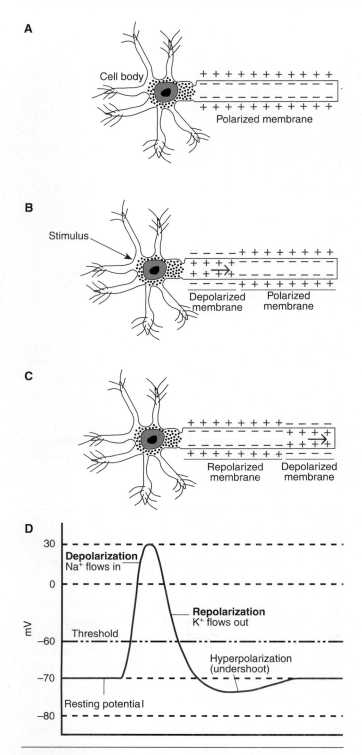

Figure 5-6 Action potential. **A.** The resting potential with a polarized membrane. **B.** The generation of the action potential with a depolarized membrane. **C.** The conduction of the action potential along the membrane. **D.** Recorded changes in the membrane potentials, threshold excitatory postsynaptic potential (EPSP), and inhibitory postsynaptic potential (IPSP).

ing or closing ion channels, the released neurotransmitter controls the excitability as well as inhibition of the interconnecting neuron.

A cell is in a **resting state** when it is not excited and not conducting an impulse. In the resting state, there is a specific level of **membrane potential** in which the distribution of positive and negative ions on each side of the membrane is unequal (polarized). Consequently, there is a difference between electrical charges on the inner and outer sides of the cell membrane (Fig. 5-6A). The specific resting membrane potential depends on the cell type but is typically between −50 and −70 mV in relation to the outside of the cell. The membrane potential is maintained by an unequal distribution of positively charged **sodium** and **potassium** ions and negatively charged **chloride** ions and proteins across the membrane. The concentration of negative ions is higher concentration inside the cell, and the concentration of positive ions is higher outside the cell.

Even during a resting state, when the nerve cell is not conducting an impulse, some ions constantly pass through the membrane. Ion channels consist of several polypeptide units arranged around a central pore. These membrane channels are usually gated (opened or closed) by electric potential or neurotransmitters. The flow of ions across the membrane depends on the density of the channels, the size of the openings, the **ion concentration gradient** (ions will move to areas of lower concentration of the ion), and the **electrical gradient** (negative ions will move toward positive charges and vice versa) across the membrane. The steeper the concentration gradient across the membrane, the greater the flow of ions from high to low concentration. The electrical gradient (membrane potential) and the concentration gradient together determine the magnitude and direction of ion flow across the membrane.

The distribution of *sodium* and *potassium* ions across the cellular membrane is adjusted constantly by the **sodium–potassium pump**, which pumps sodium out of the cell and potassium into the cell. A typical neuron has a low internal sodium and chloride concentration and a high internal potassium concentration relative to the extracellular fluid. The selective permeability of particular ion channels to specific ions is determined by pore size and charge of the interior portion of the channel.

In addition to gated ion channels, some channels, called leak channels, are active at rest. These channels are more permeable to potassium than to sodium Thus, at rest, potassium ions can easily leave the cell interior, whereas sodium cannot. The loss of positive potassium ions across the membrane creates a negative membrane potential (concentration gradient) while the cell is at rest. At the same time, negative chloride ions move into the cell across the concentration gradient, contributing to the maintenance of the negative membrane potential. Within the cell there are nonpermeant negatively charged ions that balance the chloride. The electrochemical gradient along the cell membrane keeps the external surface positive and the internal surface negative at rest (Fig. 5-6A). Maintenance of this gradient at rest is crucial for the excitability of the cell.

Nerve Excitability

Excitability is a cell's response to various stimuli and the conversion of this response into a nerve impulse or **action potential** (Fig. 5-6). Stimuli include chemical or temperature changes, electrical pulses, and mechanical stimulation. All these stimuli are converted to changes in the membrane potential of the cell. When the neuron becomes **hyperpolarized** (the cell interior becomes more negative thus, decreased excitability), it becomes less capable of triggering a large spike, called an action potential, and is thus less excitable. An action potential is triggered when the change is in the other direction of less negativity (**depolarization**) and the cell reaches threshold. Neurotransmitters released by the presynaptic cell cause one of two graded (of different magnitudes) electrical responses. If the postsynaptic cell demonstrates hyperpolarization in response to the neurotransmitter, it is called an **inhibitory postsynaptic potential (IPSP)**. An IPSP will take the membrane potential further away from the action potential threshold so that the cell becomes less likely to fire an action potential in response to other stimuli. If the neurotransmitter causes a depolarization of the membrane potential, it is called an **excitatory postsynaptic potential (EPSP)**. If the EPSP is of sufficient magnitude, the cell will reach threshold for firing an action potential.

The threshold for triggering an action potential varies from cell to cell but is typically 5–10 mV depolarized from the resting membrane potential. The depolarization of a cell membrane opens specific voltage-gated ion channels, allowing ions to flow in and out of the cell. Initially, sodium flows quickly into the cell, causing a large depolarization, to potentials > 0 mV. These sodium channels close rapidly, allowing a return to the resting membrane potential. The **repolarization** of the cell is aided by the opening of voltage-gated potassium channels that allow more potassium to flow down the concentration gradient. The membrane potential even can become slightly more hyperpolarized than the original resting membrane potential (undershoot). As the cell becomes hyperpolarized, the potassium channels also close, so that the cell can reestablish its membrane potential. All this occurs in a matter of milliseconds; hence relatively few ions flow across the membrane. In this way, the concentration gradient is not disturbed during the brief action potential, and the electrical chemical gradient that established the membrane potential in the first place remains intact.

For a period following the action potential, the cell is incapable of producing a second action potential. This is called the **absolute refractive period**. Unlike the graded IPSPs and EPSPs, action potentials are all-or-nothing responses. If the cell reaches threshold, it will always fire an action potential, and the action potential will have the same shape and magnitude every time it occurs.

Not all stimuli are strong enough to cause the cell to reach threshold for firing an action potential. However, if many stimuli with subthreshold strength occur at about the same time (or in series) and in the same place, a nerve impulse can be initiated.

Impulse Conduction

A nerve impulse is passively conducted a short distance in the axon by sodium entering the cell membrane. The interior of the axon becomes more positive than the adjacent neighboring area (Fig. 5-6B). This gradually changes the membrane potential in the neighboring area, and the impulse continues to allow positively charged ions to enter the cell membrane as it moves distally along the axon (Fig. 5-6C). Impulse conduction in a myelinated axon is the same as in an unmyelinated axon, except the impulse conduction in the myelinated axon is faster as the impulse jumps from one node of Ranvier to the other (saltatory conduction). Conduction velocities depend on the diameter of the axon; the largest diameter axons have the greatest conduction velocity. These large axons require myelination for efficient conduction and have velocities of 72–120 m/sec and diameters of 12–20 µm. In contrast, small-diameter axons (0.2–1.5 µm) are unmyelinated and have conduction velocities of 0.4–2.0 m/sec.

Most cells have their own frequencies and patterns of action potentials that serve as codes for transmitted messages. Each neuron type has a unique combination of ion channels that govern its excitability. The nervous system uses frequency coding (firing rate of action potentials) to get information about the intensity of a stimulus. For example, if one lightly presses on a patch of skin, the sensory neuron may fire at a low rate. As more pressure is applied, the firing rate of the neurons will increase to inform the CNS that the intensity of the stimulus is greater.

NEURONAL RESPONSES TO BRAIN INJURIES

Nerve cells in the human brain are less capable of further cell division and regeneration than other cell types. Limited cellular regeneration restricts the recovery of sensorimotor functions and mental processes after lesions in the CNS. The nerve cell synapses serve as good points of reference for discovering the effects of cellular injuries because, in addition to conducting an impulse, the cells transmit nutritive (trophic) substances between neurons. Trophic factors are crucial for normal cell maintenance on both sides of the synapse. A neuron may degenerate if either the presynaptic or postsynaptic terminal degenerates. Axotomy affects not only the directly injured neuron but also postsynaptic neurons and neurons that provide innervation to the injured neuron. The severity of the effect on other neurons depends on the extent to which each of the other neurons interact with surrounding noninjured neurons.

Understanding the physiologic events that cells undergo after injuries is important because the effects explain the processes of spontaneous recovery after trauma, vascular accident, tumor, and metabolic insufficiency. The two types of degenerative changes that follow axonal sectioning are the **axonal (retrograde) reaction** and **Wallerian (anterograde) degeneration** (Fig. 5-7A; Table 5-2). During axonal reactions, retrograde degenerative changes occur in the cell body in response to sectioning the axon (axotomy). This is secondary to the interruption of trophic factors that flow from the axon to the cell body and to the reprogramming of the cell body in the face of metabolic changes. Axonal injury extends from the site of injury to the cell body. In Wallerian degeneration, the degenerative changes occur in the axon region detached from the cell body. The axonal segment still attached to the cell body is the **proximal segment**, and the detached axonal segment is the **distal segment** (Fig. 5-7C; Box 5-2).

Axonal Reaction

Nerve cells undergo a series of degenerative changes in response to injury (Fig. 5-7B, Table 5-3). The microscopic structures (organelles) of the soma undergo structural changes that are evident within 24–48 hr after injury. The first cytologic signs of changes in the cell body are swelling of the organelles and dissolution of coarse clumps of **Nissl substance** into fine granules. Cellular edema, caused by an altered blood–brain barrier, obliterates structural details of the gray and white matter and triggers nuclear shrinking (pyknosis). Edema is maximal within 90–100 hr. This reactive or degenerative process in individual cells, called **chromatolysis**, begins between the axon hillock and the cell nucleus. It is followed by the degeneration of Nissl bodies and the displacement of the cell nucleus from the center to the periphery of the soma.

Depending on the severity of injury, the chromatolytic process may continue for 10–18 days. While the cell is injured and undergoing reactive or degenerative changes, cellular RNA production and protein synthesis increase, as does the formation of the plasma membrane, to regenerate the severed axon and to prevent the cell body from dying. Specifically, free ribosomes in the postchromatolysis phase synthesize increased structural proteins that are needed for restoring cellular structure and rebuilding Nissl bodies and cellular fibers. If the connection of the severed axon is properly restored, the chromatolysis ends, and the cell may return to its normal appearance. Some cells, if not seriously damaged, may respond to the natural recovery process and survive the injury. In such cases, all cell body organelles resume their normal appearance, and the nucleus again assumes a central location. However, this restoration may take months. Cells that are severely injured do not survive. They shrink and assume irregular shapes because of the degenerated organelles. They gradually atrophy and leave only debris.

Cellular swelling, if not medically treated, can lead to death by elevating intracranial pressure. By the end of a week, swelling may begin to go down, but necrotic tissues are invaded by a considerable number of new capillaries (hyperplasia) and a proliferation of macrophages (astrocytes and microglia). The period after the first week is marked by liquefaction of necrotic tissue and **phagocytosis**, in which lipid-laden macrophagic microglia cells engulf

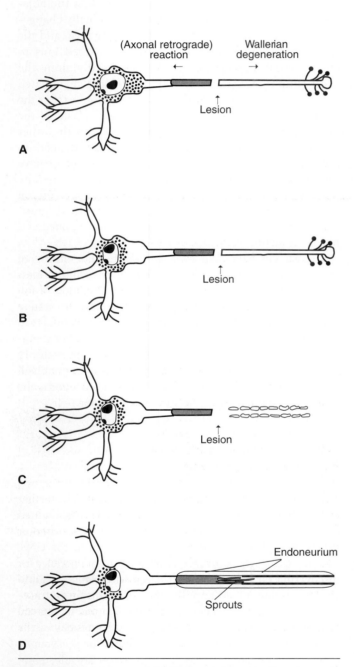

Figure 5-7 The neuronal response to injury (here, a severed axon) and the recovery process in the peripheral nervous system. **A.** Types of neuronal responses to injury. **B.** Axonal (retrograde) reaction. **C.** Wallerian degeneration. **D.** Peripheral nerve regeneration.

Table 5-2	
Neuronal Response to Injury	
Site of Degeneration	Types of Degenerative Changes
Axonal (retrograde) reaction	Chromatolysis in cell body
	Dissolution of cellular organelles
	Displacement of cell body to periphery
	Possible cellular death
	Recovery process
	Increased protein synthesis to regenerate severed axon and prevent cell body from dying
Wallerian (anterograde) degeneration	Axonal degeneration
	Myelin degeneration for sectioned axon
	Axonal degeneration beginning with its distal end
	Macrophagic process
	Recovery
	Increasing protein synthesis to promote recovery
	Forming of endoneurium tube by Schwann cells
	Closing of cleft by sprouting of cut ends of axons
	Establishing sprout connections between both axonal ends

and remove the dead tissue. Phagocytosis may take 3 or more months or more, depending on the size of the lesion. In the case of a large lesion, tissue removal is likely to leave a cavity filled with fluid and some macrophagic cells and the area is outlined by a sheet of astrocytes. The presence of such a cystic cavity in the brain of a stroke patient has made many clinicians pessimistic about the benefits of speech-language treatment and other rehabilitative efforts. However, the recovery process is highly dynamic and presumably involves multiple steps.

Wallerian Degeneration

Survival of the axon depends on cytoplasmic flow from the cell body. Deprived of the metabolic activity from the cell body, an axon cannot survive. The Wallerian reaction (Fig. 5-7C) refers to the degeneration of the axonal part that is separate from its cell body. The distal portion of the sectioned axon swells and begins to degenerate within 12–20 hr. Axons degenerate before the myelin sheath and within 2–3 days, the connected muscles become denervated. Within 7 days, the axon and its myelin are broken into small pieces, which gradually disintegrate, setting the stage for the macrophagic action of microglia cells. Phagocytosis begins in 7 days and is complete in 3–6 months (Table 5-3).

Neuroglial Responses

Neuroglial cells react to cellular injuries and brain tissue necrosis by multiplying in number (**hyperplasia**) and by increasing their size (**hypertrophy**). The infection-fighting **neutrophils** (scavenger white blood cells) arrive at the lesion site within a few days of an injury. This is followed by the migration of microglia and the proliferation of the astrocytes and other macrophages in the region of the dying cells. The breakdown of the blood–brain barrier allows monocytes (phagocytic white blood cells) to invade brain tissues. In the case of a small lesion, the astrocytes form a glial scar, called replacement **gliosis**. In large lesions, they outline the fluid-filled space, forming a **cystic cavity**.

Microglia are the scavengers of the nervous system. In case of inflammation or injury, they rapidly proliferate and migrate toward dead tissue within 24 hr. Their function is to phagocytose the cellular debris. Normally, microglia cells are small, but they become large after phagocytizing dead cells; their cytoplasm becomes less dense and their nucleus more prominent. Within 1 week, they look like typical macrophages, with pale cytoplasm and no visible processes. As the macrophages ingest the debris of myelin, cells, and lipid droplets, the nucleus is pushed to the side. The phagocytic cells dominate the injury site from the 1st week, and it may take several months to years to remove the debris of dead brain tissue (Table 5-3).

In addition, the proliferation and migration of glial cells displace presynaptic and postsynaptic terminals and cell bodies of axotomized neurons, thus impairing transmission between neurons. After normal input to the cell body is removed, new synaptic trigger zones develop on its dendritic aspect and begin to excite the cell.

Axonal Regeneration in the Peripheral Nervous System

The regeneration of fibers in the PNS has been confirmed clinically (Fig. 5-7D). The sectioned nerve endings proximal to the cell body begin regenerating within 3–4 days.

BOX 5-2

Axonal Sprouting and Axonal Regeneration

Axonal sprouting is a common observation in the nervous system affected by a lesion. Once the damaged axons degenerate and the waste is removed by scavenger cells, new growth in the affected area is visible within a short period. This is marked by the growth of boutons that are attached to normal axons. The new growth has been attributed to the trophic elements that are released by the affected neurons. While there is no evidence that this sprouting can restore the lost function, it has raised hopes for restitution through rehabilitation.

The general understanding is that sectioned axons can regenerate in the PNS but not in the CNS. Multiple factors have been identified for inhibiting axonal growth in the CNS. With the absence of an endoneural membrane, there is no guiding structure for regeneration in the CNS. In the CNS, growth of axons is inhibited by specific myelin-associated proteins involved with oligodendroglia cells. The CNS myelin is inherently a potent inhibitor of axon outgrowth, which is why myelination occurs late in development after the establishment of neuronal connections. Inflammatory responses and scar tissue also inhibit regeneration. Last, there are intrinsic differences between neurons in the PNS and the CNS, such as in protein expression. Research focusing on how to simulate the growth environment of the PNS to promote reconnectivity in the CNS has promising implications.

This regeneration is facilitated if proximal and distal ends of the severed nerve are cleaned and attached. The Schwann cells and fibroblasts contribute significantly to axonal regeneration in the PNS. In the first few days, the proliferating Schwann cells fill the interval between opposing ends of the nerve fiber. The sheath of Schwann, or neurilemma, in conjunction with the endoneurial connective tissue, forms a tube from the proximal fiber end leading to the distal end. This neurilemmal tube guides growth of the peripheral axon. As the proximal end of the axon regenerates, many sprouts (regenerated processes of axons) form. One or more axonal sprouts may grow along the tube and pass through the cleft. Some axonal sprouts that cross the scar may grow to connect to the distal portion of the axon at a rate of 4 mm a day. However, the axonal regeneration may encounter problems, one being the low probability of the regenerated axon reaching its previously attached fiber. The attachment of the regenerated axon to a different sensory or motor fiber poses additional problems. For example, the connection of a pain-mediating fiber to a touch receptor results in the sensation of pain from touch. The nerve fibers that are connected incorrectly usually atrophy (Box 5-2).

Axonal Regeneration in the Central Nervous System

Nerve growth in the CNS would have tremendous implications for the natural and assisted recovery of brain-damaged patients. The physiologic concept that most intrigues and frustrates health professionals is the minimal restoration of function after a lesion in the CNS. As a result, the prognosis for recovery of axotomized neurons in the brain is always poor. Axons severed in the CNS also undergo regrowth and sprouting similar to those in the PNS; however, unknown factors prevent damaged neurons from reconnecting to the distal axonal segments and reinnervating their target structures. One factor may be the lack

Table 5-3

Sequence of Pathologic Features in the Necrotic Process

Time	Pathologic Changes
1 day	No visible sign of tissue death
2–4 days	Elimination of structural details between gray and white matter owing to cellular edema and shrinking of cells
4+ days	Maximum swelling in necrotic tissues owing to impaired blood–brain barrier Infiltration of infection-fighting blood monocytes
1 week	Attenuation of swelling and astrocytic and capillary proliferation (hyperplasia and hypertrophy)
1 week to 3 months	Liquefaction of necrotic tissues and their phagocytosis by macrophagic microglial cells
3–6+ months	Formation of a cystic cavity Scar formation if small infarct

of the growth protein in the CNS that is present in the PNS. The proximal ends of axons in the CNS exhibit some growth (sprouting). However, this growth is not significant because the regenerated axons cannot cross the astrocytic scars. Furthermore, there are no Schwann cells and no endoneural tissue tubes (Fig. 5-5) to guide axonal growth. With no guiding structure, the regenerated axons form an axonal ball. In addition, central myelin is a potent inhibitory of axon outgrowth, which is why myelination occurs late in development. Inflammatory responses and scar tissue also inhibit regeneration. Last, there are intrinsic differences between peripheral and central neurons, such as differences in protein expression.

Despite the limited regeneration of the CNS, recovery is highly dynamic and may involve multiple steps, such as restitution of partially injured adjacent neuronal structure and functional reorganization within and across the hemispheres involving the homotopic cortex (Box 5-3).

NEUROTRANSMITTERS

Understanding neurotransmitters is important for students of communicative disorders. Neurotransmitters help regulate brain mechanisms that control cognition, language, speech, hearing, moods, attention, memory, personality, motivation, and the physiologic tuning of the brain (Fig. 5-8).

A neurotransmitter is a chemical substance released at a synapse to transmit signals across neurons (Table 5-4). There are two types of transmitters in the nervous system: **small molecule** and **large molecule (peptides)**. Small-molecule neurotransmitters include **acetylcholine**, **dopamine**, **norepinephrine**, **serotonin**, **glutamate**, and **γ-aminobutyric acid (GABA)**. The latter five are called **monoamines** because they are derived from amino acids. They are known to have short-lasting effects. Large-molecule neurotransmitters produce long-lasting effects on postsynaptic nerve cells. Most neurotransmitters have more than one receptor type and may have different effects on different synapses. Also, more than one neurotransmitter may be secreted at a single synapse. It is, therefore, difficult to identify definitively the specific behavioral effect of a given neurotransmitter at all times.

Acetylcholine

Acetylcholine was the first neurotransmitter identified and is still one of the most studied. It is synthesized from choline and acetyl-coenzyme A (acetyl Co-A) by the enzyme choline acetyltransferase. When released in synapses, it is broken down and destroyed by the enzyme **acetylcholinesterase**. Dissolution of acetylcholine is necessary to permit repetitive nerve impulses to be effective and to allow for muscle repolarization. It is one of the primary neurotransmitters of the PNS. Acetylcholine is also an important neurotransmitter of the CNS; cholinergic neurons are concentrated in the reticular formation, **basal forebrain**, and **striatum** (Fig. 5-8A).

The action of acetylcholine on muscle contraction is measured easily, whereas its effects in the CNS are more

---

BOX 5-3

Neuronal Transplant

Stem cell research has triggered an immense interest and hope for treating many degenerative and eventually fatal conditions. The basis of this hope is that the embryonic cell can be implanted in the brain to replace the lost neurons and augment the diminished physiologic or chemical activity. Stem cells are best for this replacement because they have not yet been affected by myelin-associated factors and have not grown the axonal process. The success of transplanted embryonic cells is variable and, unfortunately, has not lived up to the promise in clinical application. The microenvironment into which the cells are transplanted helps determine the cells success in surviving and contributes to clinical improvement. In addition, stem cells have the potential to become neuroblasts and thus to evolve into different types of nerve cells. Stem cells have shown potential for the treatment of Parkinson disease and in the management of spinal cord injuries. In addition, they may offer some hope for Huntington disease and Alzheimer disease. However, their utility in restoring language and higher mental functions in stroke patients remains extremely remote because the higher cortical functions relate to the intracortical connections that are precise, multiple, and established with repeated use. While stem cell replacement holds the key to the future, it has triggered an ethical controversy because many such cells are obtained from human embryos. Research is focusing on alternate sources of stem cells, such as neurons grown in controlled cultures and finding potential cells already in the system. Other cells with potential for growth and multiplication, undifferentiated from stem cells, have been identified in the human olfactory bulb, around the ventricles, in the regions of the hippocampus, bone marrow, as well as adult tissue of any kind (fat, liver, CNS tissue, etc.). The difference between embryonic and alternate cells is that the numbers of alternate stem cells per unit weight of tissue is smaller and that they have to be grown under different conditions to assume stem cell potential in contrast to embryonic stem cells.

---

difficult to decipher. Thus the direct behavioral effects of acetylcholine are more well characterized in the PNS than in the CNS. The cholinergic neurons in the forebrain (**nucleus basalis of Meynert**), together with related nuclei

ceruleus, and **lateral medullary reticular formation**. Noradrenergic neurons project to the thalamus, hypothalamus, limbic forebrain structures, and cerebral cortex. Descending noradrenergic fibers project to other parts of the brainstem, cerebellar cortex, and spinal cord.

Clinically, noradrenergic neurons are thought to be involved in generating paradoxical sleep and maintaining attention and vigilance. Drugs used for the treatment of depression act by enhancing norepinephrine transmission. When examined in postmortem brains, norepinephrine has been found to be distributed richly in the left pulvinar and right ventrobasal nuclear complex of the thalamus. This norepinephrine asymmetry at the thalamic level is intriguing because it may be related to handedness and the prevalence of one-sided vascular lesions.

Serotonin

Although serotonin is an important neurotransmitter of the CNS, 95% of it is found peripherally in blood platelets and the gastrointestinal tract. The highest concentrations of serotonin neurons are found in the **raphe nuclei** (Fig. 5-8D). The serotonergic terminals are in the reticular formation, hypothalamus, thalamus, **septum**, hippocampus, **olfactory tubercle**, cerebral cortex, basal ganglia, and amygdala. The rostral reticular serotonergic projections are active in sleep; the caudal reticular serotonin terminals, with afferents from the periaqueductal gray matter, interact with spinal enkephalin interneurons and exert some control over pain input.

Clinically, the firing rate of serotonin and noradrenergic neurons fluctuates with sleep and wakefulness and thus may be involved in the general activity level of the CNS. Serotonin is thought to be involved with the overall level of arousal and slow-wave sleep. It also contributes to the descending pain-control system.

Severe depression is thought to be associated with low serotonin. Serotonin levels were lower in individuals who died from suicide than in those who died from an accident. Antidepressant drugs appear to enhance the concentration of serotonin at the synapse by reducing its uptake.

GABA

GABA, a derivative of glutamate, is the major inhibitory neurotransmitter for the CNS. There are two classes of receptors, one that mediates fast inhibitory transmission and one that mediates slower, modulatory effects. Neurons containing GABA are widespread in the nervous system. Examples of GABA local-circuit neurons are cells found in the hippocampus, cerebral cortex, and cerebellar cortex (Fig. 5-8E). GABA serves as the inhibitory neurotransmitter from the striatum to the globus pallidus and substantia nigra, from the globus pallidus and substantia nigra to the thalamus, and from the cerebellar Purkinje cells to the deep cerebellar nuclei. GABA projections suppress the firing of projection neurons and sharpen contrast by inhibiting nearby elements.

Pharmaceutical agents that interact with GABA receptors are widely prescribed for clinical conditions such as epilepsy, anxiety, and insomnia. GABA is implicated in **Huntington chorea**, a degenerative disease characterized by involuntary movements secondary to the loss of GABA-producing neurons in the caudate and putamen (Fig. 13-6B). Decreased GABA-containing **striatonigral** (striatum to substantia nigra) projections result in a lower GABA levels to the substantia nigra. A reduction in GABA causes an elevation of the ratio of dopamine to acetylcholine, which produces abnormal movements. In contrast, a lower ratio of dopamine to acetylcholine ratio, resulting from loss of nigral dopaminergic cells, is associated with the reduced movement (**bradykinesia**) or lack of movements of **Parkinsonism**.

Glutamate

Glutamate is the main excitatory neurotransmitter in the mammalian CNS. Most of the other neurotransmitters discussed in this chapter mediate slower, modulatory effects in the CNS. Glutamate mediates fast synaptic transmissions in the CNS, much in the same way that acetylcholine mediates muscle contractions in the periphery. Glutamate is produced by all excitatory neurons in the CNS, and the majority of neurons have receptors for this compound. Its concentration in the extracellular space is regulated tightly by re-uptake pumps in the surrounding glia cells because too much glutamate causes excitotoxicity and excessive calcium influx. Brain damage secondary to stroke or degenerative disorder may be the result, in part, of excessive release or insufficient reuptake of glutamate. In addition to mediating fast transmission, glutamate can also mediate slower, modulatory effects through a different class of receptors.

Peptides

Peptides are large-molecule chemicals that can function as neurotransmitters or neuromodulators. Most neurons that contain a neuropeptide also contain one of the classic small-molecule transmitters. For example, GABA-ergic striatal neurons that project to the globus pallidus also contain peptides, such as **enkephalin**, **endorphins**, and **substance P**. This suggests that a single synapse can mediate multiple effects. Many of these peptides consist of opioidlike compounds, and their projections are important in pain management.

Drug Treatment Principles

Drug treatment modifies the action of neurotransmitters at synapses either by blocking their effects or by simulating their actions. Two important principles explain the nature of drug treatment:

- **Blocking enzymatic breakdown or reuptake of a neurotransmitter.** Increasing the amount of neurotransmitter in the synaptic cleft increases the postsynaptic response to the neurotransmitter. For example, neostigmine, an anticholinesterase drug is used to impede acetylcholine breakdown by the enzyme acetylcholinesterase, allowing the level of available acetylcholine to rise. Anticholinesterase drugs are standard treatment for myasthenia gravis, which is characterized by weakness and fatigue of voluntary muscles and is caused by a reduced number of acetylcholine receptors in the postsynaptic membrane at the neuromuscular junctions.

- **Regulating the activity of the postsynaptic membrane.** One example is atropine, which is commonly used to dilate the pupil. The drug blocks the effects of the normally released acetylcholine on the constrictor fibers of the iris, thus causing pupil dilation. Another example is curare, which prevents the excitatory effects of acetylcholine on muscle fibers. South American Indians and other tribal hunters use the drug on their hunting arrows because curare causes paralysis by inhibiting the efferent impulses to muscles. Paralysis of the respiratory muscles ensures death by suffocation.

CLINICAL CONCERNS

Brain Tumors

A **neoplasm** (or tumor) refers to an uncontrolled growth of body tissue and glia. Tissue involved with a tumor may retain some of its original functions or may revert to a primitive functional state, depending on the severity of tissue infiltration. The underlying cause may have to do with an improper expression of **oncogenes** (coding proteins involved with cellular growth) and a loss of tumor-suppressor genes. What further adds to the growth of a tumor is **angiogenesis**, the formation of new blood vessels promoting growth in tumorous tissue.

Among the notable characteristics of brain tumors are their locations and rate of growth. A tumor can be **primary** or **metastatic**. *Primary* tumors arise from glia or meninges within the CNS. *Metastatic* tumors arise elsewhere in the body and spread to the brain from the area outside the brain. Most of the spreading tumors in the brain come from cancer of the breast and lung or from melanoma (malignant skin cells that contain melanin). This spread from the remote sources occurs through the lymphatics or blood vessels.

Moreover, tumors in the brain are either **malignant** (rapidly invasive) or **benign** (noninvasive). Most malignant tumors grow fast, invade the surrounding tissue, and are fatal. These tumorous tissues are often multifocal and microscopically undifferentiated from the surrounding tissues which makes it difficult to remove them. Malignancy is determined by grading a tumor on a scale (I–IV). Tumors with a low grade are benign, and their cells are segregated and are differentiable from the surrounding cells; higher-grade tumors are more malignant, and their tissue is undifferentiated from the surrounding areas.

Astrocytomas, **ependymoma**, and **oligodendrogliomas** are the common malignant tumors of the brain. *Astrocytomas* arise from astrocytes. Glioblastoma multiform, a type of astrocytoma, is the most malignant type of brain tumor; half of patients die within 18 months. *Ependymoma* arises from the ependymal cells lining the ventricles and obstructs the ventricular functions. *Oligodendrogliomas* arise from the oligodendroglia and are often seen in the frontal region of the adult brain.

Benign tumors grow slowly and do not infiltrate. The **meningiomas**, **acoustic neuromas**, **vestibular schwannomas**, and **pituitary adenomas** are common benign tumors of the brain. Slow-growing *meningiomas* arise from the meninges, which are the protective membranes of the brain and spinal cord. Meningiomas lead to increased intracranial pressure because they often affect the **falx cerebri** (fold of dura mater separating the two cerebral hemispheres) in the parasagittal space and the cerebral convexities. *Adenomas* of the pituitary glands cause hormonal dysfunctions and produce visual symptoms by compression of the **optic chiasm**. *Acoustic neuromas* and *vestibular schwannomas* arise from the nerve sheath and are located at the cerebellopontine angle. They contribute to the impairments of audition and equilibrium. By proximity to the lesion site, facial nerve involvement is commonly seen.

Symptoms of these tumors are related focally to the brain area affected. Tumors that initially involve the silent brain regions become symptomatic in later stages. Besides focal symptoms, common clinical symptoms of a brain tumor include progressive weakness, speech or visual loss, anomia, headache, impaired concentration, forgetfulness, and altered personality. The most notable complications of a tumor are seizures and increased intracranial pressure. Increased intracranial pressure, if not treated, can be fatal as it causes midline shift and cortical herniation. Medical treatment of tumors involves surgical excision, radiation therapy (γ-knife), and/or chemotherapy.

Multiple Sclerosis

Multiple sclerosis (MS), an autoimmune and degenerative condition, has been linked to viral infections and abnormalities in the immune system, which reacts improperly to antigens, causing antibodies to attack the myelin (Fig. 5-9). The myelin sheath degenerates, but the axon remains intact. The initial sparing of axons most likely accounts for the periods of remission (recovery) that occur in many cases. Haphazard demyelination and glial proliferation occur simultaneously, and the broken-up myelin is transported by microglial cells to the regional perivascular spaces. Intense proliferation of fibrous glia exceeds the ordinary reparative process; and as a result, the glia form dense plaques, or patches, predominantly at sites in the white matter of the brain and/or spinal cord. Plaques are a few millimeters to several centimeters in diameter. This has an effect on the speed of nerve conduction. In advanced cases, the plaques cause secondary degeneration of the axons, which in the

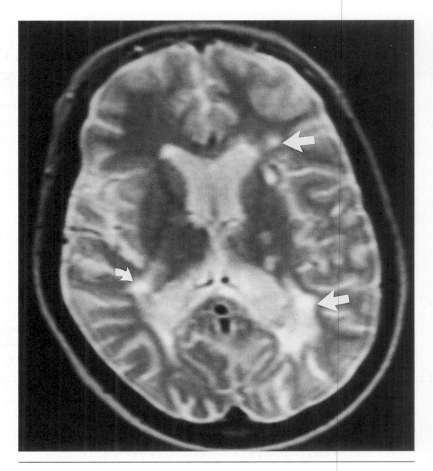

Figure 5-9 Multiple periventricular and deep white matter foci of abnormal increased signal (*arrows*) on an axial T2-weighted MRI study in a patient with multiple sclerosis.

spinal cord usually results in weakness and spasticity. In the brain, there is predilection for the plaques to occur in the region of the ventricles, brainstem, and cerebellar peduncles. In addition, the optic nerves and optic chiasm are sites of plaque formation. In time, brain plaques may cause axonal degeneration that may result in progressive neurologic symptoms.

These plaques usually begin in young adults of 30–40 years of age and are known for their slow evolution. More than 80% of patients exhibit a pattern marked by relapsing and remission of symptoms, at least in the early stages. As the oligodendroglia cells repair the damaged axonal membrane lesion site, a period of clinical symptoms is followed by recovery. However, as the disease progresses, axons also start degenerating, resulting in permanent and progressive sensorimotor disability. With a female to male ratio of 2:1, there are 30–60 cases per 100,000 people in the United States. The majority of patients survive for many years.

The symptoms are variable, depending on the part of the brain being affected. Early symptoms may be loss of vision, double vision, vertigo, loss of balance, weakness, and numbness in the limbs. Complaints of tremor, ataxia, speech impairment, dizziness, and disorders with urination appear later in the course of the disease. The diagnostic triad described by Charcot in 1862 (nystagmus, scanning speech, and intention tremor) is sometimes seen in the later stages of illness. Patients with MS are known to exhibit delayed or nonexistent evoked responses to visual, auditory, and somatic stimuli.

The exact antigen implicated in the immune attack seen in multiple sclerosis remains unknown. Nonetheless, pathogenesis seems to implicate cytokines, which are proteins that regulate the quality (intensity and duration) of an immune response within the plaque. An example is **tumor necrosis factor** α (TNF-α), which has also been identified as being associated with inflammation and demyelination; this raises hope that its inhibition might prevent and/or slow acute demyelination.

There is no known cure for multiple sclerosis; most of the treatment is symptomatic, addressing the inflammatory cascade described earlier. Treatment involves drug use for reducing pain, fatigue, and spasticity as well as antibiotics for infections. Corticosteroid drugs have been used to alleviate inflammatory symptoms, shorten attacks, and promote remission. Also, β-interferon injections are used to reduce the frequency and severity of new attacks and slow the progression of the disability by inhibiting the immune processes.

Myasthenia Gravis

Myasthenia gravis is a chronic disease characterized by fatigable muscle weakness that becomes worse with exercise and temporarily improves with rest. An impairment of impulse transmission is caused by a loss of acetylcholine receptors at the neuromuscular junction. In this autoimmune condition, antibodies bind to proteins that are normal components of one's own body. The antibodies bind with the acetylcholine receptors at motor end plates and prevent the normal effects of acetylcholine. Antibody binding also causes degeneration of the acetylcholine receptors so that lesser receptors remain on the muscle cells. The antibody-producing cells seem to recognize antigens derived from the thymus. About 50% of patients with myasthenia gravis have enlarged thymus glands.

Symptoms appear at any age. They are more prevalent in females during the first 30 years of life but, thereafter, are more prevalent in men. Onset is gradual, and muscles may be focally or generally involved. Weakness gets worse during the day and disappears after rest. The first signs of the disease often appear in constantly used muscles, such as the muscles of the eye and of respiration. Ptosis and diplopia are the most common early manifestations of the illness. Involvement of the cranial nerves also causes altered facial expression, regurgitation, choking, hypernasality, and a dropped jaw. A myasthenic crisis may occur from a sudden increase in severity of the weakness. Bulbar symptoms in which speech and breathing are involved along with generalized weakness require hospitalization and intensive care unit (ICU) management.

Diagnosis is made predominantly on clinical symptoms, the presence of serum antibodies to the acetylcholine receptor, and electrophysiologic testing. Improvement after testing with an anticholinesterase drug confirms the diagnosis. Drug treatment consists of anticholinesterase drugs, such as neostigmine (prostigmin) and pyridostigmine (Mestinon). These are known to inhibit acetylcholinesterase, allowing a higher concentration of the acetylcholine in the synaptic cleft. Overdoses of medication may result in cholinergic crises consisting of muscular fasciculation, salivation, and miosis (contraction of the pupil). Thymectomy may offer the best result in young women with disease of < 5 years in duration. Myasthenic crisis is treated best by plasmapheresis, steroids, or infusion of immunoglobulins in addition to admittance into an ICU. Prognosis is good for those patients in whom the disease is not progressive. Long periods of remission do occur, but some patients undergo a progressive course that may result in bulbar and respiratory paralysis.

CLINICAL CONSIDERATIONS

PATIENT ONE

A 60-year-old man went to see a neurologist with the complaint that he is easily tired. He needs rest even after a mild exertion. The neurologist who interviewed and examined the patient noted the following:

- A 6-month history of double vision
- Respiratory weakness with shallow breathing and limited vital capacity
- Near-normal muscular strength after rest
- Progressive weakness including slurred speech after a brief period of physical activity
- The neurologist suspected a myoneural disorder. This diagnosis was confirmed by the results of an edrophonium (Tensilon) test, in which administration of this drug improved the patient's physical strength.

Question: How can you relate this weakness after sustained physical activity to the diagnosed condition?

Discussion: In myasthenia gravis, the motor end plate is damaged by antibodies, which are directed against acetylcholine receptors and restrict muscle contraction. Because normal-appearing muscles fatigue with persistent motor tasks, such patients are subjected to stress testing. See any textbook on motor speech disorders for the effect of this condition on speech. Anticholinesterase drugs increase muscle strength by slowing the enzymatic destruction of acetylcholine at the myoneural junction.

PATIENT TWO

A 47-year-old woman with a 3-week history of double vision, numbness in the left leg, dizziness, and gait imbalance was taken to a hospital where the examining neurologist noted the following:

- A reported history of a 10-day episode of blindness and pain involving the right eye about 2 years ago
- Right optic nerve paleness
- Internuclear ophthalmoplegia (failure of adducting eyes in horizontal gaze)
- Decreased pinprick on the left lower abdomen down to the left knee
- Signs of mild cerebellar dysfunction involving the right extremities with gait ataxia
- Mild weakness of the left lower extremity

Brain MRI revealed multiple white matter hyperintensities, some perpendicular to the ventricles and one in the brainstem.

Question: Can you identify the associated disease?

Discussion: This is a case of demyelinating disease. A history of neurologic symptoms with reoccurrence exemplifies the clinical pattern of exacerbations and remissions. Multiple but random and separated hyperintense patches (plaques) of demyelination suggest this to be a case of multiple sclerosis. This condition affects speech and swallowing in its advanced stages.

PATIENT THREE

A 45-year-old woman complained of feeling tired and weak in her legs after short walks or small amount of motor activity. Her speech became unintelligible within a few minutes after talking. She was seen by a neurologist, who noted the following:

- Bilateral ptosis
- Incomplete lateral movement of the right eye
- Expressionless, droopy face
- Progressive and fatigable motor weakness
- Progressive speech unintelligibility after continuous speaking

Based on the patient's history, age, and progressive fatigue as well as improvement after the administration of a cholinergic drug (neostigmine), the neurologist suspected that this was a case of an autoimmune disorder, in which the patient's own immune system was attacking the postsynaptic receptor sites at the neuromuscular junction.

Question: This patient suffers from which of the following diseases?

a. Graduate school syndrome
b. Myasthenia gravis
c. Multiple sclerosis
d. Huntington chorea
e. Stroke

Discussion: This is a case of myasthenia gravis. In myasthenia gravis, elevated serum antibodies destroy the postsynaptic acetylcholine receptors of the myoneural junction. Thus the acetylcholine released in the synaptic cleft is not quantitatively adequate to activate the muscle

The muscle weakness is characterized by progressive fatigue. Neostigmine inhibits the enzyme that degrades acetylcholine in the synapse, thereby increasing the amount of acetylcholine for muscle function.

SUMMARY

The neuron is the fundamental unit of the nervous system. Its major characteristic is the ability to communicate within the nervous system, with other parts of the body, and with the environment. With billions of multisynaptic connections, the nerve cells serve higher mental functions that include memory, thinking, reasoning, calculation, and language. Neuroglial cells, which support and protect nerve

cells, are important in tissue repair and participate in phagocytizing cellular debris. Nerve cells communicate with one another through nerve impulses that represent all neuronal activity. The nerve impulses have a chemical component that underlies the electric potential of the cells. A neurotransmitter is a chemical substance released at a synapse that transmits signals across neurons. There are two types of transmitters in the nervous system: **small molecules** and **large molecules** (peptides). Small-molecule neurotransmitters include **acetylcholine**, **dopamine**, **norepinephrine**, **serotonin**, **glutamate**, and **GABA**. They are known to have short-lasting effects. Large-molecule peptides produce long-lasting effects on postsynaptic nerve cells.

QUIZ QUESTIONS

1. Define the following terms: action potential, astrocytes, autoimmune, axonal reaction, chromatolysis, glial cells, hyperplasia, hypertrophy, phagocyte, Wallerian degeneration

2. Define in one line each the pathophysiology of multiple sclerosis and myasthenia gravis.

3. Match each of the following numbered functions with its associated lettered neuroglia type.

   1. provide structural support for primary brain cells
   2. migrate to the site of lesion and seal the cavity or fill the cavity with scar tissue
   3. scavenger cells of the CNS that macrophage (digest) the debris in the area of infarct in the brain
   4. form the myelin sheath in the CNS
   5. line the ventricles and contribute to the blood–brain barrier
   6. form the myelin sheath in the PNS

   a. astrocytes
   b. oligodendrocytes
   c. microglia
   d. ependymal cells
   e. Schwann cells

4. Match each of the following neurotransmitters with its associated lettered neurotransmitter.

   1. acetylcholine
   2. dopamine
   3. norepinephrine

   a. As a major neurotransmitter in the PNS, it controls voluntary movements through its release by spinal or cranial motor fibers.
   b. Paucity of its secretion is associated with Parkinson disease.
   c. Neurotransmitter that plays a role in regulating sleep, attention, and moods.

4. GABA   d. An inhibitory neurotransmitter which is implicated with Huntington chorea.

TECHNICAL TERMS

acetylcholine
acetylcholinesterase
action potential
astrocytes
autoimmune
axon
axonal reaction

chromatolysis
cytologic
cytoplasm
dendrites
depolarization
dopamine
endoneurium

epineurium
excitatory postsynaptic potentials
GABA
glial cells
hyperplasia
hypertrophy
impulse
inhibitory postsynaptic potentials
locus ceruleus
macrophage
microglia
myelin

necrosis
nerve cell
Nissl bodies
node of Ranvier
norepinephrine
oligodendroglia
permeability
phagocyte
polarization
Schwann cells
serotonin
synapse
thymus
Wallerian degeneration

Diencephalon: Thalamus and Associated Structures

LEARNING OBJECTIVES

After studying this chapter, students should be able to:

- Identify major structures of the diencephalon and describe their functions

- Discuss the functional importance of the thalamus

- Identify the locations of major thalamic nuclei

- Describe the functions of major thalamic nuclei

- Describe afferent and efferent projections of major thalamic nuclei

- Relate thalamic nuclei to their corresponding cortical areas

- Discuss sensorimotor and higher mental functions of the thalamus

- Explain thalamic syndrome

GROSS ANATOMY OF THE DIENCEPHALON

The diencephalon, concealed beneath the cortex, has well-marked boundaries. On the anteroposterior axis, it extends from the **interventricular foramen** to the **posterior commissure**. The **cerebral cortex**, **lateral ventricle**, and fibers of the **corpus callosum** form the superior boundary, whereas the **third ventricle** marks the medial limit of the diencephalon. The **posterior limb of the internal capsule** is the lateral limit of the diencephalon; an arbitrary line drawn from the hypothalamic **mamillary bodies** to the **pineal gland** forms the ventral limit of the diencephalon (Fig. 6-1; see Figs. 2-11 and 2-18). The diencephalon is composed of four parts: **thalamus**, **epithalamus**, **subthalamus**, and **hypothalamus**.

The thalamus serves as an **integrator** and **gateway** for information projected to the forebrain. The *epithalamus,* the oldest part of the diencephalon, includes the *pineal gland* and is concerned with diurnal and autonomic bodily functions. The subthalamus, a small region ventral to the thalamus, is important in motor functions through its con-

nections with the brainstem, **basal ganglia**, and diencephalic structures. The *hypothalamus* is located below the thalamus. Functionally, it is part of the **autonomic nervous system (ANS)**, mediating endocrine and other metabolic states, such as body temperature, water balance, and sugar and fat metabolism. This chapter provides a simplified description of the thalamus, focusing on its anatomy and sensorimotor and cognitive functions.

THALAMUS

The thalamus, an ovoid nuclear mass, measures about 3 cm anteroposteriorly and 1.5 cm mediolaterally. It lies beneath the cortex in each hemisphere along the midsagittal line. The general location of the thalamus with respect to other surrounding structures can be seen on horizontal (see Figs. 2-15 and 2-18), coronal (Fig 6-1A; see Fig. 2-19), and midsagittal (Fig 6-1B; see Fig. 2-11) sections of the brain. Removal of the overlying roof of the third ventricle and of the lateral ventricles, including the corpus callosum and the cortical mantle, exposes the lateral extent of the dorsal thalamus. The anatomic boundaries of the thalamus are identical to those of the diencephalon, except that the ventral limit of the thalamus is marked midsagittally by the hypothalamic sulcus (Fig 6-1B; see Fig. 2-11).

Functionally, the thalamus is an important part of the basic neural circuitry, which involves thalamus–cerebral cortex–thalamic pathway. The reverberating circuits of this pathway provides means of both retaining information through time and projecting incoming information to other parts of the forebrain. The thalamus also receives constant feedback from the cortex.

Consisting of a collection of subcortical nuclei, the thalamus and its circuit serve three important functions. First, they channel the projections of sensory information entering the lower levels of the nervous system to specific cortical areas. Specific nuclei of the thalamus receive and channel the sensations of pain, taste, temperature, audition, and vision to the primary sensory areas in the cerebral cortex. Second, they integrate motor information and project information from the basal ganglia, limbic system, and cerebellum to the primary and premotor cortices (see Chapter 13). Third, with the brainstem reticular afferents and their multiple targets within the thalamic nuclei, the

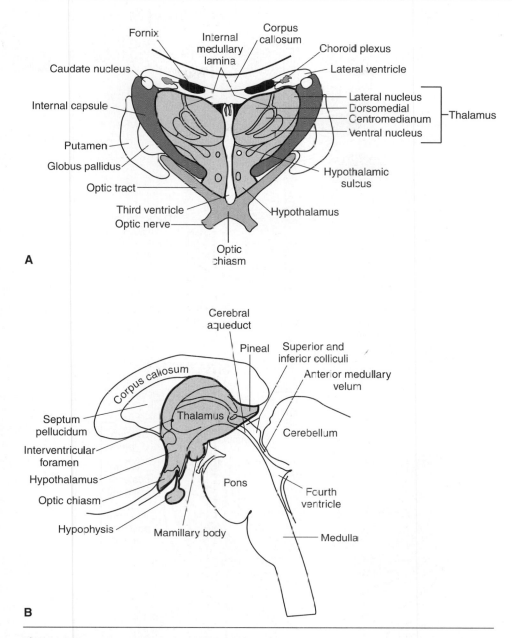

Figure 6-1 A. Coronal section of the brain showing the location of the diencephalon and its lateral and medial boundaries. B. Midsagittal section showing the general location of the diencephalon (*solid line*) and its rostral, ventral, and caudal boundaries.

thalamus and its circuit regulate functions of the associational cortex and regulate cortically mediated cognitive functions.

The thalamus is divided into many nuclei; each nucleus has bidirectional fiber connections to specific cortical areas. These thalamic connections form the thalamocortical functional units, which are involved in sensorimotor and cognitive functions. Some thalamic nuclei are known for their active participation in higher mental functions, whereas others, because of their anatomic connections, are presumed to participate in somatosensory functions, language, speech, and memory. Neuropathologic observations and histochemical techniques illustrating retrograde degen-

eration of the thalamic nuclei have helped researchers develop detailed maps of the nuclei and their projections to the cortex.

Thalamic Structure

The thalamus consists of three tiers of nuclei: **medial** (mediodorsal), **lateral**, and **ventral** (Fig. 6-2). Each tier contains multiple nuclei:

- Medial nuclear complex
  - Dorsomedial nucleus
  - Midline nuclear complex
- Lateral nuclear complex
  - Lateral dorsal nucleus

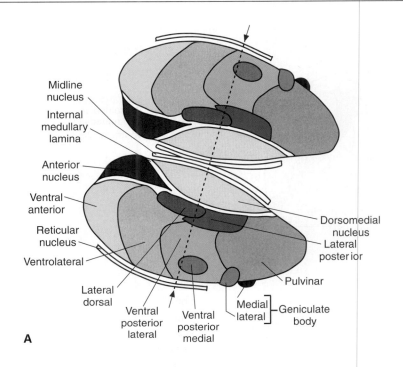

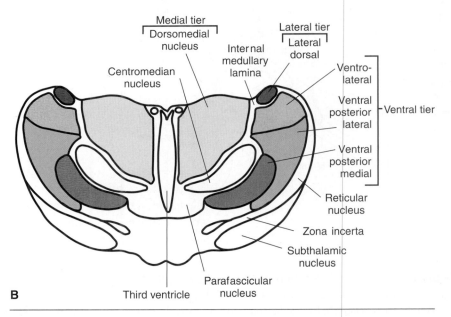

Figure 6-2 Thalamic anatomy. **A.** Dorsolateral view of the thalamus and its nuclei. **B.** Cross-section of the thalamus showing the three thalamic tiers (medial, lateral, and ventral) and their nuclei.

- Lateral posterior nucleus
- Pulvinar
- Ventral nuclear complex
  - Ventral anterior nucleus
  - Ventrolateral nucleus
  - Ventral posterior nucleus (lateral and medial)
  - Lateral geniculate body
  - Medial geniculate body

Additional nuclei are found in the thalamus:

- Anterior nucleus
- Reticular nucleus
- Intralaminar nuclei
  - Centromedianum nucleus
  - Parafascicular nucleus

The **internal medullary lamina**, a Y-shaped sheath of myelinated fibers, runs in a rostrocaudal fashion, dividing the thalamus into mediodorsal and lateral tiers (Fig. 6-1A). Rostrally, the two prongs of the internal medullary lamina surround the **anterior nucleus**; the stem of the internal medullary lamina splits posteriorly and contains the small **intralaminar nuclei**. The ventral tier of the thalamic nuclei is lateral and inferior to the lateral tier of the nuclei.

Projections and Functions of Thalamic Nuclei

The thalamus serves as the diencephalic component of the thalamic–cerebral cortex interactive system. Each thalamic nucleus receives definitive information from thalamic or extrathalamic structures (Fig. 6-3A) and screens the information before transmitting it to functionally related areas of the cortex (Figs. 6-3B and 6-4; Table 6-1). Familiarity with the afferent and efferent projections is

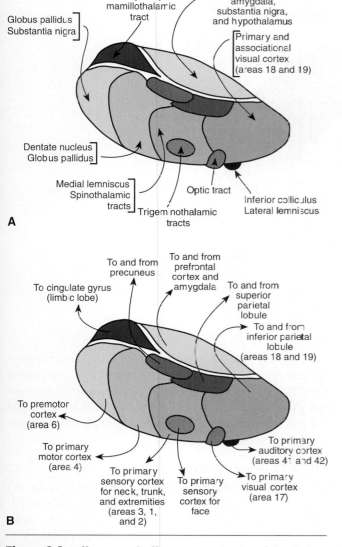

Figure 6-3 Afferent and efferent projections of the thalamic nuclei. **A.** The principal afferent projections of the major thalamic nuclei. **B.** The primary efferent thalamocortical projections of the important thalamic nuclei.

essential for understanding the importance of thalamic nuclei in sensorimotor, speech, language, and cognitive functions. These connections explain the rationale for selecting certain nuclei in stereotaxic management of intractable pain and movement disorders.

Medial Nuclear Complex

The medial nuclear complex consists of the **dorsomedial nucleus** and the **midline nuclear complex**.

Dorsomedial Nucleus

The dorsomedial (DM) nucleus is an enlarged nucleus in the human brain, occupying the area between the periventricular gray matter of the *third ventricle* and the *internal medullary lamina*. The **mammillothalamic tract**, with connections to the structures associated with memory and learning, such as the **mammillary bodies** and **hippocampus**, passes beneath this nucleus. The DM nucleus receives feedback from the primary cortical areas and distributes it to the cortical association areas. The reverberating network of this nucleus is involved with the development of emotion, judgment and reasoning, memory, language, and cognitive functions. The dorsal-level thalamic–cortical networks are also involved in sensory learning and motor learnings.

- **Afferent connection:** information is primarily received from the prefrontal cortex, hippocampus, centromedianus nucleus, orbitofrontal cortex, and hypothalamus.
- **Efferent projection:** bidirectional projections are primarily to the prefrontal and orbitofrontal cortices and limbic structures.

With projections to the prefrontal cortex and limbic structures, the DM nucleus integrates visceral information with affect, emotions, thought processes, personality, and judgment. The DM nucleus may also regulate mood, which can be pleasant, unpleasant, euphoric, or depressive, depending on the nature of the sensory input and stored experiences. Clinically, the destruction of the DM has resulted in lowering the threshold for rage. Surgical lesions in the DM have been used to ameliorate anxiety-related disorders in humans. Lesions in the DM have been associated with memory loss in patients with **Wernicke-Korsakoff syndrome**, a personality disorder caused by chronic alcoholism characterized by amnesia, disorientation, delirium, confabulations, and hallucinations. When injury to this area involves memory, it likely involves the underlying fibers of the mammillothalamic tract, which contain projections from the mammillary bodies and hippocampus, structures closely related with memory functions.

Midline Nuclear Complex

The midline nuclear complex, an important visceral nucleus, is a diffuse and less distinct cluster of nuclei above the hypothalamus in the *periventricular walls* of the *third ventricle*. The nuclei lie in the region of the **massa intermedia fibers** and bridge the gray matter across the third ventricle.

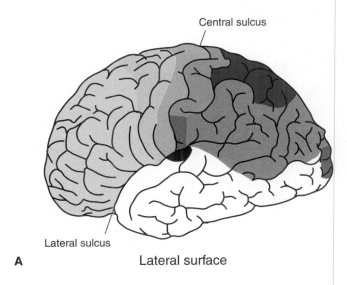

A   Lateral surface

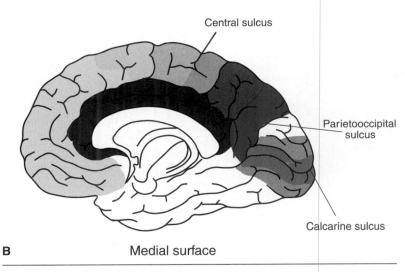

B   Medial surface

Figure 6-4 Lateral (A) and midsagittal (B) surfaces of the left hemisphere locating the areas of the thalamocortical projections shown in Figures 6-2 and 6-3.

- **Afferent connection:** The midline nuclear complex receives information from the brainstem reticular formation.
- **Efferent projection:** With projection to the cingulate gyrus and the hypothalamus, this nucleus is known to serve important visceral functions.

Lateral Nuclear Complex

The lateral nuclear complex is a narrow cellular strip on the dorsolateral surface of the thalamus. It consists of three nuclei: **lateral dorsal nucleus**, **lateral posterior nucleus**, and **pulvinar**, arranged in rostrocaudal fashion.

Lateral Dorsal Nucleus

The functions and connections of the lateral dorsal (LD) nucleus are poorly understood. This nucleus is immedi-

ately caudal to the anterior nucleus, and it has reciprocal connections with the medial **parietal lobe** (precuneus gyrus). It also receives afferents from the posterior **cingulate gyrus**. Its connections with the parietal and *cingulate* cortices suggest that the LD nucleus is likely to contribute to visceral–sensory integration.

Lateral Posterior Nucleus

The lateral posterior (LP) nucleus lies caudal to the LD nucleus, and its functions are inadequately understood. It receives information from the adjacent thalamic nuclei and is reciprocally connected to the **superior parietal lobule**. As a multisensory receiving area, the superior parietal lobule is concerned with the integration and transcoding of multiple sensory modalities underlying higher mental functions.

Table 6-1

Thalamic Nuclei: Afferent and Efferent Projections and Major Functions

Thalamic Nucleus	Afferents From	Efferents To	Major Functions
Medial nuclear complex			
Dorsomedial nucleus	Prefrontal cortex, substantia nigra, amygdala, and hypothalamus	Prefrontal cortex and amygdala	Integrates visceral information with affect, emotions, thought processes, and judgment
Midline nuclear complex	Brainstem reticular formation	Cingulate gyrus and hypothalamus	Regulates visceral functions
Lateral nuclear complex			
Lateral dorsal nucleus	Posterior cingulate gyrus (precuneus)	Precuneus region	May serve visceral–sensory integration
Lateral posterior nucleus	Adjacent thalamic nuclei and superior parietal lobule	Superior parietal lobule	Participates in integrating and transcoding multiple sensory modalities underlying higher mental functions
Pulvinar	Primary and associational visual cortex; inferior parietal lobule	Inferior parietal lobule	Contributes to language functions: formulation, language processing, lexical properties, reading, and writing
Ventral nuclear complex			
Ventral anterior nucleus	Globus pallidus and substantia nigra	Premotor cortex and primary motor cortex	Facilitates skilled movements; initiates voluntary movements
Ventrolateral nucleus	Dentate nucleus and globus pallidus (basal ganglia)	Primary motor cortex	Coordinates and integrates voluntary motor functions
Ventral posterior nucleus Lateral	Medial lemniscus and spinothalamic tracts	Primary sensory cortex Upper 2/3rds	Relays somatosensory (protopathic, epicritic) sensation from neck, trunk, and extremities
Medial	Trigeminothalamic tracts	Lower third of the primary sensory cortex	Relays somatosensory (protopathic, epicritic) sensation from face
Lateral geniculate body	Optic tract	Primary visual cortex	Relays visual information
Medial geniculate body	Inferior colliculus and lateral lemniscus	Brodmann areas 41–42; primary and association auditory cortex	Relays auditory information
Anterior nucleus	Mamillary body of hypothalamus via mamillothalamic tract	Cingulate gyrus (limbic lobe)	Mediates visceral and emotional information
Reticular nucleus	Cortex thalamus and reticular formation	Thalamic nuclei, including reticular formation	Integrates (presumably) and regulates thalamic neuronal activity
Intralaminar nuclei, centromedium nucleus	Globus pallidus; vestibular nucleus; superior colliculus; brainstem reticular formation; spinal cord (pain and sensory); and motor, premotor, and prefrontal cortices	Basal ganglia and thalamus	Modulates excitability of cortex (related to cognitive functions) and overall function of basal ganglia (related to sensorimotor functions)

Pulvinar

The pulvinar, the most posterior portion of the thalamus and the largest thalamic nucleus, lies caudally in the lateral division.

- **Afferent connection:** The pulvinar receives its major projections from the primary and associational visual cortices, superior colliculus, and the visual reflex center in the midbrain. The pulvinar is also connected with other thalamic nuclei.
- **Efferent projection:** The outgoing projections of the pulvinar terminate in the inferior association cortex of the parietal lobule. This cortical region includes important structures, such as the **angular** and **supramarginal gyri**.

With projections to the parietal lobe, the pulvinar makes contributions to higher mental functions, including language formulation, language processing, lexical properties, reading, and writing. The association of some of these linguistic functions with the pulvinar has been identified by stereotaxic exploration of the subcortex (Ojemann et al. 1968).

Ventral Nuclear Complex

The ventral nuclear complex relays information from sensory surfaces to the sensory cortex and provides feedback from the motor system effectors (muscles and joints) to the primary and secondary motor cortices. This neuronal circuitry is continuously involved in sustained cortical activity related to sensation and precise motor control. The ventral nuclear complex consists of five primary nuclei: **ventral anterior nucleus**, **ventrolateral nucleus**, **ventral posterior nucleus**, **lateral geniculate body**, and **medial geniculate body**. The boundaries of these nuclei are not clearly demarcated, and the structures are known to have many overlapping fibers. This nuclear complex serves as the relay center for specific sensory and motor information.

Ventral Anterior Nucleus

The ventral anterior (VA) nucleus lies in the most rostral area of the ventral nuclear complex.

- **Afferent connection:** It receives input from the inner segment of the **globus pallidus** via the **ansa lenticularis** and the **fasciculus lenticularis** (see Chapter 13). Other afferent fibers to the VA nucleus come from the **substantia nigra**, **intralaminar**, and midline thalamic nuclei.
- **Efferent projection:** The outgoing projections of the VA nucleus extend to the premotor cortex (Brodmann area 6) and primary motor cortex (Brodmann area 4). The premotor cortex facilitates skilled and sequential movements, and the primary motor cortex is responsible for initiating voluntary movements.

Ventrolateral Nucleus

The ventrolateral (VL) nucleus lies in the medial portion of the ventral nuclear complex, and it is important in the regulation of volitional movements.

- **Afferent connection:** As a motor relay nucleus, the VL nucleus receives fibers from the contralateral cerebellar hemisphere via the **superior cerebellar peduncle**. Additional inputs are received from the inner segment of the *globus pallidus* via the fibers of the *ansa lenticularis* and *fasciculus lenticularis* (see Chapter 13).
- **Efferent projection:** The VL nucleus projects to the primary motor cortex, which is responsible for initiating all voluntary movements. This nucleus is important in coordinating different aspects of motor functions because it integrates input from the basal ganglia (caudate nucleus, putamen, and globus pallidus) with feedback from the cerebellum before projecting the integrated information to the motor cortex.

The projections of the VL nucleus directly contribute to voluntary motor tasks; a disruption of this projection results in motor abnormalities (dyskinesia). This nucleus, because of its role in relating the basal ganglia to the motor cortex, has consistently been targeted for stereotaxic management of movement disorders.

Ventral Posterior Nucleus

The ventral posterior nucleus occupies the entire posterior half of the *ventral nuclear* mass, and it consists of two areas: **ventral posterior lateral** and **ventral posterior medial nuclei**. Both these nuclei serve as thalamic relay centers for somatosensory (protopathic and epicritic) sensation from the body and face (see Chapter 7).

Ventral Posterior Lateral Nucleus

The ventral posterior lateral (VPL) nucleus is the sensory relay nucleus that relays information related to somatic sensation from the body.

- **Afferent connection:** It receives sensations of pain, temperature, and discriminative touch from the body via the **ventral** and **lateral spinothalamic tracts** and the **medial lemniscus**.
- **Efferent projection:** The efferent fibers mediate the sensory information to the dorsal two-thirds of the primary somesthetic cortex in the postcentral gyrus (Brodmann areas 3, 1, 2), in which sensory information pertaining to all modalities is analyzed.

Ventral Posterior Medial Nucleus

The ventral posterior medial (VPM) nucleus is lateral to the **centromedianus nucleus** and medial to the VPL nucleus. It serves as the thalamic sensory relay center for the sensations of taste, pain, temperature, and discriminative touch for the head and face.

- **Afferent connection:** The VPM nucleus receives information from the secondary fibers of the **trigeminal (CNI) nerve**, which serves the face, head, and neck. It also receives projections from the gustatory (taste) nucleus in the brainstem.

- **Efferent projection:** This nucleus projects sensory information to the lower third of the primary somesthetic cortex in the postcentral gyrus region, where sensory information reaches consciousness and is analyzed.

The projection fibers from the ventral posterior complex travel through the **internal capsule** and extend to the primary somesthetic cortex in the parietal lobe. Even though cortical participation is necessary for the refinement of these sensations and their interpretation in the context of previous experiences, some awareness of pain, temperature, and discriminative touch sensations has been demonstrated at the thalamic level.

Lateral Geniculate Body

The lateral geniculate body (LGB), beneath the pulvinar, is the thalamic relay center for the sensation of vision.

- **Afferent connection:** Afferents to the LGB mediate the visual information from half of the visual field of each eye. These fibers originate from the ganglion cells in the temporal half of the retina from the ipsilateral eye and the medial (nasal) half of the retina from the contralateral eye, and they carry a point-to-point projection of the retina to the *LGH*.
- **Efferent projection:** The **geniculocalcarine fibers** from the LGB terminate in the upper and lower lips of the **calcarine fissure**, which is the **primary visual cortex**, also known as Brodmann area 17 (see Chapter 8).

Medial Geniculate Body

The medial geniculate body (MGB) is the circular area on the posterior surface of the thalamus beneath the pulvinar; it is the relay center for audition.

- **Afferent connection:** The afferent fibers to the MGE come from the **organ of Corti** in each ear via the fibers of the *lateral lemniscus* and brachium of the **inferior colliculus**.
- **Efferent projection:** The fibers leaving the MGB constitute auditory radiations (**geniculo-Heschl fibers**) traveling through the *internal capsule* and terminating in the primary auditory cortex on the superior surface of the lateral fissure, the transverse the gyrus of Heschl (Brodmann area 41, 42).

Additional Nuclei in the Thalamus
Anterior Nucleus

The anterior nucleus protrudes as an anterior tubercle in the floor of the *lateral ventricle* and is surrounded by the forks of the *internal medullary lamina*. The anterior nucleus is functionally related to the **limbic brain** (hippocampus, dentate gyrus, cingulate gyrus, and hypothalamus) and, in part, contributes to digestive, respiratory, urogenital, emotional, and endocrine functions.

- **Afferent connection:** The anterior nucleus receives information from the ipsilateral and contralateral *mamillary bodies* of the hypothalamus through the **mamillothalamic**

tract; the mamillary bodies in turn receive information from the **reticular formation**, **hippocampus**, and **septum pellucidum** via the **fornix**.
- **Efferent projection:** The efferent cortical projection of the anterior nucleus passes through the anterior limb of the *internal capsule* to the **cingulate gyrus**, a limbic structure.

Functionally, besides mediating visceral and emotional information, the anterior nucleus also regulates the hypothalamic and limbic influence on the **neocortex**. Mammillary (hypothalamic) afferents to the anterior nucleus also imply its role in memory function because the degeneration of the mammillary bodies is usually noted in alcoholics as part of **Wernicke-Korsakoff syndrome**. Electrical stimulation and its ablation induce changes in blood pressure, anxiety levels, and emotional drive.

Reticular Nucleus

The reticular nucleus consists of a thin, structurally invisible layer of nerve cells that covers the entire lateral thalamus and is located between the **external medullary lamina** of the thalamus and the internal capsule. This nuclear complex consists of neurons that are similar to those in the brainstem reticular formation and the intralaminar (centromedianus) nuclei. These scattered thalamic nuclei receive input from virtually all ascending systems as well as from other thalamic nuclei. With collateral afferents from thalamocortical and corticothalamic projections, it consists of diffuse projections to the cortex. Along with the intralaminar nucleus, the reticular nucleus is involved with attention related to wakefulness and to sensory input. This nucleus is thought to integrate and regulate thalamic neuronal activity and influence cortical functions by facilitating the thalamocortical relay.

Intralaminar Nuclei

The **intralaminar nuclear complex** consists of several nuclei interspersed in the core of the internal medullary lamina (Fig. 6-2). The centromedianum nucleus and **parafascicular nucleus**, two important intralaminar nuclei, indirectly contribute to the diffuse reticular–brain activation system.

- **Afferent connection:** The intralaminar complex receives afferents from the globus pallidus, vestibular nucleus, superior colliculus, and most importantly, the brainstem reticular formation. The centromedianum and parafascicular nuclei also receive cortical afferents from the motor, premotor, and prefrontal cortical areas. The rostral intralaminar complex receives input from the brainstem reticular formation, and pain and other sensory inputs from the spinal cord.
- **Efferent projection:** The intralaminar nuclei predominantly project to the basal ganglia (putamen and caudate) and sparsely to the entire cerebral cortex.

The intralaminar system as a whole influences the excitability of the association cortex with both its intrathalamic projections and striate collaterals to the cortex. Thus the thalamic intralaminar system is in a prime position to modulate the excitability and overall function of both the cortex and basal ganglia related to sensorimotor and cognitive functions. Intralaminar nuclei, in particular the centromedianus, are also known to evoke a cortical recruiting response when directly stimulated with electrical impulses (Bhatnagar and Mandybur 2005; Bhatnagar et al. 1989, 1990a, 1990b). The stimulation of the centromedianum nucleus has been noted to have positively affected human performance in many cortically mediated higher mental functions involving the frontal, parietal, cingulate, and orbital areas of the association cortex.

FUNCTIONAL CLASSIFICATION OF THE THALAMIC NUCLEI

In accordance with the source of the afferent fibers, cortical projections, and type of the mediated information, the thalamic nuclei can be functionally classified as either specific or nonspecific. This classification scheme simplifies the thalamic anatomy and helps in learning the nuclei and their functions.

Specific Thalamic Nuclei

The **specific sensory nuclei** receive definitive information and project it to specific cortical areas. Based on the source and nature of the transmitted information, the specific nuclei are further divided into **primary sensory**, **secondary sensory**, and **association sensory nuclei**.

Primary sensory nuclei receive specific sensory information as follows: The LGB receives visual input from both eyes and projects it to the visual cortex. The MGB receives tonotopic information from both ears and transmits it to the primary auditory cortex. The VPL nucleus receives sensations of pain, temperature, and discriminative touch from the body and relays them to the somatosensory cortex. The VPM nucleus receives sensations of pain, touch, and temperature from the face and projects them to the somatosensory cortex.

Secondary sensory nuclei receive information from specific subcortical structures and project it to well-defined cortical zones as follows: The VA nucleus receives information from the globus pallidus, substantia nigra, and intralaminar nuclei and projects it to the premotor cortex and intralaminar nuclei. The VL nucleus receives motor-specific information from the cerebellum and globus pallidus and projects it to the primary motor cortex. The anterior nucleus receives information from the mamillary bodies of the hypothalamus and sends it to the cingulate gyrus, a limbic structure. The DM nucleus sends projections from the substantia nigra, hypothalamus, and amygdala to the prefrontal cortex, which regulates personality and intellectual functions.

Association sensory nuclei receive input from other adjacent thalamic nuclei and project it to associational areas of the cortex. They include the pulvinar, with projections to the inferior parietal lobule (the area important for integration of crossed sensory modality and sensorimotor information), and the LP, with projections to the superior parietal lobule.

Nonspecific Thalamic Nuclei

The **nonspecific nuclei** receive general, diffuse information from cortical areas, basal ganglia, and reticular information and project diffusely to the cortical areas, basal ganglia, and specific thalamic nuclei. For example, the intralaminar thalamic nuclei diffusely project to the cortex and control the rhythmic electrical activity of the brain.

EPITHALAMUS

The epithalamus consists of two small structures: **habenular nucleus** and pineal gland (see Figs. 2-15 and 16-6). The cone-shaped pineal gland, an endocrine structure, renders an inhibitory influence over gonadal (sex gland) functions. It also secretes melatonin in response to the day–night cycle (as sensed by the visual system), regulates diurnal rhythms of the brain, and controls endocrinic activity related to the sleep cycle. Located lateral to the pineal gland, the habenular nuclei—with afferent and efferent projections to the anterior hypothalamus, limbic lobe, orbital cortex, and brainstem reticular formation—serve autonomic functions, such as emotional experiences and drives, and possibly the sense of smell.

SUBTHALAMUS

Subthalamic structures, although anatomically included in the diencephalon, are functionally related to the basal ganglia and are discussed in Chapter 13 (see Figs. 13-3, 13-6, and 3-23). The *subthalamus* refers collectively to several nuclei between the thalamus and the midbrain. The subthalamus includes primarily the subthalamic nucleus and secondarily the **prerubral** (**fields of Forel**, or **H fields**) **area** and **zona incerta**.

The subthalamic nucleus is connected to the globus pallidus via bidirectional fibers, and it makes substantial contributions to motor functions. A lesion in this nucleus results in contralateral hemiballism, a motor disorder characterized by involuntary violent, flinging movements that persist during wakefulness but disappear during sleep (see Chapter 13).

The fields of Forel are the prerubral region through which various motor fibers pass before terminating in the thalamus (see Fig. 13-5). The zona incerta lies in the subthalamus between the thalamic and the lenticular fasciculi. It receives projections from the motor cortex. By projecting motor information to the superior colliculus and pretectal area, the zona incerta functions as a visuomotor coordinator.

HYPOTHALAMUS

The hypothalamus contains important nuclei and a tract that forms the crossroads among the limbic system, brainstem, and thalamus. Located below the thalamus, it forms the ventrolateral walls of the *third ventricle*. It includes many specific nuclei and several structures, such as the **optic chiasm**, mamillary bodies, **hypophysis (pituitary gland)**, **infundibular stem (pituitary stalk)**, and **tuber cinereum** (see Chapter 16). The hypothalamus is a functionally unique organ because its afferents and efferents involve two modes of communication: neural and hormonal. Using the neural impulses, the hypothalamus connects with the brain and spinal structures; the hormonal efferents, mostly regulated by the pituitary gland, allow the hypothalamus to communicate with the body by releasing proteins into the blood circulation. This acts as a weak blood–brain barrier, and the proteins released influence body activity (see Chapter 17).

Closely connected with the forebrain and the limbic system, the hypothalamus serves three partly overlapping functions. First, it serves as the control center for the ANS. Second, it controls endocrinic activities through neurophysis by means of neurosecretions; the neurosecretions control important metabolic activities of the body and provide for homeostatic states. Third, it regulates body temperature, water and food intake, sugar metabolism, sexual behavior, and emotional state (e.g., feelings of well-being, anger, and aggression). Lesions in the hypothalamus result in diabetes insipidus, which is characterized by increased urinary output and excessive thirst, disturbances of temperature control and food and water intake, and hormonal abnormalities.

COGNITIVE FUNCTIONS OF THE THALAMUS

The belief that the thalamus plays only a precognitive sensorimotor role is no longer accepted. In the past 40 years, evidence from neurolinguistic and neurosurgical research has shown that some language and speech functions, along with cognitive processes, are asymmetrically lateralized at the thalamic level. In addition, a less discussed fact is that the thalamus mediates overall cortical alertness, information flow, and tuning of cortical structures. The thalamus, in conjunction with adjacent basal ganglia structures, participates in speech and language processing.

Penfield and Roberts (1959) first proposed that the thalamus, with its extensive projections, integrates speech and language functions. More recently, radiographic images have helped identify many cases of spontaneous thalamic lesions with subsequent aphasic disturbances. Using data from patients with hemorrhage in the dominant thalamus, investigators have found persisting aphasic symptoms, such as verbal paraphasia, anomia, and jargon, with otherwise

intact comprehension and repetition. Evidence supporting thalamic participation in language function has also come from intraoperative language and speech testing by the focal stimulation of the thalamic nuclei, which was used for functional mapping during stereotactic operations. Stereotactic destructive lesions in the ventrolateral nucleus and pulvinar of the thalamus for the treatment of dyskinetic behavior further supports the belief that there are language-specific functions in the left dominant thalamus (Ojemann 1983). Evaluation of language function in patients with lesions in the left VL thalamic nucleus and the pulvinar revealed transient and lasting aphasia, including naming disturbances, speech-related disorders, and reduced word fluency.

Thalamic stimulation has been found to facilitate verbal recall (Bhatnagar and Andy 1989; Bhatnagar and Mandybur 2005; Bhatnagar et al. 1989, and 1990a, 1990b). Facilitatory effects have been noted on verbal memory, lexical retrieval, and nonverbal functions from stimulation of the left centromedianus, a neurolinguistically unexplored and previously unimplicated intralaminar thalamic nucleus. Some facilitatory effects on verbal memory were also found after stimulation of the right centromedianum nucleus, but they were not as dramatic as the ones observed from the stimulation of the left centromedianus (Bhatnagar et al. 1990a).

In at least one case, the mechanical intraoperative perturbation of the left thalamus, preparatory to a therapeutic lesion placed for chronic pain, resulted in the elicitation of stutter-like syllabic reiterations (Andy and Bhatnagar, 1991). It is interesting that stimulation in the same area of the intralaminar thalamic nuclei in four neurosurgical patients also led to the amelioration of acquired stuttering (Andy and Bhatnagar, 1992). This thalamic influence on cortically mediated higher mental functions has been judged to be a facilitatory one.

THALAMIC SYNDROME

Although the most discriminating analysis of somatosensory information and its integration with tactile, visual, and auditory information occurs in the sensory cortex at the parietal lobe, crude sensations of pain, touch, temperature, vibration, and taste can be appreciated at the thalamic level. Thalamic syndrome (depending on the location and extent of the lesion) is characterized by increased or decreased thresholds for the sensations of touch, pain, and temperature on the contralateral half of the body. Thalamic pathologies may alter the perception of somatic sensation for some patients, so that a contact with a wisp of cotton can be quite painful. In other cases, the threshold to pain is high; but once that threshold is reached, the sensation is exaggerated and more painful than normal. For example, a pinprick may provoke a burning sensation of pain, and pleasant musical tones may sound like uncomfortable discord. The pain associated with thalamic syndrome is usually poorly localized and intractable to analgesic agents. Paraesthesias, such as the sensation of ants crawling on the skin, also occur.

Linguistically impaired motor speech (dysarthria), anomia, and a variable degree of reading and writing disorders have been observed to occur after thalamic lesions (Alexander 1989). Emotional responses, such as laughing and crying inappropriately, may accompany thalamic syndrome, which most commonly results from the occlusion of the thalamogeniculate branch of the posterior cerebral artery.

CLINICAL CONSIDERATIONS

PATIENT ONE

A 45-year-old man fell while taking a shower. His wife found him on the floor, fully conscious. Realizing that something was not right, she advised him to take a rest. Within a few hours, his speech was unintelligible. He also developed weakness and pain in his right arm. At this point, the woman drove her husband to the hospital emergency room, where the attending physician noted the following signs:

- Paresis in the right arm
- Severe pain in the right shoulder and arm
- Lowered pain threshold (a slight touch to the arm caused excruciating pain sensation)
- Dysphonia and imprecise articulation
- Word-finding deficit
- Good auditory comprehension

The presence of sensorimotor impairments without any sign of aphasia led the physician to suspect a subcortical lesion. The brain MRI study revealed a left thalamic cerebrovascular accident.

Question: How can you relate these symptoms with the thalamic pathology?

Discussion: A CVA in this patient affected the posterior region of the left thalamus, which affected the following:

- The weakness in the arm and speech muscles resulted from the interruption of adjacent motor fibers in the internal capsule.
- Severe pain sensation resulted from the overreaction of the primitive pain mechanism secondary to the lesion.
- Involvement of the thalamocortical (parietal lobe) projections account for anomia, which is commonly seen in patients with thalamic syndrome.

PATIENT TWO

A 55-year-old female truck driver suddenly experienced difficulty seeing while driving. She made an appointment with a neurologist, who noted the following:

- Left homonymous hemianopia, manifested as loss of vision in the temporal field of the left eye and nasal field of the right eye
- Difficulty with localizing sound sources and directions
- Some difficulty in understanding others during conversation
- Normal pure tone threshold
- Normal visual acuity
- No involvement of speech, language, or cognitive functions

The brain MRI study revealed a small lesion involving the lateral-posterior area of the right thalamus.

Question: How can you relate these symptoms with the thalamic nuclei that is most likely to be involved?

Discussion: This is an involvement of the geniculate bodies (LGB and MGB), which are located in the lateral-posterior area of the thalamus and mediate vision and audition, respectively. The involvement of the LGB resulted in the loss of the left visual field. The involvement of the MGB contributed to central auditory processing deficits, marked by a normal hearing threshold but impaired processing and reduced ability to identify the direction of sound.

PATIENT THREE

A 55-year-old man presented with slurred and slow to articulate speech and numbness but no pain sensation in his mouth. The brain MRI study revealed a small infarct in the caudal-ventral-posterior thalamic region.

Question: Of the following thalamic nuclei that mediate somatosensation from the face, which is likely to be involved?

- ventrolateral
- ventral anterior
- ventral posterior lateral
- ventral posterior medial
- lateral dorsal

Discussion: The ventral posterior medial nucleus receives trigeminal afferents mediating pain, touch, and temperature from the face and projects to the lower third of the postcentral gyrus region. Impaired articulatory precision is related to altered proprioceptive afferents.

PATIENT FOUR

A 70-year-old patient with Parkinson disease, with a deep brain stimulator involving the left VL thalamic nucleus, was seen by a speech language pathologist (SLP) for speech unintelligibility. The goal of the implant was to modulate thalamic-cortical projections.

Question: Which of the cortical areas, exclusively receiving afferents from the VL, was likely to be affected?

- Brodmann area 4
- Brodmann area 17
- Brodmann areas 9–10
- Brodmann areas 41–42
- Brodmann areas 3, 1, 2

Discussion: The primary motor cortex (Brodmann area 4) receives projections from the ventrolateral thalamic nucleus.

SUMMARY

The diencephalon, between the telencephalon and midbrain, consists of four major structures: thalamus, subthalamus, epithalamus, and hypothalamus. The thalamus, the largest and the most prominent diencephalic nucleus, serves as the sensorimotor relay center to screen all sensory and motor information before channeling it to the cerebral cortex. The thalamus is divided into many functionally specific nuclei, and each of these nuclei makes direct anatomic projections to corresponding functional areas of the neocortex. The subthalamus is important in the organization of motor functions and is functionally related to the basal ganglia. The epithalamus, the oldest part of the diencephalon, consists of the habenular nucleus and pineal gland. The pineal gland, an endocrine organ, mediates its influence on sex glands and diurnal rhythm. The hypothalamus is a major diencephalic structure for controlling activities of the autonomic and endocrine systems.

QUIZ QUESTIONS

1. Define the following terms: diencephalon, hypothalamus, subthalamus, thalamus

2. Label the major thalamic nuclei.

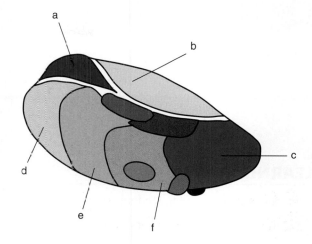

3. Match each of the following numbered thalamic nuclei with its associated lettered statement.

1. ventral lateral
2. ventral anterior
3. pulvinar
4. dorsal medial
5. anterior nucleus
6. lateral geniculate body

7. medial geniculate body

a. precentral gyrus
b. premotor cortex
c. inferior parietal lobule
d. prefrontal cortex
e. cingulate gyrus
f. primary auditory cortex (gyrus of Heschl)
g. primary visual cortex (calcarine cortex)

TECHNICAL TERMS

analgesia
diencephalon
epithalamus
hypothalamus

nonspecific nuclei
specific nuclei
subthalamus
thalamus

Somatosensory System

LEARNING OBJECTIVES

After studying this chapter, students should be able to:

- List the major modalities of sensation

- Relate receptor types to corresponding modalities of sensation

- Explain the three-neuron organization for somatic sensation

- Describe the neural pathways for the epicritic systems of the face and body

- Describe the neural pathways for the protopathic systems of the face and body

- Describe the neural pathways of conscious and unconscious proprioception

- Outline common disorders of sensation

- Explain the concepts and mechanisms of referred and phantom pain

- Relate various somatosensory disorders to plausible lesion sites

- Explain the rationale for assessing somatic sensation

SOMATOSENSATION

Somatosensation refers to the bodily experienced sensations of pain, temperature, touch, and **proprioception**. It begins with specialized receptors in the skin, muscles, joints, and blood vessels that convert sensory stimuli to neural signals and transmit them to the **parietal lobe**. Localized receptors in the skin and muscles feed into a single sensory nerve fiber, many of which combine to form a fiber bundle.

The **afferent** (sensory) **fiber bundle** joins the **spinal efferent** (motor) **fiber bundle** to form a **spinal nerve** (see Fig. 2-32). Closer to the spinal cord, however, the afferent and efferent fiber bundles separate, forming **dorsal and ventral spinal nerve fibers** (Fig. 7-1). There are two types of afferent nerve fibers that have their cell bodies in the **dorsal root ganglion** (**DRG**). Only stretch afferent neuronal terminals (A1) synapse with a lower motor neuron (LMN) den-

drite or cell body and mediate the stretch reflex. The LMN circuitry not only distributes to local (segmental and intersegmental) reflex output but also integrates other ongoing output activity descending from the higher central nervous system (CNS) levels. All other afferents terminate in the dorsal horn association nucleus.

The dorsal horn circuitry modifies and integrates the input information before distributing collaterals to the brainstem **reticular formation**, the upper sensory centers on the opposite side, and the rostral intersegmental reflex circuits. The ascending fibers carry information regarding pain, touch, temperature, and sense of position and travel through the **spinal cord**, **brainstem**, and **thalamus**. The information is then projected to the **primary sensory** (**postcentral gyrus**) and the **associational sensory** (**superior parietal lobule**) cortices in the parietal lobe. The primary cortex analyzes information for a conscious perception of the sensation. In the sensory associational region, on the other hand, the lower-order tactile sensations are analyzed, elaborated on, integrated with previous experiences, and raised to the highest conscious level for cognitive functions. The somatosensory system is discretely organized; each tract separately mediates its respective modalities of sensation, which maintains the point-to-point representation of its corresponding body surface (**somatotopic organization**). The higher cognitive functions of the parietal lobe are discussed in Chapter 19.

Knowledge of the **sensory receptors**, **ascending paths** taken by sensory fibers, **points of fiber crossing**, and **cortical areas** related to underlying conscious perception provides the groundwork for understanding somatosensory organization. This knowledge not only helps us examine the modalities of pain, touch, and temperature but also helps us relate patterns of sensory deficits to lesion sites in the central pathways.

Types of Sensation

The somatic senses are divided into three primary types: **mechanoreceptive**, **thermoreceptive**, and **nociceptive** (Table 7-1). *Mechanoreception* implies the mechanical displacement of the nerve endings and includes touch, pressure, vibration (tactile), and **kinesthesia** (limb position and movement). Touch is further divided into **fine discriminative** (**localizable**) and **diffuse** (**unlocalizable**) types.

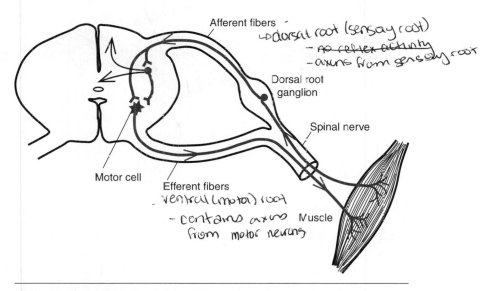

Afferent fibers
↳ dorsal root (sensory root)
– no reflex activity
– axons from sensory root

Dorsal root ganglion

Spinal nerve

Motor cell

Efferent fibers
– ventral (motor) root
– contains axons Muscle
from motor neurons

Figure 7-1 Cross-section of a spinal cord showing the afferent and efferent spinal fibers that join to form the spinal nerve.

Thermoreception includes the sensation of cold and heat. *Nociception* refers to pain related to tissue destruction.

Specialized Receptors

Various structurally different receptors, including the somatosensory end organs, are located in the skin, limb joints, blood vessels, and muscles. The receptor type for each sensory modality is not easily identifiable. Primarily, the modality of receptor type is identified by its maximal sensitivity (physiologic response) to the smallest amplitude of applied energy or sensory stimuli (such as heat, pain, and touch) and by its connection to the nerve fibers that transmit these sensations. Receptors can also be defined by their adaptiveness to stimuli. Quickly adapting receptors respond strongly when a stimulus is first applied. However, as the receptor adapts to the stimulus strength, the responses rapidly become weaker, eventually dying out. The nonadapting receptors may not respond so vigorously to the stimulus onset. Once activated, however, they continuously provide signals to the brain as long as the stimulus remains present. The basic types of sensory receptors in the body are encapsulated endings, free nerve endings, and expanded tip

endings (Fig. 7-2; Table 7-2). An additional class of receptors that mediate olfaction and taste are not discussed here.

Encapsulated Endings

Receptors with encapsulated endings are the most sensitive and rapidly adapting mechanoreceptors. Commonly distributed in subcutaneous tissues, skin, fingertips, palms, lips, and external genitals, the encapsulated receptors mediate sensations of vibration and fine discriminative and deep touch. These receptors consist of concentric layers of tissue around a nerve ending. Any deformation of the external layer compresses all of the fluid-filled inner layers, altering the contour of the capsule. The receptors in the encapsulated category are **Meissner corpuscles** and **Pacinian corpuscles** (Fig. 7-2).

Free Nerve Endings

The receptors with free nerve endings consist of fine branchings (arborization) of fiber and mediate the sensations of pain and temperature. These nonadapting receptors are distributed throughout the body, skin, cutaneous tissue, and visceral organs and respond by sending signals at a slow rate for long periods (Fig. 7-2).

Expanded Tip Endings

Merkel receptors and **Ruffini endings** consist of nerve endings with knobs that mediate touch, temperature, and pressure. Located in the dermis and joints, these *mechanoreceptors* are moderately adaptive and transmit slowly (Fig. 7-2).

Three-Neuron Organization of the Somatosensory System

All somatosensory pathways are anatomically organized in such a manner that a given sensory impulse enters the CNS, crosses the midline, and then ascends to the contralateral

Table 7-1	
Types of Sensation	
Somatic Senses	**Mediated Modalities**
Mechanoreception	Touch, pressure, vibration, and proprioception
Thermoreception	Cold and heat
Nociception	Pain

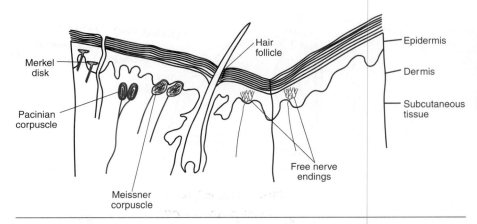

Figure 7-2 Common sensory receptors. Meissner and Pacinian corpuscles are responsible for fine discriminative touch. Both types of receptors with encapsulated endings are sensitive to touch and are rapidly adapting receptors. Merkel end organs, with expanded tips, mediate diffuse touch. Receptors with free nerve endings mediate pain and temperature.

sensory cortex. This impulse transmission involves three neurons and their fibers (Fig. 7-3). The **first-order neurons**, with their cell bodies in the spinal DRG, collect sensory information from the periphery and transmit it to the **second-order neurons** in the CNS. The second-order neurons, depending on the modality of sensation, are either in the spinal cord or in the brainstem. The second-order fibers consistently cross the midline and ascend to the opposite thalamus, which contains the **third-order neurons**. The third-order fibers project from the thalamus to the primary sensory cortex.

INNERVATION PATTERN

The spinal organization of the sensory pathway is mixed, although predominantly **ipsilateral** to the side of the afferent input. Pathways mediating discriminative touch, which form relatively late in development, have the input axon

proceeding up the ipsilateral side, and decussation is delayed to the medullary level. However, the earlier developed pathways—which mediate pain, temperature, and diffuse touch—decussate in the spinal cord and proceed rostrally on the **contralateral** side. Consequently, a spinal lesion has different implications for both of these sensation types. Such a lesion would result in the loss of discriminative touch on the body ipsilateral to the lesion and loss of pain and temperature on the side contralateral to the lesion.

ANATOMIC DIVISION OF THE SOMATOSENSORY SYSTEM

Neuroanatomically, the somatosensory system is divided into the **dorsal column–medial lemniscal system** and the **anterolateral system** (Fig. 7-4). The *dorsal column–medial lemniscal system*, also called the **epicritic system**, is phylogenetically newer. The large myelinated fibers of the dorsal column system not only conduct impulses rapidly but also represent a precise map of the body surface. Epicritic sensation, which requires a high degree of precision and intensity resolution, includes the sensations of fine discriminative touch, vibration, limb position, kinesthesia, and deep pressure. It is called the dorsal system because the fibers mediating these sensations travel in the dorsal spinal cord.

The *anterolateral system*, a phylogenetically older system, is also called the **protopathic system** (Table 7-3). The anterolateral system is further divided into the **lateral spinothalamic tract** (pain and temperature) and the **anterior spinothalamic tract** (high threshold and poorly nonlocalizable touch).

Dorsal Column–Medial Lemniscal System

The dorsal column–medial lemniscal system mediates postural position sense, fine discriminative touch, and vibra-

Table 7-2

Receptors for Somatic Sensation

Receptor Types	Suggested Mediated Modalities

Encapsulated endings
   Pacinian corpuscle
   Meissner corpuscle
	Tactile (discriminative, deep touch, vibration)

Free nerve endings	Pain and temperature (heat, cold); some tactile

Expanded tip endings
   Merkel receptors
   Ruffini endings
	Tactile (touch, pressure); temperature

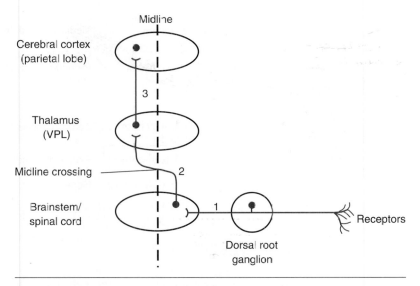

Figure 7-3 The three-neuron organization of somatosensory system. First-order neurons (*1*), with their cell bodies in the dorsal root ganglion, collect sensory information from the body surface. First-order fibers transmit sensory information to second-order neurons (*2*) in the CNS. Depending on the modality mediated, second-order neurons are in either the spinal cord or the brainstem. Second-order fibers, emanating from second-order neurons, cross the midline and terminate in the contralateral thalamus, which contains the third-order neurons (*3*) for all modalities of somatic sensation. Third-order fibers from the thalamic nuclei project to the primary sensory cortex in the parietal lobe. *VPL*, ventral posterior lateral.

tion. Position sense, which is mediated consciously and unconsciously, is divided into two types proprioception and kinesthesia. Proprioception is internal awareness of limb position in space. It is important in the acquisition of skilled movements, such as speech and writing, and it provides the cortex with a conscious awareness of the spatial position of body parts and the body during movements. Kinesthesia is internal awareness of limb movement. It is essential to the acquisition of skilled movements and provides information related to the direction and range of limb movements. Fine discriminative touch is involved with the analysis and identification of objects through tactual manipulation (**stereognosis**), the recognition of figures and numbers written on the body (**graphesthesia**), the discrimination between two or multiple points of touch, and the awareness of nondiscriminative deep touch.

Receptors

Meissner and Pacinian corpuscles, both of which are exceedingly sensitive and highly adaptive encapsulated end receptors, primarily serve epicritic sensation. They mediate discriminative touch and vibration. Additional receptors such as **muscle spindle organs** (annulospiral ends of the Ia afferents) are the most sensitive (lower threshold) receptors to vibration, kinesthesia, and proprioception.

Neural Pathways

The dorsal column–medial lemniscal system consists of two fasciculi: **fasciculus gracilis** and **fasciculus cuneatus** (Fig. 7-4; Table 7-4). Each fasciculus mediates discriminative touch from different body areas; however, both follow a similar **three-neuron sensory organization** (Fig. 7-5A). The first-order fibers, with their cell bodies in the DRG, collect sensory information from the body and enter the spinal cord. After entering the cord, the afferent axons divide into short and long branches. The short axons extend to the spinal dorsal gray horn and mediate reflexive activity. The long axonal fibers ascend ipsilaterally in the *gracilis* and *cuneatus fasciculi* and synapse on the **gracile** and **cuneate nuclei** in the medulla.

The **internal arcuate fibers**, which include the second-order fibers from the *cuneate* and *gracile nuclei,* cross the midline and form the **medial lemniscus**. The medial lemniscus, formed by the crossed dorsal column fibers, ascends and terminates on the third-order neurons in the thalamus. The projections from the third-order neurons in the thalamus travel to the sensory cortex in the parietal lobe (Table 7-4).

Fibers in the dorsal column–medial lemniscal system are arranged in a laminar fashion; the sacral fibers are the most medial in the dorsal column. Lumbar fibers travel

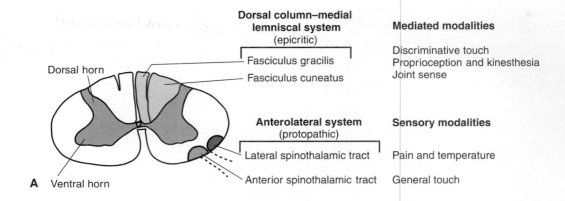

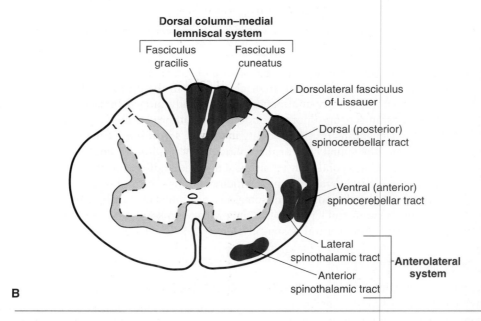

Figure 7-4 A. Anatomic division of the somatosensory system. B. Locations of the sensory pathways in the spinal cord.

Table 7-3

Primary Ascending Spinal Pathways

Spinal Pathways	Information Carried/Function
Fasciculus gracilis	Mediates discriminative touch (pressure, vibration, muscle and tendon stretch, and joint movement) from lower half of body
Fasciculus cuneatus	Mediates discriminative touch (pressure, vibration, muscle and tendon stretch, and joint movement) from upper half of body
Lateral spinothalamic tract	Transmits pain and temperature sensation
Anterior spinothalamic tract	Conveys diffuse touch; backup sensory system
Dorsal spinocerebellar tract	Transmits unconscious proprioception from distal lower limbs and joints
Ventral spinocerebellar tract	Carries unconscious proprioception from muscles of lower extremities, proximal limbs, and axial muscles
Cuneocerebellar tract	Mediates unconscious proprioception from upper limbs and joints

Table 7-4

Components of the Epicritic System: Fine Discriminative Touch

Nerve Cell Order	Associated Fibers	Target Nucleus
First-order neuron (DRG)	With cell bodies in DRG, first-order central fibers enter spinal cord to form dorsal funiculus and ascend ipsilaterally to medulla	NG and NC in caudal medulla
Second-order neuron (NG, NC)	With cell bodies in NG and NC, internal arcuate fibers cross midline in medulla and ascend as medial lemniscus to thalamus	VPL of thalamus
Third-order neuron (VPL of thalamus)	With cell bodies in the VPL, thalamocortical projections ascend from thalamus to cortex	Primary sensory cortex (body area)

DRG, dorsal root ganglion; *NC*, nucleus cuneatus; *NG*, nucleus gracilis; *VPL*, ventral posterior lateral nucleus.

parallel to sacral fibers in the dorsal column and are laterally joined by fibers from the thoracic and cervical levels. Therefore, the fibers mediating sensation from the leg are medial, whereas the fibers from the arm are most lateral.

Fasciculus Gracilis

The fasciculus gracilis transmits epicritic sensations from the lower half of the body. This includes the afferent fibers entering the dorsal column approximately from the **sacral** to **midthoracic sections** of the spinal cord (Fig. 7-5B). After projecting short axons to the dorsal horn, the first-order fibers, with neurons in the DRG, ascend medially in the dorsal column of the spinal cord. Fibers of the fasciculus gracilis terminate in the nucleus gracilis, the second-order sensory neuron in the dorsal caudal medulla. From this point, fibers of the fasciculus gracilis merge with the fasciculus cuneatus in the medial lemniscus.

Fasciculus Cuneatus

Fibers of the fasciculus cuneatus are lateral to the fasciculus gracilis in the dorsal column. The fasciculus cuneatus fibers carry epicritic sensations from the upper body and enter the spinal cord above the midthoracic level (Fig. 7-5B). These fibers ipsilaterally ascend the spinal cord dorsal column toward the brainstem and terminate at the nucleus cuneatus, the second-order neuron, lateral to the nucleus gracilis in the dorsal caudal medulla.

The *internal arcuate fibers,* the second-order fibers from the nucleus cuneatus, travel medially and cross the midline just above the pyramid in the medulla (Fig. 3-8). After the crossing (decussation), the internal arcuate fibers form the *medial lemniscus,* a fillet-shaped bundle of fibers. The medial lemniscus fibers ascend along the midline through the medulla and the pontine tegmentum (see Figs. 3-9–3-11 and 3-14). Later they migrate dorsolaterally in the midbrain to enter the **ventral posterior lateral nucleus** (VPL) of the thalamus, the third-order sensory relay nucleus (see Fig. 3-18).

Cortical Representation

Conscious sensation occurs at the cortical level; however, crude awareness of touch is also said to occur at the thalamic level. The third-order fibers from the VPL nucleus of the thalamus pass through the posterior limb of the internal capsule. They terminate in the upper two-thirds of the postcentral gyrus, the **primary sensory cortex** in the parietal lobe. The primary sensory cortex, the site that analyzes the quality of sensory information, consists of Brodmann areas 3, 1, 2. There is a specific somatotopic organization in the primary sensory cortex where the fibers from the lower extremities terminate along the superior medial aspect of the postcentral gyrus; the projections from the upper limbs terminate in the lateral region of the cortex (Fig. 7-6).

The elaboration and integration of sensory information with previously stored experiences and with information from other sensory modalities is required for recognition of an object and interpretation of its significance. This analysis and integration of stimuli is accomplished in the **somesthetic association cortex** (Brodmann areas 5 and 7), which consists of the superior and part of the **inferior parietal lobule** and which lies at the crossroads of the **temporoparieto-occipital regions**. A lesion in the association cortex results in not only cognitive impairments but also disorders of cross-modality integration, which include disturbances in **somatosensory discrimination,** tactile perception (graphesthesia and stereognosis), **sensory agnosia,** and **intersensory integration**.

Clinical Concerns

Patterns of Deficit

Lesions interrupting the ascending fibers in the dorsal column system affect fine discriminative touch sensation and position sense (proprioception and kinesthesia). Inflammation of the **peripheral nerve** and DRG or degeneration interruption of **spinal dorsal column fibers, neoplasm,** and **vascular infarcts** in the spinal cord are all common conditions that affect one's ability to process fine discriminative touch and related information.

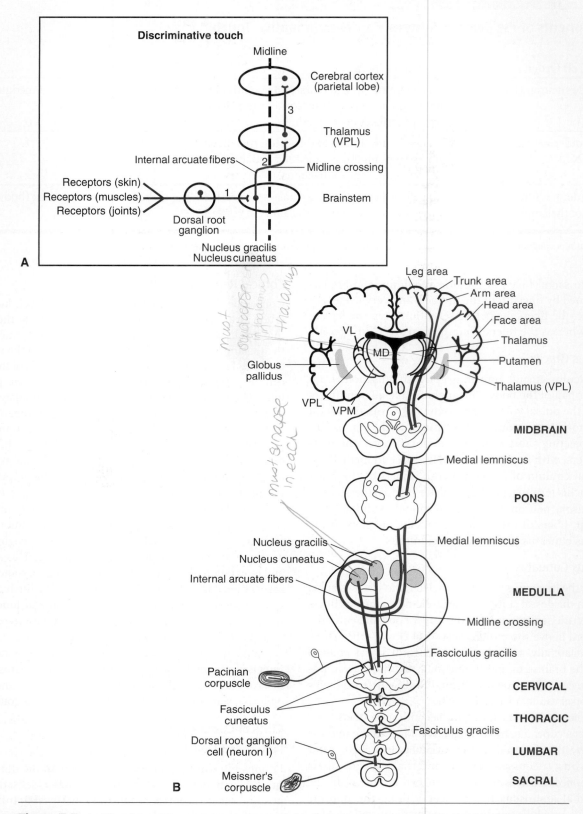

Figure 7-5 **A.** The three-neuron organization of the dorsal column–medial lemniscal system. **B.** The dorsal white column. *MD,* mediodorsal (dorsomedial); *VL,* ventrolateral; *VPL,* ventral posterior lateral; *VPM,* ventral posterior medial.

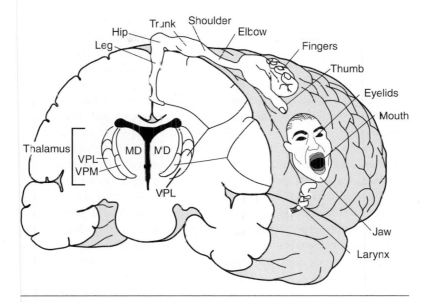

Figure 7-6 The ventral posterior lateral (*VPL*) nucleus of the thalamus is the third-order sensory nucleus. Projections from the VPL nucleus cross the internal capsule and travel to the primary sensory cortex in the parietal lobe. *MD*, mediodorsal (dorsomedial); *VPM*, ventral posterior medial.

Epicritic sensation is localizable. The pattern of loss of epicritic sensation reveals the site at which the epicritic pathway has been interrupted. This can occur at the peripheral nerve, dorsal (posterior) spinal nerve root, or dorsal column (first-order sensory neuron); at the nucleus gracilis, nucleus cuneatus, or medial lemniscus, before or after it crosses the midline of the brainstem (second-order sensory neuron); or at the VPL nucleus of the thalamus or its thalamocortical projection through the posterior limb of the internal capsule and corona radiata to the sensory cortex (third-order sensory neuron).

The pattern of deficit after a peripheral nerve injury differs from the pattern of a dorsal root or dorsal column injury. Because peripheral nerves send their axons into the spinal cord over more than one dorsal root, a peripheral nerve injury causes more widespread loss of sensation than an injury to a single dorsal root. For example, the most commonly injured peripheral nerve, the **median nerve** supplies the thumb side of the hand (Table 2-5). After complete injury to the median nerve, the sensory loss includes the thumb, index finger, middle finger, and the side of the ring finger. The compression of the median nerve near the wrist results in **carpal tunnel syndrome.** By contrast, complete injury to the sixth cervical nerve root, one of the four adjacent cervical nerve roots that receive some axons from the median nerve, creates a loss of sensation in the thumb and part of the forearm but does not affect the other fingers supplied by the median nerve because they send their axons into the spinal cord via the seventh cervical nerve root, not only the sixth.

Damage to the dorsal column of the spinal cord is rarely as selective as a peripheral nerve or nerve root injury; usually both dorsal columns are affected by injury or disease, and all modalities of epicritic sensation are impaired below the level of the lesion. Occasionally, one dorsal column is affected and the other is spared. Because axons in the dorsal column travel up toward the medulla on the same side on which they entered the spinal cord, the sensory deficit is always ipsilateral to the lesion. The key to clinically identifying the spinal cord as the site of injury is finding a level on the body below which sensation is abnormal—impaired, altered, or lost. For example, a lesion that completely interrupts the sensory pathways at the level of the T10 causes a sensory deficit in all parts of the body below the umbilicus. If the entire spinal cord and not just its sensory pathways is damaged at a given level, motor functions are also lost below the level of the lesion. For example, with a T10 injury, the patient would also be paraplegic.

Assessment

The integrity of the dorsal column–medial lemniscal fibers is assessed by various sensory tests. Commonly employed tests are **two-point tactile discrimination**, vibratory sense, position sense, stereognosis, and graphesthesia. The two-point discrimination test assesses the individual's ability to identify two close points of stimulation. Pencil tips or a special instrument, an **esthesiometer**, is used for stimulating two closely spaced points alternated with a single-point touch. The patient, with eyes closed, is asked to differentiate between the two points of touch. The distance between the two points is gradually decreased until the subject can no longer tell which is a two-point and which is a single-point touch. For stereognosis, the patient, with eyes closed, is required to identify an object by feeling its contour, weight, shape, and texture. Graphesthesia tests a patient's ability to identify, with the eyes closed, a number or letter written on the skin. Vibratory sense is assessed via a tuning fork held against a bony surface. The patient must describe when and where the vibration was felt.

The **Romberg test** is used to evaluate proprioception. With eyes closed, the patient stands with feet together. Unsteadiness in this position indicates a lack of proprioception in the lower extremities. Kinesthetic awareness is tested by moving the individual's fingers and toes while he or she reports on the direction of joint movements. Kinesthetic proprioception concerning position sense is also tested by moving the patient's arm to an angle 45° or more and then asking him or her to duplicate the shoulder angle with the other arm. Separate assessments of the upper and lower limbs can be used to evaluate the integrity of the fasciculi gracilis and cuneatus.

Anterolateral System

The anterolateral system, which mediates pain and temperature modalities, is named for the location of its fibers within the spinal white column. It follows the *three-neuron organizational framework* but differs from fibers in the dorsal column with respect to its **crossing point**. Fibers of the anterolateral system cross at various points in the spinal cord. The *first-order fibers,* with their cell bodies in the DRG, enter the spinal cord and travel one or two spinal segments up or down before synapsing on the **substantia gelatinosa** and **nucleus proprius**, the *second-order neurons* in the spinal dorsal gray column. The *second-order fibers* cross the midline of the spinal cord and travel to the VPL nucleus of the thalamus, a *third-order nucleus,* which projects to the sensory cortex (Fig. 7-7A; Table 7-5).

The anterolateral system is divided into the lateral and anterior spinothalamic tracts. The *lateral spinothalamic tract* mediates the sensations of pain and temperature. The *anterior spinothalamic tract* mediates diffuse, or unlocalized (crude), touch.

Lateral Spinothalamic Tract

Receptors

End organs with free nerve endings are the mediators of pain and temperature sensations. Some encapsulated receptors may also secondarily contribute to the modalities of pain and temperature.

Neural Pathway

The pathway carrying the sensations of pain and temperature (hot and cold) begins at the nociceptive receptors in the skin (Fig. 7-7B). The *first-order fibers,* with their nuclei in the DRG, carry sensations from the receptors in the skin and enter the dorsolateral spinal cord. After entering the cord, these fibers travel up or down a few spinal segments in the **dorsolateral fasciculus (Lissauer tract)** before penetrating the dorsal spinal gray matter. After penetration, the fibers terminate in the substantia gelatinosa and nucleus proprius. Collaterals from the substantia gelatinosa and nucleus proprius project via interneurons to motor neurons in the ventral gray horns and mediate withdrawal reflexes.

The *second-order fibers* cross the midline in the ventral white commissure to ascend in the lateral spinothalamic tract (Fig. 7-7B). Fibers carrying pain and temperature sensation from the entire body travel in the lateral spinothalamic tract and ascend toward the brainstem on the way to the thalamus. After traveling through the medulla (see Fig. 3-11), ventrolateral pons (see Fig. 3-14), and midbrain tegmentum (see Fig. 3-16), the spinothalamic fibers terminate on the *third-order neurons* in the VPL nucleus of the thalamus. **Thalamocortical fibers** travel through the internal capsule and corona radiata, then project to the upper two-thirds of the postcentral gyrus in the parietal lobe (Fig. 7-6). The primary sensory cortex (Brodmann areas 3, 1, 2) is responsible for a fine analysis of sensation and determines its quality and source.

Cortical Representation

Note that the stimulation of the primary sensory cortex does not result in the experience of pain. This primary cortex determines where the pain is (localization) but is not involved in the intensity of the pain. Pain may be characterized as sharp or dull (diffuse). The neuronal mechanism of sharp pain is well understood, as it is projected to the cortex by way of specific thalamic (VPL and **ventral posterior medial [VPM]**) **nuclei** (see Chapter 6). It involves faster conduction and is precisely localizable. However, dull pain involves multisynaptic pathways. The lateral spinothalamic tract mediating nociceptive afferents from the body, viscera, or face gives off many collaterals that terminate on the reticular nuclei in the brainstem; these reticular nuclei project to the thalamus, hypothalamus, and hippocampus.

Clinical Concerns

The emotional response to the hurtfulness of pain includes the limbic system. The nociceptive afferents from the body, viscera, or face reaching the thalamus also innervate the **intralaminar nuclei** of the thalamus (see Chapter 6). These project into the limbic system, including the hippocampus, amygdaloid complex, and associated old cortex. The experience of the affective aspect of pain—the hurtfulness of the pain—is undoubtedly associated with these projections

The descending reticular (**periaqueductal gray matter**) projections are known to modulate pain perception. The reticular projections, along with other brainstem nuclei, project to the dorsal horns of the spinal cord to inhibit the pain-mediating pathways. By regulating the transmission of pain, the reticular projections participate in mediating many somatic and visceral responses to pain, such as nausea, fainting, changes in heart rate, and alterations in the frequency and depth of respiration.

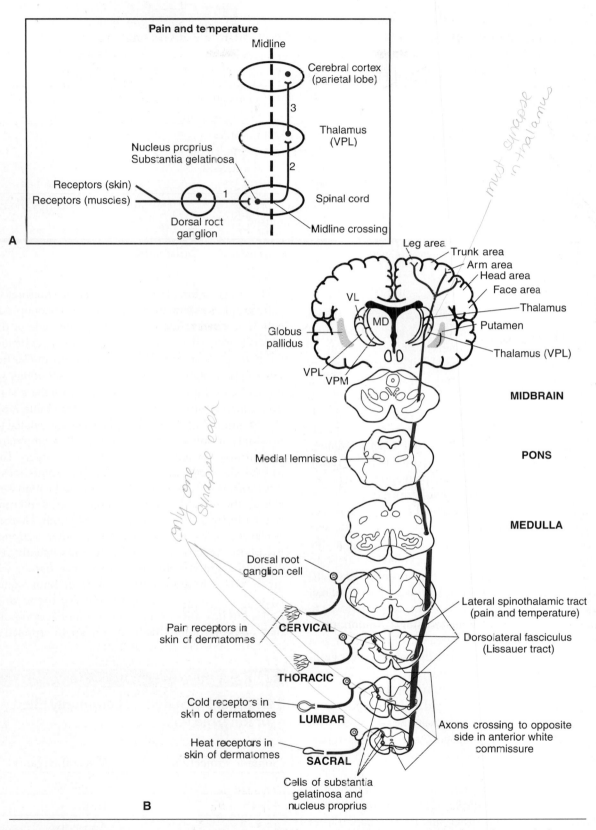

Figure 7-7 A. The three-neuron organization of the anterolateral system. B. The lateral spinothalamic tract, which carries pain and temperature sensation from body. *MD*, mediodorsal (dorsomedial); *VL*, ventrolateral; *VPL*, ventral posterior lateral; *VPM*, ventral posterior medial.

Table 7-5

Components of the Protopathic System: Pain, Temperature, and Touch

Nerve Cell Order	Associated Fibers	Target Nucleus
First-order neuron (DRG)	With cell bodies in DRG, first-order fibers enter spinal cord	NP and SG in spinal dorsal horn
Second-order neuron (NP, SG)	With cell bodies in NP and SG, second-order fibers cross midline in spinal cord, form lateral and ventral spinothalamic tracts, and ascend to thalamus	VPL of thalamus
Third-order neuron (VPL of thalamus)	With cell bodies in VPL, thalamocortical projections ascend from thalamus to cortex	Primary sensory cortex (body area)

DRG, dorsal root ganglion; *NP,* nucleus proprius; *SG,* substantia gelatinosa; *VLP,* ventral posterior lateral nucleus.

Patterns of Deficit

An interruption of the ascending fibers at any point in the neuraxis alters the perception of pain and temperature. Damage to peripheral (spinal) nerves or the DRG subsequently to compression or reduced local circulation results in a reduced pain sensitivity. A pinched nerve root from a herniated disk usually results in pain perceived in the body area connected to the compromised neural structure. All outgrowing nerve processes results in a period of hyperalgesia during the growth process. Damage to *spinothalamic fibers* also affects the transmission of pain and temperature to the sensorimotor cortex. Because pain and temperature fibers cross the midline in the *spinal gray matter,* a lesion of the lateral ventral area of the spinal cord results in loss of pain and temperature sensations from the opposite side of the body below the lesion. Similarly, a lesion at the brainstem level affects the contralateral half of the body. However, if the *DRG, nucleus proprius,* or *substantia gelatinosa* is damaged, sensation is affected on the ipsilateral half of the body.

Knowing the point of fiber crossing is important in determining which cutaneous area will be affected as a result of a given lesion. This information serves as the guiding post for choosing the anatomic site for the surgical management (**chordotomy**) of intractable pain. Patients' inability to perceive sensations in delineated body areas allow clinicians to identify the dermatomes involved with the level of the spinal cord damage. Once the affected dermatomes are determined, one can identify which afferent nerves or spinal dorsal roots are damaged (see Fig. 2.34).

Pain cannot always be solely attributed to a particular anatomic pathway. For example, **referred pain** occurs at one site but is sensed in another site. Pain sensation from viscera is poorly localized and serves as a good example of referred pain. The CNS does not contain special pathways devoted to visceral sensation; thus visceral pain impulses follow the same pathways that are used by somatic pain afferents. Therefore, the brain is likely to interpret visceral pain impulses as somatic pain signals. For example, cardiac pain is referred to the chest and/or inner side of the arm. This is because the area of reference for pain coincides with the body parts served by somatic sensory nuclei from the same spinal segments, which are T1–T8. Thus sensory nuclei from the same spinal segment mediate sensation from different visceral and somatic areas (Table 7-6).

Phantom limb is another phenomenon related to pain. If a limb or substantial part of a limb is amputated, the patient may, for many months after the surgery, continue to have shooting pain and tingling and sometimes feel as if the fingers or toes were crossed or that the limb were bent behind the back. The pain or discomfort is interpreted as originating from the missing part of the limb. There are two explanations for phantom pain. First, after sectioning, the peripheral process of afferent neurons usually regrows. Often the growth tip encounters scar tissue, where it grows into a **hypersensitive tangle** or knot (neuroma). Irritation from pressure, tightening scar tissue, or a prosthesis often results in the generation of action potentials that, on projection to the forebrain, are interpreted as pain

---

Table 7-6

Principal Dermatomes Commonly Cited for Referred Pain

Somatic Projection	Visceral Organ(s)
C3–C4	Diaphragm
T1–T8	Heart
T10	Appendix
T10–T12	Testes and prostate
T10–T12	Ovaries and uterus

in a no longer existing distal innervation zone. Second, it is difficult to forget a lifetime of learning the association between the distal, now missing, part of the limb and the touch, pain, and position experiences associated with that part.

With its somewhat unlocalizable cortical representation, pain has proven to be a mysterious perception. Its medical treatment continues to pose challenges. For example, the alleviation of pain by cutting the dorsal root (rhizotomy) or a tract (tractotomy) has usually been transient; the pain has most often returned, and with greater intensity. The ablation of the ventrobasal thalamus (a site associated with thalamic pain syndrome) generally decreases sensation from the contralateral side of the body, but it does not entirely suppress the pain. Intralaminar stimulation has, however, proven to be more beneficial and effective (Bhatnagar, et al., 1990; Bhatnagar and Mandybur, 2005). It is interesting that direct stimulation of the exposed brain has resulted in an evoked sensation of tingling, pressure, and numbness, but it has never resulted in the evoked sensation of pain. This finding has allowed neurosurgeons to operate on the brain of awake patients (Penfield and Roberts, 1959; Bhatnagar et al., 2000).

Narcotics, **nonaddictive analgesics**, and **local anesthetics** are commonly used for pain relief. The best analgesic is morphine, an extract from the opium poppy. These agents suppress pain sensitivity by inhibiting receptor functioning, blocking the transmission of pain impulses, or blocking or slowing the central pain-processing mechanism. Local anesthetic agents are used to control pain by blocking its transmission peripherally or centrally. The human brain is known to contain enkephalin a morphine-like substance. Released from the nerve endings in the CNS, enkephalin not only serves as an analgesic in the body but also regulates mood and motivation.

Assessment

The modality of pain is assessed by pricking the body surface with a pin or by pinching the skin. The patient is asked to describe the sensation. This is repeated until the area of deficit is mapped. There are three common types of altered responses to pain: **analgesia** (no sensation of pain), **hypalgesia** (decreased sensation to pain or higher pain threshold), and **hyperalgesia** or exaggerated response (increased pain sensation or lower pain threshold).

Thermal sensation is assessed by using hot and cold stimuli. Hot and cold stimuli are applied to various parts of the body and the patient is asked to differentiate them. Common pathologic responses related to thermal sensation are **athermia** or **thermal anesthesia** (total absence of sensation), **hypothermia**, **thermal hypesthesia** or hypoesthesia (raised or elevated threshold of response to thermal stimuli), and **hyperthermia** or **thermal hyperesthesia** (lower threshold to temperature, resulting in an exaggerated response).

Anterior Spinothalamic Tract

Information pertaining to two types of touch, discriminative and diffuse, travels in different neural pathways. Diffuse touch refers to a global sensation that lacks a qualitative description and does not relate to a specific location. Diffuse touch is mediated through the *anterior spinothalamic tract,* which also includes collaterals from the dorsal column. Neuronal conduction for diffuse touch sensation follows a *three-neuron organizational system,* similar to the system that mediates pain and temperature (Fig. 7-7A).

Receptors

The identity of nerve endings transducing diffuse touch is not fully resolved. All three types of receptive end organs (encapsulated endings, free nerve endings, and expanded tip endings) and the collaterals from the dorsal column contribute to this less localized touch sensation.

Neural Pathway

The *first-order* sensory fibers transmit general touch sensations from the skin to the CNS. On entering the dorsolateral spinal cord, the fibers disperse longitudinally in the **dorsolateral fasciculus of Lissauer**. They then travel up and down a few spinal segments before terminating in the *nucleus proprius* and *substantia gelatinosa,* the *second-order nuclei* in the dorsal horn. Some second-order fibers terminate in the adjacent gray matter, which serves spinal reflexes; however, most cross the midline in the ventral spinal gray matter and turn upward to form the *anterior spinothalamic tract* (Fig. 7-8). The anterior spinothalamic tract fibers ascend in this general location to the brainstem, where they move laterally, getting closer to the lateral spinothalamic tract (see Figs. 3-11, 3-14, and 3-16). Before terminating in the VPL nucleus of the thalamus, the anterior spinothalamic tract fibers give off many collaterals to the *brainstem reticular formation.* The *third-order fibers* from the thalamus travel through the internal capsule, then project into the upper two-thirds of the postcentral gyrus located in the parietal lobe. The anterolateral spinothalamic tract projects bilaterally to the sensory cortex.

Clinical Concerns and Assessment

Diffuse touch serves as the backup sensory system for the dorsal–lemniscal column and it projects to the cortex bilaterally. Because it is the secondary system, interruption of the anterior spinothalamic tract causes no obvious clinical deficit. Diffuse touch can be abolished only when the spinal cord is completely severed.

Diffuse touch is tested using a piece of cotton or a wisp of wool. The stimulus is applied to various regions of the body while the patient is asked to report whether there is any sensation of touch. A patient relying on this backup system notices a touch but cannot determine its location or describe its quality. It can be assessed effectively only when the pathway for fine discriminative touch is not functioning.

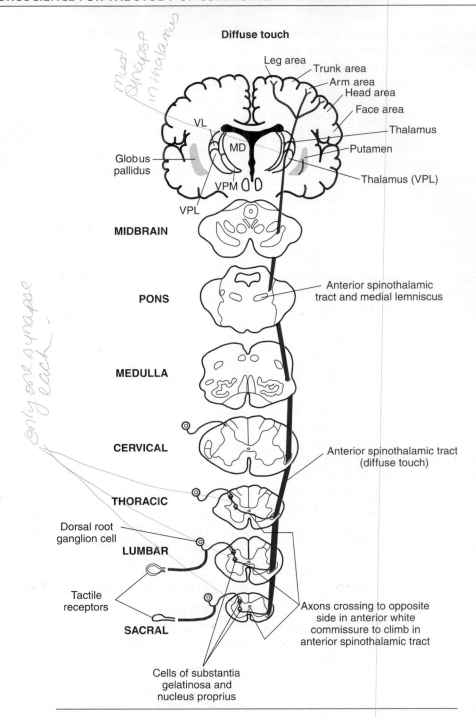

Figure 7-8 The anterior spinothalamic tract, which transmits diffuse touch from the body. *MD,* mediodorsal (dorsomedial); *VL,* ventrolateral; *VPL,* ventral posterior lateral; *VPM,* posterior medial.

TRIGEMINAL NERVE

The **trigeminal (CN V) nerve** is the principal sensory nerve for the face and head. The **maxillary**, **ophthalmic**, and **mandibular branches** of the trigeminal nerve innervate different regions of the head, face, and intraoral structures. These branches cover the face and head area and mediate cutaneous sensations from the skin of the face,

forehead, anterior half of the scalp, and most of the dura mater, orbital cavities, and mucosal membrane in the nasal and oral cavities. Fibers of the trigeminal (CN V) nerve are also joined by the fibers carrying sensation from the following nerves: **facial (CN VII)**, **glossopharyngeal (CN IX)**, and **vagus (CN X)**. Together, these nerves cover the remaining scalp, external ear, ear canal, tympanic membrane region, and pharyngeal and laryngeal areas.

The trigeminal system is comparable to the previously discussed body-sensory system. It contains different neural mechanisms for the *epicritic system,* which is responsible for fine discriminative touch, proprioception, and kinesthesia as well as the *protopathic sensations of* pain, temperature, and diffuse touch. In each system, different fibers serve epicritic and protopathic sensations from the head and face. The receptors serving the various sensations for the head and face are identical to the receptors previously discussed for the body.

Three-Neuron Organization of Trigeminal System

The trigeminal sensory system also follows the standard *three-neuron organization;* however, locations of the first- and second-order neurons for the trigeminal system are different (Fig. 7-9A). The peripherally located **semilunar (Gasserian) ganglion** of the trigeminal (CN V) nerve serves as the *first-order* neuron. This is functionally identical to the DRG of the general sensory system. Afferent fibers, except for those associated with stretch receptors, have their cell bodies in the semilunar ganglion. There are two *second-order* trigeminal sensory nuclei in the brainstem: the **chief (principal) sensory nucleus** (discriminative touch) and the **trigeminal spinal tract nucleus** (pain and temperature). The ascending first-order trigeminal sensory fibers synapse on the chief sensory nucleus, whereas the descending first-order sensory fibers terminate in the nucleus of the trigeminal spinal tract. The second-order sensory fibers from these two central nuclei cross the midline and ascend to the VPM nucleus of the thalamus. The *third-order* fibers from the VPM nucleus travel through the internal capsule, then terminate in the lower third of the postcentral gyrus, which serves as the primary sensory cortex for the face.

Fine Discriminative Touch from Face

Receptors

The encapsulated end organs mediate fine discriminative touch from the face; these receptors are discussed in the section "Dorsal Column–Medial Lemniscal System."

Neural Pathway

The *encapsulated receptors* in the skin of the face and head, are the first to receive discriminative touch sensations. The *first-order* trigeminal (ophthalmic, maxillary, and mandibular) fibers, with their cell bodies in the *semilunar ganglion,* mediate fine discriminative sensation from the head, intraoral structures, and face. The central processes of the semilunar ganglion terminate in the cells of the *chief* (principal) *sensory nucleus* of the trigeminal (CN V) nerve. The *second-order* trigeminothalamic fibers from the chief (principal) sensory trigeminal nucleus project to the thalamus. One fasciculus of fibers crosses the midline and ascends in the *medial lemniscus* (although it is considered to be part of the **ventral secondary ascending tract**) to the contralateral VPM nucleus. The second fasciculus of fibers, which con-

sists of a few uncrossed projections from the *primary sensory nucleus,* travels in the **dorsal secondary ascending tract** to the ipsilateral VPM nucleus, which plays a role in reticular-cortical arousal. The VPM nucleus of the thalamus relays sensation from the head and face. The *third-order sensory* fibers from the VPM travel through the internal capsule and project to the lower third of the postcentral gyrus, the primary sensory cortex for the face (Fig. 7-9; Table 7-7).

The neural mechanism for proprioceptive and kinesthetic sensations from the teeth, periodontium, palate, temporomandibular joint, and jaw-jerk reflex involving the muscles of mastication is slightly different. It involves the **mesencephalic nucleus,** a trigeminal nucleus that is comparable with the DRG, but it is in the pons. This mediates sensation from stretch receptors and relays it to the trigeminal motor nucleus, controlling the mechanism of jaw reflex and the force of bite.

Clinical Concerns and Assessment

Damage to both the semilunar ganglion (first-order neuron) and the chief sensory nucleus (second-order neuron) blocks the sensory projections involving fine discriminative touch and proprioception from half of the face, head, and intraoral cavity with ipsilateral effect. However, damage to only one trigeminal branch (ophthalmic, maxillary, or mandibular) is likely to affect only a selected facial or intraoral area.

Discriminative sensation from the face and head can be tested by use of the procedure described for assessing the dorsal column–medial lemniscal system. The two-point discrimination test and the test for tactile recognition of objects or letters are commonly used to determine impairments of discriminative touch. Proprioception is assessed using passive jaw movement.

Pain and Temperature from Face

Receptors

Receptors with *free nerve endings* are discussed in the section "Anterolateral System."

Neural Pathway

The central processes of the ophthalmic, maxillary, and mandibular trigeminal branches mediate pain and temperature from the nociceptive receptors in the facial and intraoral skin. The *first-order* trigeminal sensory fibers, with cell bodies in the **semilunar ganglion,** enter the midpons. They then turn downward (caudally), terminating in the **spinal trigeminal nucleus.** This tract extends up to the C4 level of the spinal cord. The **spinal trigeminal tract** (CN III) also receives general somatic sensation from the facial, glossopharyngeal (CN IX), and vagus (CN X) nerves. Together these three nerves mediate pain and temperature sensations from the structures associated with the external ear (pinna and meatus), tympanic membrane, and the mucosa of the pharynx, larynx, esophagus, and eustachian tube. The *second-order* trigeminal fibers from the spinal trigeminal

extent to which kinesthetic and proprioceptive losses are solely the result of the interruption of this tract. The Romberg test assesses cerebellar function related to proprioception; it however, also reflects the functioning of conscious proprioception (dorsal column–medial lemniscal system).

LESION LOCALIZATION–RULE 3: SPINAL CENTRAL GRAY LESION

Presenting Symptoms and Rationale

Bilateral loss of pain and temperature sensation with preserved sense of touch in the same limbs (usually the two upper limbs) implies a lesion (cavitation or syringomyelia) in the spinal central gray. A segmental level of the cavitation in the central spinal gray results in a bilaterally located deficit. This lesion interrupts the decussating fibers of the anterior white commissure, which mediates pain and temperature sensation.

CLINICAL CONSIDERATIONS

PATIENT ONE

A 35-year-old woman was involved in an automobile accident and taken to the emergency room (ER). She was examined by a neurologist who noted the following:

- A complete loss of epicritic (two-point touch and proprioceptive) sensation in right lower limb
- Paralysis of the right lower limb
- Loss of pain and temperature from the left lower limb

A spinal MRI study revealed a fractured thoracic vertebra with a fragment of bone in the spinal canal. The clinical findings indicated injury to the right half of the spinal cord at the T12 level; this is also called spinal cord hemisection and Brown-Séquard syndrome (Fig. 7-11). A re-evaluation of the sensorimotor functions 3 weeks

later revealed spasticity in the limb and a positive Babinski sign.

Question: How can you relate these clinical symptoms to the identified pathology?

Discussion: There are three important sensorimotor signs of spinal hemisection (Brown-Séquard syndrome): (1) spastic paralysis on the side ipsilateral to the lesion; (2) ipsilateral loss of proprioception, kinesthetic sense, and discriminative touch below the level of the lesion; and (3) contralateral loss of pain and temperature below the level of the lesion.

- The descending corticospinal fibers cross the midline in the caudal medulla; thus the T12 lesion caused paralysis in the limbs ipsilateral to the lesion site. Gradually and within 3 weeks, the limb became spastic with a positive Babinski sign. These symptoms of the corticospinal tract lesion indicate the damage is to the upper motor neuron (see Chapter 14).
- The dorsal column fibers ipsilaterally ascend in the spinal cord and cross the midline in the caudal medulla, thus the T12 lesion resulted in proprioceptive loss on the side of the body ipsilateral to the lesion.
- The fibers mediating pain and temperature cross to the opposite side at every spinal level before forming the lateral spinothalamic tract. Thus the T12 lesion blocked the transmission of pain and temperature from the contralateral body below the lesion site.

PATIENT TWO

A 55-year-old cook consulted with his doctor regarding the lack of pain and thermal sensation in his hands and forearms. On examination, the physician found the following:

- A few burn marks on the palms and fingertips
- No response to pinpricks and thermal stimuli in the hands and forearms
- Some weakness and atrophy of muscles of the hand

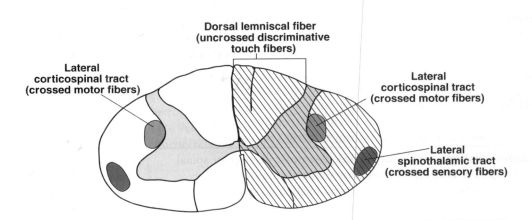

Figure 7-11 Anatomic involvement causing Brown-Séquard syndrome.

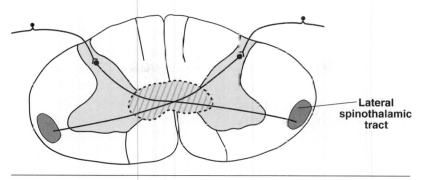

Figure 7-12 Anatomic involvement in syringomyelia.

A spinal MRI study revealed a cavity formation in the C6–C8 and T1 regions of the cord (Fig. 7-12).

Question: How can you explain these pain and temperature symptoms in relation to the identified syringomyelia?

Discussion: Formation of the syringomyelic cavity in the spinal cord from C6 to T1 affected the following structures:

- Crossing of pain and temperature fibers from the arm and hand regions; consequently, the patient did not have sensation of noxious stimuli from the arms and hands.
- Nearby α-motor neurons in the gray matter of the anterior horns; thus the weakness observed in his hands.

PATIENT THREE

A 62-year-old man who suffered stroke while asleep was taken to the ER. The attending neurologist noted the following:

- Unintelligible dysarthric speech
- Right facial paralysis
- Impaired swallowing with paresis of the right pharyngeal muscles
- Loss of pain and temperature sensation on the right face
- Loss of pain and temperature on the left half of the body
- Intact cognitive and linguistic functions

Question: Can you localize a lesion (somatosensory cortex, motor cortex, internal capsule, basal ganglia, or medulla) that was likely to produce these dissociated findings?

Discussion: These dissociated (left and right sided) symptoms suggest the involvement of the vagus (CN X), facial (CN VII), and spinal trigeminal tracts/nuclei and the fibers of the lateral spinothalamic tract fibers. Only a right medullary location of the lesion could affect these nerves and produce right facial and pharyngeal involvement.

This lesion also affected the crossed ascending fibers of the lateral spinothalamic tract, which transmitted pain temperature information from the left half of the body.

PATIENT FOUR

A 70-year-old woman complaining of episodic excruciating pain in her face was reported to have gradually become disinclined to speak and to have begun using gestures. Considering a possible case of depression or psychosis, she was taken to a neurologist, who noted the following:

- Malnourished body habitus
- No limb or facial paralysis
- No sensory loss on either side of her face
- Excruciating episodic pain involving the face any time the patient touched the ipsilateral alveolar region with the tip of tongue

A brain MRI study revealed no abnormality. The attending neurologist concluded the patient had cranial nerve dysfunction associated with a trigger zone.

Question: Can you provide an explanation for the patient's disinclination for speaking?

Discussion: This is a clear case of trigeminal neuralgia. Trigeminal neuralgia is characterized by episodes of intense (sudden and stabbing) pain. The pain was initiated by touching a trigger zone, which in this case was the alveolar region. This condition of evoked pain caused the patient to refrain from speaking and eating.

PATIENT FIVE

A 55-year-old man suffered a stroke while sleeping; he exhibited altered somatosensory problems and saw a neurologist who noted the following:

- Loss of fine discriminative touch from the right half (upper and lower extremities) of the body
- Loss of sensation from the left side of his face
- No other sensorimotor symptoms, except absence of the left corneal reflex

Question: Which of these clinical signs is most indicative of the lesion site?

Discussion: As per rules of lesion localization (see Box 1-3), the ascending (sensory) and descending (motor) fibers are present throughout the neuraxis and, therefore, are susceptible to interruption at multiple levels. The cranial nerves, however, can be affected by a lesion located exclusively in the brainstem. Thus the loss of facial sensation and the absent corneal reflex (afferent pathway = trigeminal (CN V) nerve; efferent pathway = facial (CN VII) nerve) strongly indicate that the lesion site is in the brainstem.

PATIENT SIX

A 55-year-old woman woke up perspiring; she was alarmed by experiencing numbness and clumsiness of her right hand. She was taken to a neurologist, who noted the following:

- Intact right arm strength
- No loss of sensation for pain, touch, and temperature
- Impaired tactile recognition of object in the right hand (astereognosis)
- No recognition of anything written on the right palm (agraphesthesia)
- Difficulty with orientation on a map
- Some constructional problems
- No sign of motor speech problem and or aphasia

A brain MRI study revealed a small infarct involving Brodmann area 5 extending to area 7 in the parietal lobe.

Question: Can you relate these selected symptoms with the cortical area responsible for the cortical sensory integration?

Discussion: This is a minor stroke involving the small parietal branches of the middle cerebral artery in the area of the superior parietal lobule (Brodmann areas 5 and 7). This parietal lobule serves cortical sensory integration and visual-spatial functions. Cortical sensory integration serves functions like recognition of information written on the skin and tactually identifying objects. Reading maps, identifying locations, following directions, drawing, and copying are examples of visual integration functions.

SUMMARY

Somatic sensation includes the physical experiences of pain, temperature, touch, and proprioception. It begins with specialized receptors in the body and terminates in the parietal lobe. Receptors in the skin convert sensory stimuli to neural signals and transmit the stimuli on afferent nerve fibers to the primary sensory cortex in the parietal lobe via the spinal cord, brainstem, and thalamus. This awareness is later transmitted to the sensory association cortex, where the information is analyzed, elaborated on, integrated with previous experiences, and raised to the highest level of consciousness. The somatosensory system is discretely organized; the information collected by specialized receptors is transmitted on separate axonal tracts. Each tract mediates specific modalities of sensation. Within each tract, a point-to-point somatotopic representation of the body surface (somatotopic organization) is maintained. This spatial organization of neurons, tracts, terminals, and nuclei is maintained up to the somesthetic cortex (body homunculus). Knowledge of sensory pathways, sensory receptors, points of fiber crossings, and cortical areas underlying conscious perception for different sensations provides a solid groundwork for understanding sensory organization. This knowledge enables one to relate patterns of sensory deficits with lesion sites and to solve clinical problems more effectively.

QUIZ QUESTIONS

1. Define the following terms: analgesia, anesthesia, graphesthesia, kinesthesia, proprioception, stereognosis.

2. Define the concept of referred pain.

3. Define the concept of phantom pain.

4. Match each of the following numbered attributes with its associated lettered spinal tract.

1. thermal sensitivity	a. lateral spinothalamic tract
2. crude/diffuse touch	
3. pain sensation	b. anterior spinothalamic tract
4. unconscious proprioception	
5. vibratory sense	c. spinocerebellar tracts
6. position sense	d. dorsal column–medial lemniscal system
7. two-point discrimination	

TECHNICAL TERMS

adaptation	kinesthesia
analgesia	proprioception
anesthesia	protopathic
chordotomy	referred pain
encapsulated endings	sensory receptors
epicritic	spinocerebellar
expanded tip endings	spinothalamic
free nerve endings	stereognosis
graphesthesia	tactile

Visual System

LEARNING OBJECTIVES

After studying this chapter, students should be able to:

- Outline the anatomy of the eyeball and describe the function of these structures

- Describe the structures of the retina and their functions

- Explain structural and functional differences between cones and rods

- Provide an account of photochemistry of retinal photoreceptors

- Discuss the mechanism of color vision and its disorders

- Explain the neural mechanism of dark adaptation

- Describe optical properties of normal vision

- Define common errors of refraction and their optical remediations

- Discuss the central visual pathway

- Relate visual field defects with lesion sites

- Describe the neural mechanism of visual reflexes

Not only is the visual system an important sensory modality but its disturbances provide important clues to numerous neurologic conditions. Visual perception involves a combination of four events: (1) the **refraction** of light rays by the **lens** and **cornea**, (2) the conversion of electromagnetic energy in light by the **retinal photoreceptor cells** into nerve impulses, (3) the transmission of impulses from the retinal photoreceptors to the **visual cortex** in the occipital lobe, and (4) the perception of visual images in the **primary visual cortex**. The primary visual cortex projects to the adjacent visual association region, where visual information is elaborated and synthesized with experiences in memory for its recognition. The organization of this chapter follows the order of neural events as they occur, beginning with the eyeball and ending with the primary visual cortex.

Distinguishing among three sets of terms is essential for understanding the visual system: **optic nerve** and **optic tract**, **visual** and **retinal fields**, and **monocular** and **binocular vision**. The *optic nerve* includes the nerve fibers from the retina to the **optic chiasm**. The *optic (CN II) tract* includes nerve fibers traveling between the chiasm and the **lateral geniculate body (LGB)** of the thalamus. Thalamic projections to the visual cortex travel via the **geniculocalcarine (optic radiation) fibers**. The *visual field* is the external area visible to one or both eyes without movement. The *retinal field* is the focused representation of the visual field. The retinal image is the reverse of the visual field image—that is, up becomes down and left becomes right.

The retinal field for each eye contains the portions of the visual field that are seen in common with the other eye (binocular) and a portion that is seen only by one eye (monocular). The *monocular visual field* is the lateral portion of the visual field that is perceived in only one eye (Fig. 8-1). By alternately closing the left and right eyes, one can produce a shift between right and left monocular vision. The *binocular visual field* is seen in both eyes as they simultaneously focus on a single object. Light rays from an object strike the corresponding (homonymous) retinal points in both eyes and the images from the two eyes merge into one image in the cortex. Any slight deviation in the coordination of the eyes would prevent light rays from striking corresponding (homonymous) retinal points, resulting in double (diplopia) vision.

ANATOMY OF THE EYE

Eyeball

The eyeball weighs ~7.5 g and is 2.4 cm (~1 inch) long. Five-sixths of its surface is concealed within the **orbital cavity**. The eyeball is divided into a small **anterior** and a large **posterior cavity** (Fig. 8-2A).

The *anterior cavity* contains the **ciliary body, suspensory ligaments, iris,** and **lens** (Fig. 8-2B). The principal function of these structures is to refract light rays to produce a sharply focused image on the retina. The anterior cavity is divided into **anterior** and **posterior chambers**. The anterior chamber includes the area between the *cornea* and *iris,* and the posterior chamber includes the area between the *iris* and the suspensory ligament. The anterior chamber is filled with **aqueous humor**, a fluid similar to **cerebrospinal fluid (CSF)**, that is produced behind the

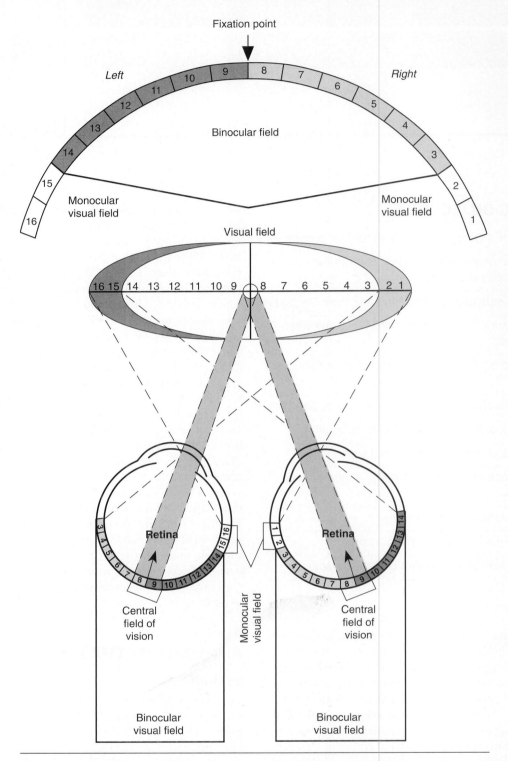

Figure 8-1 Binocular and monocular visual fields. *Shaded area,* binocular field; *open area,* monocular field.

iris in the posterior chamber by the **choroid plexus** of the **ciliary processes**.

The aqueous humor flows through the pupil to the anterior chamber, where its production is balanced by its drainage into the venous system through the **canal of Schlemm**. The fluid passes through the veins of the choroids through a valve-like mechanism, which prevents its back flow. The two major functions of the aqueous humor are maintaining normal intraocular pressure and linking the lens and cornea with the circulatory system. Any chronic increase in intraocular pressure, wherein the production of aqueous humor exceeds its reabsorption, leads to **glaucoma**,

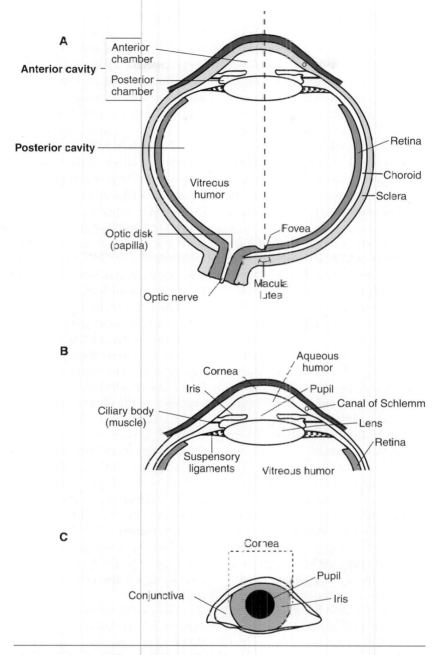

Figure 8-2 Structures of the eyeball. A. Cavities and chambers. B. Cross-section of the anterior cavity showing the ciliary muscles and suspensory ligaments and their attachments to the lens. C. Anterior view of the iris around the pupil.

which is characterized by an increased intraocular pressure (>22–25 mm Hg) and, subsequently, reduced blood flow to the retina and irritation of the retinal neurons. It is a silent disease in which the changes are progressive and cause no discomfort. Untreated glaucoma can cause blindness by restricting blood flow to the optic (CN II) nerve at the optic disc. Atrophy of the optic (CN II) nerve has serious implications for defects in the field of vision. The field defect begins from the periphery and progress to the central vision. One of the treatments for glaucoma involves controlling the secretion of vitreous humor using vasoconstricting drugs to attenuate the ciliary blood supply.

The *posterior cavity*, the area between the lens and the retina, is filled with **vitreous humor**, a jelly-like (gelatinous) substance that in part maintains normal intraocular pressure and prevents the eyeball from collapsing. The aqueous humor of the anterior cavity undergoes constant replacement, but the vitreous humor is formed once in early life and is never replaced. It has a very a slow rate of turnover, thus it takes a long time for macrophages to remove blood in case of a hemorrhage involving the vitreous humor. Floaters, commonly seen in the visual field, are protein molecules located in the vitreous humor near the retina.

The eyeball consists of three ocular layers (Fig. 8-2): outer **fibrous tunic** (**sclera**), middle **vascular tunic** (**choroid**), and inner **nervous tunic** (**retina**). The fibrous tunic, an extension of the meningeal **dura mater**, has two divisions: sclera and **cornea**.* The sclera, the white of the eye, is a dense layer of opaque connective tissue that covers the round section of the eyeball. A larger part of the sclera is concealed within the orbital cavity. The cornea, a nonvascular and transparent fibrous region of the eye, is in the exposed area of eyeball and it covers the anterior chamber (Fig. 8-2B).

The middle vascular tunic consists of the choroid, iris, **ciliary** (muscle) **structure**, and lens. The choroid contains an elastic connective tissue membrane that lines the internal surface of the sclera. The choroid is not only the source of the vascular supply to the sclera and outer retina but also contains **melanocytes** (pigment-producing cells). Normally, the choroid pigment melanocytes make the eyeball opaque by preventing stray light from entering the optic globe through the sclera. In the presence of pigment cell abnormalities related to **albinism** (which involves many alleles, and thus there are many grades of choroid pigment reduction), stray light that escapes absorption penetrates to the retina, making vision in bright light difficult and even painful. This causes photophobia, which is a fear and avoidance of light.

The iris and ciliary muscle are the connective tissue of the choroid. The **radial** (dilator) and **circular** (constrictor) fibers of the iris surround the **pupil**, an opening in the center of the iris. Working like a diaphragm and controlled by the autonomic nervous system (ANS), the iris regulates the amount of light that enters the eye by adjusting the pupil size. A contraction of the circular (construction) iris fibers in response to autonomic parasympathetic activity decreases pupil size, reducing the amount of light entering the eye, whereas constriction of radial fibers in response to autonomic sympathetic (T1–T3) activity enlarges the pupil, allowing more light to enter.

Ciliary muscle fibers, innervated by the parasympathetic projections of the **oculomotor (CN III) nerve**, form a ring (sphincter) around the optic globe. They contract to narrow the diameter of the optic globe, reducing the tension on the suspensory ligaments (**zonules of Zinn**). This releases the tension on the lens capsule and allows the elastic lens to approach or assume its natural spherical (round) shape. A denervated ciliary muscle results in a more highly refracting lens. The increased refraction of light entering the pupil is necessary for producing a sharp image in near vision.

The lens, which consists of multiple layers of protein fibers, is enclosed in a transparent capsule of connective tissue. One of the common pathologic conditions of the lens is **cataract**, an age-induced painless production of nontransparent fibrous protein. It results in the clouding of the lens or its capsule because the quality of the focused image depends on the degree of lens opaqueness. The treatment of a cataract requires the surgical removal of the opaque lens. The lens is held behind the pupil by suspensory ligaments that attach to the ciliary body. It is responsible for properly focusing images on the retina through the refraction of light rays. Abnormalities in the lens structure affect its refraction capacity, resulting in impaired focusing. The ciliary muscle and its processes regulate the changes undertaken by the lens to accommodate for near vision. Surgical replacement of the lens involves implanting a lens in the capsule in a technique that does not affect the accommodation mechanism of the lens.

The nervous tunic (retina), the innermost layer of the eyeball, consists of 10 layers of cells and is in the posterior two-thirds of the eyeball. It contains the photoreceptor cells (**rods and cones**) that transduce the absorbed light energy into neural impulses and local potentials. Other retinal cells participate in the transmission of visual impulses to the cortex.

Retina

The cellular layer known as the retina lies in the posterior portion of the eyeball. It consists of two layers: outer and inner. The outer layer, located next to the choroid, contains pigmented epithelium; the inner layer represents the neural elements. The retina, a specialized growth of the brain, contains a complex arrangement of 10 layers of cells, including nerve cells, neuronal processes, and supporting cells (Fig. 8-3). The functions of the **rods** and **cones** (**photoreceptors**), **bipolar cells**, and **ganglion cells** are discussed in this chapter.

The photoreceptors (cones and rods) form the most external cellular layer, whereas the ganglion cells constitute the proximal (internal) layer of cells in the retina. Light rays entering through the *cornea, aqueous humor, pupil, lens,* and *vitreous humor* first pass through the proximal layers of the ganglionic, **amacrine**, **horizontal**, bipolar, and other cellular components before striking the *rods* and *cones*. The electromagnetic energy in the light rays is absorbed by the photosensitive cells at the retinal level. Light rays that escape absorption at the retinal photosensor level are absorbed by the pigment cells of the surrounding choroid layer. In general the outer segments of the photoreceptors absorb the photons as (quantum of light) and convert them into electric signals, as graded potentials, that travel passively through synaptic transmission to the bipolar neurons and finally activate the ganglion cells, which process the signals as action potentials to the brain.

General properties of the photoreceptors are that they do not use action potentials. Instead, communicating with

---

*The cornea is an ectodermal structure; although, for convenience, it is here considered a dural extension.

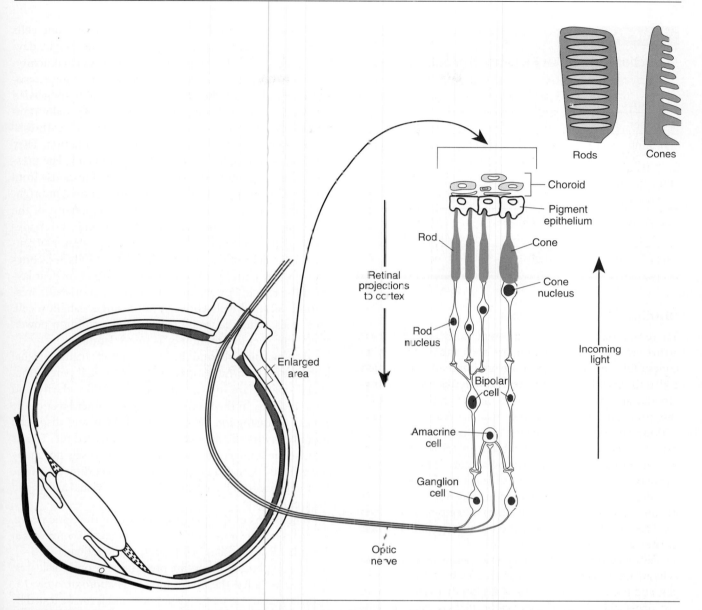

Figure 8-3 Cellular organization of the retina with its three layers of cells: photoreceptors (rods and cones), bipolar cells, and ganglion cells. Light rays enter and pass through all these layers to reach the cones and rods, which are activated to generate action potentials. Action potentials from the photosensors carrying the visual code travel back to the bipolar cells and ganglion cells. Ganglion cell projections form the optic nerve.

the retinal cells using local synaptic transmission, they respond to light energy in a graded fashion and their photosensitive lamellae (identical to cilia) are continuously replaced. The absorbed electromagnetic energy of the light rays activates the rods and cones, which transduce energy into local potentials. By inhibiting and exciting the adjacent cells, these potentials travel to the bipolar cells, which, by means of local potentials and the release of transmitters, affect the excitability of the ganglion cells. The ganglion cells are the retinal cells with voltage-gated sodium channels and are thus the first to generate action potentials. Ganglion cell axons converge at the **optic disk** (**papilla** or optic nerve head) to form the optic nerve. Posteriorly, these axons pierce the eyeball, projecting to

the **optic chiasm**, which also receives projections from the other eye.

The structure of the fundus (the retinal area seen with an ophthalmoscope) provides important clues about brain diseases; **papilledema**, a common pathology of the fundus, is caused by the edema of the axonal tips of the nerve. Marked by an elevated optic disk with poorly defined boundaries, it provides clinically significant information about disease processes, such as hypertension, diabetes mellitus and disk swelling.

The rods and cones are functionally and structurally different. They are sensitive to light rays of different wavelengths, mediate vision under different light conditions, and contain different visual pigments (Table 8-1).

Table 8-1

Functional Summary of Photoreceptors

Features	Cones	Rods
Number	30 million	100 million
Location	Fovea, central retina	Retina, except fovea
Functional conditions	Bright light	Low light
Color processing	All colors	Only gray shades
Visual acuity	High	Low

Distribution of Photosensors

There are ~130 million photoreceptors in the human retina. Of these, ~100 million are rods and 30 million are cones (Table 8-1). Cone cells are predominantly in the central retina, which consists of the **macula lutea**, a small circular area lateral to the optic disk (Fig. 8-2A). Within the macula lutea is the **fovea centralis**. With a diameter of 700 μm and covering 2° of the retina from the center, the inner retinal layer is almost absent in the fovea, leaving only its outer layer of the photoreceptors. This allows for the maximum amount of light to reach the fovea, which is also the focal point of central vision (Fig. 8-4). The number of cones per unit gradually declines in regions farther from the fovea centralis, whereas the number of rods becomes greater in the peripheral retina.

The functions of other retinal-amacrine and horizontal cells are not discussed here. Overall, they have an integrative role and use local inhibitory and excitatory potentials only.

Functions of Photosensors

As noted, cone and rod cells contain different visual pigments, are sensitive to light rays of different wavelengths, and operate under different light conditions. Cone cells have a high threshold for light and require bright daylight to function. The cones mediate sharp **visual acuity**, color vision, and tasks that require high temporal resolution. Hundreds of photons (elements of light) are needed to evoke responses from cones, which are virtually nonfunctional in the dark. Conversely, rods, with a low threshold for light, require only a few photons to function. They function in dim light and mediate night vision. The presence of fewer photons can evoke a maximal response from the rods. For this reason, rods are nonfunctional in bright daylight. With sensitivity to selective components of the color spectrum, rods differentiate black, white, and shades of gray, detect movement, and identify shapes but they cannot resolve details or mediate color vision. Rods and cones have specific patterns of connections to other nuclear layers of the retina. For example, because of poor spatial resolution, >20 rod cells converge on a single ganglion cell. Cone cells, which have a higher spatial resolution power, directly project to ganglion cells in a 1:1 ratio.

The macula lutea and the fovea centralis regulate visual acuity, color discrimination, and sharp visual perception. Visual images are focused in the macula for clarity and color analysis. In the fovea centralis, the inner layer of the bipolar and ganglion cells is pushed apart and displaced laterally, giving the appearance of a depressed pit. This is because the fovea contains neither blood vessels nor many nerve fibers, it enables light rays to project directly on the photoreceptors and allows for the highest visual acuity and color perception.

The axons of the ganglion cells form the optic nerve, which travels the inner surface of the retina and converges at the optic disk (papilla) before exiting the retina (Fig. 8-5). Because no photoreceptors are present in the optic disk area, this area is called the **blind spot**; it is approximately 15° medial to the center of the visual axis, and it can be tested by slowly moving an object in front of the retina. The object will briefly disappear as it is projected on the optic disk (e.g., the letter Z in Fig. 8-5).

VASCULAR SUPPLY OF THE RETINA

The cerebral part of the **internal carotid artery** as its passes the cranial dura gives off the **ophthalmic artery**, which passes through the **optic foramen** to enter the orbit. The ophthalmic artery branches into the **central retinal artery** and the **ciliary artery**. After traveling along the optic nerve, the central retinal artery separates to supply the inner retinal layer. The ciliary artery, on the other hand, supplies the choroidal layer and the outer retinal layer. The retina, with its acute dependence on blood supply, is highly sensitive to vascular ischemia. Therefore, retinal dysfunctions may indicate pathology involving the internal carotid artery.

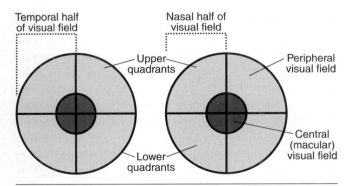

Figure 8-4 Central and peripheral visual fields and their divisions into temporal and nasal half-fields and upper and lower quadrants.

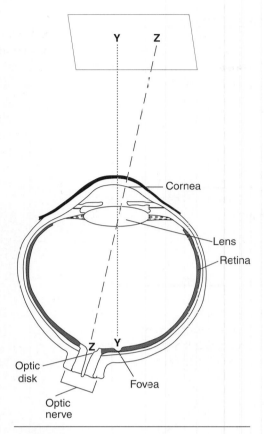

Figure 8-5 The blind spot. Fixation of the right eye on the letter Y projects the adjacent letter Z onto the optic disk, which lacks receptors.

PHOTOCHEMISTRY OF RETINA

Photochemistry entails the absorption of electromagnetic energy in light by the visual pigments of rods and cones and its conversion into neural impulses. Photopigments are colored proteins in the outer membranes (photosensitive lamellae) of rods and cones. These lamellae undergo structural changes on absorbing light. Rods and cones transmit local potentials to the bipolar cells, which in turn activate ganglion cells by means of neurotransmitters. The ganglion cells are the first cells to generate action potentials, which travel on their axons in the oculomotor nerve (CN III).

Rhodopsin, the photosensitive visual pigment in rods, is sensitive to blue to green wavelengths (400–575 nm). Located mostly in the peripheral retina, rods are sensitive to low light conditions and mediate night vision. Structurally wide and containing a greater number of lamellae—analogous to cilia-containing photosegments—the rods have a greater photosensitivity but lack visual acuity. All visual photopigments contain two elements: **opsin**, a glycoprotein, and **retinal** (visual yellow), a light-absorbing molecule that is a derivative (aldehyde) of vitamin A.

In the absence of light, the photoreceptors release glutamate at the synapses. This neurotransmitter release is attenuated in case of light exposure, which triggers a series of neuronal events related to the decomposition and regeneration of pigments. This chemical decomposition generates changes in the membrane potentials of the receptor cells. A series of biochemical events occurs in between to resynthesize the rhodopsin, which takes 7–30 min. This is also the time needed for adapting to darkness. The inability to see at night, even after this normal period of dark adaptation is called **night blindness** (nyctalopia); it is usually caused by a deficiency of vitamin A. In daylight, rods are saturated by bright light and do not respond to light.

Photopsin, the photopigment of cones, consists of retinal, opsin, and light-absorbing molecules. The photochemical processing of cones is similar to that of rods, in which phototransduction involves the decomposition of the photopigment and its resynthesis. It also involves the neurotransmitter glutamate. Its secretion increases in dark settings and decreases in light settings. Because of sensitivity to different wavelengths (for color vision), cones contain three types of photopigments (proteins), which promote maximum absorption of light from different parts of the light spectrum. The three types of opsin/cones account for the **trivalent color vision**. Three issues related to neural coding in the retina are **spectral sensitivity**, **color vision**, and **dark adaptation**.

Spectral Sensitivity

In addition to being sensitive to different light conditions, rods and cones are sensitive to different wavelengths of light. They have different **visibility curves**, known as the **scotopic** (rods) and **photopic** (cones) luminosity curves (Fig 8-6). The scotopic (night vision) curve is obtained from eyes adapted to the dark. This rod-mediated visibility curve shows great sensitivity to light rays with wavelengths of 400–600 nm, with maximum sensitivity at 507 nm, in the blue-green range. The same eye adapted to light has a photopic visibility curve that covers wavelengths of 425–700 nm and maximum sensitivity to 555 nm, in the yellow-green range.

Color Vision

Cones in the human eye are sensitive to wavelengths ranging from 400 to 700 nm. In this spectrum, the colors change from blue to red after passing through green, yellow, and orange. There are three types of cones in the retina, and each has photosensitive pigments specialized for different wavelengths (**blue cones**, **green cones**, and **red cones**). Spectral differences in the cones make them respond best to light of different wavelengths. Short-wavelength cones (S-cones) are sensitive to blue and have a maximum absorption at 445 nm. Medium-wavelength cones (M-cones) are sensitive to green and respond with a maximum absorption at 535 nm. Long-wavelength cones (L-cones) are sensitive to red and respond with maximum absorption at 570 nm.

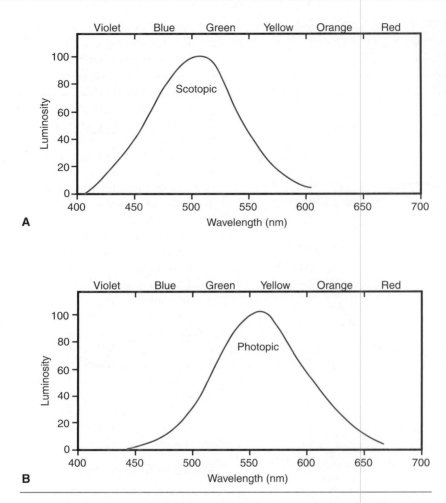

Figure 8-6 Relative sensitivity of the rods and cones to light of various wavelengths. **A.** The scotopic luminosity curve. **B.** The photopic luminosity curve.

Trichromatic color vision results from the combination of the activities of the blue, green, and red cones.

Dark Adaptation

Dark adaptation is the normal night vision possible within a few minutes after entering a darkened room. As noted, it normally takes between 7–30 min for the eyes to adjust to a dark room. This is the time needed for the rhodopsin to be reconstituted. After a person moves from bright daylight to a dark room, the cones initially remain sensitive to light and continue to process colors by resynthesizing photopigments; thus both cones and rods increase their sensitivity to light. If the low-light conditions persist, the cones, with their high threshold to light, gradually become nonfunctional. The rods, with their low threshold to light, then begin functioning. As the rods start adjusting to dim light, vision become **achromatic**. The only color that is still recognized is red, because rods are insensitive to red light (Fig. 8-6A). The red wavelength is processed exclusively by the rod-free fovea centralis. Thus one can adapt to the dark while continuing to process red color by wearing red goggles.

OPTICAL MECHANISM

The eye functions as an optical instrument. Sharp focusing of an image depends on the adequate refraction of light rays, which ensures a properly focused image on the inner surface of the retina. Familiarity with the optical principle of refraction and the **refractive properties** of the lens is essential to understanding the optical mechanism of the eye.

Refraction

Light rays travel in straight lines and slow down when entering a transparent medium from a medium of greater density. If the light rays strike a surface with a different density at an angle, they bend. This is called refraction. The degree to which light rays bend depends on two factors: the **refractive index**[†] of the medium into which the

---

[†]The refractive index of any transparent substance is the ratio of the velocity of light in air to the velocity of light in the second transparent substance. For example, a glass cube has a refractive index of 1.5: velocity of light through air (300,000 km/sec) divided by the velocity of light through glass velocity (200,000 km/sec) = 1.5.

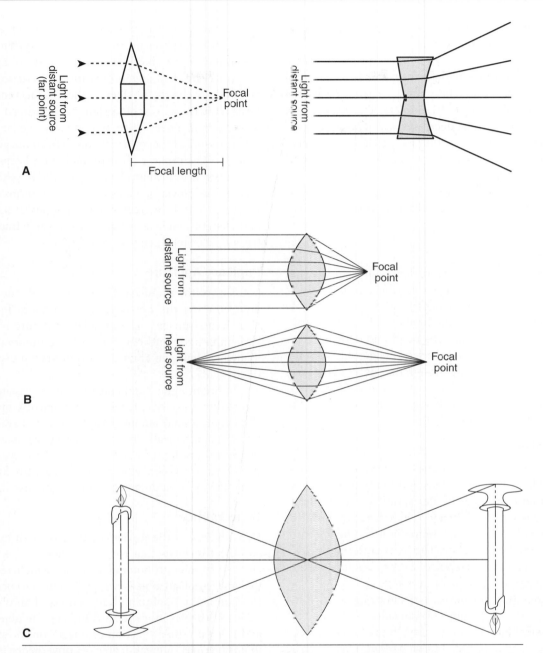

Figure 8-7 A. Refraction through convex and concave lenses. B. Two convex lenses possess similar refractive powers, but they have different focal lengths because the rays entering the upper lens are parallel, whereas rays entering the lower lens diverge. C. The eye as an optical mechanism in which the object focused on the retina is reversed in relation to the visual field.

waves enter and the **angle** at which the rays strike the surface. If traveling light waves strike a medium of a different density perpendicular to the wave front, the striking waves slow down, although they continue to travel along the same course without any deviation (refraction). However, if the waves strike an angled interface of a medium with a different refractive index (density), they bend.

Refractive power is measured in **diopter units**, and the total refractive power of the eye is 60 diopters. In the eye, refraction of light rays depends primarily on the curvature and optical density of the cornea and on the lens shape. The

cornea alone contributes about 42 of the 60 diopters to the refraction. A simple example of refraction can be seen in a biconvex lens (Fig. 8-7A). In this lens, the top and bottom sections have an angulated shape, whereas the central section is rectangular. The angulated top section of the lens bends the striking waves downward, whereas the bottom angulated section of the lens bends the waves upward. The rectangular center portion of the lens (nonangulated and perpendicular to the wave front) permits light rays to pass through without deviation. All of these light rays converge at a common point (**focal point**) to form the focused image.

The distance from the lens to the focal point is the **focal length**, and the point from which the rays originate is the **far point**.

The power of a lens is defined in terms of the focal length. The action of the ciliary muscles can increase the refractive power of a lens by 12 diopters. This elasticity of the lens (**accommodation**) decreases with age. This gradual reduction in ability to accommodate the lens for near vision is called presbyopia, which usually begins around age 40, and this ability is virtually nonexistent by age 65. This poses a problem with reading, but reading glasses or glasses with bifocal lenses are helpful in overcoming this difficulty.

Lens Types

The two most common types of lenses are **convex** and **concave** (Fig. 8-7A). Each type contributes differently to refraction. A convex lens reduces focal length by adding greater convergence to bending light rays. Light rays striking the angled edges of the lens bend and converge to a common focus point beyond the lens, where they join the undeviating waves traveling through the center of the lens. In contrast, a concave lens, with its inward-angled edge, increases the focal length by diverging rays away from the centrally entering rays of the lens.

Optics of the Eye

Focusing an image on the retinas entails three processes: **refraction** of light rays by the lens, **pupillary aperture** control, and **ocular convergence**. Refraction of the rays leads to proper focusing of the image. The refractive power of a lens is controlled by its accommodation. The aperture of the pupil opening regulates the light entering the eye. Convergence refers to the control of the eyes for tracking a moving object.

For all practical purposes, a distance of 20 ft (6 m) between the lens and the object is considered common for assessing vision. Light rays originating from an object placed 20 ft or more away are parallel to each other. They must be bent adequately to converge on the fovea centralis. Light rays from an object closer than 20 ft are generally divergent (Fig. 8-7B). This divergence of rays is too great for the cornea and resting lens to focus the image on the retina. Therefore, greater refraction is required. Because the distance between the center of the lens and the fovea centralis is considered fixed at 17 mm, the lens and the refractive mechanism must assume different shapes to refract the parallel rays reflected from a distant object and the diverging rays from a near object. This is made possible with the regulation of the lens (**lens accommodation**) curvature by the action of the ciliary muscle.

Refraction by the Lens

The curvature of a lens (as opposed to its flat surface) determines its refractive power. A lens with greater outward round curvature has more refractive power and acutely bends light rays toward the focus point. What makes the lens unique is its ability to increase or decrease its refractive power by changing its curvature. The action of the ciliary muscles change the shape of the lens (accommodation). If the refractive power of the lens is unchanged, the diverging rays from a near object would converge far behind the photosensors of the retina, resulting in an image that is out of focus. The process of accommodation keeps the image of a near object in sharp focus by modifying the lens's curvature. The power of a lens is defined in terms of the focal length. A lens with greater refracting power has a shorter focal length, whereas a lens with lower refractive power has a greater focal length.

Pupillary Aperture

The size of the pupillary aperture controls the amount of light entering the eyes and contributes to formation of clear retinal images. The pupillary aperture is controlled by sympathetic and parasympathetic innervation of the dilator (radial) and constrictor (circular) muscle fibers of the iris.

In bright light, pupil constriction is regulated by parasympathetic activity; it results in a narrow opening that allows only a small amount of light to enter. In dim light, the pupil sympathetically dilates to enlarge the opening, allowing maximum light to enter the eye. Reflexive pupil constriction also serves as a protective mechanism for the retina when the eye is suddenly exposed to intense light.

Convergence

Convergence is the inward turning of both eyes to keep an object in focus that is moving closer. This movement also contributes to binocular vision, which results when the images of an object are projected on corresponding (homonymous) points in both retinas. If an object moves closer, both eyes move inward to keep the object in focus and to retain the projection of images on the same points in both retinas. A great degree of convergence is needed to clearly see objects extremely close to the eyes. Different ocular muscles are involved in regulating the coordinated act of ocular convergence (see Chapter 15).

Retinal Image Formation

Forming an image on the retina is guided by one optical principle: The retinal image is a reversed and inverted form of what is seen in the visual field. Light reflected from the top portion of an object is projected onto the **lower retina**. Rays from the bottom portion of an object strike the **upper retina**. The projected upside down image is also a mirror image of both the left and the right sides of an object (Fig. 8-7C). Even though the retinal image is upside down and reversed, the correct interpretation of the image is learned via a process that begins at birth and is mediated by the associational visual cortex.

CENTRAL VISUAL PATHWAYS

The central visual mechanism includes the pathway from the retina of the eye to the primary visual cortex, which is located on the midsagittal surface of the occipital lobe (Fig. 8-8). Two important characteristics of the central visual mechanism are a point-to-point representation of the visual field from the retina through the LGB to the primary visual cortex and the projection from each eye to both cerebral hemispheres (basis for binocular vision). Familiarity with the pathways carrying visual information and the crossing points of the visual fibers provides the

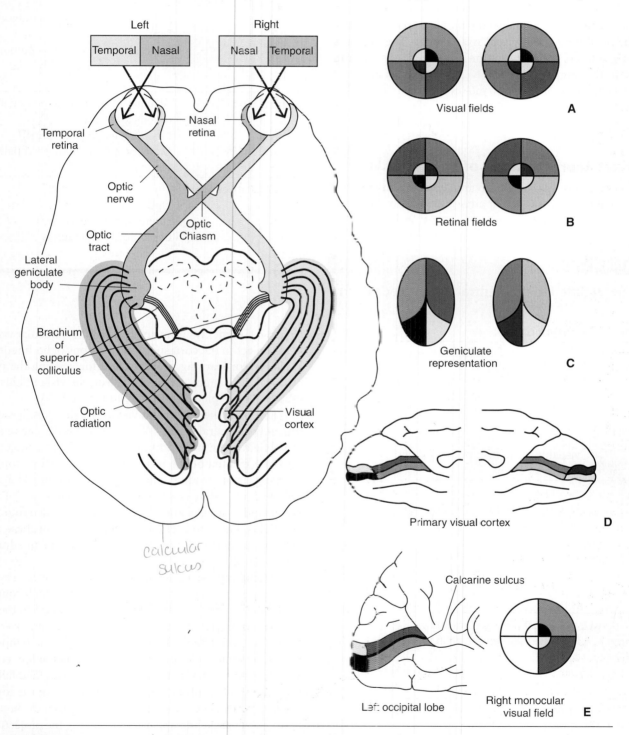

Figure 8-8 The visual pathways from the retina to the visual cortex in the occipital lobe and representation of the visual fields as processed along the optic pathway. A. The visual fields. B. The retinal fields. C. The geniculate representation. D. The cortex. E. The right monocular visual field as mapped on the left primary visual cortex in the occipital lobe.

basis for relating lesion sites with specific visual field defects (Fig. 8-8; Table 8-2).

The optic nerve (CN II) fibers from the retinal cells exit the orbital cavity through the **optic foramina** and enter the cranial cavity. Optic nerves from both eyes come together at the optic chiasm rostral to the hypothalamus (see Figs. 2-8 and 2-11). The optic tract fibers from the optic chiasm travel caudally and laterally and terminate in the **LGB**, the thalamic visual relay center. The geniculo-calcarine fibers (optic radiation) loop laterally and caudally in the **temporal lobe**, travel to the occipital cortex, and terminate in the superior and inferior opercula (lips) of the **calcarine fissure**, the primary visual cortex (Brodmann area 17), located on the midsagittal surface of the occipital lobe (Table 8-3).

Retinal Representation of Visual Fields

The eyes do not function individually, and a large part of the visual field, the binocular area, is covered by both eyes

Table 8-3

Panoramic View of Visual Processes

Process	Structures
Traveling light rays	Cornea Anterior cavity (aqueous humor) Lens Posterior cavity (vitreous humor) Retinal cells (ganglion, bipolar, rods, cones)
Retinal processing	Changes in membrane potential in rods and cones Bipolar cells (local potential) Ganglion cells (action potential) Optic nerve
Cortical processing	Optic chiasm Optic tract Lateral geniculate body Geniculocalcarine fibers Visual cortex

Table 8-2

Rules Related to the Central Visual Mechanism

Rule	Description
1	Retinal image is a reversed and inverted form of visual field image
2	Nasal retinal fibers (representing temporal visual field) cross at optic chiasm and project to opposite cortex Temporal retinal fibers (representing nasal visual field) remain uncrossed and project to ipsilateral cortex
3	Geniculocortical fibers representing lower visual field quadrant pass dorsally through cerebral white matter to reach visual cortex (upper lip of calcarine fissure) Geniculocalcarine fibers representing upper visual field quadrant pass ventrally and laterally through loop of Meyer and project to visual cortex (lower lip of calcarine fissure)
4	Upper retinal fibers (representing lower visual field quadrant) terminate in upper visual cortex Lower retinal fibers (representing upper visual field quadrant) project to lower visual cortex
5	Peripheral visual field is represented rostrally along calcarine fissure Central (foveal) visual field is represented caudally along calcarine fissure and extends beyond to occipital pole cortex

(Fig. 8-1). Light rays from an object in the binocular visual field project to the corresponding portions of both retinas. However, for learning purposes and for keeping the path of visual projections precise and clear, the visual fields for each eye are depicted separately in Figure 8-8A.

The visual field, the area viewed by the eyes, has **central** and **peripheral regions** (Figs. 8-4 and 8-8). The central visual field is the small area in the center. This is projected onto the macula of the retina and is responsible for the sharpest vision, reading, and object recognition. The central field of vision is surrounded by a large peripheral visual field. The visual field for each eye is divided into two half fields: **nasal** and **temporal halves**. Each of these half fields is further divided into **upper** and **lower quadrants** (Fig. 8-4).

Retinal representation of the visual field for each eye is also divided into nasal and temporal halves, which contain upper and lower quadrants. As noted, the image in the visual field is projected to the retina in **reversed** and **inverted form** (Fig. 8-8B; Table 8-2). Light rays from the temporal half of the visual field project to the nasal half of the retina. Similarly, rays from the nasal half of the visual field fall on the temporal half of the retina. Light rays from the top of the object strike the lower retina, and rays from the bottom of the object strike the upper retina. Taking the projections for both eyes into consideration, light rays from an object in the right visual field fall on the nasal retina of the right eye and the temporal retina of the left eye. Light rays of an object from the left visual field strike the nasal half of the retina in the left eye and the temporal half of the retina in the right eye.

Retinal Representation to Optic Chiasm

Optic nerve fibers from the retinal ganglion cells enter the cranial cavity to reach the optic chiasm. Two rules account for the partial crossing of fibers at the chiasm. First, fibers from the nasal halves of the retinas (representing temporal visual fields for each eye) cross the midline to project to the opposite visual cortex. Second, fibers from the temporal half of each retina (representing nasal halves of the visual fields) remain uncrossed and project to the ipsilateral visual cortex. This accounts for projection of the right visual field to the left hemisphere and projection of the left visual field to the right hemisphere (Fig. 8-8; Table 8-2).

Retinal Representation to the Lateral Geniculate Body

Each optic tract (**postchiasmic fibers**) carries visual information from both eyes. The left optic tract mediates the right visual field for each eye. The left optic tract contains the projections from the temporal half of the left retina (nasal visual field for the left eye) and the nasal half of the right retina (temporal visual field for the right eye). Similarly, the right optic tract transmits the left visual field for each eye and includes the projections from the nasal half of the left retina (temporal visual field for the left eye) and temporal half of the right retina (nasal visual field for the right eye). This arrangement of contralateral projections from each eye is consistent with contralateral sensory and motor organization. The optic tract projects to the LGB of the thalamus.

Each LGB receives a point-to-point projection from the homonymous (left or right) halves of the field of both eyes (Fig. 8-8C). The visual information is distributed on both sides of the LGB. Fibers from the upper retinal quadrants (representing lower visual field quadrants) terminate in the medial portion of the LGB, whereas fibers from the lower retinal quadrants (representing upper visual field quadrants) project to the lateral portion of the LGB.

Retinal Representation to the Visual Cortex

Geniculocalcarine fibers, or **optic radiations**, constitute the last phase in the transmission of visual information to the visual cortex (Fig. 8-8D). Geniculocalcarine fibers enter the retrolenticular portion of the posterior internal capsule on their way to the primary visual cortex (Fig. 9-9). The geniculocalcarine fibers divide into the **dorsal** and **ventral** bundles of fibers. The dorsal bundle of fibers, traveling straight to the cells in the visual cortex above the calcarine fissure, carries information from the upper retinal quadrants (representing the lower visual field quadrants). The ventral bundle of fibers forms the **loop of Meyer**. These geniculocalcarine fibers first move rostrally and then make a lateral excursion around the inferior (temporal) horn of the lateral ventricle before traveling to the cells in the visual cortex below the calcarine fissure. These fibers mediate projections from the lower retinal quadrants (representing the upper visual field quadrants) (Table 8-2).

Primary Visual Cortex

The primary visual cortex (Brodmann area 17) is bilateral and lies on the midsagittal surface of the occipital lobe (Fig. 8-8; see Fig. 2-10). It is divided into two opercula (lips), which are separated by the calcarine fissure. Each visual cortex receives information from both eyes. The lower (inferior) lip of the visual cortex, on the *lingual gyrus,* receives projections from the lower portion of the retina (representing the upper quadrant in the visual field). The upper (superior) lip of the visual cortex receives projections from the upper retina (representing the lower quadrant in the visual field). The central visual field, representing the macular region of the retina, occupies a comparatively large area in the caudal part near the occipital pole, amounting to > 50% of the primary visual cortex. The peripheral visual fields are represented in the anterior portions of the calcarine cortex (Fig. 8-8E; Table 8-2). The primary visual cortex is characterized by a wide layer 4. It contains an extra band of myelinated fibers and is known to send cortical feedback projections to the LGB. This myelinated structure seems to be the site of large geniculocalcarine input.

VISUAL CORTEX DEVELOPMENT

In early development, visual pathways from both eyes compete for equal access to synaptic spaces in the visual cortex, in particular for the connectivity in layer 4. This competing input from both eyes is essential for normal vision and proper depth perception.

The critical period plays an important role normal axonal connections, when the axonal afferents from both eyes have equal access to the overlapping cortical regions and compete for the available synaptic spaces. This is measured in terms of the number of synapses. The connections that succeed during the critical period become permanent. If for some reason axons from one eye are not functional during this developmentally critical period—from 5–6 years of age—they lose the claim for the synaptic spaces in the visual cortex. This gives prominence and dominance exclusively to axons from the other eye for controlling all the available synaptic space in the brain.

VISUAL REFLEXES

Visual reflexes are concerned with the changing of **pupil size** and **lens shape**. The ocular muscle fibers regulating these reflexes are innervated by the parasympathetic fibers of the oculomotor nerve (CN III), which regulate pupillary constriction and lens accommodation. Pupil dilation, on the other hand, is regulated by the sympathetic efferents (Fig. 8-10).

Pupillary Light Reflex

In the pupillary light reflex, the eyes react to bright light by constricting the pupils. The neural mechanism for these pupillary changes involves the **pretectal area**, the **Edinger-Westphal nucleus**, and fibers of the oculomotor nerve (Fig. 8-9A). The activated retinal ganglion cells send projections to the brain. These fibers leave the optic tract before the LGB and synapse on cells in the pretectal area. The pretectal area, a small unspecified area between the **superior colliculi**, bilaterally projects to the Edinger-Westphal nucleus, which is the visceral nucleus of the oculomotor (CN III) nerve. The preganglionic fibers from the Edinger-Westphal nucleus join the oculomotor fibers and innervate

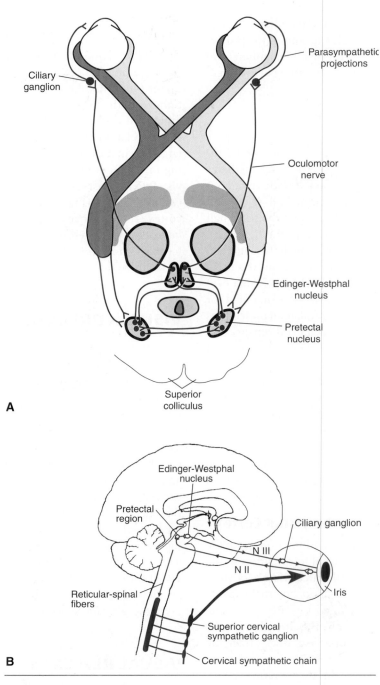

Figure 8-9 **A.** Parasympathetic innervation of the iris for pupil constriction in light. **B.** Sympathetic innervation of the eyeball for pupil dilation in dark. *N*, nerve.

the ipsilateral **ciliary ganglion** in the orbit. The postganglionic fibers from the ciliary ganglion provide parasympathetic projections to the circular (constrictor) fibers of the iris. The constriction of the circular fibers narrows the aperture of the pupil, a condition called **miosis** (Fig. 8-10A).

Both pupils constrict in response to light entering one eye. The pupillary reaction in the eye exposed to light is the **direct response**, whereas the reflexive pupillary change in the other eye is the **consensual response**. In complete darkness, constriction of the radial (dilator) fibers of the iris results in pupil dilation, or **mydriasis** (Fig. 8-10B).

The pupil dilatory function involves both inhibition of the Edinger-Westphal nucleus and facilitation of sympathetic activity. Sympathetic projections exit from T1 to T3 and travel in the cervical sympathetic chain to the **superior cervical ganglion**, which sends postganglionic projections to the radial fibers of the iris muscle in the eyeball (Fig. 8-9B).

Oculomotor nerve (CN III) lesions alter the pupillary light reflex. Interrupted afferent projections from one eye affect the light reflex in both pupils. This is tested by checking to see if light projected into each eye elicits both direct and consensual responses. Presence of the consensual response without a direct pupil response suggests a lesion involving the projection from the Edinger-Westphal nucleus to the same eye. An interruption of the sympathetic fibers causes paralysis of the dilator fibers of the iris and results in a permanently constricted pupillary diameter (miosis) The resulting condition is part of **Horner syndrome**, which is characterized by an ipsilaterally constricted pupil (**miosis**), drooping eyelid (**ptosis**), and loss of facial sweating (**anhidrosis**).

Accommodation Reflex

The accommodation (or near) reflex regulates the refractive power of the lens (Fig. 8-11A). The distance between

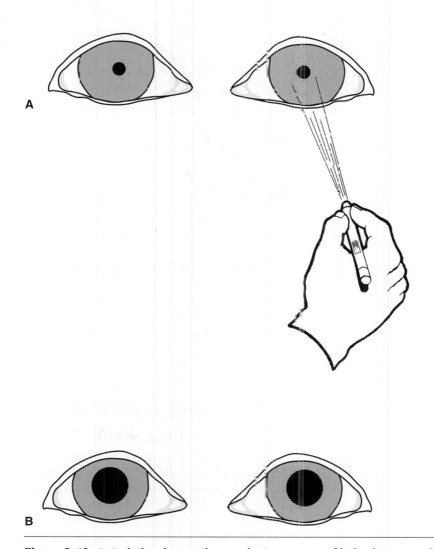

Figure 8-10 A. In light, the pupil controls the amount of light that enters by reflexively constricting, which results in a narrower opening. B. The pupil reflexively dilates in the dark, allowing maximum light to enter the eye.

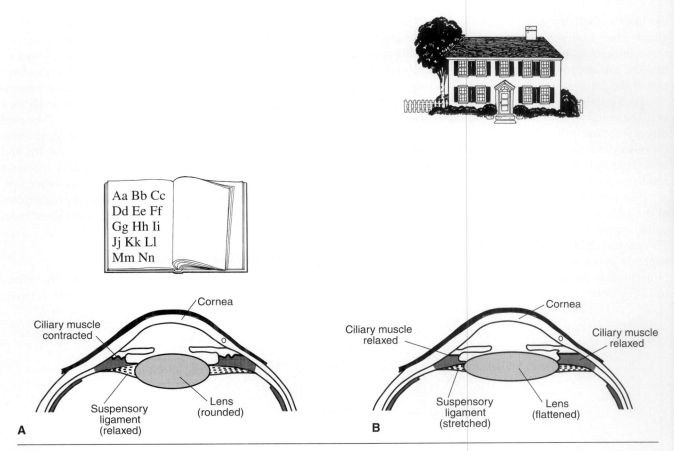

Figure 8-11 Lens accommodation for near (**A**) (<20 ft) objects and distant (**B**) (>20 ft) objects.

the lens and the retina remains the same as an object moves closer to the eyes. Keeping an object in focus requires increased refractive power of the lens, which occurs when the lens assumes a more nearly rounded (spherical) form. This reflexive modification of the lens curvature is controlled by the contraction of the ciliary muscles through the suspensory ligaments. The parasympathetic contraction of the ciliary muscles pulls the ciliary processes forward and reduces tension in the suspensory ligaments. With no pulls from ligaments, the lens, because of its elasticity, assumes a more rounded form, thus acquiring greater refractive power. This is needed for clearly viewing objects that are close (<20 ft) to the eye (Fig. 8-11A). The relaxed state of ciliary muscles exerts tension on the suspensory ligaments that pull on the lens, flattening the lens. This reduces the refractive power, permitting far vision (Fig. 8-11B).

The neural mechanism of the accommodation reflex is slightly different from the light reflex. It involves the primary visual cortex in addition to the LGB and the **mesencephalic reflex** center (Fig. 8-9A). As the image of an object moving closer begins to blur, the visual cortex sends projections to the superior colliculus, which mediates visual information to the pretectal area. The pretectal nuclei send crossed and uncrossed fibers to the Edinger-Westphal nucleus, which projects preganglionic parasympathetic fibers in the oculo-

motor (CN III) nerve to the ciliary ganglion. The postganglionic projections from the ciliary ganglion cause constriction of the ciliary muscle. Consequently, the lens, released from the tension of the suspensory ligaments, becomes round and acquires greater refractive power. The accommodation reflex has two additional components: eye convergence and pupillary constriction (discussed earlier). Children have greater ability to accommodate the lens than do adults; starting at about age 45 years, the lens gradually loses the flexibility to control the refractive power (**presbyopia**).

CLINICAL CONCERNS

Errors of Refraction

The refractive power of the eye is largely determined by the cornea and lens. In an **emmetropic** (normal) **eye**, there is a normal relationship between axial length and the eye's refractive power, so that light rays from objects beyond 20 ft can converge on the fovea without any lens accommodation (Fig. 8-12A). When the relationship between the refraction and the focal length is not optimal or correct, parallel light rays from distant objects converge either behind the retina or in front of it. Refractive problems cause blurred vision, visual

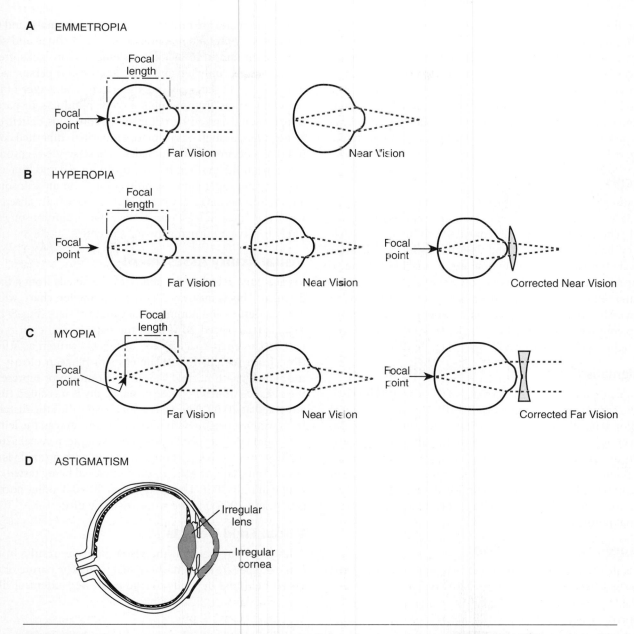

A EMMETROPIA

Focal length

Focal point

Far Vision

Near Vision

B HYPEROPIA

Focal length

Focal point

Far Vision

Near Vision

Focal point

Corrected Near Vision

C MYOPIA

Focal length

Focal point

Far Vision

Near Vision

Focal point

Corrected Far Vision

D ASTIGMATISM

Irregular lens

Irregular cornea

Figure 8-12 The normally refractive eye, common refractive errors, and their corrections. **A.** In a normal (emmetropic) eye, light rays from a near or far object are adequately refracted so that the rays converge directly on the retina, enabling formation of a clear image **B.** In a farsighted (hypermetropic, hyperopic) eye, an image from a near point is focused behind the retina. The resulting condition can be corrected with convex lenses. **C.** In a nearsighted (myopic) eye, an image from a far point is focused in front of the retina. This refractive condition can be corrected with concave lenses. **D.** Refractive errors of astigmatism result from irregular curvatures of the cornea, lens, or both. Consequently, horizontal and vertical points from various visual fields are focused at two different focal points on the retina, resulting in distorted vision.

fatigue, and possibly headaches. There are three common types of refractive errors: **hypermetropia** (farsightedness), **myopia** (nearsightedness), and **astigmatism**.

Hypermetropia

As noted, the focal point in a hypermetropic or hyperopic eye falls behind the retina (Fig. 8-12B). The two factors which contribute to this focusing error are the axial length of the eyeball is short and the refractive power of the lens is inadequate. Hypermetropic patients are farsighted (can see distant objects normally). This is because light rays from distant objects are parallel (less divergent) and are adequately refracted for converging on the fovea. The problem is in focusing near objects. Young hypermetropic patients may compensate for this refractive error by lens accommodation. Contracting the ciliary muscle removes tension from the suspensory ligaments and results in a convex lens with greater refractive power. However, after a limit, known as the **near point** of vision, the near objects can no longer be brought into focus. Furthermore, continuous use of accommodation may cause hypertrophy of the ciliary muscle. Hypermetropic error may be corrected by placing a convex lens in front of the eye, which adds greater refractive power needed for converging the light rays on the retina (Fig. 8-12C).

Myopia

Because the focal point in the myopic eye falls in front of the retina (Fig. 8-12D), these patients cannot see distant objects well. The two factors which contribute to myopia are that the eyeball has a long axis and the lens has strong refractive power. Individuals with myopia are nearsighted, because light rays from near objects are divergent and thus require greater refraction and/or a longer axis for converging on the retina. Myopic errors of refraction may be corrected by placing a concave lens before the eye. The concave lens diverges the light rays and adds focal length (Fig. 8-12E).

Astigmatism

Astigmatism is a refractive error caused by irregular shape of the cornea, lens, or both (Fig. 8-12F). Horizontal corneal and/or lens diameters do not have the same refractive power as vertical diameters. Consequently, different portions of light rays passing through the lens focus at different points on the retina. Astigmatic errors of refraction can be corrected by a combined cylindrical and spherical lens because it can bring all light rays into focus at the same retinal point.

Disorders of Color Vision

Several forms of color blindness or confusion have been described in clinical populations. Three major kinds of color

vision anomalies are **protanomaly**, **deuteranomaly**, and **tritanomaly**. A *protanopic* patient lacks red cones and sees only green and blue. A *deuteranopic* person lacks green cones and sees only red and blue. A *tritanopic* person lacks blue cones and sees only red and green. The degree of impairment varies from complete color blindness to partial impairment, marked by color confusion. This deficit can be acquired, though it is primarily inherited. Inherited color blindness occurs mostly in males, whose single X chromosome, from the mother, has the opsin for red and blue colors. The photopigment for blue color is on an autosome, and tritanomaly is rare. Color blindness is usually absent in women because at least one of their two X chromosomes is likely to have a normal gene for the cones.

Visual Acuity Assessment

Visual acuity refers to the ability to see details from a fixed distance. This is measured by use of a **Snellen chart**, which contains letters and numbers in a variety of sizes (Fig. 8-13). The chart is placed 20 ft from the patient, and each eye is tested. The chart specifies the distances, written as a fraction, from which the characters can be seen clearly by individuals with normal vision. The numerator represents the distance from which the visual acuity is measured (usually fixed at 20 ft). The denominator specifies the distance from which a person with normal vision can read the letters and numbers of a specific size. For example, a visual acuity of 20/80 means that, although a person with normal vision could read that line at 80 ft, the individual being tested can read it at only 20 ft. The designation 20/20 denotes normal acuity and 20/400 is the worst visual acuity.

Visual Field Defects

A lesion at any point in the visual pathway results in the loss of a specific point in the visual field. The nature of the visual field loss depends on the point and extent of fiber

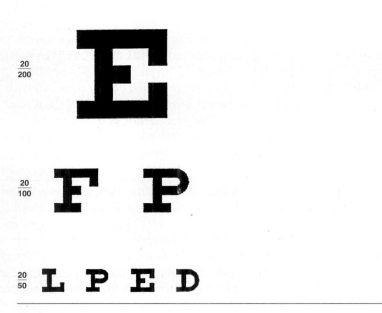

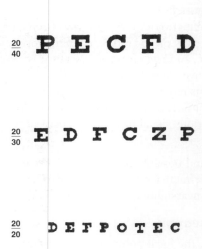

Figure 8-13 Snellen chart.

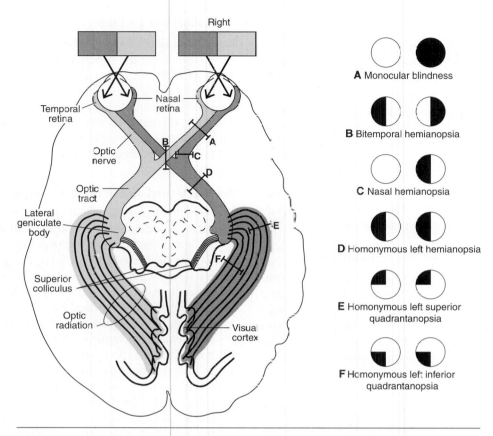

Figure 8-14 Common lesion sites in the visual pathways and the associated patterns of visual field losses.

interruption. The straightforward nature of the visual projections makes it easy to relate the locations of injury to specific patterns of field losses and vice versa. There are two types of field defects: **homonymous** and **heteronymous**. *Homonymous* refers to similar regions of visual field defects for each eye. This means either the right half of the visual fields for both eyes or the left half of the visual fields for both eyes is involved. *Heteronymous* refers to two different parts of the visual field being impaired. For example, the left half of the visual field for one eye may be affected, whereas the right half of the visual field for the other eye is affected; this is known as **bitemporal hemianopia**. Injuries at selected points along the visual pathway result in predictable patterns of visual field defects (Fig. 8-14; Table 8-4).

Table 8-4

Visual Field Loss and Associated Anatomic Sites

Lesion Site	Visual Field Loss
Optic nerve	Monocular blindness
Optic chiasm (usually secondary to a pituitary gland tumor)	Bitemporal hemianopsia (tunnel vision)
Lateral edge of optic chiasm, interrupting fibers from ipsilateral temporal retina	Nasal hemianopsia in one eye
Optic tract (postchiasmic or geniculocalcarine fibers)	Homonymous hemianopsia
Temporal lobe pathology interrupting outer (ventral) geniculocalcarine tract fibers	Upper (superior) quadrantanopsia
Temporoparietal lobe pathology interrupting inner (dorsal) geniculocalcarine tract fibers	Lower (inferior) quadrantanopsia

Monocular Blindness

A complete severing of the optic (CN II) nerve at any point between the eyeball and the optic chiasm results in total blindness in that eye. This occurs because none of the optic (CN II) nerve fibers from the retina is spared (Fig. 8-14A). However, the actual implications of **monocular blindness** are slightly different because of binocular vision. If one eye is blind or closed, the other eye is still capable of covering the entire visual field, except for a small, temporal crescent-shaped peripheral field for the blind eye. Thus even after severance of the optic (CN II) nerve, one is functionally blind only for this monocular portion of the field, although there may be additional problems with depth perception.

Bitemporal, or Heteronymous Hemianopia

Bitemporal hemianopia is loss of vision in the temporal visual fields. It is associated with pathology of the optic chiasm (Fig. 8-14B). A chiasmatic injury, usually induced by a tumor of the **pituitary gland**, interrupts fibers from both nasal retinas. It produces blindness in the temporal visual fields for both eyes, commonly called tunnel vision.

Nasal Hemianopia

Nasal hemianopia refers to loss of vision in the nasal field of only one eye. The associated pathology encroaches on the lateral edge of the optic chiasm and selectively interrupts the fibers from the ipsilateral temporal portion of the retina. The result is nasal hemianopia in the corresponding eye (Fig. 8-14C).

Homonymous Hemianopia

Homonymous hemianopia is loss of vision in homonymous—either right or left—fields for both eyes. An interruption of fibers at any point in the course of the optic tract, LGB, or geniculocalcarine fibers results in homonymous (same field in both eyes) visual field losses (Fig. 8-14D). For example, a lesion in the right optic tract interrupts visual fibers from the retinas of both eyes, resulting in a left visual field defect for both eyes.

Homonymous Left Superior Quadrantanopsia

Homonymous left superior quadrantanopsia is loss of vision in the superior left quadrants of the visual fields for both eyes. The geniculocalcarine fibers divide into the ventral (outer) and dorsal (inner) fascicles while traveling to the visual cortex. The outer fascicle of fibers carries information from the inferior retinal quadrants of the retina (representing the upper or superior quadrants in the visual fields); these fibers sweep around the inferior horn of the lateral ventricle in the temporal lobe in the loop of Meyer. A temporal lobe lesion on the right side of the brain selectively interrupting the outer fibers of the geniculocalcarine tract causes blindness in the left upper quadrants of the visual fields of both eyes (Fig. 8-14E).

Homonymous Left Inferior Quadrantanopsia

The inner fibers of the geniculocalcarine tract, carrying information from the superior or upper retinal quadrants, travel directly through the temporoparietal substance. Therefore, a right-sided temporoparietal lobe lesion interrupts the geniculocalcarine tract inner (dorsal) fibers; this interrupts the transmission of visual information from the right upper retinal quadrants, resulting in vision loss in the left lower (inferior) visual field quadrants for both eyes (Fig. 8-14F).

Primary and Association Visual Cortices

A lesion involving the visual cortex in one hemisphere results in blindness in the opposite field of vision (hemianopia or hemianopia). The extent of the blindness depends on the size of the lesion. The central (macular) vision is usually saved, which is attributed to the collateral circulation from the middle cerebral artery. Bilateral visual cortical involvement results in cortical blindness, which is masked by blindness but with preserved ability to follow light.

The **visual association cortex** (Brodmann areas 18 and 19) wraps around the primary cortex on the medial and lateral surfaces and is reciprocally connected with the temporoparietal cortex and thalamic pulvinar. With afferents from the primary visual cortex, the visual association cortex synthesizes and elaborates visual perception and serves higher visual functions, such as recognition of an object form, face, and color, appreciation of its significance in the context of personal experiences, assignment of meaning, and visual memory. The association cortex is also important in the ability to read, write, and understand written information.

Stroke and traumatic injuries confined to the visual cortical areas have provided information about its role in many visually based higher mental functions that represent perception integrated with meaning. There is a difference between **apperceptive agnosia** (failure to recognize an object secondary to a perceptual deficit) and **associative agnosia** (failure to recognize an object or attach meaning with preserved perception). A lesion involving the association cortex (Brodmann areas 18 and 19) and/or extending to the inferior temporal lobe areas (Brodmann areas 20, 21, and possibly 37) may result in **visual agnosia**, in which one cannot recognize an object or written name despite normal visual perception. A lesion in the association cortex, usually bilateral, can result in **prosopagnosia**, an impaired ability to recognize faces. A lesion extending to the lateral occipitotemporal (fusiform) gyrus region results in **achromatopsia**, an impaired ability to recognize colors and objects. A noted linguistic disorder associated with occipital lesions is **alexia without agraphia**, in which the patient cannot comprehend written information but can still write. The underlying pathology involves an infarct of the corpus callosum and infarct in the occipital cortex. (Higher visual cognitive functions are discussed in Chapter 19.)

Optic aphasia, a common neurolinguistic syndrome seen in cases with occipital associative cortical lesion is characterized by an impaired ability to name visually presented objects, although the semantic knowledge associated with object is retained. For example, a patient cannot name an object presented visually, but he or she can name the actions associated with the object. A bilateral lesion at the junction of the parieto-occipital region has also been associated with the loss of voluntary control of eye movements (with preserved reflexive movements); this is also called Balint syndrome.

LESION LOCALIZATION—RULE 4: VISUAL PATHWAY LESION

Presenting Symptoms and Rationale

- **Blindness in one eye** suggests an optic nerve lesion anterior to the optic chiasm. Each optic nerve contains fibers from both nasal and temporal regions of the retina of one eye.
- **Bitemporal hemianopia** (one does not see things laterally in the visual fields) results from a lesion compressing or otherwise interrupting crossing fibers (from the nasal retina of each eye) in the optic chiasm. Fibers mediating visual information from the temporal (outer) visual fields (perceived in the nasal part of the retina) cross the midline at the optic chiasm.
- **Homonymous hemianopia** is associated with a lesion of the optic tract anywhere between the optic chiasm and the occipital lobe. Fibers from the two eyes representing the same (homo) visual fields (e.g., the temporal visual field of the left eye and the nasal visual field of the right eye) travel together in the optic tract.
- **Visual agnosia**, **alexia** (failure to comprehend written material), **homonymous hemianopia**, and **spared macular vision** are all associated with a lesion of the visual cortex (Brodmann area 17) and visual association areas (Brodmann areas 18 and 19). Involvement of the visual cortex receiving optic tract fibers accounts for contralateral hemianopia. Involvement of the primary and associational visual cortices, which are supplied by the posterior cerebral artery, results in agnosia and alexia.

CLINICAL CONSIDERATIONS

PATIENT ONE

A 65-year-old man gradually began having visual difficulty. He could see things well if they were right in front of him but did not see them if they were to his left or right. He was worried about developing tunnel vision like his diabetic neighbor, who had retinal degeneration. His ophthalmologist found nothing wrong with his retina and visual acuity. However, the examination revealed bitemporal hemianopia. A brain MRI study revealed a tumor of the pituitary gland.

Question. How can you relate the clinical symptoms to the pituitary gland tumor?

Discussion: The pituitary gland tumor affected the retinogeniculate fibers from both nasal retinas at the optic chiasm. This resulted in a bitemporal hemianopia.

PATIENT TWO

A 60-year-old right-handed architect was admitted to the hospital after a stroke. After the first 3 weeks of acute and intensive care, he exhibited severe aphasia. The attending speech language pathologist (SLP) noted the following:

- Fluent verbal output that carried little meaning
- Moderate anomia
- Paraphasic (mostly unrelated) errors and perseverations
- Moderate reading and writing problems
- Normal hearing thresholds but difficulty in understanding others
- Normal sensory or motor functions, except an upper right visual field defect

A brain MRI study revealed an infarct in the left posterior superior temporal gyrus (Brodmann area 22) and in parts of the inferior parietal lobe.

Question: How can you relate the clinical symptoms of aphasia and visual field deficit to a left temporal lobe lesion?

Discussion: The subcortical extension of the temporal lesion affected the left geniculocalcarine visual radiation fibers. These fibers carried information from the lower retinal quadrants, representing the upper quadrants of the visual field. The left temporal lesion also resulted in Wernicke aphasia.

PATIENT THREE

A 65-year-old man with a history of hypertension had a minor stroke involving the brainstem. He lost consciousness for 5 min. He was taken to the hospital, where the attending neurologist noticed the following:

- Normal sensory and motor functions
- Asymmetry in pupil size; the left pupil was 2–3 mm larger in the dark

Question: How can you account for these clinical symptoms in light of a brainstem lesion?

Discussion: The larger left pupil dilation could result from either a right sympathetic or a left parasympathetic lesion. The crucial clinical point is the context in which the asymmetry was noticed: dark or light. The presence of pupillary asymmetry in the dark implies that the sympathetic system did not function well for the smaller (right) pupil. Thus the patient had a right sympathetic lesion. However, if this pupillary asymmetry had been present in the light, it would indicate a left parasympathetic disruption.

PATIENT FOUR

A 55-year-old woman with a history of hypertension and cardiac problems woke up very confused and did not recognize the rooms and other locations in her house. She was taken to a neurologist who noted the following:

- Impaired left–right orientation
- Left spatial hemineglect
- Failure to draw objects
- Poor writing, marked by displaced and irregularly sized graphemes
- Inability to see people and objects on the left side with both eyes

The neurologist predicted that the patient had a right temporal-parietal lesion. The temporal-parietal infarct was confirmed via a brain MRI study.

Question: How can you explain the relationship between the visual field deficit and the right hemispheric lesion?

Discussion: This is a case of left homonymous hemianopia, which refers to blindness in the left half of the visual fields for both eyes. Lesions anywhere from the LGB to the calcarine cortex can produce this type of visual field loss. In this case, a stroke involving the temporal-parietal cortex interrupted the visual radiation pathway.

PATIENT FIVE

A 70-year-old man complained of gradually losing his ability to see from his left eye; this posed as a problem only when he drove. The attending neurologist noted the following:

- Complete blindness in the left eye
- Absence of pupillary light reflex on the left side
- Normal light reflex in the right eye

An MRI revealed a large tumor of the left optic nerve anterior to the optic chiasm.

Question: How can you relate the visual field deficit with the diagnosed tumor?

Discussion: This is a case of monocular blindness secondary to the prechiasmatic involvement of the afferent fibers of the optic nerve. This interruption of the fibers had also affected the light reflex unilaterally.

PATIENT SIX

After dazzling graduate students with a *Power Point* presentation in a completely dark and silent room, the instructor turned the lights on to see if the students were still there. This not only startled the students, but also caused an instant constriction in their pupillary diameters.

Question: Can you explain the neural mechanism involved with changes in students' pupillary apertures?

Discussion: Pupillary muscles receive both sympathetic and parasympathetic projections. Sympathetic projections travel to the radial (dilator) muscles via the superior cervical ganglion, whereas the parasympathetic projections innervate the circular (constrictor) muscles of the iris via the Edinger-Westphal nucleus and the oculomotor nerve (CN III). This pupillary construction was a parasympathetic response to light and was caused by the contraction of the circular fiber of the iris.

SUMMARY

The visual system is concerned with image perception, which involves four events: (1) the lens and cornea of the eye refract light rays (2) retinal photoreceptor cells then convert the electromagnetic energy of the light rays into changes in the membrane potential; (3) through integrating processing by other retinal neurons, the retinal ganglion transmits generated action potentials to the thalamus with relay to the visual cortex. (4) Finally, visual images are perceived in the primary visual cortex and interpreted in the associational visual cortex. Optical disturbances affect image formation, whereas lesions interrupting visual fibers result in different visual field losses.

QUIZ QUESTIONS

1. Define the following terms: astigmatism, binocular vision, focal length, lens accommodation, optic disk, pupillary constriction, retinal field, visual field.

2. Describe the refractive abnormality displayed by patients with myopia and hypermetropia.

3. Name each quarter and side of the visual fields for each eye in the figure.

4. Name each of the visual field defects shown in the figure.

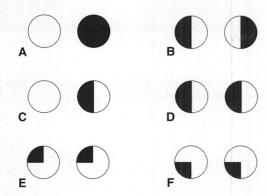

5. Match each of the following numbered structures to its associated lettered statement.

1. sclera
2. canal of Schlemm
3. rods
4. cornea
5. choroid
6. iris
7. lens
8. ciliary body
9. fovea centralis
10. macula lutea
11. cones

   a. drains aqueous humor from the anterior cavity into the venous system
   b. outer layer of connective tissue that covers the eyeball
   c. transparent covering of the anterior chamber and is continuous with the opaque sclera
   d. supplies blood to the retina and contains melanocytes to make the eyeball opaque to stray light
   e. regulates pupil size and the amount of light entering the eye
   f. automatically innervated smooth muscle fibers that can reduces tension on the lens capsule
   g. refracts light to properly focus images on the retina
   h. corresponds to the central retinal field and contains a yellowish pigment
   i. retinal region of the focal point of central visual axis, occupied by cones
   j. photoreceptors that mediate visual acuity and color vision
   k. photoreceptors that mediate night vision and are sensitive to moving images but not color

TECHNICAL TERMS

aqueous humor
astigmatism
binocular vision
bitemporal hemianopia
blind spot
cones
far point
focal length
focal point
fovea
homonymous hemianopia
hyperopia
iris
luminosity curve
macula lutea

miosis
monocular vision
mydriasis
myopia
near point
optic disk
photopsin
refraction
retina
rhodopsin
rods
scotopic vision
visual acuity
visual field
vitreous humor

Auditory System

LEARNING OBJECTIVES

After studying this chapter, students should be able to:

- Describe the basic properties of sound and their measurements

- Discuss the structures of the outer, middle, and inner ear

- Discuss the functions of the outer, middle, and inner ear

- Describe the physiology of the cochlear mechanism

- Discuss the mechanism for localizing sound sources

- Describe the central auditory mechanism

- Explain distinctive functional characteristics of the auditory system

- Discuss the cortical and reticular role in auditory processing

- Discuss the effects of cortical and subcortical lesions on hearing

- Differentiate between conductive and sensorineural hearing losses

- Describe the common audiometric/special hearing tests and discuss their clinical importance

- Explain the neuronal pathways mediating auditory reflexes

- Discuss the role of the descending auditory pathway

Hearing is essential to the acquisition of spoken language. It serves as a foundation for verbal communication, the most common form of social interaction. Hearing impairment, either congenital or adventitiously acquired, restricts effective communication by affecting the transmission and/or perception of sound. The process of **audition** (hearing) begins when sound waves strike the **tympanic membrane**. The resulting vibration of the tympanic membrane converts the pressure waves into mechanical energy, setting the middle ear bones (**ossicles**) into motion. This mechanical energy is further transformed into a hydraulic form of energy in the cochlear fluid of the **inner ear**. The

patterned hydraulic waves in the inner ear stimulate the **cochlear hair cells**, which send the impulses through the fibers of **vestibulocochlear (CN VIII) nerve** to the **cochlear nuclei** in the brainstem. The nuclei in the **cochlear complex** project the nerve impulses to multiple synaptic points in the brainstem and the **thalamus**. The combined signals from both ears are analyzed for sound localization in the brainstem according to their intensity and frequency patterns.

Auditory impulses finally travel to the primary auditory cortex, which is located on the on the superior surface of the temporal lobe in the **Heschl gyri**. The primary cortical area is involved with the sound pattern analysis that is needed for auditory discrimination and perception. The perceived auditory impulses further travel to the **Wernicke (language association cortex) area** in the left hemisphere, where the auditory signals are analyzed and interpreted into language-specific meaningful messages for the comprehension of spoken language. This chapter provides a functional description of the anatomy and physiology of hearing from the ear to the **primary auditory cortex**.

SOUND, PROPERTIES, AND MEASUREMENTS

Sound is created when a force sets an object into motion so that molecular vibration in the medium propagates a pressure wave. It is the movement of the molecules in the medium that transmits sound, which is characterized by two major attributes: **frequency** and **intensity**. **Time**, either the elapsed period or the sound onset phase, is also an important property of sound.

Frequency refers to the speed of particle vibration or the number of complete cycles; it is expressed in cycles per second, or **Hertz (Hz)**. Frequency determines the **pitch** of the sound or tone. The human ear can detect sounds within a range of 20–20,000 Hz. The important frequencies for human speech are in the range of 250–8,000 Hz. Low-frequency sound waves are perceived as having a low pitch, whereas high-frequency sound waves are perceived as representing a high pitch. However, the relationship between frequency and pitch is not always linear.

Intensity of sound is represented by the amplitude of the sound waves. It refers to the strength of molecular movement and is correlated with perceived loudness. The strength of molecular movement is measured in terms of its sound pressure in **dynes per square centimeter**, or **µPa** (micro Pascals). Because the range of sound pressure to which the human ear is sensitive is quite large, this pressure is measured in **decibels (dB)**. A decibel is defined as the log of the ratio between the **measured sound pressure (P_x)** and a well-defined **reference sound pressure (P_r)**. The formula for calculating the **sound pressure level (SPL)** in decibels of a given sound is as follows: SPL (dB) = 20 log P_x/P_r

Conventionally, the reference sound pressure is 0.0002 dyne/cm², or 20 µPa, which corresponds to the sound pressure required to make a 1000-Hz sound just audible to the human ear. If P_x equals P_r, the SPL is 0 dB. A measure of 0 dB decibels does not mean the absence of sound but rather that the measured sound pressure is the same as the reference sound pressure. If the measured sound pressure is 100 times the reference sound pressure, the intensity of the measured sound pressure in would be 40 dB, because the log 100 = 2.

The human ear is sensitive to an SPL intensity range of 0–140 dB. Prolonged and repeated exposure to sounds >90–100 dB may cause permanent structural damage to the cochlear hair cells and sounds of >140 dB cause pain.

Changes in intensity are perceived as changes in loudness. As intensity increases, there is a perceived increase in loudness. However, there is not always a 1:1 relationship between loudness and intensity. This is because the human ear is not equally sensitive to all sound frequencies. More intensity is required at some frequencies for a listener to just detect the presence of that sound than at other frequencies

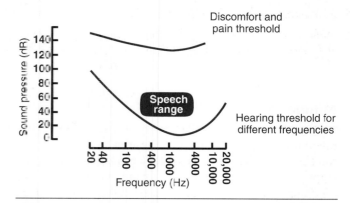

Figure 9-1 Thresholds of hearing sensitivity for various frequencies.

(Fig. 9-1). For example, the average normal-hearing listener needs 45.5 dB to hear a 125-Hz sound but requires only 8.5 dB to hear a 2000-Hz sound.

The best known reference for decibels is known as **hearing level (HL)**, which indicates sound intensity in relation to average normal hearing. A HL of 0 dB denotes an intensity level that is barely heard by the human ear.

ANATOMY AND PHYSIOLOGY

External Ear

The **external ear**, which is not as well developed in humans as it is in dogs and cats, includes three structures (Fig. 9-2): the cartilaginous **pinna, external auditory meatus,** and **tympanic membrane**. The *pinna* contributes to detecting the direction of sound by channeling collected sound

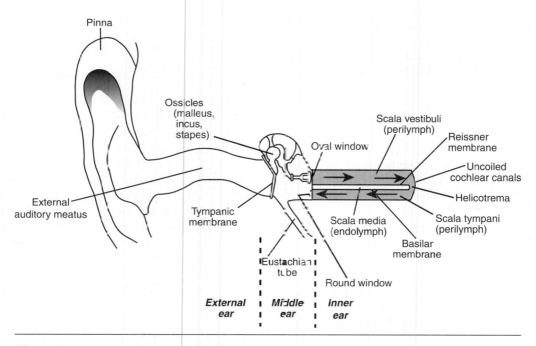

Figure 9-2 Anatomy of the external, middle, and inner compartments of the human ear.

waves into the *external auditory meatus*. The *tympanic membrane* is attached to the external auditory meatus at the end and separates it from the *middle ear*. The canal serves as the resonator, allowing peak resonance for the frequencies that are important for most human voices.

Middle Ear

The **middle ear** is an air-filled cavity between the tympanic membrane and the cochlea of the inner ear. It contains three interconnected small ossicles (the **malleus**, **incus**, and **stapes**) that are suspended by ligaments and serve as a mechanical lever system. These ossicles connect the *tympanic membrane* to the **oval window** of the inner ear. The *malleus*, the first bone, is attached at approximately the midpoint of the tympanic membrane. The *incus*, the second bone, is between the malleus and the stapes. The footplate of the *stapes*, the third bone, sits in the oval window of the *cochlea*. The **eustachian tube**, which runs from the middle ear to the **nasopharynx**, ventilates the middle ear by equalizing middle ear pressure with the atmospheric pressure in the external ear.

The middle ear has three primary functions: transmitting sound pressure variations by converting acoustic energy into mechanical energy, equalizing air pressure, and reflexively controlling energy transmission to the inner ear by regulating movements in the ossicular chain.

Transmission of Sound Pressure Variations

The transmission of vibrations from the *tympanic membrane* through the ossicles to the *oval window* involves a decrease in amplitude but an increase in force. This amplification in the force of movement results from two mechanical properties: the ratio of the area of the tympanic membrane to the oval window and the lever action of the ossicles. The area of the oval window (3.5 mm^2) is only about 14% of the effective area of the tympanic membrane (50 mm^2). The lever action of the ossicles provides a mechanical advantage of 1.3 times. Because pressure equals force per unit area, the discrepancy in the size of the tympanic membrane and the oval window, along with the lever action of the ossicles, allows the middle ear to increase sound pressure by approximately 18 (14 × 1.3) times on the cochlear fluid. This amount of amplification is required to overcome the greater impedance of the cochlear fluid compared to air.

The mass and stiffness of the middle ear structures pose a clear restriction on their speed of motion, which limits the range of sound frequencies that can be efficiently transmitted through the middle ear. We hear only the sound frequencies that are not dampened by such motion limitations imposed by the mass and stiffness of the middle ear system.

Pressure Equalization

The eustachian tube connects the middle ear cavity to the nasopharynx. Opening during swallowing, sneezing, and other reflexive activities, the eustachian tube equalizes the air pressure in the middle ear with the atmospheric pressure on the other side of the tympanic membrane. This pressure equalization is needed to ensure efficient transmission of sound from the tympanic membrane to the oval window. Any infection of the membranous lining of the eustachian tube or a middle ear infection may restrict the opening of the eustachian tube to the nasopharynx. The air trapped in the middle ear is absorbed and negative middle ear pressure results, which has a damping effect on ossicular movements. As a result, the high pressure outside the tympanic membrane pushes it inward, and the usually flat membrane becomes concave.

Reflexive Control of Ossicle Movement

Energy transmission through the middle ear and movement of the ossicles are influenced by two muscles in the middle ear cavity: **tensor tympani** and **stapedius**. The function of these muscles is to reflexively protect the auditory mechanism from structural damage by controlling ossicular motion when a person is exposed to high-intensity sounds. The stapedius muscle, controlled by the **facial (CN VII) nerve**, restricts ossicular movements by changing the dimension of the stapes movement. The stapes foot plate is oval, thus having both a long and a short rotation axis. The contraction of stapedius shifts the axis from long to short, reducing the amount of perilymph displacement.

The *tensor tympani* muscle which is controlled by the **trigeminal (CN V) nerve**, also participates in restricting ossicular movements. Combined, both muscles involve at least three neurons (one interneuron) to reflexively stiffen the ossicular system and attenuate the transmission of energy for high-intensity sounds from the external ear to the inner ear (attenuation reflex); the usual latency time of this reflex is 50–150 msec. However, this latency is too long to protect the inner ear from a loud noise. Even with prolonged exposure to loud music, sound intensity is attenuated by only 10 dB. This attenuation is largely caused by the action of the stapedius muscle and affects low-frequency sounds only. The overall extent of noise attenuation by the tensor tympani is small. Because it inserts on the malleus, it probably reduces the flexibility of the tympanic membrane.

Inner Ear

The inner ear consists of the **bony labyrinth** and the **membranous labyrinth**. The bony labyrinth is a series of cavities in the petrous portion of the temporal bone. The interconnecting canals and cavities of the bony labyrinth contain the three **semicircular ducts** and the cochlea. The membranous labyrinth is formed by the fluid filled **saccule**, **utricle**, and semicircular ducts. The inner ear consists of a dual-functional mechanism for serving the special sensory modalities of audition and **equilibrium**. Both of these functions are served by the interconnected fluid-filled membranous labyrinth ducts (Fig. 9-3). The saccule, utricle, and semicircular ducts mediate equilibrium (see Chapter 10), whereas the **cochlear duct (scala media)** of the labyrinth serves hearing.

Cochlear Structure

The cochlea is a snail-shaped structure coiled 2.5 times around the **modiolus**, the central bony core of the cochlea

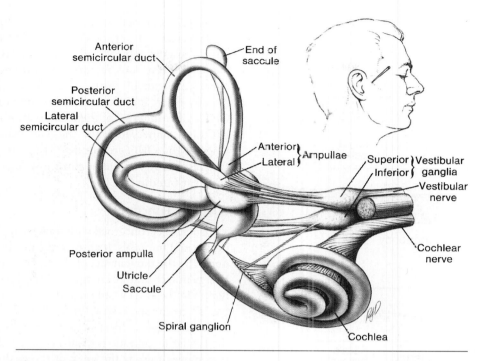

Figure 9-3 The vestibular labyrinthine and circuitous cochlea and the cochlear and vestibular nerves.

(Fig. 9-3). To provide a lengthwise orientation to the cochlear anatomy, it is shown sectioned in Figure 9-4 and uncoiled in Figures 9-2 and 9-5. The cochlea consists of three fluid-filled scalae (cavities): the **scala vestibuli**, scala media, and **scala tympani**. On lengthwise orientation, the *scala vestibuli* is the uppermost compartment, which follows the inner contour of the *cochlear duct* and joins the *scala tympani* at the apex of the cochlea though the **helicotrema**, a small aperture. The scala tympani lies at the bottom and follows the outer contour of the cochlea. The *scala media*, which ends near the cochlear apex, is between the scala tympani and scala vestibuli.

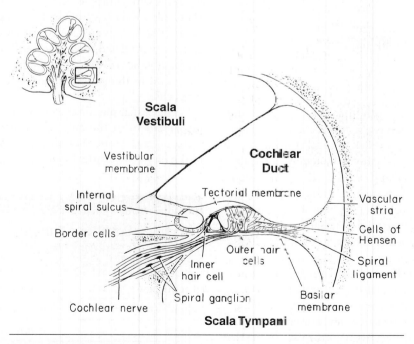

Figure 9-4 The cochlear duct on a radial section of the cochlea showing the cavities of the scalae vestibuli, media, and tympani and the structures of the cochlear duct. The location of the section is given in the *inset*.

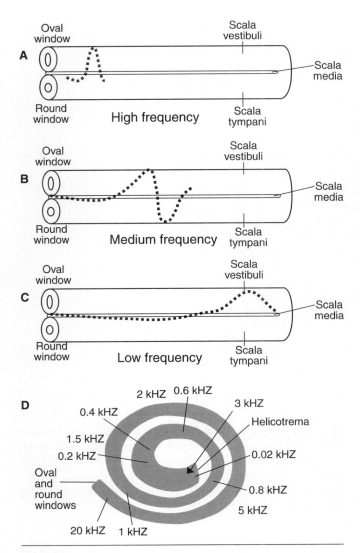

Figure 9-5 Traveling wave patterns of high-, medium-, and low-frequency sounds and the corresponding basilar membrane displacements.

As part of the bony labyrinth, the scalae vestibuli and tympani are filled with **perilymph**, a fluid with a high sodium (Na^+) concentration, similar to cerebrospinal fluid (CSF) in composition. The scala media, a membranous labyrinth, is filled with **endolymph**, a fluid with a high concentration of potassium (K^+), similar to intracellular fluid in composition. **Reissner (vestibular) membrane** separates the scala media from the scala vestibuli, whereas the **basilar membrane** separates the scala media from the ventrally located scala tympani.

The scala media (*cochlear duct*) contains a sensory structure called the **organ of Corti**, which contains hair cells, the primary receptor cells. In humans, the hair cells are arranged into three to four rows of **outer hair cells (OHCs)** and one row of **inner hair cells (IHCs)**, which run along the length of the *basilar membrane*. There are approximately 12,000 OHCs and 3,000 IHCs. Projecting from each OHC

are 40–150 **stereocilia**, in a W-shaped pattern, and projecting from each IHC are 50–70 stereocilia, in a V-shaped pattern. The **cilia** (apical ends) of the OHCs project to the overlying gelatinous **tectorial membrane**, which extends over the organ of Corti. The cilia of the IHCs do not directly insert into the tectorial membrane. The IHCs and OHCs differ in terms of their innervation. The bases of the IHCs are innervated by the cochlear nerve endings, whereas the OHC are connected to the projections from the descending auditory pathways, including the **olivocochlear bundle (OCB)**.

Cochlear Function

The cochlea is concerned with transferring sound vibrations into neural impulses. It absorbs the mechanical energy produced by the movements of the stapes and transduces this energy into hydraulic energy, which passes though the perilymph in the scala vestibuli and scala tympani. Because the basilar membrane is structurally flexible, it responds to the pressure in the cochlear perilymph by its displacement. As the basilar membrane is displaced at its base, the deformation moves toward the apex of the cochlea as a traveling wave. As the pressure wave moves, its velocity slows but the amplitude increases toward the apex, eventually reaching maximum. Different sound frequencies produce different traveling wave patterns, with a peak amplitude at different regions of the cochlea (Table 9-1). The peak amplitude of the traveling wave for high-frequency sound occurs near the base of the basilar membrane.

As the frequency of the stimulus decreases, the peak amplitude of the traveling wave moves toward the helicotrema. A signal consisting of many frequencies causes a sound wave to travel with multiple peaks along the basilar membrane. Hair cells are most stimulated at the point of the maximum peaks (Fig. 9-5), which suggests that the cochlear frequency selectivity is related to the mechanical properties of the basilar membrane. However, the frequency selectivity may also be related to the structural and electrical properties of the hair cells.

The basilar membrane movement produces mechanical displacement of the cilia of the hair cells relative to the tectorial membrane. The shearing effect on the apical ends of the hair cells results in an increased cilia permeability to

Table 9-1

Cochlear Locations Tuned to Specific Frequencies

Frequency	Site of Maximum Amplitude
High	Near oval window
Medium	Middle
Low	Near helicotrema

potassium ions (K⁺). The inward movement of the ions depolarizes the hair cell, which triggers the release of a neurotransmitter. The neurotransmitter, in turn, depolarizes the cochlear nerve terminals and causes action potential discharges, which travel to the brainstem through the fibers of the vestibulocochlear nerve (CN VIII).

Electrical Transduction

The chemical properties of action potentials include the ionic properties of the hair cells and transmission of the charged particles through the cell membranes (see Chapter 5). There is an ionic gradient between the endolymph and intracellular potential of the hair cells. The endolymph, which has a high concentration of potassium ions, has a potential of +80 mV. The intracellular potential is −70 mV; hence there is a 150-mV gradient difference across the cilia of a hair cell. This difference is considered essential for normal functioning of the hair cell. As the basilar membrane moves against the **tectorial membrane**, deformation of the stereocilia of the hair cells increases potassium ion permeability and opens K⁺ sensitive pores in the tips of cilia.

The mechanical deformation of the receptive ends during the wave motion in the cochlea opens ion-specific channels, allowing the movement of potassium into the cell bodies through the cilia in the scala media. With this K⁺ influx, the depolarized hair cell opens the voltage-sensitive calcium (Ca²⁺) channels, causing calcium ions to move into the cell. The movement of calcium into the hair cells initiates the release of **glutamate** (a fast excitatory neurotransmitter) from the synaptic vesicles of the hair cells, which is picked up by glutamate receptors in the cochlear nerve terminals. The action potential discharges that are generated in the nerve terminals travel through the fibers of CN VIII to the cochlear nuclear complex located at the **pontomedullary junction**.

Neural Coding of Auditory Information

In the transmission of audition, all the properties of sound (e.g., timing, intensity, frequency) are fully retained throughout the path to the brain. The mechanism used to code these attributes is not well understood; however, it is likely that information is coded in a variety of ways and may include some redundancy. For instance, the cochlear frequency represented by the stimulation of hair cells at specific regions along the basilar membrane may be only one way of coding this auditory information. The frequency could also be coded in part by the number of cochlear units responding adequately to a specific frequency and/or the synchronous firing patterns of auditory nuclei. Sound intensity could possibly be coded by the number of related neural units stimulated along the basilar membrane, by the intensity of discharging rates of fibers, or by the number of axons involved in the transmission. Furthermore, the central pathway may regulate which fibers are active in transmitting auditory signals, the properties of the sound (intensity, frequency), and information related to binaural or monaural interactions (Kingsley 1999).

Retrocochlear Auditory Mechanism

The retrocochlear portion of the auditory system transmits auditory signals from the hair cells in the organ of Corti to the brainstem cochlear nuclei (Fig. 9-6). The hair cells transmit nerve impulses to the peripheral (unmyelinated)

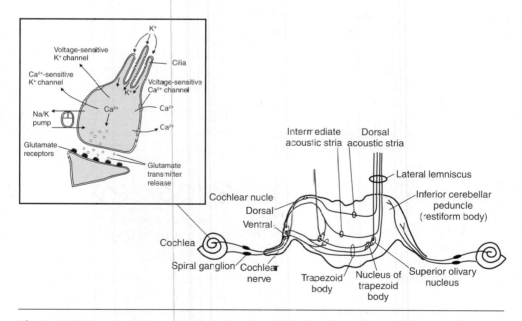

Figure 9-6 Retrocochlear neural mechanism. Peripheral processes of the spiral ganglions project to hair cells in the cochlea. *Insert,* the impulse transduction by which the glutamate release depolarizes the cochlear nerve terminals.

axons of the unipolar **spiral ganglia** (first-order neuron). The central (myelinated) processes of the *spiral ganglion cells* form the acoustic branch of vestibulocochlear (CN VIII) nerve and pass through the **internal auditory meatus**, a canal in the petrous portion of the temporal bone that opens into the cranial cavity at the side of the junction of the pons and medulla. The afferent axons synapse in the cochlear nuclei (Figs. 9-4 and 9-6). There are ~ 30,000 spiral ganglia cells in the modiolus, which can be divided into types I and II. Type I cells, which amount to about 90% of the total spiral ganglion cells, respond to a narrow range of frequency by being connected to only a few select hair cells in the cochlea, indicating a selectivity of processing. On the other hand, the axonal processes, originating from type II cells in the spiral ganglion, synapse with 10 or more hair cells, sug-gesting their sensitivity to a wider range of frequencies and with less precision.

CENTRAL AUDITORY PATHWAYS

The physiology of the sensory system includes a three-neuron pathway (see Chapter 7). However, this organization is not fully applicable to the auditory system. The auditory cortical projections involve multiple synaptic relay points between the cochlear nuclei (second-order neurons) and the thalamus (third-order neurons).

The **central auditory pathway** extends from the **cochlear nuclear complex** and all its nuclei up to and including the primary auditory cortex (Fig. 9-7; Table 9-2). The my-

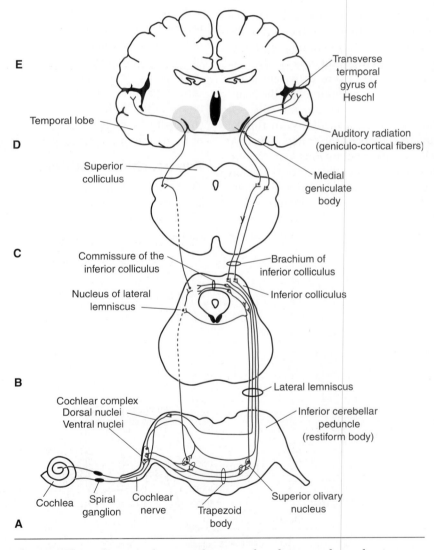

Figure 9-7 Auditory pathways. The central auditory pathway begins as secondary fibers arising from the cochlear nuclear complex and forming crossed and uncrossed stria. These fibers synapse on the superior olivary nucleus and ascend through the brainstem to the auditory cortex. **A.** Medulla. **B.** Pons. **C.** Inferior colliculus level. **D.** Medial geniculate body of thalamus. **E.** Transverse gyrus of Heschl.

elinated fibers of the vestibulocochlear (CN VIII) nerve enter the brainstem laterally at the pontomedullary junction and synapse on the cochlear nuclear complex. Structures in the central auditory pathway are the cochlear nuclei, **superior olivary nuclei**, **lateral lemniscus**, **inferior colliculus (IC)**, **brachium of inferior colliculus**, **medial geniculate body (MGB)**, **auditory radiations** (geniculocortical fibers), and primary auditory cortex in the transverse gyrus of Heschl (Tables 9-2 and 9-3).

Transmission in the central auditory pathway is regulated by two basic rules: one relates to preserving information and the other relates to information processing. Preserving information involves the retention of the tonotopic connection from the cochlear hair cells to the primary auditory cortex. The processing rules refer to the contralateral nature of projections and the incorporation of monaural and binaural information. The **contralateral** nature refers to the preponderance of projections that originate in one ear and travel to the auditory cortex on the opposite side; thus projections to the auditory cortex on the same side (**ipsilateral**) are clinically less significant.

Table 9-2

Summary of the Auditory System

Auditory Functions	Structures
Signal conversion in neural impulses	Cochlea (hair cells)
First-order nerve cells	Spiral ganglia
Signal transmission to CNS	Auditory nerve
CNS structures involved with transmitting and processing auditory signals	Cochlear nuclear complex Trapezoid body Superior olivary nucleus Inferior colliculus Brachium of inferior colliculus Medial geniculate body Primary and secondary auditory cortices

CNS, central nervous system.

Table 9-3

Auditory Structures and Associated Processing Disorders

Structures	Clinical Characteristics
Outer and middle ear	Interruption of sound transmission by air (conductive hearing loss); marked by air–bone gap, fluctuating hearing loss, softly spoken speech, and hearing well in noise
Cochlear hair cells	Interruption of sound transmission to same degree by air and bone (sensorineural hearing loss); marked by difficulty in hearing and understanding speech particularly in noise, speaking loudly, and loudness recruitment
Auditory nerve and structures	Preserved hearing sensitivity but unable to understand speech and some difficulty hearing in noise
Cochlear nuclear complex	Altered hearing sensitivity leading to impaired hearing (deafness) in ipsilateral ear
Superior olivary nucleus	Profoundly impaired ability to identify sound sources; minimal effect on hearing sensitivity
Lateral lemniscus	Impaired ability to process speech in noise, identify sound source, and grasp crucial linguistic information in discourse; minimal effect on hearing sensitivity
Inferior colliculus	Reduced ability to process and screen patterns of speech; impaired integration of audition with visual-motor functions for reflexive responses
Medial geniculate body	Reduced ability to incorporate attention in screening auditory information, regulating information processing speed and activating audition-triggered visceral functions; minimal effect on hearing sensitivity
Gyrus of Heschl Unilateral lesion	Impaired ability to discriminate and process complex time-based sound patterns typifying phonemic units of human speech; minimal effect on auditory sensation
Bilateral temporal lesions isolating Wernicke area	Severely impaired ability to comprehend speech (pure word deafness) owing to imperceptions of speech stimuli; preserved speech production, naming, reading, and writing functions

Cochlear Nuclear Complex

Fibers of the vestibulocochlear (CN VIII) nerve enter the brainstem at the pontomedullary junction dorsolateral to the **inferior cerebellar peduncle** (**restiform body**). They terminate in the cochlear nuclear complex (second-order neuron), which is divided into **dorsal** and **ventral nuclei** (Figs. 9-6 and 9-7; see Fig. 3-11). The dorsal cochlear nucleus lies dorsolateral to the restiform body, whereas the ventral cochlear nucleus is ventrolateral to the restiform body. The entering fibers of the vestibulocochlear nerve also divide into dorsal and ventral branches and synapse onto the respective cochlear nuclei. Specialized cochlear cells, such as bushy and multiform, have been identified in the cochlear complex (Kinsley 1999). Some of these cells may provide a sustained response to tones mediating important sound attributes such as phase and timing, whereas others may be responsive to changes in sound pressure level.

An important principle governing the functional representation at the cochlear nuclear complex and through the auditory pathway is the discrete tonotopic organization. There is a one-to-one relationship between the tonal representation of the hair cells in the organ of Corti and the cells in the cochlear nuclear complex. The fibers from the apex of the cochlea, which carry low-frequency information, terminate at the superficial layers of the cochlear nucleus, whereas fibers from the base of the cochlea, which carry high-frequency information, penetrate deeper in the nucleus and thus preserve the tonal correspondence. This discrete tonotopic representation is retained throughout the ascending fibers of the central auditory pathway and all its nuclei up to the auditory cortex.

Cochlear Projections

The cochlear nuclear complex sends multiple projections to both the ipsilateral and contralateral ascending auditory pathways. The exact nature of these projections is not as clear as it seems to be in brainstem diagrams. Although most auditory fibers cross the midline to project to opposite cortical areas, a small number of fibers ascend ipsilaterally. The cochlear projections that cross the midline travel in three bundles: **dorsal acoustic stria**, **intermediate stria**, and **trapezoid body**. Again, there is a function for each of these channels in mediating a specific auditory attribute; however, our knowledge of those attributes is incomplete. The cells along the crossing fibers of the trapezoid body form the nucleus of the trapezoid body. The fibers of the dorsal acoustic stria cross the midline and terminate in the contralateral **lateral lemniscus** without sending projections to any of the **olivary nuclei**. The collaterals from the fibers of the intermediate acoustic stria may project to the ipsilateral and/or contralateral superior olivary complex, and the main body of fibers joins the contralateral lateral lemniscus. The fibers of the trapezoid body, by far the most important and largest stria, cross the midline to terminate in the **superior olivary nucleus**, which is located laterally in the dorsal pons. The auditory fibers that are ipsilateral either send projec-

tions to the ipsilateral superior olivary nucleus or bypass it on their way to the ipsilateral lateral lemniscus.

Superior Olivary Nucleus

The superior olivary nucleus, a collection of nuclei in the pons, is the first structure to receive auditory inputs from both the ipsilateral and the contralateral cochlear nuclei. It contains binaural cells (lateral superior olive and medial superior olive) that are uniquely equipped to calculate differences in the time and intensity of auditory stimuli from both ears. The superior olivary nucleus contains two large dendrites extending from the opposite sites of the soma. The medial dendrite receives projections from the contralateral cochlear nuclei, whereas the lateral dendrite receives input from the ipsilateral cochlear nuclei. This structural arrangement allows the superior olivary nucleus to compare, millisecond by millisecond, the auditory signals arriving from both ears. By integrating time differences of as little as 400 μsec and the slightest intensity differences received from both ears, the superior olivary nucleus contributes to the spatial localization of the sound. This ability to localize sound is remarkable, as the path difference between the ears is only 5 inches or so.

Lateral Lemniscus

The lateral lemniscus, the primary ascending auditory pathway, extends from the superior olivary nucleus to the inferior colliculus of the midbrain (see Fig. 3-14). Its fibers climb laterally in the pontine tegmentum. The cell bodies along the fibers form the nucleus of the lateral lemniscus. The lateral lemniscus receives crossed and uncrossed projections from the dorsal, ventral and intermediate striae. Thus it retains a bilateral representation with added representation from the opposite ear. This bilaterality of projections explains why pathology of the central auditory pathway at any level does not lead to a profound hearing impairment in one ear.

Inferior Colliculus

On their way to the midbrain, the fibers of the lateral lemniscus pass dorsolaterally in the pontine tegmentum, potentially making numerous connections, before synapsing on nuclei in the inferior colliculus in the midbrain (Fig. 9-7; see Fig. 3-15). Virtually all of the lateral lemniscus fibers synapse on the nuclei in the IC; the remaining few fibers pass without synaptic relays to it. Both inferior colliculi are connected through the **commissural fibers** of the inferior colliculus, permitting further crossing and integration of monaural and binaural properties of the auditory input. This integration has additional implications for the localization of a sound source. While the cellular organization in the IC is known to retain frequency-specific regions with increased neuroanatomic complexity and projectional diversity, the central and pericentral cells of the inferior colliculus respond to complex patterns of auditory stimuli, indicating a higher level of signal analysis and information processing. The primary output of the inferior colliculus is to the thalamus, as its projections travel through the IC's brachium to the MGB (Figs. 9-7 and 9-8; see Figs. 2-21 and 3-16).

A largely ignored part of the inferior colliculus is that along with the superior colliculus and sensorimotor afferents, it is a part of the tectal neuronal circuitry in the brainstem, which provides the organism with a three-dimensional neurologic map of the external environment. According to this neurologic map, eye movements and/or head turns and body turns occur in response to visual stimuli (superior colliculus), loud or unexpected directional sounds (inferior colliculus), or sudden or unexpected tactile stimuli. These startle reflexes are quite rapid and can occur even if the thalamus or cerebral cortex is nonfunctional. The outer layers of the superior colliculus receive ganglion cell axons from the retina in an organized map of the environment, by which a stimulus activates specific areas of the retina. Ascending auditory signals send collateral information into the IC, providing a similar spatial orientation. The IC projects fibers to the deep layers of the superior colliculus, where the common output for the visual and auditory startle reflexes uses tectobulbar and tectospinal pathways to reach the spinal and brainstem motor apparatus.

The IC also sends fibers to the midbrain reticular formation. With a reticular integration, the circuitry of the tectum also has a cognitive role to play by incorporating attentional processes for selecting, screening, analyzing, inhibiting, and/or enhancing the processing of auditory information and for audition-based learning. This also explains how audition contributes to the automatic survival mechanism.

Medial Geniculate Body

The MGB is the thalamic relay nucleus for the transmission of auditory information. Located in the laterocaudal portion of the lower layer of thalamic nuclei, it receives its tonotopic input from the ipsilateral inferior colliculus (Figs. 9-7 and 9-8; see Fig. 3-16). There is no known crossing of impulses directly at the level of the MGB. Nonetheless, the possibility remains for some information to cross to the other side through thalamic commissural (massa intermedia) fibers. The fibers of the MGB (auditory radiations or geniculocortical) pass ventrally (sublenticular) and caudally (retrolenticular) to the lenticular portion of the **internal capsule** (Fig. 9-9). They terminate in the ipsilateral primary auditory

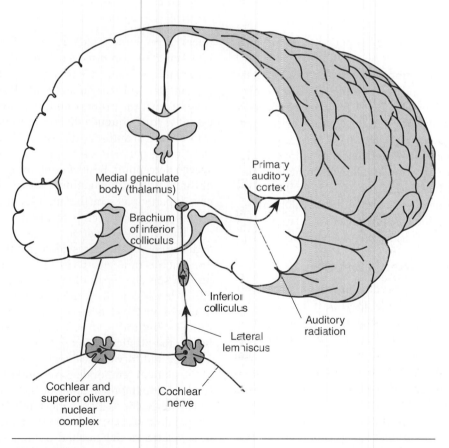

Figure 9-8 Auditory pathways from the cochlear nucleus to the primary cortex through synaptic connections with the inferior colliculus and medial geniculate bodies. The course of the geniculocortical fibers illustrates the lateral transition of these fibers through the internal capsule to the gyrus of Heschl.

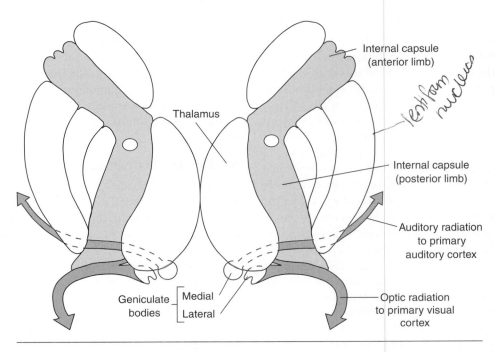

Figure 9-9 Horizontal view of the auditory projections from the medial geniculate bodies to the primary auditory cortex depicting the transition of the geniculocortical fibers below the posterior limb of the internal capsule.

cortex, the gyrus of Heschl in the superior temporal lobe (Fig. 9-8).

With its strategic location between the basal ganglia and the thalamic nuclei and its multiple and diverse projections, the MGB is plausibly involved with issues beyond the transmission of information to the cortex. Owing to its projections to the adjacent putamen (basal ganglia), amygdaloid nucleus (limbic lobe), and tertiary regions of the temporal and parietal cortex and its afferents from the brainstem reticular-activating system, the MGB is likely to help integrate attentional processes with auditory information. The MGB may also use auditory afferents to regulate visceral functions, emotional expression, and the pain mechanism.

Primary and Auditory Association Cortex

The primary auditory cortex (Brodmann area 41), located in the transversely oriented gyrus of Heschl, is buried in the lateral sylvian sulcus on the dorsal surface of the superior (first) temporal gyrus; it is marked by the structural property of the koniocortex with a well-developed **inner granular layer** (layer IV), similar to the visual and somatosensory cortices. This area is surrounded by the **secondary (association) auditory area** (Brodmann area 42), which extends onto the lateral surface of the superior temporal gyrus.

Receiving impulses through crossed and uncrossed fibers from both ears, the *primary auditory cortex* is known to retain the cochlear tonotopic representation. The geniculocortical fibers mediating higher frequencies terminate in the posteromedial region of the gyrus of Heschl, and the fibers transmitting lower frequencies synapse in the anterolateral region. The area between these two regions receives fibers carrying the middle range of frequencies. This tonal representation was discovered through experiential studies on animal brains and has not been demonstrated in the human brain (Bhatnagar and Andy 1988). Research on cats suggests that the primary auditory cortex is not absolutely essential for frequency discrimination; rather, it has vital importance in auditory discriminations that are based on the timing patterns of auditory events, such as human speech perception. Besides containing an organization map of three-dimensional auditory space, the primary auditory cortex participates in the analysis of sound patterns that are essential for speech perception.

The *secondary auditory cortex,* along with the primary auditory cortex, processes other essential properties of audition, such as timing patterns and spatial attributes typical of human speech. A pathologic involvement of the auditory cortex leads to acoustic aphasia and is characterized by an impaired ability to perceive and discriminate speech. The primary auditory cortex has also been known to retain functional plasticity (Box 9-1).

The auditory cortical region is surrounded by the area of the **planum temporale (temporal planum)** and is hidden by the overlying operculum of the temporal, parietal, and frontal lobes (Fig. 9-10). In most individuals, the left planum temporale area is larger than in the right brain, a fact that has been related to the cerebral dominance. (Geschwind and Levitsky, 1968.)

An extensive axonal bundle connects the auditory cortex to Wernicke area (Brodmann area 22), the language association cortex. This **association cortex** includes part of the planum temporale and posterosuperior first temporal gyrus; it is concerned with recognizing language stimuli,

Plasticity in the Auditory Cortex

The brain's ability to reorganize in response to an injury is highly prevalent only in younger brains. However, neuronal plasticity continues to a certain extent even in adult brains. By installing an electrode in the **nucleus basalis of Meynert** below the globus pallidus in a rat brain, Kilgard and Merzenich (1998) reinforced the cholinergic projections to activate cortical auditory neurons. The rats were exposed to a 9-kHz tone in 8- to 40-sec intervals. This exposure was paired with a brief electric stimulation of the nucleus basalis of Meynert. The rats' auditory cortexes were later examined for tonotopic representation using a single neuron recording. Most auditory neurons in experimental rats were found to respond to tones near 9-kHz. The neurons responsible for the other tones were confined to a small area in the remaining auditory cortex. This clearly supports the idea of plasticity in the adult brain.

Use of an externally applied current for mapping the cortex has revealed a progressive reorganization in the human adult brain. Stimulation for a prolonged period resulted in a functional reorganization: a deficit elicited in the beginning of the procedure was noted to have faded away from the same cortical tissue (Lesser et al. 1986). In an experiment of a motor-nerve transaction, the stimulation of a cortical area that controlled muscles innervated by a specific nerve was later noted to control other muscles (Donoghue and Sanes 1988).

interpreting their meanings with respect to previous auditory memories and linguistic experiences, and comprehending spoken language. The Wernicke area, as part of the larger language interpretative cortex, also receives visual and somesthetic information and contributes to language formulation (Fig. 9-10).

AUDITORY REFLEXES

Auditory reflexes coordinate head and eye movements toward sound and influence vestibular functions. This reflex mechanism primarily involves three anatomic pathways. The **first pathway** includes the projections from the inferior colliculus to the superior colliculus and tectum, integrating the auditory and visual systems and controlling extraocular movements. This also includes reticulospinal projections from the lateral lemniscus region, which are involved with the startle and attention reflexes. The **second pathway** from the *superior olivary nucleus* to the **medial longitudinal fas-**

ciculus projects to the nuclei of the following cranial nerves: **oculomotor (CN III)**, **trochlear (CN IV)**, and **abducens (CN VI)**. Impulses traveling on these two pathways regulate directional ocular movements in response to auditory stimuli. The **third pathway** includes the auditory projections to the vestibular nuclear complex and cerebellum and participates in equilibrium.

VASCULAR SUPPLY TO THE AUDITORY MECHANISM

The oxygen supply to the neuronal circuitry of audition comes from an intricate arterial network of the brainstem. The inner ear cochlear mechanism, semicircular canals of the vestibular mechanism, and spiral ganglia and their central and peripheral processes receive their vascular supply from the **basilar artery**, in particular the internal auditory (labyrinthine) artery, which is a branch of the **anterior inferior cerebellar artery (AICA)** (see Fig. 17.1). Any vascular interruption involving the AICA is likely to result in a monaural hearing loss and dysfunction of the facial nerve (CN VII). Depending on the extent of the lesion, ocular movements may also be impaired secondary to the involvement of the abducens nerve (CN VI).

The ascending auditory path involving the superior olivary nucleus and the lateral lemniscus fibers receives its blood through the smaller bilateral circumferential branches of the basilar artery. Branches of the **superior cerebellar artery (SCA)** provide blood to the IC. An occlusion of the lateral basilar branches or SCA is likely to affect fibers ascending from both ears, resulting in a binaural attenuation of hearing sensitivity. The thalamic MGB relies on the thalamogeniculate artery for its blood supply. The blood supply to the primary and secondary auditory cortex is through the branches of the middle cerebral artery (see Chapter 17).

DISTINCTIVE PROPERTIES OF AUDITORY SYSTEM

There are four distinctive auditory system characteristics: bilateral auditory representation, sound source localization, tonotopic representation, and descending auditory projections for the tuning of the receptors.

Bilateral Auditory Representation

Bilateral cortical auditory representation is credited to the multiple crossings of auditory information through ascending interconnections at the levels of the cochlear nuclei, lateral lemniscus, and IC. The primary auditory cortex in each hemisphere receives input from both ears. The major input to the primary auditory cortex is from the opposite ear, with fewer projections from the ipsilateral ear. A lesion at any point along the central auditory pathway extending from the pons to the auditory cortex does not result in complete hearing loss in the opposite ear; it causes only a mild

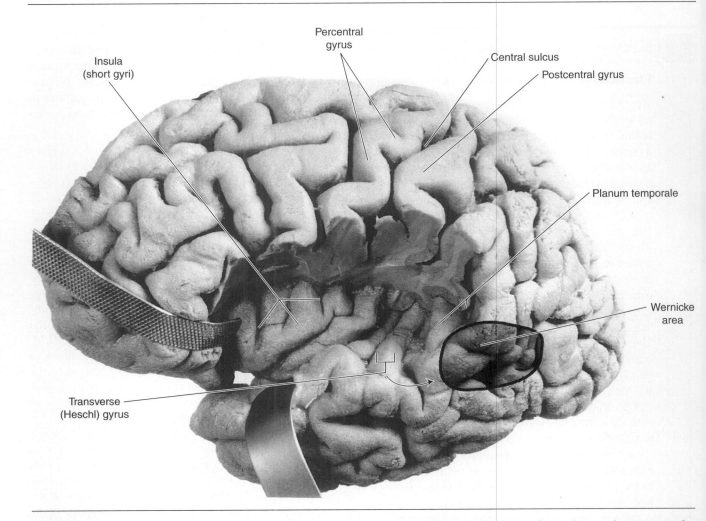

Figure 9-10 The exposed primary auditory cortex and planum temporale with the tissues from the overlying operculi of the frontal and parietal lobes removed. The projections from the primary auditory cortex to Wernicke area (association language cortex) are also shown.

loss of hearing, if any. However, a bilateral cortical ablation or lesion involving the primary and association auditory cortex (Brodmann areas 41 and 42) results in profound loss of auditory discriminative and speech perceptive skills.

Sound Source Localization

The interaural difference between the time and intensities of acoustic impulses is important in localizing the sound source. When each ear receives a particular sound at dissimilar times, the difference is known as the interaural time delay. The ear nearest the source receives the information first. The time difference between the ears can be estimated by dividing the difference in path length by the speed of sound. The intensity difference is the differentially perceived loudness of a sound. Because the sound is less intense in the ear farther from the source, individuals can use the loudness difference to determine a sound's location.

The sound-localizing mechanism begins at the level of the superior olivary nucleus in the brainstem. It is the first nucleus to receive crossed and uncrossed projections from both ears, and it uses the time delay and intensity difference to determine the exact location and direction of sound sources.

Tonotopic Representation

Discrete tonal representation at the cochlear level is maintained throughout the central auditory pathway. Despite the multiple interconnections and crossings in the ascending pathways, the tonal representation from the hair cells in the cochlea is retained throughout the auditory system. Tones are even represented in the primary auditory cortex, where a single neuron responds best to certain sound frequencies.

Descending Auditory Projections

Parallel to the ascending projections to the auditory cortex, descending auditory fibers are known to exist from the primary auditory cortex to the cochlear hair cells and conduct impulses in the reverse direction. These descending fibers provide feedback circuits to refine the perception of pitch and loudness and to sharpen the reception of specific frequencies through the process of lateral inhibition. The recurring connections of the descending fibers begin from the primary auditory cortex and make synaptic relays to the thalamus, brainstem (inferior colliculus), and superior olivary nucleus before terminating in the cochlear hair cells. The descending connections (crossed and uncrossed) consist of the fibers of the following tracts: corticogeniculate, corticocollicular, colliculo-olivary, olivocochlear, and colliculocochlear. These not only sharpen the signals by improving the signal-to-noise ratio but also enhance cues for sound localization and contribute to the quality of the perceived sound.

Olivocochlear fibers contribute to better hearing in noisy situations through the suppression of competing background sounds. These fibers attenuate the transduction of certain sound frequencies through the regulation of the contractile properties of the OHCs by changing their length and influencing their responsiveness. By reducing their bend during a basilar membrane movement, the olivary-cochlear projections contribute to a reduction in hearing sensitivity by 20–25 dB (Kingsley 1999).

CLINICAL CONCERNS

Hearing Impairments

Clinically, hearing impairment is categorized into four types: **conductive**, **sensorineural**, **mixed**, and **central**. Pathologies of the outer and middle ear, which affect sound transmission to the cochlea, cause a **conductive hearing loss**. Lesions affecting the sensory receptors in the organ of Corti and/or the fibers of the vestibulocochlear nerve (CN VIII) cause a **sensorineural hearing loss**. Mixed hearing loss includes both conductive and sensorineural impairments. Hearing loss associated with a lesion in the brainstem or higher is called central hearing loss (Table 9-3).

Conductive Hearing Loss

Middle ear pathologies affect sound transmission to the cochlea and cause a conductive hearing loss. Conductive hearing impairment, generally less severe, is characterized by fluctuating hearing loss, good word–speech recognition ability at high intensities, softly spoken speech, impaired auditory reflex, and, most important, an air–bone gap. **Otitis media** is a common cause of conductive hearing loss in children. Middle ear fluid accumulation secondary to eustachian tube malfunction not only causes a fluctuating hearing impairment but, if not treated, can have implications for normal speech and language development.

The most common cause of conductive hearing loss in adults is **otosclerosis**. This is a dominant autosomal condition, in which a pathologic growth of bone near the oval window impedes the movement of the stapes. Surgical removal of the stapes and insertion of a Teflon prosthesis can restore hearing in most cases of otosclerosis.

Sensorineural Hearing Loss

Sensorineural hearing loss (SNHL) is associated with pathology in the stereocilia (hair cells) and/or the auditory nerve. SNHL is permanent, irreversible, and can range from moderate to complete in the affected ear. Clinically, it is characterized by difficulty in understanding speech, particularly in noise and tinnitus; cochlear involvement is also marked by recruitment (abnormally rapid growth of loudness after the hearing threshold is reached). Patients usually speak loudly in addition to their reduced self-monitoring ability.

A cochlear implant procedure has been used in some cases to treat SNHL. It involves the implantation of an electronic device containing 12–22 pairs of electrodes in the cochlea; a microprocessor is used to separate sound into different frequencies or range of frequencies, which regulate the amplitude of different electrodes.

Exposure to noise is a common cause of SNHL. Prolonged and repeated exposure to intense environmental noise (industrial environment, loud rock music, and engine noise) can damage hair cells. The noise-induced effect is noticeable generally for high frequencies. Toxicity owing to the accumulation of certain antibiotics in an infant's endolymph can also be damaging to hair cells. Other cause includes **Ménière disease** and **presbycusis**. Ménière disease, a chronic condition associated with edema and the hydrops (excessive accumulation) of the endolymphatic membranous labyrinth, is marked by progressive and fluctuating hearing loss, ringing in the ears, and vertigo (sensation of spinning). Presbycusis is an age-induced hearing impairment that affects perception and discrimination of sound. This progressive hearing loss primarily affects the high frequencies and results from the de-generation of hair cells in the first turn of the cochlear duct.

Disease, irritation, or pressure on the nerve trunk can structurally affect the vestibulocochlear (CN VIII) nerve fibers and cause hearing impairment. It results in tinnitus and can cause mild to profound hearing impairment. The clinical picture is similar to general SNHL, except that patients usually hear well but exhibit difficulty understanding speech, which increases in noise. Extensive damage to the nerve can result in unilateral deafness.

Tumors of the sheath (**Schwann cells**) of the vestibulocochlear nerve (CN VIII) are also associated with hearing impairment. Such tumors (**vestibular schwannoma** or **acoustic neuroma**) are located at the cerebellopontine angle and are clinically associated with hearing impairment and disequilibrium. In later stages, tumorous growth can involve the intracranial roots of the trigeminal nerve (CN V) and facial nerve (CN VII), which results in the loss of pain and temperature sensation from the ipsilateral face (spinal tract of trigeminal nerve), facial weakness (facial nerve), loss of taste from the anterior part of tongue (chorda tympani of the facial nerve [CN VII]), and cerebellar symptoms (unstable gait and ataxia).

Mixed Hearing Loss

In mixed hearing loss, patients exhibit lowered sensitivity to both air- and bone-conducted stimuli. A typical **audiogram** reveals an air–bone gap, with bone conduction being better.

Central Auditory Impairment

The central auditory system includes the lower brainstem (cochlear nuclei, superior olivary nucleus, and lateral lemniscus), upper brainstem (inferior colliculus and medial geniculate body), and the primary auditory cortex. Clinically, the most identifying feature of central auditory dysfunction is the near-normal sensitivity to auditory stimuli but impaired processing of linguistic and metalinguistic signals.

Lower Brainstem Involvement

With input from the ipsilateral inner ear, a pathologic involvement of the cochlear nuclear complex can cause deafness by altering the hearing sensitivity in the ipsilateral ear. It interrupts the projections to the superior olivary nucleus and affects the ability to localize the source and direction of the sound, which is based on the binaural summation of input from both (ipsilateral and contralateral) cochlear nuclei. An involvement of the superior olivary nucleus may have only a minimal effect on hearing sensitivity, but has a profound effect on the ability to identify and discriminate the source of sound. Similarly, a unilateral involvement of the lateral lemniscus is not likely to cause a severe hearing impairment in either of the ears. However, it causes subtle processing symptoms, such as impaired processing of speech in noise and retaining of crucial linguistic information in a conversational setting.

Upper Brainstem Involvement

With increased neuroanatomic complexity, reticular integration, and projectional diversity, the central and pericentral cells of the inferior colliculi play an important role in screening and responding to complex auditory patterns. Their involvement affects the transmission of auditory signals and the integration of audition with visual–motor functions for reflexive responses. It also has implications for the metacognition of self-awareness in three-dimensional space. With multiple crossed and uncrossed input and diverse projections, the MGB has an important role in integrating complex auditory patterns with the reticular arousal system (Bhatnagar et al. 1989, 1990). Pathology of the MGB might restrict a patient's ability to select and attend to auditory information, regulate the processing speed, and activate emotional and visceral functions associated with audition. The attenuated integration of attention might also result in delayed and subnormal linguistic processing.

Cortical Involvement

Patients with unilateral cortical lesions usually have near-normal hearing thresholds. However, they exhibit impaired ability to perceive and discriminate speech. Both hearing sensitivity and speech perception are known to be profoundly impaired after bilateral cortical lesions. The secondary auditory cortex, along with the primary auditory cortex, also processes other essential properties of audition typical of human speech, such as timing patterns and spatial attributes. A pathologic involvement of the primary and secondary auditory cortices leads to acoustic aphasia. Patients with acoustic aphasia display an impaired ability to discriminate speech sounds and phonemes, a skill essential for learning and understanding language.

Involvement of the language association cortex (Brodmann area 22) results in aphasic deficits. This produces a full-blown **paragrammatic syndrome** (**Wernicke aphasia**), which is characterized by impaired comprehension of spoken and written language, reduced ability to write, word-finding deficits, euphoric behavior, and poor self-monitoring skills. Lexical retrieval disorder is marked by verbal confusion, verbal paraphasia, and frequent neologisms that render verbal output in a disjoined form of speech, which is usually referred to as jargon aphasia. Words can be spoken fluently, although speech remains largely meaningless (see Chapter 19).

Pure Word Deafness

Pure word deafness, a language syndrome, is associated with a temporal lesion. This uncommon and infrequent disorder is manifested by a severe loss of language comprehension, though speech production, naming, reading, and writing are spared. The associated pathology involves a bilateral temporal lesion, which causes an isolation of the primary auditory cortices from the Wernicke area by interrupting the fibers bilaterally radiating from the gyrus of Heschl (see Chapter 19).

Right hemispheric temporal lesions affect the processing of environmental sounds, nonverbal memory, and musical and prosodic interpretation. Supporting evidence has come from research on patients undergoing temporal lobotomy for medically intractable epilepsy; tonal processing was not disrupted after a left temporal lobectomy.

Evaluation of Hearing Disorders

There are many diagnostic tests of hearing. **Tuning fork tests** are the simple bedside tests of hearing and are used commonly by neurologists and other medical professionals in the hospital environment. **Pure tone audiometry** is the most commonly used test for evaluating hearing sensitivity. **Tympanometry, evoked otoacoustic emissions**, and **auditory brainstem response (ABR) audiometry** are specialized tests of hearing.

Tuning Fork

Tuning forks are often used to informally differentiate a conductive hearing loss from a SNHL. **Rinne** and **Weber** are two commonly used bedside auditory tests (Fig. 9-11).

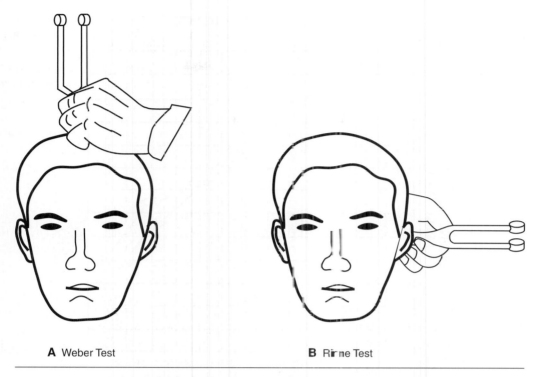

A Weber Test   **B** Rinne Test

Figure 9-11 Tuning fork testing. A. In the Weber test, louder sound in the ipsilateral ear indicates a conductive hearing loss; a louder sound in the contralateral ear suggests a sensorineural loss. B. In the Rinne test, the patient's ability to hear through air conduction indicates a conductive hearing loss.

Rinne Test

In the Rinne test, the stem of a vibrating tuning fork (512 Hz) is placed on the mastoid process and the patient listens to the tone by bone conduction. When the intensity of the stimulus decreases and the tone from the fork can no longer heard by the patient, the fork is placed in front of the ear so the patient can attempt to hear the sound by air conduction. A patient with normal hearing or SNHL should again hear the tone (positive Rinne), because hearing through air conduction is better than through bone conduction. A patient with a conductive hearing loss will not hear the tone again (negative Rinne).

Weber Test

In the Weber test a vibrating tuning fork is placed on the scalp at the vertex, and the patient is asked to lateralize the sound—specifically the patient determines whether the tone is more pronounced in one ear. In patients with normal hearing or bilaterally symmetrical hearing loss, the sound is sensed at the midline. Those with a unilateral conductive hearing loss hear the sound primarily in the affected ear. Patients with a unilateral SNHL hear the sound mainly in the unaffected ear.

Pure Tone Audiometry

Pure tone audiometry is used to establish the threshold of hearing across the frequency range that is most important for human communication. A pure tone audiometer generates pure tones at various frequencies and intensities. The calibration of the audiometer takes into consideration the differential sensitivity of the human ear to various frequencies by making 0 dB HL at each frequency equal to the lowest intensity level in SPL decibels required by the average normal listener to hear that frequency. Hearing threshold is the lowest intensity level required for an individual to respond at a given frequency. In audiometry, hearing is tested by determining air- and bone-conduction thresholds. The results of testing are plotted on an audiogram, a graphic representation of the patient's bone- and air-conduction responses to each frequency (Fig. 9-12).

Hearing loss refers to an increase in intensity above the normal sensitivity required to reach the threshold. For example, a 50-dB loss at 1000 Hz means that the patient requires 50 dB of sound pressure above normal sensitivity to obtain the threshold. In the case of a conductive hearing loss, the threshold for bone conduction is better than that for air conduction. This threshold difference is referred to as the air–bone gap. Hearing sensitivity by bone and air is equal in SNHL (Fig. 9-12).

Tympanometry

Tympanometry, a specialized and reliable auditory test, evaluates the compliance of the tympanic membrane and middle ear pressure under the conditions of changing air

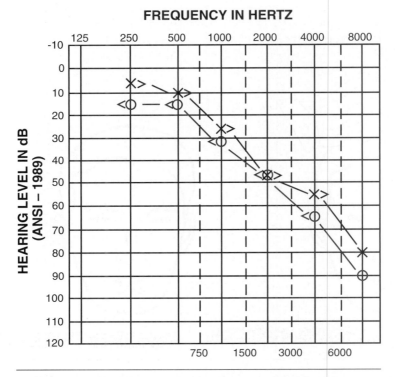

Figure 9-12 Audiogram demonstrating bilateral sensorineural loss; air conduction and bone conduction thresholds average at the same decibel level. *Black line,* left ear; *red line,* right ear.

pressure (relative to atmospheric pressure) in the external auditory meatus. Impaired tympanic membrane compliance is a clinical indicator of middle ear pathology (e.g., pressure changes in fluid, ossicular immobility, and eustachian tube dysfunctioning).

Otoacoustic Emission

The outer cochlear hair cells in normally hearing individuals are known to spontaneously produce clinically low-intensity signals (otoacoustic emission). Otoacoustic testing measures these spontaneous signals, which are used to evaluate the functioning of the conductive mechanism of the middle ear and cochlear hair cells. Otoacoustic emission can also be evoked by introducing brief acoustic stimuli in the external canals. Absence of these minute subclinical signals indicates dysfunctioning of the OHCs and the conductive mechanism to and from the cochlea.

Auditory Brainstem Response Audiometry

Auditory brainstem response (ABR) audiometry measures neuronal activity (synchronous neural firings) from the brainstem auditory pathway within 10 msec after the onset of controlled stimuli, such as click sounds. Within this period, five negative wave peaks are identified from the event-based electrical activity recorded from scalp electrodes (see Fig. 20-15). Each of these response classes indicates a different anatomic point in the auditory pathway (see Table 20-5). By taking into consideration the altered interpeak

latency or changes in the peaks of amplitude, one can identify lesion sites in the vestibulocochlear (CN VIII) nerve or brainstem. ABR audiometry is a reliable and clinically powerful test; it does not require the patient's participation and can be performed on infants and uncooperative patients (see Chapter 20).

CLINICAL CONSIDERATIONS

PATIENT ONE

A 65-year-old university professor complained of difficulty hearing with her left ear accompanied by ringing, nausea, and dizziness. She was taken to a hospital. On testing, she exhibited the following signs:

- Hearing loss in the left ear
- Tendency to fall to her left side
- Loss of pain and temperature sensation on the left side of the face and right side of the body
- Difficulty swallowing

A brain MRI study revealed a small infarct in the dorsolateral medulla on the left side.

Question: How could a dorsal medullary lesion cause problems with hearing and equilibrium and account for the sensory loss and difficulty swallowing?

Discussion: The cochlear and vestibular branches of the vestibulocochlear (CN VIII) nerve enter the brainstem at the junction of the medulla and pons. Occlusion in the posterior inferior cerebellar artery affected the second-order (vestibular and cochlear) nuclei of CN VIII, the descending tract of the trigeminal (CN V) nerve, lateral spinothalamic tract, and motor nucleus of the vagus (CN X) nerve. The involvement of the left cochlear nucleus affected the hearing threshold in the left ear. The involvement of the left vestibular nucleus accounted for her falling to the left. The involvement of the trigeminal system resulted in analgesia and thermal anesthesia on the left side of the face. The interruption of the crossed fibers of the lateral spinothalamic tract resulted in the loss of pain and temperature sensations from the right side of the body (see Chapter 7). The involvement of the adjacent vagus (CN X) nerve nucleus and fibers resulted in swallowing problems.

PATIENT TWO

A 50-year-old man lost hearing in his right ear and had right-sided imbalance. At first, he compensated by using his left ear when using the telephone. As his equilibrium-related difficulty worsened, he began hearing a high-pitched ringing in the right ear and noticed right facial weakness. He decided to see his physician. The examining physician observed the following symptoms:

- Right-sided facial weakness
- Mild unsteadiness while walking
- Right ear hearing loss of 45 dB, which increased to 65 dB for higher frequencies, established by pure tone audiometry
- Marked reduction in right ear speech discrimination

Positive Rinne findings and poor speech discrimination in the right ear ruled out a conductive hearing loss. A brainstem MRI study confirmed a right acoustic schwannoma at the cerebellopontine angle. Surgical removal of the tumor relieved the pressure and largely restored the impaired functions.

Question: How can you account for this clinical picture by relating the symptoms to the involved pathways?

Discussion: A Schwann cell tumor (schwannoma) at the cerebellopontine angle compressed both branches of vestibulocochlear (CN VIII) nerve roots. This resulted in right ear hearing loss and a right-sided equilibrium problem. The neoplasm also compressed the facial cranial (CN VII) nerve root, creating Bell palsy, or facial paralysis secondary to facial (CN VII) nerve injury. Unsteadiness while walking resulted from the involvement of the vestibular nerve.

PATIENT THREE

A 25-year-old teacher fell in front of her students while teaching and was taken to the emergency room (ER) where the attending neurologist noted the following:

- Headache and vomiting
- Profound hearing loss in the right ear, determined by pure tone audiometry
- Disequilibrium with a tendency to fall to the right
- No other sensorimotor or cognitive impairment

A magnetic resonance arteriography study indicated a thromboembolic occlusion of an artery originating from the AICA.

Question: How can you explain these symptoms?

Discussion: The labyrinthine (internal auditory), a branch of the AICA, supplies blood to the inner ear, which includes the cochlea, spiral ganglion cells, and vestibular apparatus.

PATIENT FOUR

A 27-year-old woman with a 3-week history of an auditory problem and double vision was taken to the hospital where the examining neurologist noted the following:

- A reported history of a 10-day episode of impaired vision and understanding of spoken language
- Right optic nerve pallor (paleness)
- Tendency to run into things because of her inability to see objects on the floor
- Mild signs of cerebellar dysfunction involving the right extremities with gait ataxia

A speech-language pathology consultation revealed the following:

- Auditory incomprehension marked by inattentiveness to details, missing information, inconsistencies in response, and difficulty in making sense out of speech in noise
- No signs of impaired language (aphasia), cognitive dysfunction (dementia), or unintelligible speech (dysarthria)

An audiologic consultation revealed the following:

- Difficulty with sound localization
- Mild bilateral hearing loss on pure tone audiometry
- Better comprehension of words in quiet atmosphere
- Near-normal acoustic reflexes at normal hearing levels
- Normal evoked otoacoustic emission responses, suggesting a structurally intact cochlea
- Near-normal brainstem auditory evoked responses, testifying to a normal functioning of the auditory pathway

The attending neurologist considered that the patient had multiple sclerosis, which was confirmed by the presence of multiple white matter hyperintensities (demyelinated plaques) on brain MRI studies, which revealed one in the cerebellum and two in the posterior lateral thalami involving the geniculate bodies.

Question: Based on your anatomic knowledge, can you relate the auditory symptoms with the identified pathology sites?

Discussion: This is a case of a central auditory processing deficit, in which the patient has performed well on traditional diagnostic tests but continues to have difficulty in processing linguistic signals. Bilateral involvement of the MGB has restricted the patient's ability to screen auditory information and regulate the speed of information processing. The attenuated integration of attention might have also been involved in abnormal linguistic processing. The involvement of the MGB affected visual processing. The cerebellar hyperintensity contributed to disequilibrium.

SUMMARY

Audition begins in the external ear, when collected sound waves strike the tympanic membrane. The resulting vibration of the tympanic membrane converts sound waves into mechanical energy, causing the middle ear bones to move back and forth. This mechanical energy is further transformed to a hydraulic form of energy in the cochlear fluid of the inner ear, which activates the sensory hair cells in the cochlea and transforms the hydraulic energy to electrical nerve impulses. The nerve impulses are transmitted by the vestibulocochlear nerve (CN VIII) fibers to the cochlear nuclei in the brainstem. The cochlear cells project these nerve impulses to multiple synaptic points in the brainstem and thalamus before transmitting the impulses to the primary auditory cortex in the temporal lobe. The auditory impulses travel from the primary and secondary auditory cortex to the Wernicke (associational language) area, where the auditory signals are analyzed and interpreted into meaningful language-specific messages.

QUIZ QUESTIONS

1. Define the following terms: audiogram, binaural, inferior colliculus, lateral lemniscus, medial geniculate body, monaural, primary auditory cortex, trapezoid body.

2. List the function of the superior olivary nucleus.

3. Match each of the following numbered terms with its associated lettered statement.

   1. conductive hearing loss
   2. sensorineural hearing loss
   3. Rinne test
   4. Weber test

   a. a tuning fork is placed on the scalp at the vertex and the subject reports if it is heard better in one ear
   b. the butt of a tuning fork is first placed against the mastoid process while the subject listens
   c. pathologies affecting the sensory receptors in the organ of Corti and/or their projections to the cochlear nuclear complex
   d. impaired sound transmission in the middle ear

TECHNICAL TERMS

audiogram
audiometry
association cortex
conductive hearing loss
decibel
hearing loss
inferior colliculus

lateral lemniscus
medial geniculate body
primary auditory cortex
sensorineural hearing loss
superior olivary nucleus
trapezoid body

Vestibular System

LEARNING OBJECTIVES

After studying this chapter, students should be able to:

- Discuss the importance of the vestibular system in equilibrium
- Describe the anatomy of the vestibular system
- Describe the projections of the vestibular complex
- Explain the physiology of equilibrium
- Describe the mechanism of nystagmus
- Discuss the vestibular mechanism that controls rotational and ocular movements
- Explain methods used for assessing the integrity of the vestibular mechanism
- Discuss common vestibular dysfunctions

The vestibular system, with sensitivity to angular and linear acceleration, regulates the position of the head and neck in space and monitors righting motor (postural) reflexes and upright posture. It also coordinates eye movements and controls eye fixation during body and head movements. All of these functions are controlled subconsciously by integrating information received from receptors in the semicircular membranous ducts of both inner ears. Closely associated with the sensory afferents, the vestibular system constantly integrates incoming visual information and proprioceptive signals from the body, which contribute to the execution of complex, skilled, and coordinated activities, such as dancing, skating, and acrobatics.

ANATOMY OF THE VESTIBULAR SYSTEM

The major components of the vestibular system are the semicircular ducts, vestibule (saccule and utricle), and vestibular nuclei (Figs. 10-1 to 10-4). Other functionally associated structures are the medial longitudinal fasciculus (MLF), brainstem reticular formation, midbrain tectal and

tegmental areas, and cerebellar nuclei. The sensory receptors (hair cells) in the semicircular ducts respond to rotations of the head and changes in body position. They project impulses to the brainstem vestibular nuclei, which in turn transmit the information to the medial longitudinal fasciculus, cerebellum, spinal motor neurons, and brainstem reticular network to coordinate posture and eye, head, and neck movements.

Semicircular Ducts and Vestibular Sacs

The three semicircular ducts in the inner ear are connected to the vestibule (utricle and saccule). These structures of the membranous labyrinth are filled with endolymph, which is secreted by the stria vascularis of the cochlea. The semicircular ducts are at right angles to one another and are named according to their relative positions: anterior posterior, and lateral (Fig. 10-2). Spatially different positions enable the receptors in the ducts to detect acceleration of the body in the planes. Each semicircular duct contains an enlarged end area called the ampulla (saccular dilation), which contains cristae. The cristae are made of sensory hair cells (cilia) covered by a gelatinous, mass-filled capsule, called the cupula, which extends upward to the ampullary roof (Fig. 10-3B). The hair cells are sensitive to angular head movements. When the head turns, the endolymph in the semicircular duct flows toward the cupula. This builds pressure on one side, bending the cupula and distorting the cilia. Distortion of the cilia generates action potentials, which are projected to the vestibular nuclei in the brainstem.

Inside the vestibule are two sacs, the utricle and saccule, which are continuations of the membranous tubes of the semicircular ducts. Both ends of the semicircular canals are connected to the utricle. The maculae of the utricle and saccule also contain sensory receptors (hair cells). A thin layer of gelatinous mass, the otolithic membrane, covers these hair cells (Fig. 10-3C). The otolithic membrane contains calcium crystals, which add mass to the membrane. The maculae lie in the horizontal plane when the head is held horizontal, so that the otolithic membrane sits directly on the hair cells. In this case, if the head is tilted or linearly accelerated, the membrane lags behind, bending the cilia. The subsequent increase or decrease in the firing rate of cells results in a sense of body acceleration. The

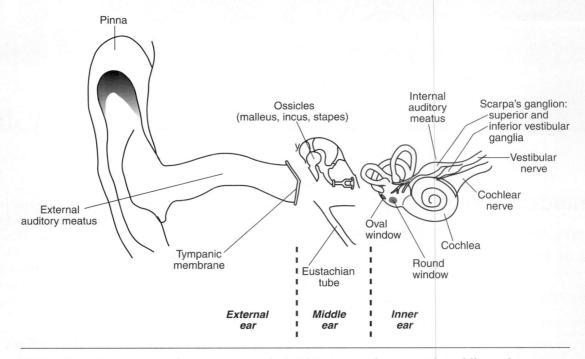

Figure 10-1 Frontal view of the anatomic relationship among the external, middle, and inner parts of the ear.

gravitational pull of the otolithic membrane also adds to the mass and bends the cilia, which changes the membrane potentials of the receptor cells, resulting in action potentials (impulses) that contribute to the sensation of up and down.

The **vestibular labyrinths** and the receptors of both sides interact in harmony when the vestibular system is functioning normally. The **vestibular receptors**, like **cochlear terminals**, do not exhibit significant adaptations. Thus the endings in the utricular and saccular maculae signal steady-state gravitational information and some dynamic changes (in **inertia** during linear acceleration and deceleration of head movements).

Vestibular Nerve and Nuclei

The vestibular nerve is formed by the fibers of the first-order sensory neurons in the vestibular (**Scarpa**) ganglia. The peripheral processes of Scarpa ganglion connect to the hair cells in the utricle, saccule, and semicircular canals; and its central projections form the vestibular nerve (Figs. 10-3 and 10-4). The vestibular ganglion of Scarpa consists of **superior** and **inferior ganglia**; each of these receives specific vestibular fibers. These vestibular ganglia are located in the cavity of the petrous bone (the bony labyrinth), and their central processes enter the through the **internal auditory meatus** to reach the junction of the medulla and pons.

The vestibular nerve fibers, which carry information concerning body **equilibrium** to the vestibular nuclei, join the auditory afferents to form the **vestibulocochlear (CN VIII) nerve** before they emerge from the internal auditory meatus to enter the **pontocerebellar junction** of the

brainstem. Beside the vestibular and cochlear fibers, the fibers of the **facial (CN VII) nerve** also pass through the internal auditory meatus. Thus a lesion at this point has significant implications for a series of symptoms that include **vertigo**, **tinnitus**, **sensorineural hearing loss**, and **facial (Bell) palsy**.

Upon entering the brainstem, the vestibular and auditory (CN VIII) nerve fibers of separate on their way to project to different groups of nuclei. Vestibular fibers terminate in the **vestibular nuclear complex** in the lateral-dorsal area of the medulla; the vestibular nuclear complex consists of the **superior vestibular nucleus**, **lateral vestibular nucleus**, **medial vestibular nucleus**, and **inferior vestibular nucleus** (Fig. 10-4). The auditory nerve fibers project to the **cochlear nuclei**, which are located at the pontomedullary junction (see Chapter 9).

Vascular Supply to the Membranous Labyrinthine

The **labyrinthine artery**, which originates from the **anterior inferior cerebellar artery (AICA)**, supplies blood to the membranous labyrinth, including the cochlear structure, the semicircular canals, and their first-order neurons (Fig. 17-1). Involvement of these arteries affects the functioning of the membranous labyrinth and produces the symptoms of hearing impairment, nystagmus, dizziness, and unsteady gait. The thrombotic involvement of the AICA also results in symptoms involving multiple cranial nerves (spinal tact of CN V plus the facial [VII], vagus [X], and hypoglossal [XII] nerves).

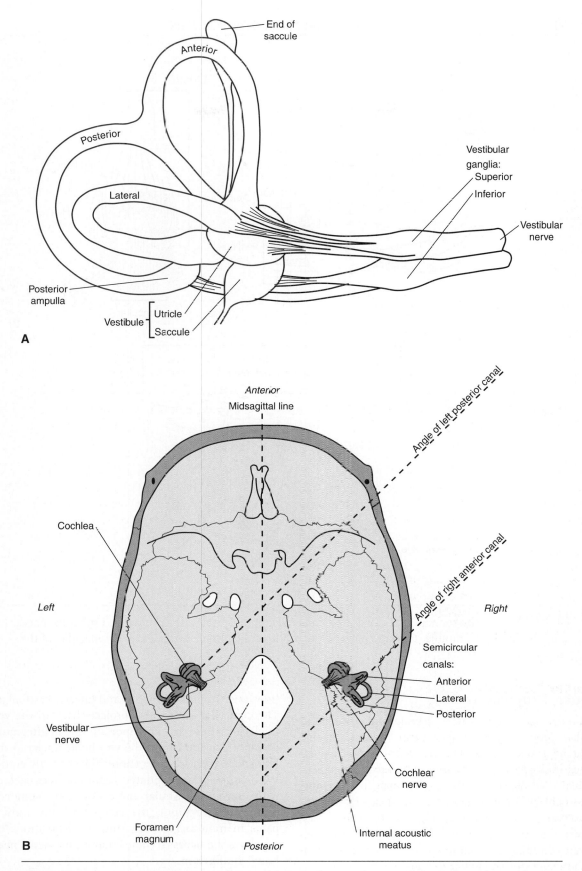

Figure 10-2 A. Structures important for equilibrium: the membranous labyrinth made up of inter-connected tubular ducts, the semicircular ducts containing the endolymphatic fluid, the utricle, the saccule with an extension (not shown), and the cochlear duct. The vestibular ganglia and vestibular nerve are also shown. B. Orientation of the anterior, horizontal, and posterior semicircular canals in the base of the skull. The planes of vertical orientation for the anterior and posterior canals form similar angles in relation to the midsagittal line

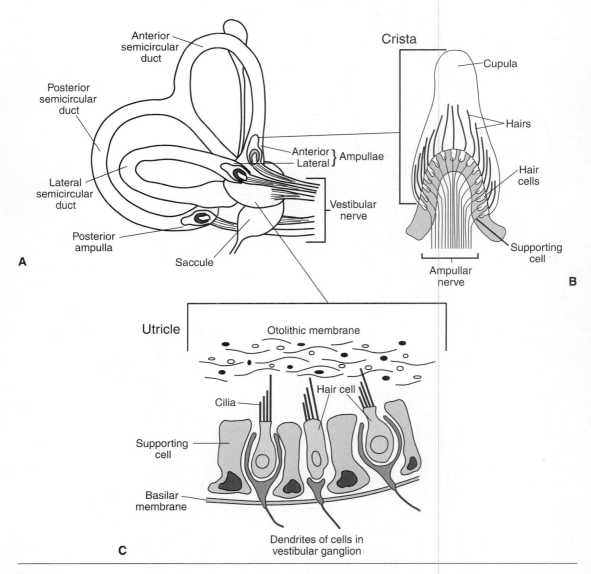

Figure 10-3 **A.** The semicircular canals and enlarged ampullae house the cristae. **B.** Hair cells, nerve, and cupula in the ampulla. **C.** Hair cells and the otolithic membrane arrangement of maculae of the saccule and utricle.

Vestibular Projections

The vestibular nerve fibers enter the brainstem at the pontomedullary junction, and most of them terminate in the vestibular nuclear complex. The vestibular complex then distributes multiple secondary projections to the cerebellum, spinal cord, **nuclei of the extraocular (oculomotor [CNIII], trochlear [CN IV], and abducens [CN VI]) nerves,** and other parts of the brainstem (Fig. 10-4). Of the fibers that bypass the vestibular nuclei, many instead enter the cerebellum through the **juxtarestiform body,** located medial to the **inferior cerebellar peduncle.**

Projections to the Cerebellum

The major projections from the vestibular nuclei go to the older cerebellar structures, including the **flocculonodular lobe**, **vermis**, and **fastigial nucleus**. Most of these projec-

tions arise from the superior and inferior vestibular nuclei. The cerebellar cortex also projects back to the vestibular nuclei and thus plays an important role in integrating additional information from the vestibular nuclei to the vestibulospinal tract for the maintenance of body equilibrium. With constant and updated vestibular feedback coupled with cerebellovestibular projections and spinocerebellar proprioceptive input, the cerebellum not only participates in monitoring body and head positions but also regulates the necessary muscular adjustments needed for body equilibrium.

Projections to the Medial Longitudinal Fasciculus

The fibers of the MLF are in the midline of the pons, medulla, and midbrain. The MLF fibers, with input from the medial vestibular nuclei, bilaterally project impulses to the

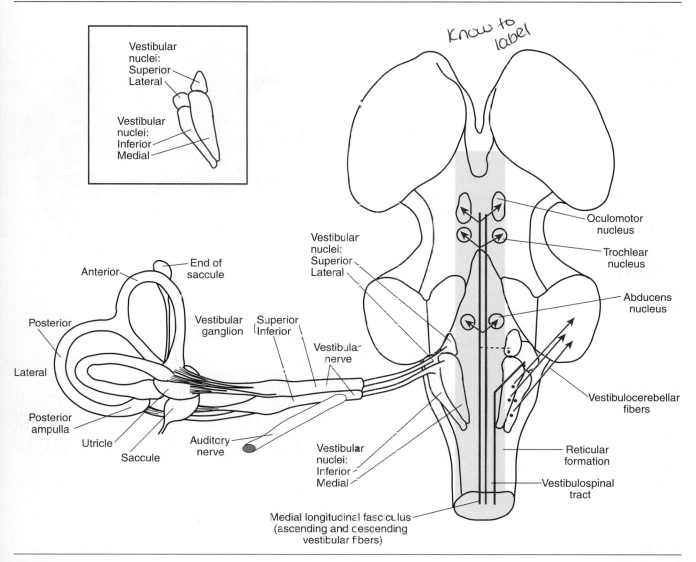

Figure 10-4 Semicircular canals, vestibular ganglia, and their projections to the vestibular nuclei in the brainstem.

motor nuclei of the oculomotor (CN III) nerve, trochlear nerve (CN IV), abducens (CN VI) nerve, and **spinal accessory (CN XI) nerve**. As part of the pontine gaze center, these cranial nerves regulate vertical and horizontal movements of the eyes and coordinate them with head movements through the innervation of the ocular and neck muscles. Crossed and uncrossed projections from the MLF activate and coordinate appropriate extraocular muscles for controlling conjugate eye movements and regulating visual fixation. The right conjugate movement, for example, involves the coordination of the **lateral rectus** (in the right eye) and **medial rectus** (in the left eye) for avoiding double vision. Descending medial longitudinal projections also regulate neck posture.

Projections to the Spinal Cord

Fibers originating from the lateral vestibular nucleus descend through the medulla, enter the ventral column of the spinal cord, and terminate at different spinal levels as they supply the motor units of the axial muscles and the limbs. The primary function of the vestibulospinal projections is to maintain the muscle tone that is needed to counteract the pull of gravity. This is done as the vestibulospinal projections activate the antigravity muscles. Sensory fibers from the spinal cord terminate in the caudal dorsal part of the vestibular nucleus, completing the feedback circuit between the brainstem and spinal cord, a circuit that is necessary for equilibrium maintenance.

Additional Vestibular Projections

Additional vestibular fibers—with projections to the brainstem reticular formation, and ascending reticular activating system—mediate several important functions, including tonal control, maintenance of body equilibrium, and regulation of visceral–automatic activities (e.g., dizziness, nausea, and vomiting with excessive labyrinthine stimulation).

NEURAL MECHANISM FOR CONTROLLING EYE MOVEMENTS

There are two neural mechanisms for controlling eye movements: **vestibular-ocular** and **voluntary**. The vestibular-ocular network regulates the reflexive control of conjugate and vertical eye movements through the crossed and uncrossed projections of the medial longitudinal fasciculus (Fig. 10-4). The frontal eye field (Brodmann area 8), which is located in the **middle frontal gyrus**, regulates voluntary control of **saccadic eye movements**, ensuring that the eyes turn toward objects of interest and danger (Fig. 10-5).

Vestibular Control of Conjugate Eye Movement

We constantly move with the slow or quick movements of our heads. If our eyes were fixed to the head with no compensatory mechanism for head movements, it would be difficult for us to see clearly. Everything that we see would appear out of focus and distorted by fluctuating movements if not for the important vestibulo-ocular connections that serve as the neurally controlled gyroscopic compensatory mechanism for stable eye movements. Lesions of the MLF (usually the result of multiple sclerosis or a stroke) produce dysconjugate eye movements.

When triggered by rapid head movement, the vestibular (semicircular canals) component of the inner ear sends signals to the medial vestibular nucleus, which provides input to the abducens (CN VI) nucleus within the **pontine horizontal gaze center**. This input, inhibiting ipsilateral conjugate eye movement while facilitating contralateral eye movement, ensures a smooth conjugate ocular movement. With its ascending projections to the trochlear (CN IV) nuclei in the vertical gaze center, the vestibular input also regulates any vertical ocular movement (Fig. 10-4).

If for any reason, normal or pathologic, the vestibular input is reduced, the eyes as a rule deviate to the side of the reduced vestibular input. This is commonly seen in case of a lesion involving the vestibular mechanism and with stimulation of the external auditory canal with cold water. Even in case of a head movement to the opposite side, the activation of the ipsilateral eye compensates and keeps the visual image fixed on the retina, thus avoiding any visual blurring.

Mechanism for Controlling Voluntary Eye Movement

Gaze control involves coordinated movements of the eyes for maintaining objects on the central retina (**fovea**) for clarity. These movements are saccadic and include quick and smooth. The quick movements cover up to 400–450° per second and track stable objects. Smooth movements cover 50–60° per second and keep a moving target focused on the retina. Voluntary control of eye movements comes from the frontal eye field (Brodmann area 8) by way of the **superior colliculus** in the **midbrain**. With afferents from

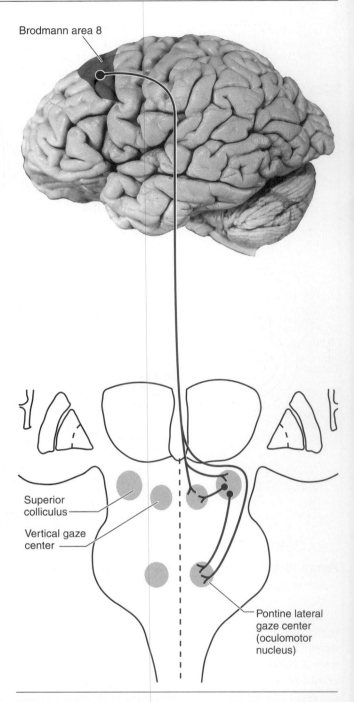

Brodmann area 8

Superior colliculus

Vertical gaze center

Pontine lateral gaze center (oculomotor nucleus)

Figure 10-5 The mechanism responsible for controlling eye movements.

the **parietal lobe** (Brodmann area 7), prefrontal cortex, and the deep layers of the superior colliculi, the frontal eye area activates the brainstem gaze (vertical and horizontal) centers (Fig. 10-5).

The parietal afferents, with links to the visual association cortex, lead us to explore novel visual stimuli, whereas the frontal afferents regulate the direction of the gaze. The afferents from the superior colliculus, representing the integration of the visual, auditory, and reticular reflexive functions, provide the basis for integrating attention with visual pursuit in saccadic ocular movement. The superior colliculus, though, might be involved with the simpler attributes of the stimuli.

PHYSIOLOGY OF EQUILIBRIUM

Two physiologic mechanisms control equilibrium: **dynamic** and **static**. Dynamic (kinetic) equilibrium regulates the maintenance of body and head positions during rotational and angular acceleration and deceleration. Static equilibrium regulates straight-line (linear) movements of the head in space and regulates both head and body position during rest.

Dynamic Equilibrium

The hair cells of the cristae in the semicircular ducts regulate dynamic equilibrium. The angular and rotational head movements serve as the stimuli for the receptor cells in the semicircular ducts. Particularly, each group of receptors responds to movement that is oriented in the plane of the duct. When receptors in the duct of one side are excited, receptors in the corresponding semicircular duct of the opposite side are simultaneously inhibited (Fig. 10-2). On rotation of the head, the moving endolymph in the canal deforms the cristae. Deformation of hair cells generates action potentials, which travel to the brainstem (Fig. 10-3).

The **unipolar neurons** in the vestibular ganglion that innervate the cristae are constantly active, firing even without a stimulus. This neuronal firing either increases or decreases when cristae are deformed by rotational and angular movements. The frequency of firing increases when the crista bends toward the utricle. The firing rate decreases when the crista bends away from the utricle.

Sensation of Rotation

Three important events in body rotation represent the three stages of movement of the endolymph in the semicircular canals; they are best demonstrated with a rotating (Bárány)

chair. Each stage relates to the specific state of endolymph inertia and produces a different rotatory sensation.

Stage 1

When a person rotates to the right (clockwise), the endolymph in the horizontal canal tends to move in the opposite direction (counterclockwise) of the head movement (Fig. 10-6A). This occurs because of the stationary state of the fluid (inertia). The cristae project into the endolymph and also move to the left (counterclockwise) with the endolymph. The directional bending and movement of the cristae influence the impulses that are transmitted to the brainstem vestibular nuclei. The brainstem vestibular nuclei interpret this rotation sensation to be clockwise, which is opposite of that of the endolymph movement. The slow phase of bilateral eye movement is always in the direction of the deviation of the cristae.

Stage 2

After 20 sec of moderate rotation, the endolymph loses its inertia, gathers momentum, and starts moving in the direction of the rotation of the body (Fig. 10-6B). The endolymph and cristae have acquired a new state of inertia related to the turning body, and the hair cells are no longer distorted. Because the endolymph at this stage is rotating at the same speed and direction as the body, the sensation of rotation at this point is minimal with eyes closed.

Stage 3

When the rotation of the chair suddenly stops (Fig. 10-6C), the body stops, but the endolymph continues moving clockwise. This results in a counterclockwise sensation of rotation. This directional change occurs because the fluid-containing horizontal ducts have stopped rotating, but the fluid, having attained rotational inertia, continues to move. The cristae bend clockwise with the clockwise movement of the endolymph, and this activates the sensation of rotating

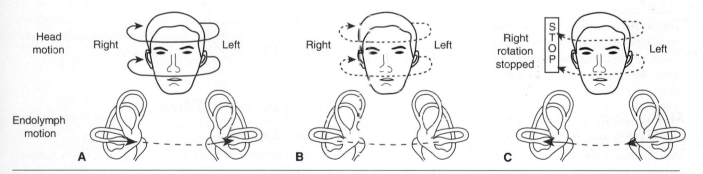

Figure 10-6 The three stages of endolymph movement in relation to the sensation and direction of body rotation with the eyes closed. These head rotations involve endolymph in the horizontal (lateral) semicircular canals. **A.** At the beginning of rotation, the counterclockwise movement of the endolymph induces a clockwise sensation of rotation. **B.** With constant rotation after a period of head turning, the endolymph and bony canals rotate at same rate, and sensory cells in the ampullae are not stimulated; thus there is no longer any sensation of rotation. **C.** With halted rotation, the clockwise rotation suddenly stops and the endolymph continues to flow clockwise because of inertia; this induces a sensation of counterclockwise rotation. *Arrows,* direction of motion.

in the direction opposite of the one sensed in stage 1. All the reflex effects are hardwired into the system, so that the adjustment of the antigravity muscles of the neck, trunk, and legs force the body to turn and follow the head.

Static Equilibrium

Static equilibrium, which depends on the utricle and saccule, monitors and maintains a balanced position of the head and body in space against gravity during rest and during straight-line head movements. The mechanism for these sensory receptors is similar to that of the semicircular ducts. The deformation of the apical ends of the receptors, by the movements of the otolithic membrane, generates action potentials that are transmitted to the brainstem. Gravity acting on the otolithic membrane causes the macula to respond quickly to any tilting movement of the head; prolonged fluctuating activation of the maculae produces motion sickness.

The vestibular ducts supplement the control of static equilibrium through predictive functions. An example of such a function is detection of a slight change in head position that prevents a fall while a person is running. The postural reflexes automatically adjust the tone of antigravity muscles. In contrast, the utricle cannot detect loss of balance until it actually occurs. Being off balance must be detected quickly if the person is to initiate appropriate adjustments.

Nystagmus

The function of the vestibular reflexes is to maintain a stable, conjugate visual fixation point. If the head rotates in any plane slowly, the vestibular reflexes produce the exact opposite conjugate eye rotation, maintaining the fixation point. These slow rotatory eye movements and the reflex wiring involve the vestibular nuclei and the **archicerebellum**. If the slow rotation reaches the limit of eye rotation, a rapid correction (saccadic movement) brings the conjugate fixation to a new point in the environment. Then the slow compensatory counter-rotation begins again, maintaining the new fixation point followed by a rapid corrective movement. This saccadic network is also used by the visual system in shifting the fixation point in the **visual startle reflex** and by the auditory system in the **auditory startle reflex**.

The rhythmic movements of the eyeballs in **nystagmus**, the most common vestibular reflex, is a normal compensatory reflex. It consists of two phases: a slow phase in which the eye slowly drifts away from the central field of gaze toward the periphery, and a fast phase in which the eye, with a sudden jerk, returns to the central field of gaze. Nystagmus is identified according to the direction of its quick phase (e.g., left nystagmus occurs when the quick component is to the left).

These are normal compensatory reflexes. If the head rotation continues, the sequence of slow–fast–slow reflexes continues. The slow phase moves both eyes in the opposite direction of the head rotation and thus maintains a stable eye fixation point. The fast phase allows the eyes to find a new fixation point. Any visual stimulation is blocked during the fast phase so that no blurred vision is experienced.

The absence of nystagmus with continued head turn is abnormal, and so is its emergence without any head rotation. A new method of assessing nystagmus is electronystagmography (ENG), which is based on electro-oculography and involves placing skin electrodes at the outer canthi (outer angle of each eye) to register horizontal or vertical nystagmic movements.

Induced Vestibular Eye Movements, or Nystagmus

The influence of the vestibular system on eye movements is best illustrated by rotating a person in a rotating chair. The rotation induces ocular nystagmus, a rhythmic eye movement with slow and fast components (Fig. 10-7). During clockwise rotation of the vestibular ducts (with counterclockwise flow of endolymph in the horizontal semicircular ducts), the eyes move slowly counterclockwise. The fast component of nystagmus is clockwise in the direction of rotation (Fig. 10-7A). During a counterclockwise rotation (Fig. 10-7B), the fast component of nystagmus is counterclockwise.

Nystagmus can originate in the occipital lobe or in the vestibular apparatus. **Opticokinetic nystagmus** is vision dependent and not vestibular instigated. It can be activated by visual fixation on a moving pattern and can be induced in any dimension—horizontal, vertical, and oblique. Vestibular nystagmus is independent of visual input.

However, visual input can be used to suppress vestibular nystagmus, which is best illustrated by ice skaters and ballet dancers. Professional figure skaters and ballet dancers have developed the capacity to control their eye movements independent of vestibular feedback. Neither shows any reactive nystagmic movements during and after body rotations. To prevent reactive nystagmus, ballet dancers and figure skaters learn to use visual feedback to suppress vestibular input by quick head rotations laterally over the shoulders. This facilitates continued eye fixation on the same object while the body continues to turn more slowly. Untrained persons do not have this compensatory mechanism and fall after only a few body rotations.

CLINICAL CONCERNS

Motion Sickness

Motion sickness, the most common disorder of the vestibular system, is characterized by vertigo, the subjective sensation of body rotation. It is also associated with dizziness or light-headedness, nausea, and vomiting. In some instances the symptoms are disabling. This is true especially after repeated up and down movements, such as in an airplane in rough weather or on a boat in high waves. Fortunately, most people adapt to these circumstances, and those who do not

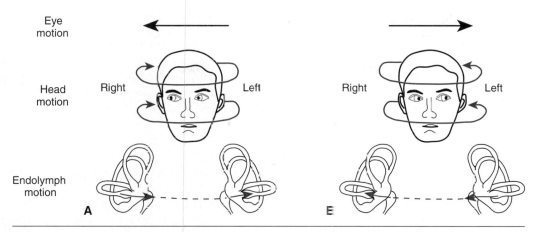

Figure 10-7 Nystagmic movements. A. With right nystagmus, in the beginning of a slow clockwise head rotation, inertia induces a counterclockwise change of pressure in the endolymph of the lateral semicircular duct, with consequent bending of the cupula to the left. Nystagmus in this instance is termed right, or clockwise, which is the direction of the readjusting, fast phase. B. With left nystagmus, in the beginning of counterclockwise head rotation, inertia induces a clockwise flow of the endolymph in the lateral semicircular canal. This results in the vestibulo-ocular reflex, causing a quick jerk of the eyes counterclockwise. *Black arrows,* nystagmus direction; *solid red,* movement direction; *dashed red,* endolymph direction.

can be treated with an antihistamine, such as dimenhydrinate (brand name: Dramamine).

Vertigo

Vertigo, the sensation of spinning through space (**subjective vertigo**) or of the environment spinning around oneself (**objective vertigo**) can be very disabling. It is mostly associated with impaired function of the vestibular apparatus and is commonly found in people who suffer from **Ménière disease**, a condition of obscure origin characterized by abnormally high endolymphatic pressure and later by mixing of endolymph and perilymph secondary to a rupture in the vestibular apparatus. Ménière disease also involves the organ of hearing and includes tinnitus (ringing, humming in the ear), hearing loss, and eventual deafness. Either acute or chronic **labyrinthitis** may also cause vertigo.

Labyrinth Dysfunction

Labyrinthitis is the irritation of the intercommunicating semicircular ducts and vestibule of the vestibular apparatus secondary to a viral infection or inflammation. It is a common labyrinth dysfunction and often a cause of vertigo. Impairment of the labyrinth on one side (unilateral) causes a short period of vertigo, disequilibrium, nystagmus, and some nausea and vomiting. The patient tends to fall toward the side of the lesion. This is likely to result from impaired downward pressure on one foot secondary to unopposed vestibulospinal activity on the normal side. The disequilibrium that occurs after bilateral destruction of the labyrinth is generally transient, although it sometimes persists and recurs for many months. Vestibular impairment in animals has been found to be more incapacitating than in

humans. One reason may be that most animals rely less on visual input for equilibrium than do humans.

Benign Positional Vertigo

The condition of benign vertigo, which is caused by changes in head position, is commonly seen in the elderly population. The underlying causes include oversensitive vestibular cilia and otolithic degeneration.

CLINICAL DIAGNOSTIC TESTS

The **acceleration–rotation chair** and **caloric stimulation** are commonly used to evaluate vestibular functions.

Acceleration–Rotation Chair

The integrity of vestibular projections to the cranial nerve nuclei that regulate extraocular muscles and to motor nuclei of the spinal cord can be examined by stimulation of the labyrinth in a rotating subject. The rotation test, also called the **Bárány test**, is performed on a patient seated in a rotating chair with his or her head tilted forward at 30°. The head tilt accommodates the semicircular canals being tested in the horizontal plane. After turning clockwise for 20 sec, the chair is suddenly stopped (Fig. 10-7C). Because of inertia, the endolymph moves in the direction of rotation (clockwise) and its pressure causes the cupula to bend in the same (clockwise) direction. The movement of the endolymph induces nystagmus (quick phase) in the direction opposite (counterclockwise) to the motion of the endolymph. This postrotatory effect is used to evaluate vestibular functions.

Caloric Stimulation

The vestibular end organ functions can also be independently assessed by caloric stimulation of the semicircular ducts. This involves the irrigation of both ear canals with water of different temperatures because caloric stimulation of the vestibular end organ induces nystagmus. This assessment is particularly important in patients with symptoms of dizziness and vertigo. Caloric assessment can be performed using warm (40°C) or cold (30°C) water. In a normal patient, cold water in the external auditory meatus induces nystagmus to the side opposite the canal/ear tested, whereas warm water causes nystagmus to the same side. In the case of a unilateral lesion involving the vestibular pathway, there will be either reduced or absent nystagmus in the ear on the side of the lesion. In a normal subject, both ears are likely to respond equally.

Ice water is used in cases of coma to differentiate bilateral frontal lobe lesions from brainstem lesions in unconscious patients after a head injury. In the ice water test the external canal is filled with cold water for 20 sec. A frontal lobe lesion is suspected if the eyes slowly and tonically deviate to the side of the ear being instilled and no nystagmus is noted. If coma is produced by a brainstem lesion, the instillation of cold water causes no response of the conjugate gaze.

CLINICAL CONSIDERATIONS

PATIENT ONE

A 50-year-old woman had sudden episodes of ringing in the ears, dizziness, vomiting, and vertigo. Every time she got up, she felt unsteady. She was taken to the hospital and on testing exhibited the following:

- No vestibular response in the left ear on caloric testing
- Head posture tilted to the left
- Severe vertigo
- Deafness in the left ear
- Loss of pain and temperature sensation on the left side of the face

A brain MRI study revealed an infarct in the dorsal lateral region of the left medulla and caudal region of the left pons.

Question: How can you relate the vestibular symptoms with the left pontine lesion?

Discussion: The infarct in the left dorsolateral medullopontine region affected the following structures:

- Damage to the vestibular nuclear complex was confirmed by the absence of nystagmus on caloric testing of the left ear.
- Damage to the left vestibular complex interrupted vestibular projections to the cervicospinal cord, which

regulates head posture. Interruption of these fibers caused the head to tilt to the left.
- Damage to vestibulospinal projections also interrupted vestibular projections to the extensor muscles of the limbs on the ipsilateral side. Consequently, the patient was falling to the left.
- Destruction of the vestibular nucleus caused the sensation of vertigo.
- Damage to the vestibulocochlear (CN VIII) nerve and cochlear nucleus caused impaired hearing in the left ear.
- Because the auditory fibers cross in the brainstem, it is likely that there was also diminished hearing in the right ear.
- The lesion also affected the spinal nucleus of the trigeminal tract, which is within the infarct region. This affected the mediation of pain and temperature from the left side of the face.

PATIENT TWO

A 45-year-old schoolteacher woke up feeling dizzy. She experienced unsteadiness, the sensation of the room spinning, and difficulties hearing in the right ear. She consulted a neurologist who noted the following:

- Profound hearing impairment in the right ear
- Unsteady posture
- Gait ataxia with a tendency to fall to the right side
- Left nystagmus
- No sign of limb or pharyngeal paralysis
- Intact language and speech functions

A magnetic resonance angiogram revealed the absence of a branch of the basilar artery on the right side.

Question: Based on your understanding of the vestibular vascular supply, can you provide an explanation for these selective symptoms?

Discussion: This is a case of stroke involving a small brainstem artery. The presence of sudden hearing impairment, unsteadiness, dizziness, and gait ataxia implicates ischemia in the territory of the AICA. This artery, which supplies blood to the inferior cerebellum, also gives off the labyrinthine artery, which supplies the membranous labyrinth (organ of Corti and semicircular canals), spiral ganglion, and vestibular ganglion.

PATIENT THREE

A 35-year-old student had suffered two disabling attacks of vertigo associated with right ear ringing sensation within 3 months. She was seen by a neurologist, who noted the following:

- Definite hearing loss during the attacks
- Sensation of tinnitus
- Repeated attacks of vomiting and nausea

- Normal somatosensory functions outside of these attacks

The brain MRI study was normal. The neurologist suspected it to be a case of ruptured membranous labyrinth.

Question: Can you comment on the pathophysiology of these symptoms?

Discussion: This is a case of Ménière's disease, in which excessive fluid accumulation or possibly rupture involving the membranous labyrinth causes deafness, vertigo attacks, unsteadiness, and tinnitus. The repeated and periodic attacks of hearing impairment and dizziness are also associated with vomiting and nausea.

SUMMARY

The vestibular system is a reflexive sensorimotor system that controls equilibrium. With sensory receptors in the semicircular canals of the inner ear, nuclei in the brainstem, and direct connections to other brainstem systems, the vestibular apparatus helps humans maintain a balanced upright posture, coordinate head and body movements, and control eye fixation on a point in space, even during body and head movements. The vestibular system is closely associated with the visual and proprioceptive systems; it constantly integrates incoming visual and proprioceptive cues, which contribute to the execution of highly complex, skilled, and coordinated activities like dancing, skating, and acrobatics. The functional importance of the vestibular system becomes evident in patients whose body balance is impaired by Ménière's disease or tumors of vestibulocochlear (CN VIII) nerve.

QUIZ QUESTIONS

1. Define the following terms: equilibrium, inertia, labyrinth, nystagmus, vertigo.

2. A 28-year-old woman was seen for a complaint of dizziness, nausea, and vomiting. On examination she exhibited a tendency of falling to the right, left nystagmus, deafness in the right ear, analgesia on the left body, hoarseness, and swallowing difficulty. Discuss the structures in which a lesion (semicircular canals, brainstem, cochlea, or tumor at the cerebellopontine angle) might account for this syndrome?

3. Why do ballet dancers and professional ice skaters not exhibit rotational nystagmus?

TECHNICAL TERMS

cristae	macula
cupula	medial longitudinal fasciculus
dynamic equilibrium	nystagmus
endolymph	semicircular ducts
equilibrium	static equilibrium
inertia	vertigo
labyrinth	vestibule

Motor System 1: Spinal Cord

LEARNING OBJECTIVES

After studying this chapter, students should be able to:

- Discuss the anatomy of the spinal cord
- Describe the functions of the spinal structures
- Discuss the importance of the motor unit in movement
- List the major ascending and descending spinal tracts
- Describe the functions of the major sensorimotor tracts
- Explain the role of muscle spindles in reflexive motor functions
- Discuss the importance of the Golgi tendon organ
- Describe the physiology of basic spinal reflexes
- Explain the importance of the lower motor neurons
- Discuss lower motor neuron syndrome
- Explain the common pathologies affecting spinal cord functions
- Describe the sensorimotor symptoms associated with spinal cord injuries

Motor activity is a hierarchically organized function under the control of reflex mechanisms and neural networks in a rostral segment of the central nervous system (CNS) (Fig. 11-1). From the lowest to the highest, these arbitrarily identified anatomic levels are the **spinal cord, cerebellum, brainstem, basal ganglia,** and **motor cortex.** Each ascending level in the hierarchy makes a specific contribution to the final motor activity, which also is influenced in part by the activity of higher motor centers. For example, the midbrain systems modulate reflexes organized at the medullary or spinal level. The forebrain systems regulate the midbrain and spinal motor activity. Motor responses begin in the spinal cord as simple reflexes, whereas the higher motor centers participate in the regulation of skilled and patterned movements. Neuronal impulses from higher levels also initiate, inhibit, or facilitate motor functions at the brainstem and spinal cord, thus partially regulating all motor behavior.

This cortical control provides a type of parallel processing with rostral domination of hierarchical motor organization and simultaneous control of the segmental output itself. Because some time is involved in the conduction of **afferent** information, local (spinal) reflexes often are activated first, and motor mechanisms at higher hierarchic levels are activated slightly later. The best example of reflexive movement is mistakenly stepping on a tack with your bare foot. This triggers a leg-**withdrawal reflex,** which is already in progress before the forebrain can inhibit or modify the action. However, the higher motor systems can inhibit such a withdrawal reflex if the stimulus is expected and another response has been learned. For example, if someone has to pick up a hot cup, the withdrawal reflex can be inhibited while the hot cup is being moved to a supporting surface, even though the fingers are being burned.

The hierarchically defined motor functions and the nature of the specific contributions by each level are discussed in Chapters 11–14. The spinal cord is the first level in the regulation of sensorimotor functions. Stereotypical motor responses (reflexes), which are largely independent of voluntary motor control, are generated in the spinal cord and can be triggered by cortical and/or environmental stimuli. The spinal cord also relays sensory information to the cerebrum, which is vital to learning skilled and coordinated motor activity.

SPINAL PREPARATION

Spinal cord functions are most easily demonstrated by a **spinal preparation,** which involves separating the cord from the regulating influence of the brain by cutting the cord. This separation allows for examination of spinal reflexes independent of the inhibitory or facilitatory influence exerted by higher motor centers. Immediately after the spinal cut is made, the flexor and extensor reflexes become completely inactive, but they gradually re-emerge.

INNERVATION PATTERN

The general motor function in the spinal cord and brainstem is organized ipsilateral to its output and reflex input. With the crossing of **corticospinal fibers** at the **medulla,**

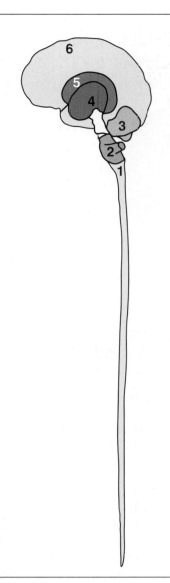

Figure 11-1 Six ascending levels of motor organization. *1*, spinal cord; *2*, brainstem; *3*, cerebellum; *4*, diencephalon; *5*, basal ganglia; *6*, cerebral cortex.

the spinal **α-motor neurons** and their **axons (final common pathway)** extend to innervate the muscles ipsilaterally (Figs. 11-2 and 11-4). Consequently, **lower motor neuron (LMN)** signs in the brainstem and spinal cord are ipsilateral to the damage of the cell body or its axon.

GROSS ANATOMY OF THE SPINAL CORD

The spinal cord extends from the base of the skull to the lower back and is approximately 43.5 cm long and 1 cm in diameter. It is divided into five regions: **cervical, thoracic, lumbar, sacral,** and **coccygeal.** A total of 31 pairs of **spinal nerves** emerge from the spinal cord (see Fig. 2-33). These nerves have mixed functions; they carry sensory information from peripheral receptors to the CNS and

transmit motor information from the CNS to the muscles. The nerves are named after the region of the spinal cord to which they are attached and are numbered in sequence. There are 8 pairs of cervical spinal nerves (C1–C8), 12 pairs of thoracic spinal nerves (T1–T12), 5 pairs of lumbar spinal nerves (L1–L5), 5 pairs of sacral spinal nerves (S1–S5), and usually 1 pair of coccygeal spinal nerves (see Chapter 2).

In adults, the spinal cord diminishes toward the lumbar region and ends as the **conus medullaris** at the L2 vertebra. The nerve root fibers from the L3 to S5 spinal segments stretch downward to reach the corresponding skeletal level before exiting the vertebral-spinal canal. The pia mater covering of the spinal cord extends beyond the conus medullaris in a thin **filum terminale,** which extends to and attaches to the coccyx. The spinal dura mater and subarachnoid space, filled with **cerebrospinal fluid** (CSF), extend beyond the conus medullaris to terminate in the sacrum by attaching to the coccyx (see Fig. 2-33).

The fact that the spinal cord does not extend into the fluid-filled subarachnoid space of the lumbosacral area has important clinical implications. This dural sac, at levels below the L1 vertebra (much lower in children because they have less disparity between the length of the cord and vertebral canal), is used for extracting CSF for diagnostic purposes (spinal tap or puncture) and for administering therapeutic and anesthetic drugs without risking damage to the spinal cord (see Chapter 20).

Internal Anatomy

Seen in cross section, the spinal cord consists of an outer ring of **white matter** and a butterfly-shaped central **gray area** (Fig. 11-2). The white matter contains ascending and descending fibers, whereas the gray matter contains nerve cell bodies and a small unmyelinated network of fibers (neuropils). The **dorsal horns** contain the secondary sensory nerve cells that receive sensory information from the body through the **dorsal root ganglia (DRG)** fibers. The **ventral horns** contain motor nerve cells, which project through the anterior roots to activate muscles, glands, and joints. The gray columns on each side of the cord are connected through the **commissures,** which consist of crossing fibers. The axonal processes of the motor neurons form the **ventral nerve root** fibers and send motor impulses from the CNS to the muscles. After traveling through the pia mater, subarachnoid space, arachnoid membrane, dura mater, and intervertebral foramina, the fibers from both the dorsal and anterior roots merge to form a **spinal nerve** (Fig. 11-2; see Fig. 2-32).

After a spinal nerve exits the intervertebral foramina, it divides into dorsal and ventral rami. The **dorsal ramus** fibers of each spinal nerve are concerned with the muscles and skin in the posterior part of the body. The **ventral ramus** fibers of the spinal nerve supply anterior body parts, including the upper and lower limbs. Before projecting to target muscles and body parts (see Fig. 2-35), the ventral rami of the spinal nerves, except the nerves from T2 to

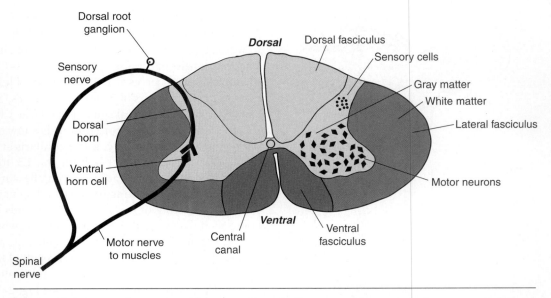

Figure 11-2 Internal anatomy of the spinal cord. The central gray matter is surrounded by white matter, which consists of three fasciculi (funiculi): dorsal, lateral, and ventral.

T11, form a network of nerve fibers called **plexuses**. Rami of the nerves from T2 to T11 directly innervate body parts.

The size and shape of the spinal cord are not uniform along its length (Fig. 11-3). The cord in the cervical and lumbar areas is broad and flattened in contrast to its shape in the thoracic areas. Widening at the cervical and lumbar segments of the cord results from the concentration of nerve cells and their fibers, which is necessitated by the sensory and motor control of the upper and lower extremity muscles. The upper extremities, especially the hands, possess more specialized sensory and motor functions than the legs, trunk, and viscera and therefore require a greater concentration of peripheral nerve fibers. Thus the size of the gray column at the cervical level is larger than at the lumbar level.

Segmental Organization

The spinal cord is anatomically and functionally organized in transverse segments extending from the cervical to the sacral region. This organization of the spinal cord indicates segmental sensorimotor innervation of the body (**dermatomes** and **myotomes**) with various distributional shapes and sizes (see Fig. 2-34). The **dermatome** (area innervated by the afferent fibers of the neurons in a single DRG) and **myotome** (muscle or muscles innervated by the axons exiting the cord via a single ventral root) may overlap each other, but because of muscle migration during development, they are not always the same.

Motor Unit

The **LMN** and **motor unit** are two important components of spinal motor control circuitry (Figs. 11-2 and 11-4). The LMN cell body provides the output pathway via its axon, which travels through the ventral root and periph-

eral nerves to innervate a skeletal muscle, where it forms multiple axon branches to activate many muscle fibers. The LMN is also the **final common pathway** because the **efferent** impulses from the motor cortex pass through this motor neuron before they can produce a muscle movement.

The motor unit consists of four components: **motor cell body**, **efferent fibers**, **motor end plate** (branching off the axonal fiber in **myoneural/neuromuscular junctions**), and **innervated muscle fibers**. A motor unit can fire repeatedly, resulting in sustained shortening of the muscle fiber elements. Damage to the LMN cell or the beginning axon eliminates the entire function of a motor unit. Damage to one of the terminal axon branches weakens the unit projections. Generalized skeletal muscle disease (e.g., **muscular dystrophy**) or reduced nerve–muscle transmission/activity (e.g., **myasthenia gravis**) weakens or eliminates the unit's force generation and causes muscle degeneration.

Motor units can be small or large, and a muscle can contain many motor units, depending on the nature of its motor control. For example, the small hand flexor muscle used for delicate and coordinated motor control can have 10–30 muscle fibers per motor unit, whereas large muscles like the **quadriceps** can have as many as 3,000 muscle fibers per motor unit.

TRACTS OF THE SPINAL CORD

The white matter of the spinal cord consists of three major bundles of longitudinal axons (fasciculi): **dorsal**, **lateral**, and **ventral columns** (Fig. 11-2). In most instances, each fasciculus contains bundles of ascending and descending fibers. The tracts are difficult to pinpoint on a cross section

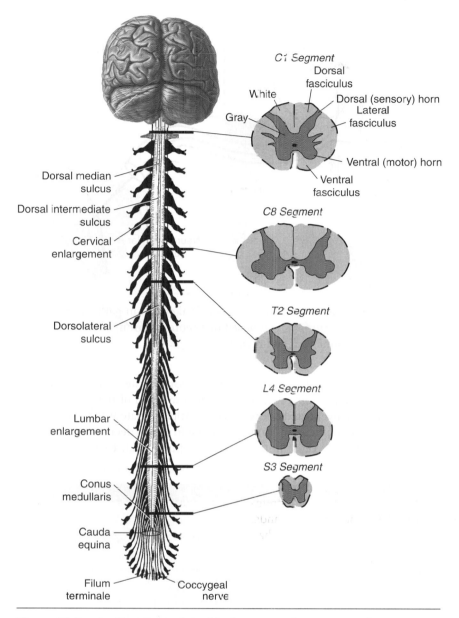

Figure 11-3 The dorsal spinal cord and its internal anatomy in five cross sections. The increase in cord size at the cervical and lumbar levels corresponds to the nerve supply for the upper and lower extremities, respectively.

of the spinal cord; however, their approximate locations can be determined from clinical evidence. The dorsal fasciculus consists largely of ascending (sensory) fibers, whereas the lateral and anterior fasciculi contain both descending (motor) and ascending (sensory) fiber bundles (Table 11-1). General locations of the various sensorimotor spinal tracts are demonstrated in Figure 11-5.

Descending Tracts

Corticospinal Tracts

Fibers of the corticospinal motor tract arise from pyramidal cells (the largest are **Betz cells**) in the cortex. Most of these cells are in the **precentral gyrus** (primary motor cor-

tex, Brodmann area 4); however, some of these cells are in other areas of the brain, including the **premotor cortex**, **primary somesthetic cortex** (Brodmann areas 3, 1, 2), and **supplementary motor cortex** (Brodmann area 6). On their way to the spinal cord, the **corticospinal fibers** cross the midline at the caudal end of the medulla and form the **lateral corticospinal tract** in the spinal cord. There are two corticospinal tracts; the other one is the **anterior corticospinal tract** (Fig. 11-6; see Chapter 14).

Lateral Corticospinal Tract

Lateral corticospinal fibers provide a mechanism by which the cerebral cortex intervenes in the control of skeletal

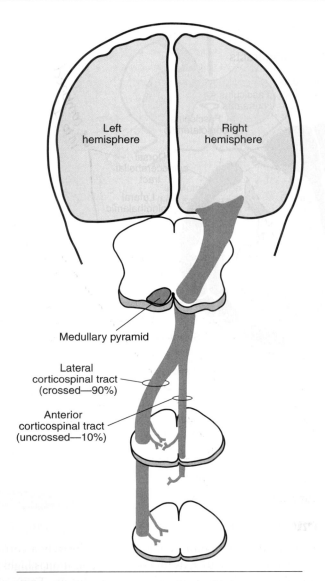

Figure 11-6 Corticospinal fibers predominantly project to the contralateral half of the body.

The vestibulospinal tract projects the vestibular impulses to the spinal LMNs. By regulating extensor muscle tone, these fibers control the reflexive adjustment of the body and limbs to keep the head stable. Originating from the nerve cells in the vestibular nucleus and incorporating projections from the inner ear and cerebellum, the vestibulospinal fibers extend throughout the length of the cord, giving off collaterals to α- and γ-motor nuclei.

Originating from the pons (**pontine reticulospinal tract**) and medulla (**medullary reticulospinal tract**), the reticular projections regulate coordinated motor functions. Reticular stimulation has been found to facilitate or inhibit voluntary and reflexive movements by altering muscle tone through the γ-motor system.

Autonomic Pathways

The **hypothalamus** is the central integrator and distributor of important autonomic projections to the brainstem and spinal visceral nuclei, and it regulates motor functions of the sympathetic and parasympathetic systems (see Chapter 16). Brainstem reticular nuclei, including the **locus ceruleus**, also relay projections that regulate spinal autonomic motor functions. Cells in the brainstem project to the cervical and thoracic segments, and they are primarily excitatory to the **phrenic motor neurons** and thoracic motor neurons participating in inspiration, vomiting, and coughing reflexes (see Chapter 16).

Ascending Tracts

The ascending fibers of the spinal cord transmit sensory information from various body parts (Fig. 11-5). The sensory impulses are pain, thermal sense, touch, proprioception, and kinesthesia (see Chapter 7). Projections from the sensory cortex refine the cortical motor efferents to the spinal cord.

The **fasciculus gracilis** is composed of axons arising from the spinal DRG in the sacral, lumbar, and lower six thoracic levels (Fig. 11-5). The fibers of the fasciculus gracilis mediate the sensations of discriminative touch, joint movement, and vibration from the lower half of the body.

Consisting of large fibers, the **fasciculus cuneatus** mediates the sensations of fine discriminative touch, joint movement, and vibration from the upper half of the body. Its fibers enter the cord from the upper six thoracic and all cervical levels (Fig. 11-5). Along with the fasciculus gracilis, the fasciculus cuneatus fibers terminate in the medullary relay nuclei of cuneatus and gracilis. Secondary fibers from these nuclei (internal arcuate fibers) decussate to form the medial lemniscus, which ascends to the **ventral posterolateral nucleus** of the thalamus and then to the primary sensory cortex (see Chapter 7).

The anterior spinothalamic tract is a backup sensory system. Its fibers mediate the sensation of crude and nonlocalizable touch (Fig. 11-5; see Fig. 7-8). After emerging from the cells in the spinal gray matter, these fibers cross the midline through the anterior commissure within several segments of the cord before ascending in the anterior spinothalamic tract. They terminate in the ventral posterolateral nucleus of the thalamus, and from there they project to the primary sensory cortex.

The fibers of the lateral spinothalamic tract transmit pain and temperature sensation (Fig. 11-5). Fibers of this tract, like those of the anterior spinothalamic tract, arise from the spinal dorsal horn nuclei and ascend in the lateral fasciculus to the thalamus and then to the cortex (see Chapter 7).

Spinocerebellar Tracts

The fibers of the ventral spinocerebellar tract mediate unconscious proprioception from the muscles of the lower extremities and proximal limbs, and they coordinate the movement and posture of the lower extremities (Fig. 11-5; see Fig. 7-10). The uncrossed fibers of the dorsal spinocerebellar tract mediate unconscious proprioception from the distal regions of the lower limbs. The cuneocerebellar fibers mediate unconscious proprioceptive information from the upper limbs to the cerebellum (see Chapter 7); these are concerned with fine and delicate control of the upper limbs.

MOTOR NUCLEI OF THE SPINAL CORD

The spinal gray matter contains thousands of motor nerve cells, which are either **anterior motor neurons** or **interneurons (internuncial cells)**. The anterior motor neurons include **α- and γ-motor neurons** (Fig. 11-7). The efferent fibers of α- and γ-motor nerve cells form the ventral roots of spinal nerves that innervate skeletal muscles. These are called **LMN** to distinguish them from the corticospinal neurons of the motor (and sensory) cortex, which are called **UMN**. The interneurons function as association cells interconnecting cell bodies within sensory and motor neuron pools. The dendritic and axonal projections of the internuncial cells connect adjacent spinal cord cells.

The cervical spinal cord gray matter also contains two specialized motor nuclei. One supplies the **phrenic nerve**, which innervates the diaphragm and participates in respiration (see Chapter 16). The other motor nucleus contributes to the spinal roots of the **spinal accessory (CN XI) nerve**, which regulates head and shoulder movements (see Chapter 15).

The α- and γ-motor neurons receive motor impulses directly from the motor centers in the forebrain and brainstem. The supraspinal projections to α- and γ-motor neurons, which initiate voluntary motor activities, are represented by balanced inhibitory (−) and excitatory (+) cortical outputs to the spinal motor neurons.

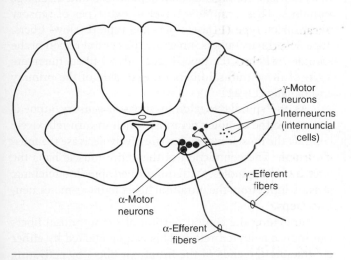

Figure 11-7 α-Cells, γ-cells, and internuncial cells in the anterior gray column of the spinal cord.

α-Motor Neurons

α-Motor neurons are the major motor neurons of the spinal cord. Their axons, with a diameter of 9–16 μm, rapidly conduct impulses. They pass through the ventral spinal root before innervating the **extrafusal fibers** of the skeletal muscles that are responsible for the voluntary and reflexive movements of the head, trunk, and extremities. On average, one α-neuron fiber innervates > 200 muscle fibers. These motor neurons are also the final common pathway because all efferent impulses from the CNS must pass through these cells before activating muscles.

γ-Motor Neurons

γ-Motor neurons, which lie alongside the α-cells in the spinal ventral horns, are smaller, half as numerous, and have smaller-diameter axonal processes. These neurons are slow impulse conductors. The primary role of γ-LMN neurons is to regulate the length of the spindle fibers and thus modulate the excitability of the annulospiral primary (Ia) endings. This regulates the stretch reflex muscle tone and allows the CNS to regulate its own state of excitability.

γ-Motor neurons are controlled by synaptic input from the brainstem reticular formation and the vestibular system. The γ-efferent fibers leave through the ventral nerve root and contract the end (contractile) portions of the intrafusal muscle fibers, stretching the central parts of the muscle spindles. On being stretched, the muscle spindles send a volley of afferent projections to the corresponding α-motor neurons, causing the reflexive contraction of the extrafusal fibers of the muscle.

Interneurons

As functionally specialized cells, the interneurons are diffusely present throughout the spinal cord and brain. There are ~30 times as many interneurons as motor neurons. With most being inhibitory, the interneuron cells serve as filters, integrating all sensory and motor functions of the CNS. The **Renshaw cell** receives axonal collaterals from nearby motor neurons, inhibiting the activity of the same or related adjacent motor neurons. This recurrent inhibition by the Renshaw cell facilitates and sharpens the activity of the projecting motor neuron from which it receives the collaterals.

MOTOR FUNCTIONS OF THE SPINAL CORD

The basic motor function of the spinal cord is a reflexive motor response. A **reflex response** is a stereotyped movement to sensory stimulation. The neuronal circuitry for reflexes is present at each segmental level throughout the spinal cord. It consists primarily of **muscle spindles, afferent fibers, α-motor neurons, efferent fibers**, and **muscle tissue** (Fig. 11-8).

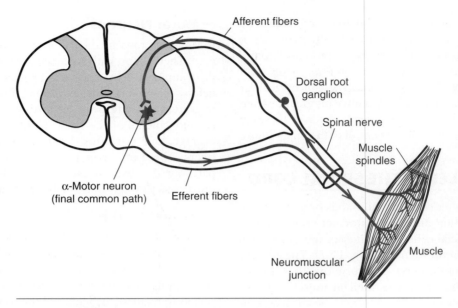

Figure 11-8 Neuronal circuitry for a spinal reflex.

For the most part, reflex functions of the spinal cord are independent of cortical voluntary control, although they are influenced indirectly by descending impulses from the motor cortex and brainstem motor centers. The input from higher motor centers participates in providing a homeostatic state of motor control, resulting in smooth motor movements. If released from higher levels of motor control, as in the case of a lesion, the spinal cord reflexes become hyperactive.

Muscle Spindles and Their Role in Motor Activity

There are two types of specialized receptors in muscles: **muscle spindles** and **Golgi tendon organs** (Fig. 11-9). Muscle spindles detect the degree and rate of change in muscle length and help maintain muscle tone. Golgi tendon organs monitor the degree of muscle tension during muscle contraction and reflexively inhibit muscle contraction, permitting the muscle to stretch and thus prevent injury caused by excessive contraction.

Muscle Spindles

As a complex sensorimotor organ, the muscle spindle is a small structure and consists of three to five specialized **intrafusal fibers** that are parallel to the surrounding extrafusal (striate) muscle fibers. The center of an intrafusal fiber is wrapped by a fast-conducting **annulospiral primary (Ia) sensory ending**. If stretched, it generates an afferent response in the afferent fiber from the spindle. The afferent impulses travel to α-motor neurons in the spinal cord via fast-conducting type Ia nerve fibers with a velocity of approximately 100 m/sec, causing the muscle to contract (Fig. 11-9A).

Muscles consist of extrafusal and intrafusal fibers. **Extrafusal fibers** make up the large mass of the skeletal (striated) muscle. They are attached to bone by fibrous tissue extensions called tendons and are controlled by α-motor neurons. Striated muscles are composed of **myosin filaments**, which are responsible for the contractility (shortening) of the muscle. **Intrafusal fibers**, which contain muscle spindles, are attached to the extrafusal fibers and are controlled by γ-motor neurons. Both ends of the intrafusal fibers contract; but the central region, which is devoid of myosin filaments, does not contract.

The γ-motor neurons control both ends of the intrafusal fibers. A contraction of both ends of these fibers causes the central portion of the fiber to stretch passively. A similar stretch of the spindles can occur if the entire muscle (skeletal) mass is stretched. Whenever the central portion of the intrafusal fiber stretches, the annulospiral primary sensory endings become depolarized and discharge impulses. These impulses travel in two types of sensory nerve fibers: **type Ia** (fast) fibers and **type II** (slow) fibers. Type Ia (primary) fibers innervate the central region of the spindles, whereas the type II (secondary) fibers innervate areas of the intrafusal fibers on each side of the primary ending (Fig. 11-9A).

As the spindles stretch, a surge of sensory input is directed to the α-motor neurons, which in turn reflexively contract the muscle mass to progressively decrease the muscle length. The contraction of the entire muscle halts the stretch of the spindles. With diminished spindle stretching, sensory input from the intrafusal fibers to the α-motor neurons stops.

Stretching the central portion of the intrafusal fibers can induce a stretch reflex. This can be elicited by either contracting the ends of the intrafusal fibers by activating γ-nerve impulses or lengthening the surrounding striate muscle. The latter is illustrated by the classic knee-jerk (stretch or myotatic) reflex. When the patient's leg is in a

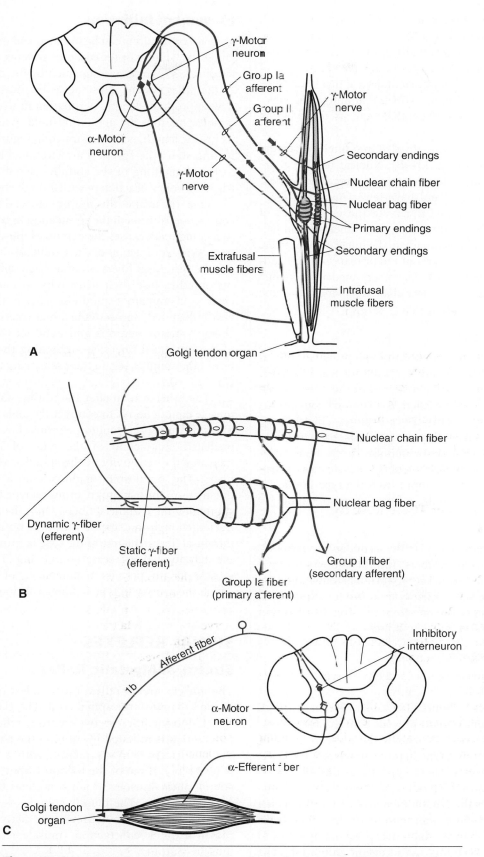

Figure 11-9 A. The relation of extrafusal and intrafusal muscle fibers to muscle stretch (muscle spindle) and tension (Golgi tendon) receptors. B. Nuclear bag and nuclear chain fibers. C. Golgi tendon organs, which mediate autogenic inhibition.

relaxed state, a tap of the patellar tendon at the knee with a reflex hammer immediately stretches both the extrafusal and intrafusal fibers of the quadriceps muscle. After a brief delay, the stretch is followed by a reflexive contraction of the same muscle. The response entails a spinal cord reflex triggered by sensory impulses in the annulospiral nerve endings of the intrafusal fibers that were stretched by the knee tap.

The intrafusal fibers are divided into **nuclear bag** and **nuclear chain fibers** (Fig. 11-9B). Nuclear bag fibers are long and have many nuclei in their center. The nuclear chain fibers are smaller and have fewer nuclei. Primary (type Ia) sensory endings innervate the central part of both the nuclear bag and nuclear chain fibers. Secondary (type II) sensory endings innervate the nuclear chain fibers only at sites beyond each end of the primary sensory endings. The intrafusal nuclear bag fibers mediate **dynamic sensory responses**, and nuclear chain fibers mediate **static responses**.

Dynamic Responses

Dynamic responses are mediated through primary (type Ia) sensory endings that terminate on the nuclear bag fibers of the muscle spindle. With a stretch of the muscle mass and/or the muscle spindle, there is a simultaneous distortion of the primary sensory nerve endings. This causes a surge of dynamic sensory input to the α-motor neurons of the spinal cord. The α-motor impulses from the anterior horn cells activate a contraction of the muscle mass, shortening the muscle. Sensory input from the type Ia nuclear bag fibers stops when intrafusal fibers cease stretching.

Static Responses

Static responses are generated in the secondary sensory endings of the nuclear chain fibers. Intrafusal fibers respond to stretch, a response which is proportional to the intensity of the stretch. The static sensory input from the intrafusal chain fibers maintains the muscle at the stretched position longer, from several minutes to hours.

Golgi Tendon Organs

Golgi tendon organs are the second type of sensory muscle receptors (Fig. 11-9C). They innervate the tough tissues that attach muscles to bones. The Golgi afferent impulses regulate muscle tension and prevent damage from excessive muscle contraction. Whenever the muscle stretch or contraction is excessive, type Ib projections from the Golgi tendon organs have an effect opposite to that of type Ia projections from muscle spindles. Excessive tension in the muscles stimulates the tendon organ type Ib fibers, which activate the intervening interneurons of the spinal cord. The interneurons in turn inhibit the spinal motor nuclei to the muscle. This accounts for autogenic inhibition. The Golgi-mediated reflex is protective, preventing the generation of a too-sudden or excessive force that could damage the muscle or its insertion.

Movement Initiation

Muscle contractions can be initiated and modified through either the γ-motor or the α-motor systems. Increased activity of one system is accompanied by increased discharges in the other system. This causes the muscle to assume a new, appropriate length. A situation in which both α- and γ-motor neurons are at subthreshold, with the muscle at its resting length, is demonstrated in Figure 11-10A. In the resting state, the spindles are stretched adequately. Any further stretching of the spindles depolarizes them and triggers a volley of action potentials to the α-motor neurons.

One way to alter this resting state and initiate a muscle contraction is through the stimulation of α-motor neurons. Activating them causes the extrafusal muscle fibers to contract. With contraction of the extrafusal fibers of the muscle, the intrafusal fibers become slack, and consequently, the spindles lose their sensitivity to muscle length. To correct this impaired spindle sensitivity, the **rubrospinal**, **vestibulospinal**, and **reticulospinal tracts** reflexively discharge γ-motor neurons and contract the end portions of the intrafusal fibers, straightening the spindles. As a result, the spindles regain their sensitivity to muscle length (Fig. 11-10A).

The other way to alter the resting state and initiate a muscle contraction is to contract the ends of the intrafusal fibers by way of the γ-motor neurons (Fig. 11-10B). The γ-mediated contraction of the ends of intrafusal fibers increases the sensitivity of the spindles and their afferent fibers. The annulospiral endings send a volley of action potentials to the α-motor neurons on type Ia sensory fibers, shortening the extrafusal fibers. Once the muscle has contracted enough to decrease the stress on the center of the intrafusal fibers, the rate of the type Ia firing decreases, and the extrafusal fibers cease contracting. The new desired muscle length permits maintenance of equilibrium in which the activity in type Ia fibers is below threshold.

SPINAL REFLEXES

Stretch, or Myotatic, Reflex

The muscle stretch reflex, the simplest of all, involves a single synapse in the spinal cord. The classic example of this monosynaptic, or two-neuron, reflex is the knee-jerk, which is initiated by tapping the patellar tendon of the quadriceps femoris muscle with a reflex hammer (Fig. 11-11). A tap of the tendon (input) leads to a brief stretch of the muscle, which stimulates the sensory endings of spindles. The muscle spindles send afferent projections to α-motor neurons, the activation of which causes a quick contraction (muscle jerk) of the same muscle (output).

The common element in all stretch reflexes is that the stretched muscle contracts after a brief delay. The principal receptors are the muscle receptors that respond to

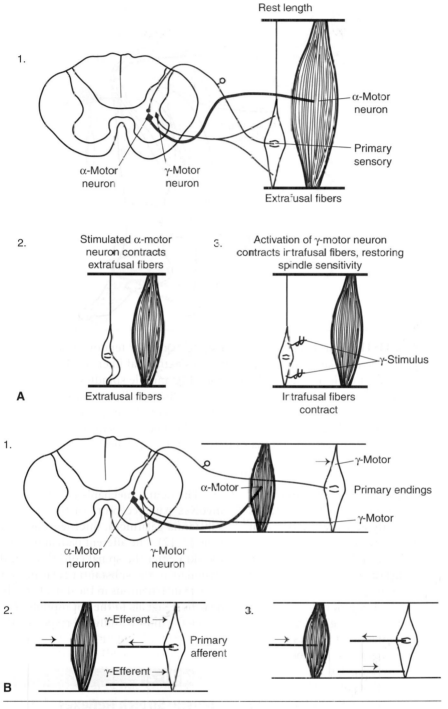

Figure 11-10 The α- and γ-motor neurons in movement initiation and the maintenance of sensitivity to stretch in the muscle spindles. A. α-Mediated voluntary contraction of the extrafusal muscle fibers leaves intrafusal fibers and their spindles without sensitivity to stretch. This condition is corrected by the reticular and vestibulospinal projections to the γ-motor neurons, which contract intrafusal fibers and restore spindle stretch sensitivity. B. In γ-initiated movement, γ-cells activate intrafusal fiber ends, deforming the annulospiral endings of the spindle afferent fibers, which synaptically activate α-motor neurons, causing contraction of the extrafusal muscle cells.

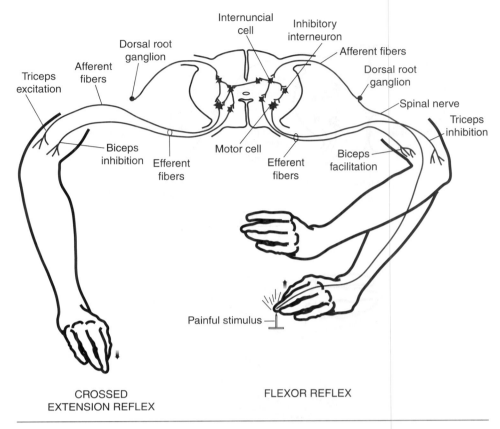

Figure 11-13 Neuronal circuitry for the crossed extensor reflex marked by the contraction of the muscle on one side accompanied by the extension of the opposing muscle or muscles. This reflex involves interneurons that diverge sensory information. This crossed sensory information activates motor neurons to extend the agonistic muscle, whereas the interneurons inhibit the motor nucleus for the antagonistic muscle, ensuring a smooth extension of the limb.

NEUROTRANSMITTERS

Four important neurotransmitters are released by the activity of brainstem projections to the spinal cord: **acetylcholine**, **norepinephrine**, **serotonin**, and **epinephrine**. Acetylcholine is the major chemical messenger of the peripheral nervous system (PNS). Released by the efferent spinal fibers in the **myoneural junction**, acetylcholine regulates voluntary or reflexive motor movements. A diminished effect of acetylcholine occurs in **myasthenia gravis** and similar disorders associated with muscle weakness. Weakness can be caused by either excessive action of the enzyme **acetylcholinesterase** or a reduced number of acetylcholine receptors at the myoneural junction. Acetylcholine also regulates autonomic functions. Except for the sympathetic postganglionic cells, acetylcholine is the primary neurotransmitter of the autonomic nervous system, which controls major visceral functions (see Table 16-1).

The pontine reticular **nucleus ceruleus** and **lateral medullary reticular formation** transmit epinephrine and norepinephrine to the spinal cord (see Fig. 13-1). Their influence is thought to be inhibitory, enhancing the signal-to-noise ratio in the spinal sensorimotor conduction system. These neurotransmitters are slow acting and have a long-lasting effect.

Located in the brainstem, the caudal reticular **raphe nuclei** send serotonin projections to the lower brainstem and spinal cord. The projections to the spinal cord synapse in the ventral and dorsal horns and in the sympathetic lateral columns. In addition, they synapse on spinal **enkephalin interneurons** and provide some control over pain transmission.

CLINICAL CONCERNS

Trauma, tumors, infections, impaired blood circulation, and degenerative conditions are common causes of spinal cord lesions. The testing of sensory and motor functions is the most reliable clinical method for determining the integrity of the spinal cord. The contraction of striate muscles during reflexes provides a clinician with important information about the complex internal mechanism of the entire motor system. Muscle reflexes are examined clinically on

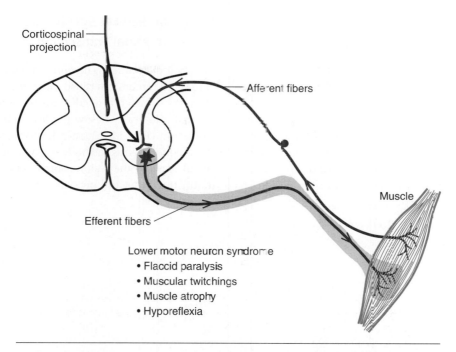

Lower motor neuron syndrome
- Flaccid paralysis
- Muscular twitchings
- Muscle atrophy
- Hyporeflexia

Figure 11-14 Injury to the motor unit (lower motor neuron syndrome).

both sides of the body to determine whether muscular movements are symmetrical and the quality of movements is normal. Reduced (**hypoactive**) or increased (**hyperactive**) quality of muscle reflexes indicates pathology in the nervous system. Spinal reflex functions are controlled via balanced excitatory (+) and inhibitory (−) supraspinal projections to the motor neurons. The corticospinal system is predominantly excitatory to motor neurons in the spinal cord. Loss of this system reduces recruitment of motor neurons and thus produces weakness. This muscle paresis is gradually converted over several weeks into spasticity, which includes hyperexcitability of many stretch reflexes (UMN syndrome). In contrast to brisk (hyperactive) reflexes with interrupted supraspinal fibers, lesions involving spinal motor neurons and/or their efferent spinal fibers lead to reduced or absent muscle reflexes (**hyporeflexia** or **areflexia**, respectively).

There are two types of spinal cord disorders: segmental and longitudinal (pathway specific). **Segmental disturbance** implies a lesion at a specific spinal level; below that level, sensory and motor functions are impaired. The severity of the deficit depends on the site and extent of the lesion. **Longitudinal disturbance** selectively affects specific nerve cells and their axons. The longitudinal involvement of axonal bundles may impair both sensory and motor systems.

Lower Motor Neuron Syndrome

The term lower motor neuron (LMN) refers to a motor neuron and its axon in the brainstem or spinal cord. A LMN cell body provides the output pathway to peripheral function via its axon, which traverses the ventral root and peripheral nerves to innervate a skeletal muscle. LMN lesions of either the spinal cell bodies in the ventral horn (e.g., poliomyelitis,

amyotrophic lateral sclerosis, vascular damage, and spinal cord tumor) or of the axon (in the ventral root or peripheral nerve) result in **denervation** of the **skeletal muscle fibers** and loss of muscle power (weakness) and precise control.

Small lesions can result in the loss of one or several motor units. Large lesions or peripheral nerve destruction can result in complete muscle weakness and total flaccidity. Such a lesion results in **LMN syndrome** (Fig. 11-14; see Table 14-1), in which muscle fibers are disconnected from motor efferents and thus cannot receive descending cortical impulses and reflexive sensory input. Deprived of their trophic efferents, the affected muscle fibers gradually degenerate. Clinical signs of LMN include **flaccid paralysis**, **absent reflexes**, **muscular fibrillation**, and eventual severe atrophy (wasting) of the muscle involved; these signs occur unilateral to the lesion.

With no projections of motor impulses from the motor neuron, the muscle fibers are completely paralyzed for both reflexes and voluntary motor movements; this paralysis is characterized by flaccid muscle tone. Denervated muscle fibers pass through several stages: a brief period of hyperexcitability and spontaneous firing (**fibrillation**), followed by silence of firing and shrinking of the muscle (**atrophy**). Fibrillation is the contraction of individual denervated muscle cells, which contract under the influence of acetylcholine circulating in the blood. If they are not reinnervated within 6 months or so, the skeletal muscle cells die and are replaced permanently by scar tissue. This is more severe than reduced muscle mass from disuse, which often is seen in **UMN syndrome**.

If the LMN survives, the normal membrane potential eventually is restored and the unit returns to its normal condition, except for when the motor system excites the cell body past threshold. Destruction of the LMN cell body or its axon results in denervation of the muscle fibers or motor unit. Destroyed LMN cell bodies are not replaced. However, destroyed LMN axons (PNS) may regenerate, and if they are directed properly past scar tissue and through their former peripheral nerve path, they can reinnervate to their former muscle fiber targets. Skilled peripheral nerve surgery, inhibition of scar tissue formation, and efforts to maintain denervated muscle fibers until reinnervation occurs are all necessary for the success of reinnervation.

Common Spinal Syndromes
Complete Spinal Transection

Vertebral dislocations, myelitis (inflammation of the spinal cord), and tumors can cause spinal transection. Immediately after the transection, all sensory and motor functions are lost bilaterally below the lesion but are spared above the lesion (Fig. 11-15; see "Lesion Localization" later in this chapter). Thus the body regions affected depend on the spinal level of the lesion. Spinal shock abolishes sensorimotor functions and persists for weeks. After a while, the

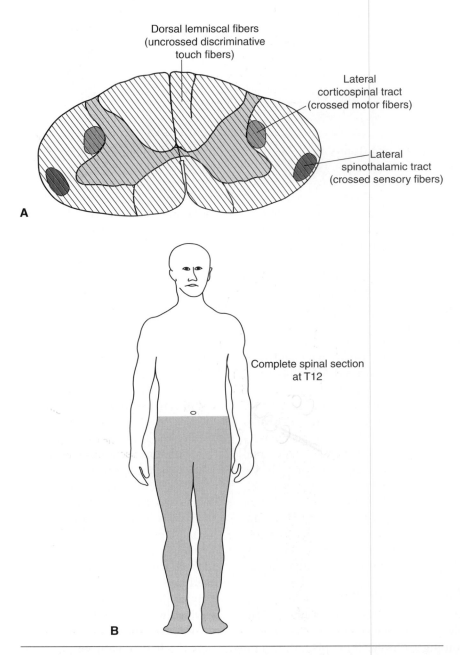

Figure 11-15 Complete transection of the thoracic spinal cord (A), resulting in bilateral paralysis and sensory loss below the level of the lesion with spared functions above the level of lesion (B).

reflex activity gradually returns at levels below the lesion. However, with the interruption of the corticospinal tract, after several weeks the patient exhibits UMN syndrome, which includes loss of delicate manipulative capabilities in the forearm and fingers, hyperactive stretch reflexes, Babinski sign, and clonic movements in which a passively moved limb undergoes rapid and repeated contraction and relaxation. With spastic legs, the patient eventually assumes an extended posture, which is characterized by extended lower limbs. If the lesion is above the level of innervation of the upper limbs, he or she often also assumes a flexed posture (see Chapter 14).

Brown-Séquard Syndrome: Spinal Hemisection

Lateral hemisection of the spinal cord produces the following three clinical conditions; understanding them requires knowledge of the locations and crossing points of the sensorimotor pathways (Fig. 11-16).

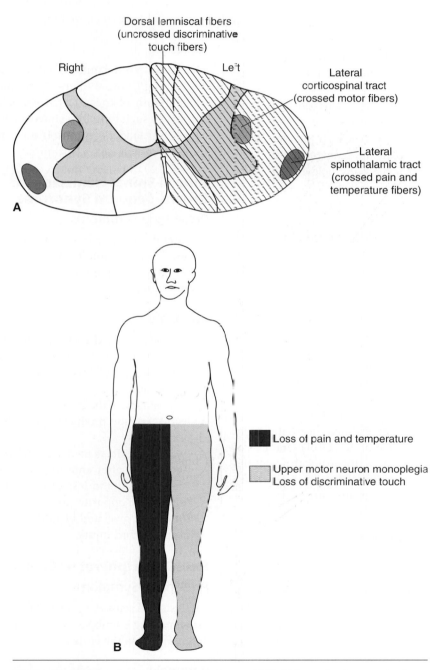

Figure 11-16 A spinal cord hemisection at T12 (**A**) results in a typical sensorimotor deficit pattern characterized by ipsilateral paralysis, ipsilateral sensory loss (discriminative sensation), and contralateral pain and temperature loss (**B**).

- **Signs of a lesion in the corticospinal tract on the ipsilateral half of the body.** In the case of a right-sided lesion at C4, there is spastic paralysis in the right arm and leg (UMN symptoms). Babinski and Hoffman signs are also present. The Babinski sign is abnormal extension of the big toe in response to a scraping stimulus to the sole of the foot (Fig. 14-5). The Hoffmann sign is when the thumb and other fingers flex from the flicking of the nail or distal phalanx.
- **Ipsilateral sensory loss.** Destruction of the dorsal lemniscal column, which contains tactile and proprioceptive axons ascending ipsilaterally to relay to the contralateral forebrain, results in loss of vibratory and discriminative sensation in the ipsilateral half of the body. The ascending dorsal lemniscal fibers cross the midline in the caudal medulla (see Chapter 7).
- **Contralateral pain and temperature sensation loss.** With fibers of the lateral spinal thalamic tract crossing immediately after entering the spinal cord, an interruption at the right C4 level affects pain and temperature from the left (contralateral) side of the body below the level of the lesion (see Chapter 7).

Syringomyelia

Syringomyelia is a developmental condition marked by a cyst or cavity within the central portion of the spinal cord. It is characterized by two clinical symptoms: loss of pain and temperature sensation and impaired motor control. The central (gray) region is the site of degeneration, and the crossing of sensory (pain and touch) fibers is interrupted, which results in a bilateral pattern of pain and temperature loss (Fig. 11-17A). If the cyst extends into the spinal motor nuclei in the involved segments, bilateral signs of LMN syndrome in the involved muscles include flaccid paralysis, hyporeflexia, and hypotonia.

The sensorimotor symptoms depend on the level of the spinal cord implicated. For example, a cavitation in the central spinal area at C4–C6 produces bilateral loss of pain and temperature for the arms, forearms, thumbs, and index fingers. A large cavitation involving C3–T4, in addition to the loss of pain and temperature, affects the shoulders and chest (Fig. 11-17B).

Subacute Combined Degeneration

Subacute combined degeneration is associated with pernicious anemia (when the number of red blood cells and the amount of hemoglobin in blood is less than normal), which results from malabsorption of vitamin B_{12}. The bilateral subacute degeneration of the spinal cord mostly involves the fibers in the dorsal lemniscal column and corticospinal tract. Involvement of the dorsal column fibers results in bilateral loss of position and vibratory sense, whereas the interruption of the corticospinal fibers produces a weakness of limbs bilaterally. The presence of paresthesia (numbness and tingling) indicates peripheral nerve involvement. As the disease progresses to the cerebral cortex, higher mental functions are affected.

LESION LOCALIZATION

Rule 5: Complete Spinal Cord Lesion
Presenting Symptoms

Paralysis and sensory loss bilaterally below the level of the lesion with spared functions above indicate a complete spinal cord trans-sectional injury.

Rationale

The spinal cord contains all ascending (sensory) and descending (motor) fibers. A complete lesion affects the transmission of these functions below the lesion point and spares such functions above the lesion point. Impaired bowel and bladder control and autonomic reflexes are commonly seen in a spinal cord injury.

Rule 6: Spinal Hemisection: Brown-Séquard Syndrome
Presenting Symptoms

Ipsilateral loss of position and vibratory sensation below the level of the lesion, ipsilateral body paralysis, and contralateral loss of pain and temperature indicate a spinal hemisection.

Rationale

1. Transection of the fasciculus gracilis and fasciculus cuneatus results in the loss of position and vibration sense along with discriminative touch on the side of the lesion.
2. Involvement of the fibers of the corticospinal tract below its decussation produces spastic hemiplegia on the side of the lesion.
3. Because the fibers mediating pain and temperature cross the midline after entering the spinal cord, their interruption results in loss of pain and temperature sensation on the opposite side.
4. Impaired bowel and bladder control is commonly seen in spinal cord injury.

Rule 7: Peripheral or Central Lesion
Presenting Symptoms

Paralysis and sensory (pain and temperature) loss affecting the same single limb suggest a lesion either in the peripheral nerve or in the cortex.

Rationale

The descending and ascending sensory fibers supplying a single limb are together only in the peripheral (nerve, plexus) area or in the somatosensory cortical area.

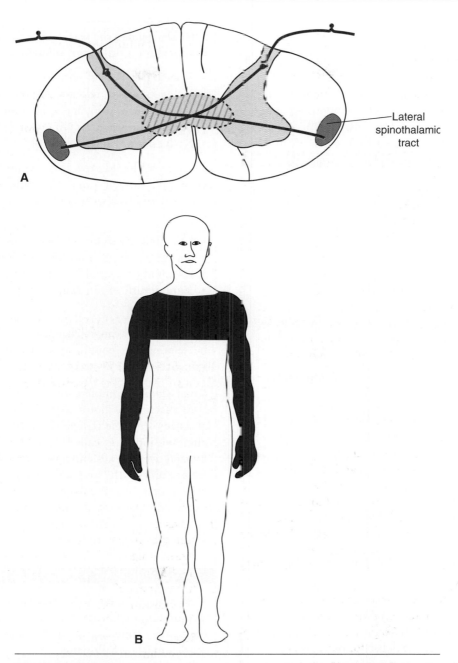

Figure 11-17 A syringomyelic cavity in the cervical gray matter (A) interrupts the crossing of pain-mediating spinothalamic fibers, causing a bilateral loss of pain and temperature and possibly bilateral flaccid paralysis of the muscles of the upper limbs (B).

CLINICAL CONSIDERATIONS

PATIENT ONE

A 3-year-old girl woke up with pain in her right leg. She had no control of her right leg and could not walk. She was taken to the hospital and examination revealed the following:

- No voluntary movement in the right leg
- Diminished tone in the leg muscles
- Absent knee-jerk and Achilles reflexes

A spinal MRI study revealed no abnormality. Clinical analysis of the CSF withdrawn through spinal tap revealed increased white blood cells, indicating an infection.

Question: How can you explain these clinical signs?

Discussion: An acute viral infection, which was diagnosed by the chemical analysis of the CSF. The infection had affected spinal LMNs from L1–L5 in the lumbar region and thereby caused weakness of the leg.

PATIENT TWO

A 30-year-old window washer fell from her ladder and injured her back at the T11–T12 level. She had bilateral flaccid paralysis of the legs and was rushed to the hospital, where she was observed for a few days. In an examination completed a few weeks later, she demonstrated the following symptoms:

- Spastic paralysis in the left leg
- Positive Babinski sign in the left leg
- Loss of position sense (proprioception) and discriminative touch in the left leg
- Loss of pain and temperature in the right foot

A spinal MRI study revealed a crushed appearance of the cord at T11–T12 on the left.

Question: How can you relate these symptoms to a crushed cord at the T11–T12 level?

Discussion: This is an example of Brown-Séquard syndrome, which is associated with spinal hemisection and is characterized by three signs:

- Paralysis on the side of the lesion
- Loss of fine discriminative touch and position sense on the side of the lesion
- Impaired sensation of pain and temperature on the side opposite to the lesion

Flaccid paralysis followed by spastic paralysis indicates spinal shock secondary to an UMN lesion, which was confirmed by the positive Babinski sign in the left foot. The loss of position sense and discriminative touch from the left toes and leg indicates the involvement of the dorsal column–medial lemniscal fibers; the loss of pain from the right leg suggests interruption of the left spinothalamic pathway. Mediating pain and temperature sensation from the right side of the body, this pathway crosses in the spinal cord at the level of entry. In this case, the initial loss of functions indicated injury to both sides of the spinal cord, but permanent injury was restricted to the left side only.

PATIENT THREE

A 16-year-old gymnast lost control of her body while exercising and fell flat on her back. Unconscious for several minutes, she was rushed to a nearby hospital.

After she awoke, she was unable to move. A neurologic examination revealed the following:

- Flaccid paralysis of both lower limbs
- No deep tendon reflexes in either leg
- Loss of touch, pain, and temperature sensation below the midthoracic (T6–T7) region
- No bladder or bowel control

A spinal MRI study revealed a complete spinal section at the midthoracic level. The patient's clinical picture changed within a week and she began to exhibit these signs:

- Hyperreflexia in both lower limbs
- Spastic paralysis of both lower limbs
- Impaired control of bowel and bladder functions
- Some return of touch and pressure sensation in the lower limbs

Question: How can you account for this clinical picture by relating the symptoms to a complete midthoracic spinal section?

Discussion: A complete midthoracic transection of the cord affected the motor control of the lower limbs. The absence of muscle reflexes for a few days immediately after the injury is called spinal shock. The return of hyperactive reflexes and spasticity, indicating an UMN lesion, reflects the loss of descending inhibitory influences. In UMN involvement, Babinski sign is also expected. The loss of consciousness in this case was attributed to a cortical concussion because it is not a feature of spinal cord injury.

PATIENT FOUR

A 45-year-old man was taken to a neurologist with a complaint of a progressively worsening weakness of both lower limbs for the past 2 months. The neurologist noted the following:

- Paralysis (flaccid) in both lower limbs and fasciculation in the muscles
- Reduced reflexes involving both limbs
- Loss of pain and temperature involving both extremities
- Impaired bladder function

A spinal MRI study revealed a large intraspinal, centrally placed tumor at the level of the conus medullaris.

Question: How can you relate these symptoms to the lesion site?

Discussion: The location of the tumor within the spinal central gray matter had affected the following structures, which are associated with the reported clinical symptoms:

- The tumor blocked the crossing fiber tract that carries pain and temperature. This subsequently resulted in a bilateral loss of pain and temperature from both lower extremities.
- The tumor also encroached on the adjacent LMN tracts and neurons bilaterally, affecting lower limb muscle strength.
- A lumbar involvement is usually associated with bowl and bladder functions.

PATIENT FIVE

A 54-year-old man, who was involved in a head-on automobile accident, experienced difficulty breathing; he was taken to the emergency room (ER), where the following signs and symptoms were noted:

- Paralysis of both right upper and lower limbs
- Loss of discriminative sensation from the right half of the body
- Profound breathing problem marked with inability to inhale
- No difficulty in exhaling
- Unintelligible speech marked with weakly articulated one-word utterances

A spinal MRI study revealed a partial spinal lesion on the right involving C3–C5. The attending neurologists concluded that the partial lesion had affected the epicritic system, corticospinal tract fibers, and phrenic nerve.

Question: How can you relate these clinical symptoms to the lesion site?

Discussion: A lesion anywhere in the neuraxis is likely to affect the descending corticospinal fibers and ascending sensory fibers. However, a lesion only at the cervical spinal cord level is likely to interrupt the phrenic nerve fibers that innervate the diaphragm, the primary muscle of inspiration. In this case, the phrenic nerve injury had caused respiratory paralysis with marked difficulty in inhalation. A right cervical lesion also caused ipsilateral paralysis (subsequent to the interruption of the crossed fibers of the corticospinal tract) and ipsilateral loss of discriminative sensation (subsequent to the involvement of the uncrossed ascending fibers of the dorsal lemniscal system).

SUMMARY

Motor function is hierarchically organized at four arbitrarily identified neuraxial levels, with the spinal cord being the lowest. Motor nuclei of the spinal cord are the final common pathway for both spinal reflex and cortical projections to muscle fibers. Consequently, the spinal cord is crucial in reflex muscle contractions and voluntary movements. The environmentally triggered reflex responses regulated by the spinal cord include the stretch (myotatic) reflex, withdrawal (flexor) reflex, and crossed extensor reflex. Even though these reflexes are independent of voluntary motor control, intact cortical projections to the spinal cord are important in the regulation of these reflexes. Constantly relayed sensory information, which is vital to coordinated motor activity, is integrated at every level of the nervous system. Spinal lesions that interrupt both cortical and spinal reflex projections to limb muscles result in LMN syndrome. The clinical picture of this syndrome is characterized by flaccid paralysis, absent reflexes, and atrophy of muscle fibers.

QUIZ QUESTIONS

1. Define the following terms: atrophy, hyporeflexia, lower motor neuron, muscle spindles, myoneural junction, stretch reflex.

2. Name the parts of a motor unit.

3. List the clinical characteristics of LMN syndrome.

4. List the spinal locations of the motor neurons that innervate the muscles of respiration. (Also see Chapter 2.)

TECHNICAL TERMS

afferent
α-motor neuron
atrophy
axon
crossed extensor reflex
efferent
extrafusal fibers
γ-motor neuron
Golgi tendon organ
hyporeflexia
interneuron

intrafusal fibers
lower motor neuron
motor unit
muscle spindles
myoneural junction
reciprocal inhibition
reflex
skeletal muscle
stretch reflex
withdrawal reflex

Motor System 2: Cerebellum

LEARNING OBJECTIVES

After studying this chapter, students should be able to:

- Discuss the importance of the cerebellum in motor activity

- Outline the major anatomic structures of the cerebellum

- Describe the function of each principal cerebellar structure

- List cerebellar afferent and efferent projections and discuss their functions

- Describe the neuronal circuitry of a cerebellar functional unit

- Discuss the major symptoms of cerebellar dysfunction

- Outline diseases and pathologies of the cerebellum

The primary level planning of a movement sequence involves the **premotor cortex** and the **supplementary motor cortex**. The fine details of this plan are managed by the **motor cortex**. However, ongoing modifications to the motor plan require participation of the cerebellum, a structure that functions as an error-control device and coordinates all relevant input and output systems during movement, particularly rapid, alternating, and sequential movements. The more precise the activity, especially rapid movements, the more cerebellar functional participation, either normal or abnormal, becomes evident. The need for the cerebellum would be minimal if there were no sequential and rapid movements.

In its regulation of movement, the cerebellum constantly monitors all cortical motor output to muscles by receiving input from the motor cortex, brainstem reticular reflex networks, and spinocerebellar (information on body and limb position and joint movement) system. The cerebellum then compares the efferent commands for intended movements with the sensory information received in terms of anticipated and ongoing motor programs. It considers targeted movement in relation to body position, muscle preparedness, muscle tone, body equilibrium, distance, and duration. If any sensorimotor discrepancy is detected between body position and motor impulse, the cerebellum sends corrective outputs in two directions.

Ascending feedback, related to what is going on and what modifications have to be made in terms of limb preparation, travels to the motor cortex via the ventrolateral thalamus. **Descending feedback** (via the **rubrospinal tract** and **reticulospinal tract**) to the **lower motor neurons** (LMNs) modulates muscle tone and reflexes at each moment during the ongoing movement. The ascending and descending functions occur simultaneously. The ascending output is informational; it is used by the thalamus and cortex the next time the movement is made. In the case of sensorimotor discrepancy, the cerebellum can increase or decrease the rate of movement and stop movements at any time.

The cerebellum is vital to the control of rapid muscular activities, such as speaking, running, typing, playing the piano, and dancing; these activities require the highest level of constantly changing muscle synergy and movement range and velocity. The cerebellum contributes specifically to **muscle synergy**, **muscle tone**, **movement range**, **velocity**, and **strength** and **maintenance of body equilibrium** by contributing both built-in and learned modifications to the motor plan. Muscle synergy refers to the **coordination** and **smoothness** in **time** and **space** of the ongoing movement, essential for fine and skilled movements. Transitions and alterations in trajectory are smoothed out by the anticipatory checking of momentum and damping of oscillations. Muscle tonal regulation involves maintaining constant tension in healthy muscles and ensuring that the muscles are prepared. Equilibrium likewise ensures that the stable posture needed for executing motor movements is maintained.

The cerebellum is not concerned with the conscious appreciation of sensations and cognitive processing. It, however, participates in **motor learning**, **motor memory**, and **movement execution** by automatically regulating and integrating information with sensorimotor mechanisms without reaching conscious awareness. In the case of cerebellar malfunctioning, a cortically controlled movement results in hitting the target, but its trajectory is jerky and requires corrections.

INNERVATION PATTERN

The relevant cerebellar sensorimotor organization is **ipsilateral** to both the **input source (muscle spindles)** and **output (LMN) target** (Fig. 12-4). This is in contrast to the forebrain motor mechanism, whose organization is contralateral (see Chapter 14). The developmentally older **ventral spinocerebellar system** and newer **dorsal spinocerebellar system** send input to the ipsilateral side to reach the cerebellum (see Chapter 7). Consequently, the effect of a cerebellar lesion is evident on the body **ipsilateral** to the lesion site. The explanation for this ipsilateral organization is that the cerebellum is wired for extremely fast functional feedback from incoming signals; this might also underscore the ability of the cerebellum to modify ongoing movements.

CEREBELLAR ANATOMY

The cerebellum, located dorsal to the junction of the pons and medulla (see Figs. 2-9 and 2-30), occupies most of the posterior fossa under the **tentorium cerebelli**. It consists of the **cerebellar cortex**, two **hemispheres**, the **internal white substance**, four **pairs of nuclei** embedded within the cerebellar white matter, and three **cerebellar peduncles**. The cerebellar surface is folded into small folia to accommodate its large size (see Fig. 2-27). Each cerebellar hemisphere is divided into three transverse lobes: **floccular nodular**, **anterior**, and **posterior** (Fig. 12-1A; see Figs. 2-28 and 2-29). Longitudinally, the cerebellum is divided into **median (vermal)**, **paramedian (paravermal)**, and **lateral hemispheres** (Fig. 12-1B).

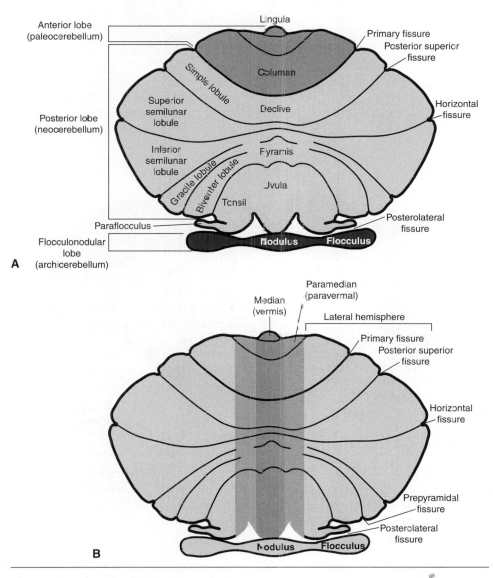

Figure 12-1 The cerebellum. A. The region caudal to the posterolateral fissure is the archicerebellum (flocculonodular) lobe. The area rostral to primary fissure is the anterior lobe. The area between the primary and the posterolateral fissures is the posterior lobe (neocerebellum). B. The cerebellum can be divided longitudinally into the vermal, paravermal, and lateral cortices.

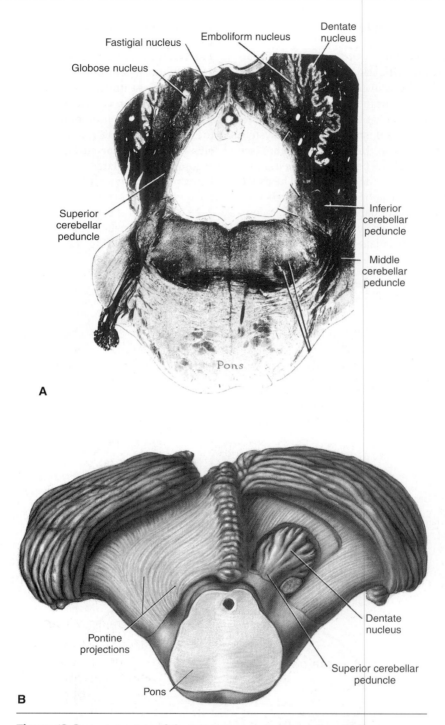

Figure 12-2 **A.** A section of the pontine tegmentum and cerebellum showing the deep cerebellar nuclei: dentate, emboliform, fastigial, and globose. **B.** An anatomical illustration of a dissected dentate nucleus with a portion of the cerebellum.

Four large nuclei are embedded in the white matter of each cerebellar hemisphere. Listed from lateral to medial, they are the **dentate nucleus, emboliform nucleus, globose nucleus**, and **fastigial nucleus** (Fig. 12-2). The dentate, the largest of the group, has a convoluted appearance in cross section. Most fibers traveling through the **superior cerebellar peduncle** originate from the dentate nucleus; this path-

way participates in the coordination of limb movements, along with the motor cortex and **basal ganglia**. Emboliform and globose nuclei also regulate the movements of ipsilateral extremities, whereas the fastigial nucleus is concerned with body posture.

Similar to the cerebral cortex, the cerebellum has a well-defined sensory and motor representation of the body.

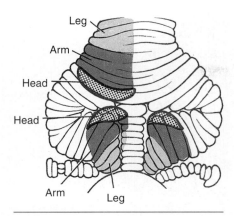

Figure 12-3 Somatotopic localization of the sensorimotor functions in the cerebellar cortex of a monkey. The sensorimotor representation of the body is known to be ipsilateral in the anterior lobe and bilateral in the posterior cerebellum.

It has two sensory body representations: tactile stimulation activates potentials ipsilaterally in the anterior lobule and bilaterally in the paramedian lobules (Fig. 12-3). An activation of a specific sensorimotor area in the cerebral cortex evokes a similar response from the same somatotopic region in the cerebellum. Motor representation tends to overlap the area covered by sensory mapping.

Transverse and Longitudinal Cerebellar Regions

The cerebellum contains three transverse regions (Fig. 12-1A; Table 12-1): **archicerebellum** (floccular nodular lobe), **paleocerebellum** (anterior lobe), and **neocerebellum** (posterior lobe). The archicerebellum (or **vestibulocerebellum**), the oldest part of the cerebellum, includes the **nodulus** and paired **flocculi**. This lobe is related to the **vestibular component** of the vestibulocochlear nerve (CN VIII), and it receives vestibular projections The

Table 12-1

Cerebellar Lobes and Their Functions

Cerebellar Lobe	Functions
Archicerebellum (floccular nodular lobe)	Equilibrium
Paleocerebellum (anterior lobe)	Muscle tone, equilibrium, & body posture
Neocerebellum (posterior lobe)	Limb coordination

flocculi- and nodulus-containing lobe regulates muscle tone via the **vestibulospinal tract** (see Chapters 10–11) and is concerned with equilibrium.

The paleocerebellum is equated with the **anterior lobe**, which includes the **superior vermis**, the **paravermal zone**, and the parts of the cerebellar hemispheres that receive data from the general sensory receptors. The paleocerebellum receives impulses from proprioceptive stretch receptors (spindles) in the muscles of the arms, legs, trunk, and face. It is most concerned with muscle tone and walking posture. The cerebellar projections through the **reticulospinal**, **rubrospinal** (**red nucleus** to spinal cord), and vestibulospinal tracts modify muscle tone (see Chapter 11).

The neocerebellum, developmentally newer and the largest part of the cerebellum, includes the remaining lateral region of the cerebellar hemisphere. Located between the primary and the posterolateral fissures, it forms the posterior lobe, which receives afferent projections from the contralateral sensorimotor cortex. The afferent fibers make up most of the crossed **middle cerebellar peduncle**. After the necessary sensorimotor integration processing, the neocerebellum projects to the contralateral motor cortex and spinal cord by way of the dentate nucleus and red nucleus. The neocerebellum is concerned with the coordination of the cortically directed skilled, movements, such as speaking, writing, and dancing.

There are three **longitudinal cerebellar regions** (Fig. 12-1B): vermal, paravermal, and lateral hemispheres. The most medial region is the treelike **vermis**, which contributes to body posture by regulating axial muscles (see Fig. 2.28). On either side of the vermis is the **paravermal region**, which regulates movements of ipsilateral extremities. The remainder of the cerebellar hemispheres form the lateral zone, which, along with the red nucleus and motor cortex regulates or adjusts skilled movements of the ipsilateral extremities.

Cerebellar Connections

The **inferior peduncle** (**restiform body**), **middle peduncle** (**brachium pontis**), and **superior cerebellar** (**brachium conjunctivum**) **peduncles** connect the cerebellum to the brainstem (Fig. 12-4; see Figs. 2-29 and 2-30). All afferent and efferent fibers traveling to and from the cerebellum pass through these three bundles (Table 12-2). Fibers that travel through the inferior and middle cerebellar peduncles are afferent; they mediate almost all sensorimotor input to the cerebellum. Fibers of the superior cerebellar peduncle are largely efferent; they transmit output from the cerebellum to the brainstem and on to the thalamus, motor cortex, and spinal cord.

Afferent Pathways

Afferents to the cerebellum originate from the spinal cord, brainstem, and motor cortex (Fig. 12-4). The 40:1 ratio of afferent to efferent cerebellar fibers underscores the significance of sensory input to the cerebellar regulation of syn-

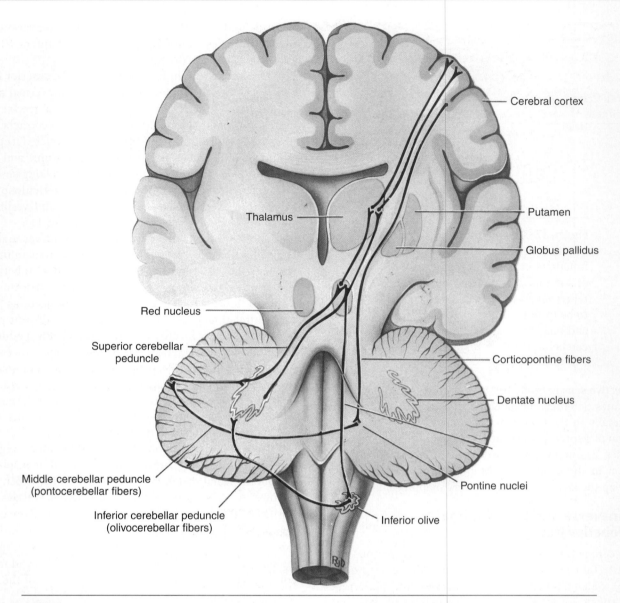

Figure 12-4 The principal afferent and efferent cerebellar projections traveling through the inferior, middle, and superior cerebellar peduncles. The olivocerebellar fibers traveling through the inferior cerebellar peduncle transmit brainstem and spinal projections to the cerebellum. Traveling through the middle cerebellar peduncle, the corticopontine and pontocerebellar fibers form the major cerebellar afferent system. Efferent fibers of the superior cerebellar peduncle decussate in the mesencephalon beneath the inferior colliculus level before ascending to contralateral motor cortex and descending to the brainstem reticular nuclei and spinal cord.

ergy in motor functions. The inferior cerebellar peduncle is an important afferent pathway through which ascending inputs from the distal limbs gain a rapid entry to the ipsilateral cerebellum. The fiber bundles that enter through the inferior cerebellar peduncle are the **vestibulocerebellar**, **dorsal spinocerebellar**, **reticulocerebellar**, **olivocerebellar**, and **cuneocerebellar tracts**.

The **vestibulocerebellar fibers** carry information from the cristae of the semicircular ducts and vestibule to the cerebellum. Most vestibular fibers are bidirectional (travel in opposite directions) and form an ipsilateral communication system between the vestibular system and cerebellum (flocculonodular lobes and fastigial nuclei). These afferents keep the cerebellum informed of the vestibular output from the inner ear, which is essential for maintaining upright posture. They also permit the coordination of ongoing body movement during movement of the head.

Fibers of the dorsal spinocerebellar tract carry muscle and joint stretch afferent information (unconscious proprioception) from the muscle spindles, Golgi tendon organs,

Table 12-2

Afferent and Efferent Cerebellar Connections

Cerebellar Peduncle	Afferent Fibers	Efferent Fibers	Function
Inferior	Spinal cord, reticular formation, olivary nucleus, and stretch receptors of the upper limbs		Mediates sensorimotor information from the spinal cord and brainstem
	Vestibular projections travel through juxtarestiform body.	Fastigio-vestibular fibers	Mediates vestibular information
Middle	Cerebral cortex via the pontine nuclei		Relays ongoing sensorimotor information from opposite cerebral hemispheres
Superior		Projections from the dentate, emboliform, and globose cerebellar nuclei	Transmits cerebellar outputs to the brainstem, then to the thalamus, motor cortex, and spinal cord.
		Spinocerebellar feedback	Mediates ongoing movements

and free nerve endings (in the joints) from the ipsilateral lower limbs (see Fig. 7-10). These ipsilateral fibers keep the cerebellum informed of momentary changes in the tension, range, and strength of muscle movement and provide error signal feedback during ongoing movement (see Chapter 7).

The **brainstem reticular nuclei**—with afferents from the cerebral cortex, spinal cord, vestibular complex, and red nucleus—project bilaterally to the paleocerebellum through the reticulocerebellar tract. Also included in the inferior cerebellar peduncle is a specialized motor cortex originating system, the **cortico-olivary system**. The cortico-olivary fibers terminate ipsilateral to the motor cortex in the **inferior olivary nucleus**. This nucleus is a major source of climbing fibers, which provide direct feedback to the **cerebellum**. The olivocerebellar fibers decussate to enter the contralateral inferior cerebellar peduncle, terminating ipsilateral to the spinal cord input, which is consistent with other inputs. Additional afferents, fibers of the cuneocerebellar tract, mediate proprioception from the stretch receptors of the upper limbs and neck to the ipsilateral cerebellum.

Afferent fibers entering the cerebellum via the **middle cerebellar peduncle** contain massive afferents from the cerebral motor cortex that synapse in the ipsilateral pontine nuclei. Forming the largest of the afferent fibers to the cerebellum, the middle cerebellar fibers enter the cerebellum as the **mossy fibers**. The pontine nuclei, with inputs from the tectum, also mediate visual and auditory information, which provide directional context for ongoing movement. Fibers from the pontine nuclei cross the midline, enter the contralateral middle cerebellar peduncle, and terminate in

the opposite cerebellar hemisphere (Fig. 12-4). Thus the right side of the motor cortex provides input to the left side of the cerebellum, which is also the side that receives ascending input from the left side of the body (see "Neuronal Circuitry of a Cerebellar Functional Unit" later in this chapter).

Efferent Pathways

The cerebellar efferents arise from three **deep cerebellar nuclei**—the dentate, emboliform, and globose—and course through the superior cerebellar peduncle (Fig. 12-4). Although the superior cerebellar peduncle also contains some afferents to the cerebellum from the axial muscles, joints, and proximate parts of the limbs, it is largely efferent. Carrying cerebellar efferents to the brainstem, thalamus, and motor cortex, the fibers of the superior cerebellar peduncle decussate at the level of the **inferior colliculus** (Fig. 12-4; see Fig. 3-15); some of the crossed fibers terminate in the contralateral red nucleus, although most continue and project to the thalamus on their way to the motor cortex. The cerebellar efferent fibers from the red nucleus also project to the spinal cord, motor cortex, reticular formation, and vestibular nuclear complex.

Motor Nuclei of Brainstem and Spinal Cord

Some cerebellar projections from the red nucleus travel to the neurons of the contralateral motor nuclei in the brainstem. Cerebellar projections to the spinal cord also innervate contralateral γ-motor neurons. Both of these provide the means by which the cerebellum modulates muscle tonal reflexes during ongoing movements (see Chapter 11).

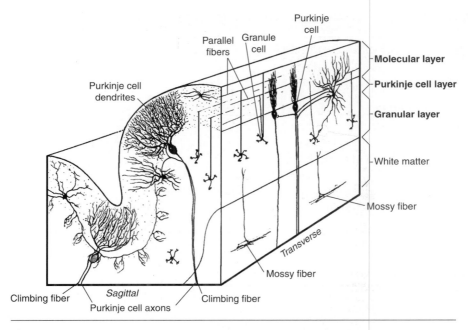

Figure 12-5 The cerebral cortex in transverse and sagittal planes showing the arrangement of the cellular layer and fibers.

Motor Cortex

Cerebellar efferent fibers traveling to the contralateral cortex via the red nucleus and the **ventrolateral** (VL) nucleus of the thalamus inform the motor cortex of the corrections to be made during ongoing movements. The corrective cerebellar output to the cortex is integrated with the basal ganglia feedback to the motor cortex in the ventrolateral thalamus (see Chapters 6 and 13).

Reticular Formation

Much cerebellar output is directed to the brainstem reticular formation, which projects to the cranial nerve nuclei for speech and to the spinal motor neurons. Reticulospinal and rubrospinal projections regulate the ongoing control of the muscle tone reflex during movement.

Vestibular Nuclear Complex

The cerebellum is connected to the vestibular complex via bidirectional fibers. Originating from the fastigial nucleus, cerebellar projections exit through the inferior cerebellar peduncle and terminate in the vestibular complex. These efferents not only coordinate ongoing motor activity during movement of the head but also project to other levels of the brainstem and upper spinal cord.

CEREBELLAR CORTEX

Structure

The cerebellar cortex is uniform in all areas and consists of three cellular layers: **molecular**, **Purkinje**, and **granular** (Fig. 12-5). The molecular layer, the most external layer, is primarily composed of parallel fibers (axons) running in a medial–lateral direction and synapsing with each successive **Purkinje cell** dendrite, much like telephone wires running through cross pieces of successive telephone poles. The middle layer is the Purkinje cell layer, which consists of a thin row of large nerve cells. Purkinje cell axons penetrate the granular cell layer, and most of these fibers terminate in deep cerebellar nuclei. It is important that all impulses leaving the cerebellar cortex pass through a Purkinje axon. The granular cell layer, the innermost cortical cellular layer, is made up of small, closely packed granule cells. Granular cells have short dendrites that synapse onto the mossy fiber axons. The granular cells also project to the molecular layer and provide extensive axonal parallel fibers that synapse on the dendritic spines of the Purkinje cells.

Neuronal Circuitry of a Cerebellar Functional Unit*

The microcircuitry of the cerebellum follows a uniform functional and anatomic pattern in all areas of the cerebellum: archicerebellum, paleocerebellum, and neocerebellum. All input axons, with branches to both the deep nuclei and cerebellar cortex, mediate excitatory (+) information to the outer cellular layer, where they excite a stripe of Purkinje cell dendrites. Axons of the Purkinje cells, on the other hand, project to inhibit (−) the activity of the deep cerebellar nuclei, which serve as the final cerebellar output. These neuronal circuits process all of the afferent information and form the outgoing cerebellar feedback essential for regulating muscle synergy and tone.

---

*This section is based on Guyton (1976).

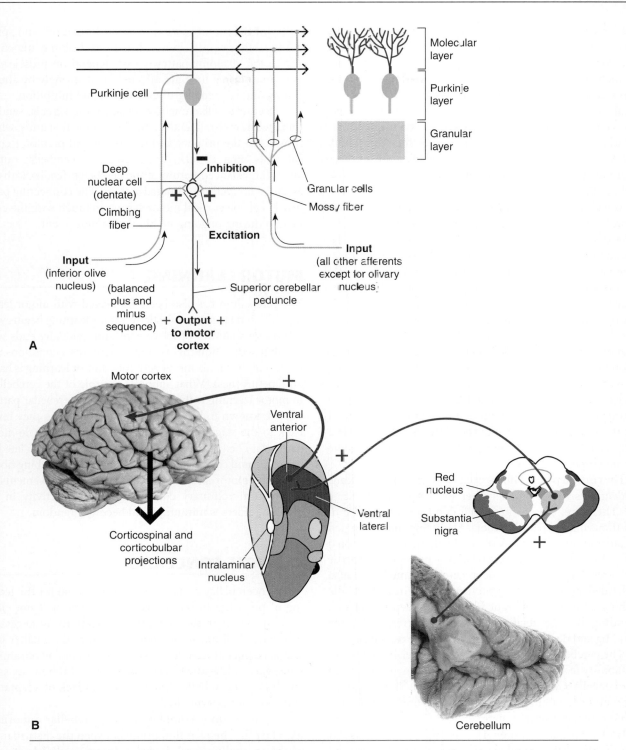

Figure 12-6 A. A cerebellar functional unit. B. The principles of the cerebellar efferents to the motor cortex.

The neuronal circuitry of a functional unit consists of **cerebrocortical cellular layers, deep nuclei, and afferent** and **efferent** fibers (Fig. 12-6A). There are millions of functional units, each with identical neuronal circuitry in the cerebellar cortex. Each cerebellar unit includes a Purkinje cell, which constantly inhibits the deep cerebellar nuclei that form the cerebellar outputs.

All afferents to the cerebellum travel via either the **climbing fibers** or **mossy fibers**. Climbing fibers are most directly related to the cerebellar Purkinje cells. These include all olivocerebellar projections (inferior cerebellar peduncle) to the cerebellar cortex. Highly developed in primates and humans, the cortico-olivary cerebellar projections of the climbing fibers provide the motor and premotor cortexes with a means of determining the activity status of the cerebellar region at any moment, an important aspect for regulating muscle synergy. The climbing fibers are extremely powerful and excitatory to the Purkinje cells and to deep nuclei cells. After sending powerful **excitatory collaterals** to these cells (Fig. 12-6A), the climbing fibers travel to the cerebellar cortex, where they synapse on the dendrites of Purkinje cells, which immediately fire their inhibitory (GABAergic) synapses to the deep cerebellar nuclei. This important afferent system is known for the direct excitability of the Purkinje cells.

Mossy fibers, which make up all other sources of afferent projections to the cerebellum, are related most directly to the sensory input systems concerned with the correlations and modulations that precede cerebellar output. First, the mossy fibers, like climbing fibers, branch to supply excitatory input to both the deep nuclei and the cortex. In the cortex, information is relayed to the outer cortical layer by granular cells, which posses excitatory axons that enter the outer cortical layer and split, sending long axons (parallel fibers) in opposite (medial and lateral) directions for long distances along the folia. The outer cortical layer also receives dendritic projections from the Purkinje cells. This explains why the climbing fibers directly activate the Purkinje cells, whereas the mossy fibers indirectly interact with the Purkinje cells. While the climbing fibers cause a highly specific output, the mossy fibers cause a less specific but tonic type of response.

The cortical parallel fibers excite a large strip of Purkinje cell dendrites. Each parallel fiber excites many Purkinje cells. Therefore, one Purkinje cell dendrite receives input from thousands of parallel fibers. Mediating the summated excitatory input, the axons of the Purkinje cells, as noted earlier, form inhibitory (GABAergic) projections to the deep cerebellar nuclei. The deep cerebellar nuclei are also bombarded by the prior excitatory inputs from both the climbing and mossy afferent fibers. The deep nuclei fire, depending on the relative timing and strength of the ascending and descending inputs, to provide cerebellar output. The cerebellar cortex also contains an elaborate series of inhibitory feedback circuits consisting of small cells, such as basket cells, Golgi cells, and spindle cells. These regulate the general excitability of the cortex and prevent it from a general cerebellar seizure state.

Under normal physiologic conditions, the cerebellar output to the cortex, basal ganglia, reticular formation, and spinal cord is excitatory, continuously balanced by afferent excitation and Purkinje inhibition. For skilled and digital activities that require rapid and alternating movements, the timing is most important in the sequence of excitatory and inhibitory neuronal events. If there is any alteration in the sequence of excitatory (+) and inhibitory (−) events and/or the timing interval between the neuronal event changes, the deep cerebellar nuclei sends faulty output signals to the brainstem. In turn, this alters muscle synergy, tone, and equilibrium and affects the integrity of the neuronal cir-

cuitry of the motor cortex, reticular formation, and spinal cord. Consequently, motor functions become uncoordinated. Rapid motor patterns that depend on muscle synergy and normal tone are affected most strongly by altered timing and sequencing of facilitation and inhibition.

Deep cerebellar nuclei constantly fire signals, sending them to the contralateral VL nucleus of the thalamus, which projects to the primary and the motor and premotor cortical areas (Fig. 12-6B). Any decrease in cerebellar output alters the balanced nature of the cerebellar feedback that is essential for well-coordinated activity. The connecting pathway keeps the cortical motor system in touch with the cerebellum during ongoing manipulative movement.

MOTOR LEARNING

The cerebellum has also been implicated with motor learning, which relates to its plasticity. Motor learning begins with a conscious control of movement and gradually ends with the skill acquisition that no longer requires a conscious regulation of the tactile motor activities. Motor learning is based on repetitiveness. What supports the role of the cerebellum in motor learning is that the patients with cerebellar pathology are known to lose movement automaticity; they revert back to the stage of conscious controlling of tactile motor patterns. This acquisition of skilled learning is related to increased and complex activity involving the climbing fibers. Once the motor skill is learned and tactile movements do not require voluntary control, the axonal activity in the climbing fibers is minimum and becomes random.

CLINICAL CONCERNS

The neocerebellar cortical region is essential for the learning of precision in sequential movements. It is not clear, though, whether the synaptic connectivity is necessary in the cerebellum, somewhere else, or both. Smaller unilateral cerebellar lesions can be compensated by retraining. However, unless they occur in young children, massive and bilateral cerebellar lesions result in lack of adaptation and cause long-term effects.

Vision cannot compensate for cerebellar abnormality, a fact that helps differentiate between the disturbances of the cerebellum and **dorsal column–medial lemniscal ascending system** (see Chapter 7). For example, the **Romberg test** is used to evaluate proprioception. A patient stands with arms extended in front, feet together, and eyes closed. If one of the patient's arms drifts downward and/or the patient begins to tilt to one side because of unsteadiness, the cause may be a cerebellar (input or output), vestibular, or proprioceptive abnormality. However, if the patient's eyes are open and the arm drifts or unsteadiness persists, the abnormality is in the cerebellum, not in the dorsal column–medial lemniscal system, since vision does not compensate for cerebellar malfunctioning. Further distinction between vestibular and cerebellar abnormalities requires additional clinical skill because lesions involving both systems produce unsteadiness and a tendency to fall to one side. The caloric test in each ear and vertigo testing can help determine the underlying cause.

Signs of Cerebellar Dysfunction

There are three general characteristics of cerebellar symptoms: (1) an ipsilateral character to the signs, which is more true of lateralized cerebellar lesions; (2) deficits related to motor functions with no sensory loss and paralysis; and (3) gradual recovery, unless there is a progressive or massive cause.

Minor cerebellar lesions produce subtle changes in motor activities that may be clinically difficult to evaluate. A large lesion in the cerebellum and its input or output systems invariably is marked by a reduced smoothness and accuracy of movement and includes **dyssynergia** and **motion** or **action tremors**. Patients with cerebellar pathology cannot precisely control their body parts during movement; although they otherwise seem normal in regard to strength and somatosensation. Cerebellar dysfunction is most pronounced in activities that require rapid, alternating movements. Furthermore, since the cerebellar organization is ipsilateral to both the input source and output target, cerebellar lesions produce ipsilateral motor disturbances.

Cerebellar dysfunction is tested by **tandem walking**, the **finger-to-nose test**, **alternating movements**, **hopping**, **limb rebounding**, and **diadochokinetic movements**. As with many other cerebral degenerative conditions, there is no treatment for degenerative cerebellar lesions. Common cerebellar impairments include ataxia, dysdiadochokinesia, dysarthria, dysmetria, intention tremor, hypotonia, rebounding, and disequilibrium.

Ataxia

Skilled movement entails approaching the target with smoothness in time and space. This smoothness also requires continuous correction for the momentum of the moving parts; the cerebellum is essential for this correction. Ataxia is lack of order and coordination in muscle activities. Coordinated motor activities are decomposed into segments—for example, while walking and turning, a patient stops before making a turn and then turns in slow motion (**bradykinesia**). The subject then resumes walking awkwardly and slowly. There is mild muscular weakness (**asthenia**) ipsilateral to the side of the cerebellar damage. **Asynergia**, an impairment in the direction and force of a given movement, is a local condition usually involving paired muscles.

Dysdiadochokinesia

Dysdiadochokinesia is a failure in the sequential progression of motor activities displayed by clumsiness in rapid and alternating movements. The ability to alternate movements is tested best by asking a subject to repeat a sequence of alternating movements that include tapping, articulating the phonemic sequence |pa ta ka|, or performing rotating movements.

Dysarthria

An impaired ability to make the needed modifications and alterations in ongoing oral–facial movement produces a drastic effect on speech. This results in dysarthric speech, which is commonly seen in cases of bilateral cerebellar lesions. Speech in ataxic dysarthria is slow, slurred, and disjointed: each word or syllable is spoken individually, which is known as scanning verbal output.

Dysmetria

Dysmetria denotes an error in the judgment of a movement's range or the distance to the target. Examples of dysmetric error are motor movements that fall short of the target (undershooting) and extend past it (overshooting). Dysmetria results from the failure to incorporate the range and distance of stationary and moving targets.

Intention Tremor

Intention tremor results from impaired ability to dampen accessory movements during a skilled movement sequence. Evident during a movement, the tremor becomes more severe as the target is approached—as demand for the function of the cerebellum becomes more important. Perhaps a better term for this clinical phenomenon is motion tremor, as the tremor disappears during rest. Intention tremor is different from resting tremor, which is a characteristic of Parkinson disease in which the patient exhibits a pill-rolling tremor only while resting (see Chapter 13).

Hypotonia

Tone is the slight tension that is constantly present in the muscle and easily detected during passive manipulation of the limbs. The functional cerebellum is trained via the γ-efferent influence on the stretch reflex to continuously optimize the motor tone of each muscle contributing to a movement. This includes opposing muscle groups that contract simultaneously to provide joint stability. In hypotonia, normal muscle tension (resistance to passive stretch) is decreased and the muscle becomes floppy. Hypotonia ipsilateral to the side of cerebellar dysfunction is a common sign of cerebellar pathology and is often accompanied by asthenia, a condition in which the muscles are likely to tire quickly.

Rebounding

Rebounding reflects impaired motor tone adjustment as well as a loss of rapid and precise corrective response, as the patient loses the ability to predict, stop, or dampen movement. For example, if a flexed arm is held back and suddenly let go, a person with cerebellar pathology cannot detect the sudden limb release. The hand movement does not stop, and the patient is likely to strike his or her own face.

Disequilibrium

Impaired vestibular processing in the cerebellum results in disequilibrium that predominantly affects the legs. Affected people walk as if they were drunk. The gait is unsteady, and the body wavers toward the side of the lesion.

Cerebellar Pathologies

Cerebrovascular Accident

The **vertebrobasilar artery** provides blood to all three cerebellar arteries—**posterior inferior**, **anterior inferior**, and **superior cerebellar arteries**—with each covering a specific cerebellar region (see Chapter 17). **Thromboembolic** or **hemorrhagic** involvement of the vertebrobasilar artery system interrupts blood circulation to the cerebellum. The **posterior inferior artery** not only supplies the inferior surface of the cerebellum and the flocculonodular lobe but also supplies the inferior cerebellar peduncle and dorsal and lateral surfaces of the medulla. Its involvement in a cerebrovascular accident (CVA) produces symptoms related to damage of the vestibular and cochlear nuclei, spinocerebellar tracts, and various cranial nerves, such as the spinal tracts of the trigeminal, facial, glossopharyngeal, and vagus nerves (see Fig. 17.1) (CN V) (CN VII) (CN IX) (CN X).

Toxicity

Toxicity consequent to chronic alcoholism may cause progressive subacute cerebellar degeneration. It occurs past middle age and is characterized by gross cerebellar atrophy and the loss of all cellular elements in the anterior lobe, most crucially the Purkinje cells. The most significant symptom is a wavering (wide-based shuffling) gait similar to that of an intoxicated person. In half of the cases, the disturbance is limited to the lower extremities. In other cases, there is incoordination, dysmetria, and dyskinesia in the upper extremities as well. Speech may be monotonous, slurred, or explosive, which disappears as the blood alcohol level attenuates with time. However, the remaining cerebellar deficits, once established, may not improve even with proper nutrition and vitamin treatment.

Progressive Cerebellar Degeneration

Many types of ataxias are the result of cerebellar degeneration, including hereditary ataxia. **Friedreich ataxia**, the most common, is an autosomal recessive genetic degenerative condition characterized by combined sensory and motor dysfunctions. Most commonly affected are the cerebellar afferent pathways (the olivocerebellar or spinocerebellar pathways) and efferent pathways (dentatorubral pathways). This condition usually appears between ages 10 and 20 years and is characterized by ataxia (incoordination and unsteadiness in walking), dysarthria, tremor, weakness, loss of proprioception, nystagmus, dysmetria, and scanning speech. There is no medical treatment for Friedreich ataxia.

CLINICAL CONSIDERATIONS

PATIENT ONE

A 1-year-old began to experience weakness in his legs. His movements were clumsy when he was playing and running. He was taken to the family physician, who noted the following signs:

- Broad-based gait
- Unsteadiness in walking
- Weakness in the lower limbs and loss of delicate movements
- Release of primitive reflexes, such as positive Babinski sign
- Loss of proprioception and discriminative touch from both lower limbs
- Positive Romberg sign (the patient could not stand straight with his eyes closed)

A brain MRI study revealed pathologic changes in the spinal cord involving the dorsal and lateral funiculi at the lumbar level. Friedreich ataxia was suspected.

Question: How can you explain these symptoms?

Discussion: The observed degenerative changes in the spinal cord had the following effects:

- Involvement of the corticospinal tract fibers resulted not only in weakness but also in the appearance of other pyramidal signs: loss of delicate movements and release of primitive reflexes.
- Damage to the spinocerebellar fibers prevented the transmission of unconscious proprioception to the cerebellum, which resulted in incoordination and unsteadiness.
- Damage to the fasciculus gracilis resulted in loss of discriminative sensation from the legs.

PATIENT TWO

An 18-year-old male complained of headaches, nausea, and vomiting for several months. He was first treated with aspirin. He returned to the hospital as his condition worsened and exhibited the following:

- Drowsiness
- Ataxia
- Spells of falling down
- Marked dysarthric speech

A brain MRI study confirmed a cerebellar tumor.

Question: How can you explain these symptoms?

Discussion: The gradual progression of the symptoms indicated a neoplastic (tumor) growth. The presence of a mass affected all cerebellar functions, including coordination, equilibrium, and motor speech. A surgical excision of the tumor is likely to relieve all of the symptoms, including dysarthria.

PATIENT THREE

The speech quality of a 52-year-old speech language pathologist (SLP) professor with a drinking problem had deteriorated gradually. This provoked complaints from her students, who found her to be unintelligible. She was seen by a neurologist who noted the following:

- Disorientation and confusion
- Subdued personality
- Wide-based gait pattern
- Unstable posture with impaired balance
- Poor performance on finger-to-nose-test
- Moderately unintelligible speech

An SLP consultation revealed the following:

- Irregular alternate motion rate
- Vowel prolongation
- Distorted consonants
- Loudness variations
- Irregular articulatory breakdown (slowly articulated and periodically overexaggerated articulation)
- Amnesia for recent information
- Word finding deficit

A brain MRI study revealed areas of degeneration in the orbital-frontal region as well as in the area located dorsal to the brainstem.

Question: How can you account for the professor's somatosensory symptoms and speech-related disorders in light of the MRI findings?

Discussion: Cerebellar cells are highly susceptible to alcohol toxicity. This case represents the degenerative effects of a long-term alcohol-induced toxicity, which had affected the following:

- Lateral cerebellar region that resulted in ataxic dysarthria subsequent to the incoordination of the articulators.
- Midline (vermian) structure that contributed to the unsteady gait and impaired balance.
- Frontal lobe involvement that accounted for her personality changes; disorientation, confusion, and amnesia could have been related to nutritional deficiency as a result of persistent alcohol use.

SUMMARY

The cerebellum does not initiate motor movements, nor does it alter sensation. It functions as a servomechanism, constantly monitoring all body motor activities and comparing intended movements (planned by the motor and pre-motor cortex) against the updated sensory information it receives. By calculating discrepancies between sensory and motor states, it regulates the quality of motor movements generated elsewhere in the motor cortex, brainstem, or spinal cord. With its ability to make alterations for greater precision and smoothness during ongoing movement, the cerebellum is essential for learning skilled movements. The cerebellum contributes to muscle synergy, tone, and equilibrium. Signs of cerebellar dysfunction include paresis, hypotonia, ataxia, asymmetry, intention tremor, dysdiadochokinesia, dysarthria, and disequilibrium. Patients with cerebellar pathology lack the ability to control and regulate motor functions. Small lesions of the cerebellar cortex may cause minimal impairments that can be compensated for. However, massive cerebellar damage involving the deep nuclei or the superior cerebellar peduncle can cause permanent and lasting deficits unless it occurs at a very young age. Cerebellar impairments do not affect reasoning, thinking, memory, or the comprehension of language.

QUIZ QUESTIONS

1. Define the following terms: asthenia, asynergia, ataxia, diadochokinesia, dysarthria.

2. Match each of the following numbered conditions with its associated lettered statement.

   1. incoordination of muscular activity during voluntary movements
   2. overshooting or undershooting when approaching a moving target
   3. incoordination with rapid alternating movements
   4. muscle weakness

   a. ataxia
   b. dysmetria
   c. asthenia
   d. dysdiadochokinesia

TECHNICAL TERMS

archicerebellum
asthenia
asynergia
ataxia
climbing fibers
deep cerebellar nuclei
dysdiadochokinesia
dysarthria

dysdiadochokinesia
hypotonia
intention tremor
mossy fibers
neocerebellum
paleocerebellum
Purkinje cells
rebounding

Motor System 3: Brainstem and Basal Ganglia

LEARNING OBJECTIVES

After studying this chapter, students should be able to:

- Discuss reticular influence on spinal motor functions
- Discuss the pathophysiology of decerebrate rigidity
- Describe the role of the basal ganglia in motor functions
- Discuss the structurally and functionally related structures of the basal ganglia
- Explain the neuronal circuitry for common basal ganglia circuits (loops)
- Outline the afferent and efferent projections of the basal ganglia circuits
- Describe the inhibitory or excitatory influence of the afferent and efferent projections of the basal ganglia circuits
- List the clinical signs of basal ganglia impairments
- Describe the major movement disorders associated with basal ganglia lesions
- Discuss the primary neurotransmitters of the basal ganglia, their projections, interactions, and functions
- Discuss neurologic conditions associated with the basal ganglia circuitry, such as Parkinson disease, Wilson disease, Huntington chorea, and progressive supranuclear palsy

The vertically organized hierarchical motor system, which also serves speech and other visceral motor activities, is regulated by motor inputs from various sources. Direct motor pathways originate in the primary motor cortex (Brodmann area 4) and descend in the pyramidal tract (corticobulbar-spinal) to the motor neurons in the brainstem and spinal cord. In addition to cortical input, the brainstem and spinal motor neurons also receive projections from extrapyramidal sources that include the basal ganglia, cerebellum, vestibular nuclear complex, and brainstem reticular formation. Together these inputs refine the cortical motor directives to the lower motor neurons in the brainstem (midbrain, pons, and medulla) and spinal cord (see Chapter 11).

BRAINSTEM MOTOR MECHANISM

The brainstem reticular network plays a significant role in modulating the output function of a reflex network, tonal function, and sensorimotor activity. The brainstem sensorimotor mechanism is composed of the **red nucleus** (see Chapter 12); **cranial nerve nuclei** (see Chapter 15); and most important, the **reticular formation**. The brainstem reticular system, which receives pyramidal, extrapyramidal and spinal inputs, contributes to muscle tone and postural control.

Structurally, the brainstem reticular formation is composed of a diffuse core of neurons and a few specific clusters of sensory and motor cells that extend from the caudal diencephalon to the upper cervical segments (Fig. 13-1A). Reticular neurons have an extensive network of overlapping serial and parallel dendrites and axons and receive inputs from the motor cortex, basal ganglia, and cerebellum. Interspersed within the reticular core are the cranial nerve nuclei that regulate visceral and motor functions, including motor speech activity. Functionally, the reticular cells, along with the cranial nerve cells, form the pivotal point for many functions of the brainstem and lower motor levels. The brainstem reticular formation, which is involved with cortical arousal, also regulates tonal modulation and activation of spinal and cranial motor functions, as well as pain perception. With multiple and extensive projections, the reticular formation also regulates many vital, integrated activities, such as vomiting, coughing, cardiovascular functions, swallowing, and respiration, the last two being the most important for speech functions (see Chapter 16). Arranged in four columns, the specific reticular nuclei are the **reticularis gigantocellular**, **pontis oralis** and **caudalis**, **lateral reticular**, **ventral reticular**, **paramedial reticular**, **raphe**, **ceruleus**, and **interstitial nuclei** (Fig. 13-1B).

Anatomically, the most outstanding feature of the reticular formation is that its projections interact with virtually all ascending and descending pathways, thus influencing all neurally coded information at every level of the nervous system. The reticular formation receives extensive input from the spinal cord, brainstem, cerebral hemispheres, cranial nerves, basal ganglia (BG), and hypothalamus and projects to nearly every level of the nervous system.

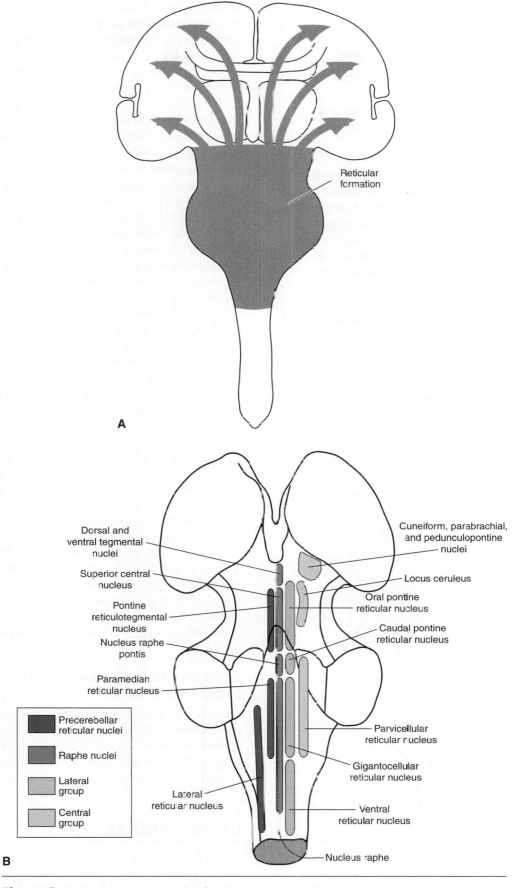

Figure 13-1 A. Brainstem reticular formation. B. Reticular columns and nuclei.

Reticular Motor Functions

The reticular formation controls both stereotyped and vital activities that can function independently from cortical inputs. These activities are performed unconsciously by the brainstem, as displayed by children with anencephaly, who are born without the neocortex but are still able to eat, suck, expel unpleasant food, cry, yawn, swallow, vomit, breathe, sleep, awaken, and turn their eyes and head toward an object.

Muscle Tone Regulation

Spinal motor output, reflexive activity, and muscle tone are under the constant control of the descending brainstem reticular networks. Muscle tone results from the action and modulation of the stretch reflex, which in a gravitational environment provides the basis for postural (antigravity) support. To control muscle tone, the brainstem reticular formation is divided into the reticular facilitatory and reticular inhibitory areas, which affect the excitability of the **α-lower motor neurons** (α-LMNs) (Fig. 13-2). The upper and lateral parts of the brainstem (midbrain, pons, and medulla) form the reticular facilitatory area. A

small lower and medial region of the medulla forms the reticular inhibitory area. Stimulation of the **reticular facilitatory area** induces an excitation of LMNs and leads to increased tone in the muscles of the extremities. Conversely, stimulation of the **reticular inhibitory area** controls motor neuron activity by reducing the muscle tone. Under normal conditions, the reticular projections to the spinal motor neurons represent a balance between reticular excitation (+) and inhibition (-). The brainstem lesions cause motor impairments by altering the reticular outputs and subsequently changing the muscle tone.

Physiologically, the reticular facilitatory area is intrinsically excitatory; it requires no other source to drive it. Its intrinsic excitation and constant neuronal firing are controlled by the inhibitory signals that descend from the forebrain (motor cortex and BG) centers. In contrast, the reticular inhibitory area is not intrinsically excitable; it requires another source to drive it. Efferent commands from the BG and motor cortex activate this inhibitory area, which, on stimulation, causes the inhibition of muscle tone.

Clinically, a lesion above the vestibular nuclear complex disconnects the forebrain (motor cortex and basal ganglia) from the brainstem reticular formation and results in a **decerebrate rigidity**, which is marked by extensor posturing of all limbs. Functionally, this lesion has two effects: release of the reticular facilitatory area from higher inhibitory control and inactivation of the reticular inhibitory area. Released from higher inhibitory impulses, the excessive facilitatory impulses increase muscle tone and induce muscle rigidity. On the other hand, a transection of the brainstem below the vestibular nucleus also releases the spinal cord from the tonic reticular (reticulospinal tract) and vestibular (vestibulospinal tract) impulses. This leads to flaccid paralysis and hypotonia. This extreme form of hypotonia results from a complete shutdown of efferent activity to and from α-LMNs, as for example during the early stages of spinal shock. Together, the reticular formation and vestibular complex also support the body against gravity and maintain equilibrium. This clinical condition of decerebrate rigidity is commonly visible in children with cerebral palsy.

Summary of Brainstem Reticular Motor Mechanism

The reticular formation contains a network of neurons in the brainstem, including sensory and motor nuclei and specialized reticular cells. The reticular formation uses integrated sensory and motor input to regulate spinal motor activity and muscle tone.

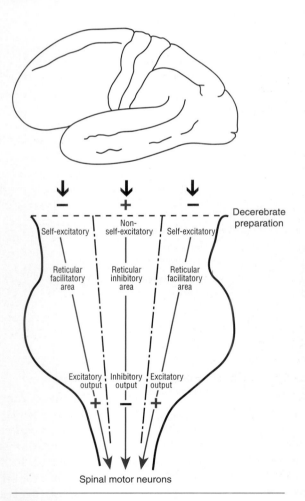

Figure 13-2 Intrinsically self-sustained reticular facilitatory areas and a non-self-sustained reticular inhibitory area.

BASAL GANGLIA

The **basal ganglia** (BG) nuclei do not initiate motor activity; rather, they regulate cortically initiated motor activity, including speech. Current understanding of the

BG is based on observations of motor disorders resulting from the pathology. Under normal physiologic conditions, the BG nuclei refine cortically generated movements by suppressing competing movements extraneous to precise and target motor activity. The BG nuclei also help adjust associated automatic motor movements (arm swinging during locomotion, follow-through during throwing, facial expressions, and basic emotional vocalization) and participate in learned reflex control, which relates to the automatic aspects of skilled motor activity after overlearning and adds grace to motor movements.

In general, the circuitry of the basal ganglia provides species-specific learned motor control and built-in reflex control patterns as a component of highly skilled movement sequences. The motor cortex is very much involved in the early acquisition of all skilled movements. Many aspects of learned movements later, with practice, become motor automatisms and require some regulating role by the BG, which also contributes to motor learning and higher mental (cognitive, perceptive, and linguistic) functions (Bhatnagar and Mandybur 2006).

The BG nuclei do not directly control spinal motor neuronal activity. Instead, they use multiple parallel or serial channels to modify cortical motor activity within an period of ~100 msec, the estimated time difference between the activation of the cortical motor nuclei and the response by the target spinal motor nuclei. The BG nuclei primarily project their modifying ascending input to the cortical motor areas on the ipsilateral side by way of the thalamus; secondarily, they project their descending input to the contralateral brainstem reticular reflex network.

There are no LMNs or upper motor neurons (UMNs) in the BG (see Chapters 11 and 14); therefore, BG lesions do not produce the paralysis that is seen after a lesion involving LMNs or UMNs. Rather, BG lesions result in a loss of inhibitory control, and thus patients exhibit an inappropriate release of patterned behaviors of involuntary motor movements (**chorea**, **dystonia**, **athetosis**, **ballism**, and **tremor**), **bradykinesia** (slow movement owing to a decrease in spontaneity), **hypokinesia** (movement with slow and limited excursion), **akinesia** (impaired movement initiation), and **altered posture**. All of these also affect motor speech quality and cause the speech to become dysarthric.

BG disorders involve the impairment of one or more neurochemical substances and their receptors, most notably γ-aminobutyric acid (**GABA**), **dopamine** (inhibitory), and glutamate (facilitatory). Huntington chorea and Parkinson disease are BG conditions that result from deficiencies in the synthesis of different neurotransmitters. Both diseases are characterized by involuntary movements, dysarthric speech, and cognitive impairments.

Innervation Pattern

The BG motor organization is contralateral to its sensory input and motor output. The BG nuclei communicate to the motor cortex on the same side; hence influence the activity of the brainstem and spinal nuclei on the opposite side. Consequently, the effect of a BG lesion is evident on the side of the body contralateral to the lesion (Fig. 13-3).

Anatomy

The BG nuclei consist of three primary subcortical nuclear masses: **caudate nucleus**, **putamen**, and **globus pallidus** (see Figs. 2-15 and 2-16). Furthermore, the **substantia nigra** and the **subthalamic nucleus** are functionally connected to the BG (see Figs 3-17 and 3-18). These primary and secondary structures participate as a whole in motor functions with the motor cortex, cerebellum, and brainstem reticular formation.

The caudate nucleus is a C-shaped structure with an elongated mass, large head, and narrow tail (see Fig. 2-17). The head of the caudate is embedded in the lateral wall of the anterior horn of the lateral ventricles. The tail of the caudate nucleus extends along the wall of the lateral ventricle and continues along the surface of the inferior horn in the temporal lobe. The putamen, located lateral to the globus pallidus, is connected anteriorly with the head of the caudate nucleus; this is because they share a common embryologic origin. Lateral to the putamen are the **external** and **extreme capsules**, **claustrum**, and **insular** cortex. The globus pallidus, which consists of internal (medial) and external (lateral) components, is between the **posterior limbs** of the **internal capsule** and putamen (see Figs. 2-15 and 2-16).

The BG nuclei primarily involve at least six neurotransmitters and their receptors: **glutamate**, **dopamine**, **GABA**, **acetylcholine**, **substance P**, and **enkephalin**. Glutamatergic projections are excitatory. **Melanin pigment**–containing nerve cells in the substantia nigra (pars compacta region) secrete dopamine, an inhibitory neurotransmitter released through synaptic terminals in the striatum (caudate nucleus and putamen). Some cells in the striatum also secrete acetylcholine, a local neurotransmitter, which in part also regulates functions in adjacent neurons. Most of the striatal cells synthesize substance P and GABA, both of which inhibit the substantia nigra. Furthermore, the serotonin projections from the midbrain to the striatum participate in the metabolic activity of the BG by regulating the striatal GABAergic neurons.

Basal Ganglia Circuitry

The anatomy and physiology of the BG nuclei can be understood best if the nuclei are viewed as a series of inhibitory or facilitatory parallel-running, interconnected loops with each loop processing corticostriatal information differently to modulate cortically generated efferents (Fig. 13-3). As a rule, afferents to the BG enter the striatum, whereas the integrated efferents of the BG leave through the globus pallidus and project to the cortex via the thalamus. The BG nuclei also receive reticular afferents from the thalamus (centromedian nucleus) and send bidi-

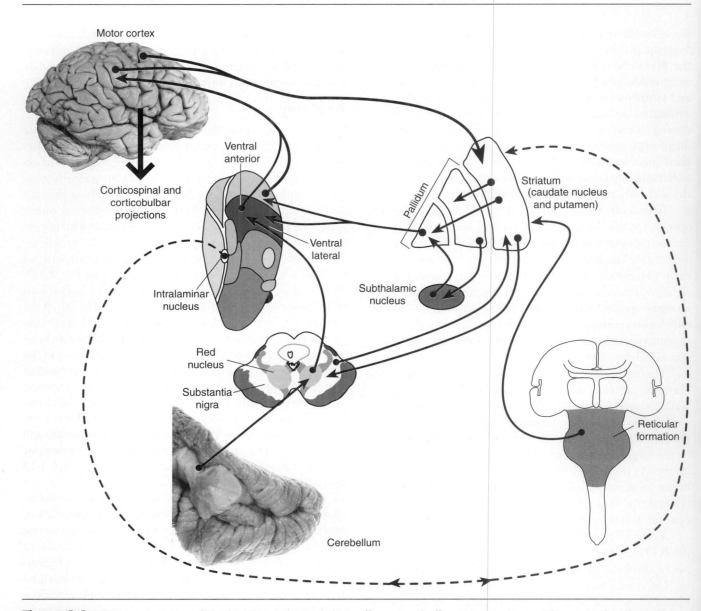

Figure 13-3 The components of the basal ganglia and their afferent and efferent projections. The major basal ganglia loops are as follows: *1*, cortex → striatum → globus pallidus → thalamus (ventrolateral and ventral anterior) → cortex; *2*, striatum → substantia nigra → striatum; *3*, globus pallidus → subthalamic nucleus → globus pallidus; *4*, thalamus (intralaminar nuclei) → striatum; *5*, cerebellum → red nucleus → thalamus (ventrolateral and ventral anterior) → cortex. Arrows mark projections to targets.

rectional projections to the reticular reflex networks. The primary projections of the BG involve the central route of cortex → striatum → globus pallidus external → globus pallidus internal → thalamus (ventrolateral and ventral anterior) → cortex (Fig. 13-3).

Anatomy of Basal Ganglia Circuitry

There are four major loops or circuits of the BG; these circuits also influence motor speech and cognitive functions that are important to students of human behaviors (Fig. 13-3). Each circuit makes a specific inhibitory or facilitatory contribution to a cortical motor output (UMN) pathway. The first loop, the largest and most central loop,

transmits motor impulses from the sensorimotor and prefrontal cortex to the neostriatum (caudate and putamen) and globus pallidus (external and internal), which send integrated BG projections back to the neocortex via the ventrolateral (VL) and ventral anterior (VA) nuclei of the thalamus. The remaining three circuits serve as subsidiaries to the first and central BG loop. Together, the subloops influence the motor cortex via the circuitry of the globus pallidus and thalamus. The second loop is concerned with the conduction of bidirectional projections of the striatum, connecting it to the substantia nigra. The third loop transmits bidirectional projections connecting the globus pallidus external to the subthalamic nucleus, and afferents from the motor cortex also project back to the globus pallidus external to join the first loop circuitry. The fourth loop transmits bidirectional projections connecting thalamic intralaminar nuclei and the pontoreticular region with the striatum. In addition, there is a secondary (non-BG) loop that connects the cerebellum with the contralateral motor cortex by way of the red nucleus and the VL thalamic nucleus.

All neuronal loops receive their primary inputs from multiple cortical and subcortical areas and participate in motor activity by projecting their outputs to the neocortex and brainstem. Each of these anatomic loops has been observed to make a specific contribution to motor activity. A detailed description of the afferent and efferent projections of the BG loops follows.

Striatum

The striatum, made up of the caudate nucleus and putamen, uses GABAergic projections to inhibit the functions of the globus pallidus and substantia nigra.

Afferents

The striatum receives input from the cortex (corticostriate fibers), substantia nigra (nigrostriate fibers), thalamus (thalamostriate fibers), and brainstem reticular formation (reticulostriate fibers) (Fig. 13-3). The glutamate-carrying corticostriate fibers project from all parts of the primary and associational (premotor and supplementary) motor cortical areas to the caudate nucleus and the putamen. The corticostriate connections are reciprocal, and there is no greater representation of the cortex in one area of the striatum than another. These projections from the cortex enter the caudate nucleus and putamen through the internal capsule. There is a notable overlapping of fibers from various parts of the cortex to the striatum, and the greatest number of projections is from the prefrontal and other associational areas.

Nigrostriate fibers from the pars compacta region of the substantia nigra have axonal terminals filled with dopamine, which facilitates some and inhibits other striatal neurons (Fig. 13.6B). Substantia nigra lesions, which deplete dopamine production, are thought to cause the motor impairments, tremor, and rigidity that are associated with Parkinson disease.

Facilitatory projections from the intralaminar (centromedian and parafascicular) nuclei and the pontoreticular area mediate ascending somesthetic (proprioceptive), reticular, vestibular, and auditory information to the neostriatum. This input provides important feedback with respect to the cortical arousal and physiologic preparedness by fine-tuning the BG and cortical pathways.

Efferents

The striate efferent fibers radiate from the putamen to the external and internal segments of the globus pallidus (striatopallidal fibers); their influence is inhibitory to the globus pallidus (Fig. 13-3). Striatopallidal fibers, which originate from the GABAergic and acetylcholine neurons in the striatum, terminate in the external and internal segments of the globus pallidus. The second striatal efferent projection is to the substantia nigra. Striatonigral fibers, also inhibitory, terminate in the pars reticulata region of the substantia nigra. The striatonigral fibers, which include fibers from both the caudate nucleus and the putamen, transmit GABA and substance P through their terminals. The striatonigral and nigrostriatal fibers, both inhibitory, are reciprocal in organization.

Globus Pallidus

The globus pallidus, serving as the striatal and BG output to the thalamus, consists of external and internal components (Figs. 13-3).

Afferents

Afferents entering the globus pallidus arise from the striatum and the subthalamic nucleus. All striatal afferents to the globus pallidus are GABAergic and thus inhibitory, except the afferents from the subthalamic nucleus, which are glutamatergic and, therefore, facilitatory.

Efferents

As the output nucleus of the BG, the globus pallidus projects to the thalamus via the pallidothalamic fiber bundle. The major BG output to the thalamus, which is GABAergic and inhibitory, arises from the internal segment of the globus pallidus and terminate in the VL and VA nuclei of the thalamus (see Chapter 6). These pallidal projections are transmitted through two fasciculi: ansa lenticularis and lenticular fasciculus (Fig. 13-4).

Three anatomic structures that pertain to the pallidothalamic fibers can be confusing: field H of Forel (prerubral area), field H_1 of Forel, and field H_2 of Forel. These three *fields of H* are where the pallidothalamic fibers cross the internal capsule, turn laterally to move upward, and enter the thalamus (Fig. 13-4). Fibers of the ansa lenticularis loop around the internal capsule and enter field H of Forel (*prerubral field*) in the subthalamic region. They turn rostrally and laterally, forming part of the thalamic fasciculus, in field H_1 of Forel. Conversely, the lenticular fasciculus fibers pass through the internal capsule and appear as field H_2 of Forel. The *lenticular fasciculus* fibers join the *ansa lenticularis* fibers at field H_1 of Forel and merge to form the thalamic fasciculus. The thalamic fasciculus fibers terminate in the VL nucleus of the thalamus, which projects to the motor cortex. The ventrolateral and ventral-anterior thalamic nuclei also receive cerebellocortical projections from the dentate nucleus of the cerebellum. Thus at the thalamic level, the cerebellocortical projections intermingle with the BG projections to the cortex.

The fibers from the external region of the globus pallidus also send inhibitory (GABAergic) projections to the subthalamic nucleus (Fig. 13-3). In addition, descending

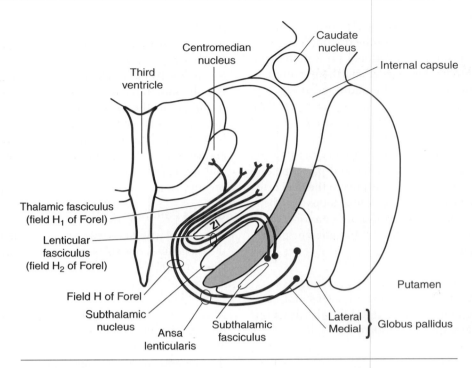

Figure 13-4 Origin and course of the pallidothalamic (ansa lenticularis and lenticular fasciculus) projections. The fibers of the ansa lenticularis travel around the internal capsule and enter the prerubral field (field H of Forel). The fibers of the lenticular fasciculus leave the inner globus pallidus and course through field H_2 of Forel and join the fibers of the ansa lenticularis to form the thalamic fasciculus (field H_1 of Forel). The thalamic fasciculus terminates in the ventrolateral and ventral anterior nuclei of the thalamus

BG output travels to the reticular reflex network in the midbrain tegmentum (Fig. 13-3). Interruption of these projections to the subthalamus and reticular network has been associated with disorders of associated movements, such as arm swinging during locomotion and follow-through during throwing.

Subthalamus

The subthalamus, a lens-shaped structure, is ventral to the thalamus and between the internal capsule and hypothalamus. It contains the subthalamic nucleus, zona incerta, and tegmental fields of Forel (field H of Forel). The subthalamic nucleus is situated next to the inner surface of the internal capsule and above the medial part of the substantia nigra (see Figs. 3-18 and 3-23). Its dysfunction is associated with ballism, and signs appear on the side opposite of the lesion.

Afferents

The BG GABAergic (inhibitory) afferents to the subthalamic nucleus emerge from the external segment of the globus pallidus (Fig. 13-3). Additional projections come from the motor cortex and the substantia nigra.

Efferents

Subthalamic efferents include glutamatergic (facilitatory) projections, primarily to the internal globus pallidus (Fig.

13-3). With its efferent projections, the subthalamic nucleus can modulate all output from the striatal system.

Substantia Nigra

The substantia nigra, a mesencephalic horizontal band of neurons, consists of the **pars compacta** and **pars reticulata** regions. The pars compacta region is packed with dark-pigmented neuromelanin-containing cells that produce dopamine or dopamine precursors to inhibit the functioning of neurons in the striatum. Degeneration of the neuromelanin-containing cells in the substantia nigra has been associated with Parkinson disease.

Afferents

The major input to the substantia nigra comes from the striatum via the striatonigral fibers; these GABAergic striatal projections inhibit the functioning of neurons in the substantia nigra (Fig. 13-3). The substantia nigra also receives some secondary projections from the subthalamic nucleus and pontoreticular formation.

Efferents

The substantia nigra projects back to the striatum through its terminals, which contain dopamine. Dopamine inhibits most of the striatal functioning (Fig. 13-3). The substantia nigra's afferent and efferent projections involve different neurotransmitters. The projections from the substantia nigra are also to the brainstem reticular formation.

Physiology of Basal Ganglia Circuitry

The physiology of the BG is discussed in terms of its ascending feedback to the motor cortex. The BG nuclei influence the activity of the motor cortex by facilitating, inhibiting, or disinhibiting (release from inhibition) components of its circuitry and their projections using neurotransmitters, such as glutamate, dopamine, GABA, acetylcholine, and substance P (Fig. 13-5). As noted, glutamate and acetylcholine are two facilitatory neurotransmitters, whereas GABA and dopamine are intrinsically inhibitory. The circuitry modulation regulates the net inhibitory output of the BG to the thalamus, which contains intrinsically facilitatory output to the motor cortex.

In a normal physiologic state, the neostriatum receives facilitatory (+) afferents from the motor (premotor, motor, and supplementary motor) and association cortical areas, the thalamic intralaminar centromedian nucleus, and the pontoreticular formation. These afferents are glutamatergic. Neostriatal influence on the globus pallidus (external and internal), subthalamic nucleus, and substantia nigra is inhibitory (-). The inhibitory efferents are transmitted through the neostriatum's GABAergic and substance P projections. The dopaminergic projections from the substantia nigra (pars compacta) inhibit the function of most of the striatal neurons, which are inhibitory to the other structures such as the globus pallidus.

The globus pallidus external, which receives inhibitory GABAergic projections from the striatum, is further inhibitory to the globus pallidus internal and to the subthalamic nucleus, which in turn facilitates the internal globus pallidus using glutamatergic impulses. The facilitatory drive from the subthalamic nucleus produces greater inhibition of the ventrolateral nucleus of the thalamus by the globus pallidus, which leads to a lesser activation of the motor cortex. The globus pallidus, integrating all the extrinsic and

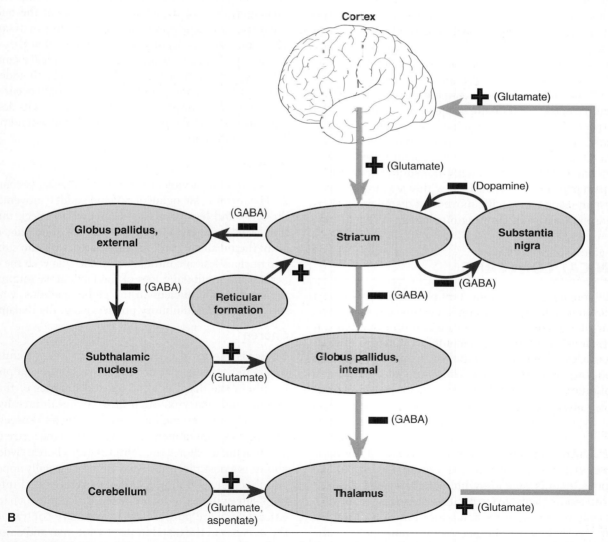

Figure 13-5 The inhibitory and excitatory basal ganglia loops along with their probable neurotransmitters. *GABA*, γ-aminobutyric acid.

intrinsic impulses of the BG circuitry, is inhibitory to the thalamus, which integrates the inhibitory BG output with corrective and facilitatory cerebellar (aspartate) output and sends intrinsically facilitatory glutamatergic projections to the cerebral cortex (Fig. 13-5).

The functional quality of the striatal activity depends on the effectiveness of the balance provided by the inhibitory dopaminergic projections and the facilitatory afferents from the cortex, reticular formation, and centromedian nucleus. An imbalance in the facilitatory and inhibitory circuits disinhibits the BG output, resulting in an altered cortical activation associated with a variety of movement disorders, such as bradykinesia, akinesia, and tremor.

Basal Ganglia Neurotransmitters

The function of the BG depends on a balanced interaction involving the major neurotransmitters glutamate, dopamine, acetylcholine, GABA, enkephalin, and substance P. As noted earlier, all of these neurotransmitters, except glutamate and acetylcholine, are inhibitory and are vital to the regulation of motor movements. Dopaminergic neurons from the substantia nigra project to the striatum (caudate nucleus and putamen) and inhibit facilitatory cholinergic (acetylcholine) as well as inhibitory GABAergic neurons, which project intrinsically to the globus pallidus and the substantia nigra in the BG. Terminals with substance P and enkephalin project to the globus pallidus and substantia nigra. Enkephalin projections in the BG and in surrounding structures, such as the thalamus, primarily participate in controlling pain and may inhibit movements. One way to accomplish movement refinement is by activating substance P, a neurotransmitter that stimulates pain perception. Impairment within a neurotransmitter system results in specific movement disorders, such as Parkinson disease and Huntington chorea.

CLINICAL CONCERNS

The BG nuclei serve an important role in refining motor activity and help in regulating some cognition and personality. The involvement of various neurotransmitters differentially affects the quality of motor functions. BG diseases result in a loss of inhibitory control and inappropriate release of patterned motor behavior, which includes dyskinesia (involuntary movements, such as tremor at rest, chorea, athetosis, dystonia, and ballism), bradykinesia (slow movement), hypokinesia (movements with limited range), disturbance of posture, and altered muscle tone (Table 13-1).

The involuntary movements of dyskinesia interrupt the motor activities of the speech musculature (dysarthria) and the limbs. At this time, only limited chemical and surgical treatment is available for BG disorders; the goal of such treatments is to restore the inhibitory function of the BG largely by obliterating the pathologic component of the circuitry. While supplementing dopamine secretion with L-dopa has been used with limited success, adrenal medulla transplant and deep brain stimulation (DBS) of the subcortical structures appears to be an additional avenue of treatment and is undergoing active investigation.

DBS has become more popular in the treatment of movement disorders, especially Parkinson disease; essential tremors; and generalized dystonia. Surgical intervention on the brain for such movement disorders has been available for > 50 years, but only recently have technological advances allowed for reversible stimulation of specific sites deep within the brain. The technique requires precision guidance of a narrow stimulating electrode that is permanently implanted with a pacemaker-like programmable battery pack. This treatment is used mainly when medications fail to control symptoms adequately so that the patient can have a more meaningful life. Effectiveness can range from improved gait and increased movement to nearly 100% of tremor relief.

Athetosis

Athetosis refers to the slow, involuntary twisting of predominantly axial and speech muscles accompanied by varying degrees of hypertonia. Athetosis of the buccofacial muscles affects motor speech and results in dysarthria. These movements occur in a sequence so that they blend together to form a continuous action. A typical example of athetosis is torsion of the hand, arm, neck, shoulder, and pelvic girdle. Athetotic movements commonly occur after a lesion involving the globus pallidus that affects its descending projections to the reticular network and ascending projections to the cortex, or both.

Ballism

Ballism, the most violent form of dyskinesia, is characterized by forceful, swinging, jerky, and sudden movements of the arms and legs. It may also involve the neck musculature. The swinging movements involve one side of the body (hemiballism) and are associated with the subthalamic nucleus lesion contralateral to the side with the dyskinesia. This results in a loss of the facilitatory output from the subthalamic nucleus to the globus pallidus, which in turn sends more inhibitory projections to the thalamus.

Chorea

Chorea is a series of rhythmic and quick yet graceful involuntary movements. The choreic movements occur predominantly in the distal extremities and muscles of the face, tongue, and pharynx. Such movements induce hypotonia in the muscles and affect swallowing and speech. Two common extrapyramidal diseases that characterize chorea are **Sydenham** chorea and **Huntington** chorea. Sydenham chorea is a postinfectious condition that usually appears in childhood several months after a streptococcal infection with subsequent rheumatic fever. The clinical characteristics, which are purposeless involuntary contractions of the muscles in the distal limbs, hypotonia, and emotional lability, become apparent between ages 5 and 13 years. Improvement occurs over weeks or months, and exacer-

Table 13-1

Movement Disorders and Diseases

Lesion Site	Involuntary Movements	Pathological Conditions
Globus pallidus and corpus striatum (putamen)	Athetosis: constant slow twisting movements in muscles of upper extremities	Toxicity, striatal degeneration, and hypoxia owing to carbon monoxide poisoning
Subthalamic nucleus	Ballism: wild swinging movements that usually involve one side of body	Stroke or denervation
Striatum (primarily caudate nucleus)	Chorea: rhythmic and quick involuntary movements of the muscles in proximal extremities	Huntington chorea
Caudate nucleus (dopaminergic deficiency owing to degenerative changes in substantia nigra)	Dyskinesia: sustained accessory movements with a desired motor act Akinesia: difficulty in initiating a movement Bradykinesia: slowness of movement Hypokinesia: quick movements of smaller range Tremor: rhythmic pill-rolling movements of fingers at rest accompanied by akinesia and rigidity	Parkinson disease

bations of the disease can occur without recurrence of infection.

Huntington chorea, a more common clinical condition of adult onset, is inherited through an autosomal dominant gene. This progressive neurologic condition is characterized by quick and jerky movements of the face, tongue, neck, and arm, and includes cognitive deficits (dementia), dysarthric speech, and personality and mood changes. It is associated with degenerative changes in the caudate nucleus and frontal and parietal lobes. With no cure or treatment, it invariably leads to death.

Tremors

Tremor, the most common form of dyskinesia, consists of constantly alternating motor activity in one or more parts of the body. The tremor, which results from the alternate contraction of opposing muscles, occurs in a rhythmic sequence of 4–6 contractions per second. Clinically, tremors are divided between resting and intentional, or action types. Resting tremor, associated with Parkinson disease, results from the degenerative changes in the substantia nigra and involves akinesia and rigidity. Intentional, or action, tremor is evident during voluntary movements and ceases in the resting state. This tremor is associated with cerebellar lesions.

Electrically, tremor may be considered a low-threshold discharging system. This is supported by clinical obser-

vations demonstrating the elimination of abnormal discharges, either by a lesion or through therapeutic DBS. Common symptoms associated with tremor include a masked face, infrequent blinking, slow movement, disturbed equilibrium, stooped posture, impaired speech, and impaired swallowing. Dyskinetic movements disappear in sleep when the brainstem reticular activating system is suppressed. Anxiety exaggerates dyskinetic movements.

Associated Movement Disorders

Loss of BG inhibition through direct descending projections to the reticular network at least in part affects automatic aspects of the associated movements, which include arm swinging during locomotion, follow-through in club swinging, facial expressions, and emotional vocalization.

Basal Ganglia Diseases
Parkinson Disease

Parkinson disease, the best-understood, chemically based BG disease was discovered by James Parkinson, a British physician, in 1817, who described it as a "progressive condition marked with involuntary tremulous motion with lessened muscular power, with a propensity to bend the trunk forward and to pass from a walking to a running phase.' Sensation and intelligence are not impaired. Originally called paralysis agitans, the primary symptoms of Parkinson disease are tremor at rest, cogwheel muscular rigidity (muscles are stiff and respond with cogwheel-like jerks to the use of constant voluntary force in bending the limb), bradykinesia (slowed execution of body movements), and loss of postural reflexes. The additional clinical signs are akinesia (slow beginning or inability to initiate a movement), shuffling gate, expressionless face, stooped (flexed) posture, micrographia (writing with smaller print), and dysarthria. Diagnosis is made on clinical grounds, usually in the 6th decade; the onset of symptoms occur between 40 and 70 years of age, with peak at 75–84 years. It affects men and women in equal proportions.

Parkinsonian symptoms relate to pathologic changes in the dopamine-producing nerve cells in the pars compacta region of the substantia nigra (Fig. 13-6A). Degeneration or depigmentation of these cells causes a dopamine deficiency. Patients with Parkinson disease lose nigral dopaminergic neurons, which normally manufacture dopamine and send it to the striatum, which has two types of dopamine receptors: D1 and D2 (Fig. 13-6B). Both of these receptors respond differently to dopaminergic projections. The nigrostriatal projections facilitate (+) D1 but inhibit (-) D2 receptors. The GABAergic projections from both D1 and D2 receptors are inhibitory to the globus pallidus. D1 striatal neurons project to the globus pallidus internal and the D2 neurons send efferents to the globus pallidus external, which in turn send inhibitory impulses to the globus pallidus internal and the subthalamic nucleus. Thus with the loss of dopaminergic neurons, dopaminergic deficiency in the nigrostriatal fibers have a differential effect on both of the receptors.

The nigrostriatal dopaminergic loss results in a disfacilitation (decreased facilitation) of D1 and disinhibition (decreased inhibition) of D2 receptors. Thus the loss causes reduced inhibition of the globus pallidus by D1 neurons. Furthermore, the disinhibition of D2 neurons results in a net increased inhibition of the neurons in the globus pallidus. This shift of chemical balance results in a state of disinhibition of the cortical motor system and is associated with the akinesia and tremors commonly in Parkinsonian dyskinesia.

Dopamine deficiency is overcome by giving the patient large quantities of L-dopa, a biosynthetic precursor of dopamine that is capable of crossing the blood–brain barrier (BBB). This drug stimulates the synthesis of dopamine in the surviving cells of the substantia nigra and avails to the striatum. However, L-dopa is found to control some symptoms for only a few years. It does not ameliorate the symptoms, arrest the disease, or revert the degeneration of the dopaminergic nigral cells. Approximately 80% of the cells must die off before significant symptoms occur. The few remaining cells may compensate if large amounts of L-dopa can bypass the rate-limiting enzyme for the neurotransmitter. L-Dopa decarboxylase, which is not specific for dopaminergic neurons, may synthesize dopamine from non-dopaminergic cells, such as serotonergic cells in the brain.

This biochemical understanding of the BG circuitry is the basis for using stereotaxic surgery. This technique alleviates Parkinsonian symptoms by inducing interruptions or eliminating pathologic discharges in the BG circuitry and is accomplished by targeting a selective structure, such as the inner segment of the globus pallidus or thalamus. The net effect of pallidotomy has been to reduce the inhibitory BG output to the thalamus and brainstem structures, subsequently reducing the bradykinesia and facilitating movement. Lesioning in the thalamus, however, somehow effects the tremor circuitry.

It is of interest that stimulation of the very same structures in the thalamus, pallidum, and subthalamus afford the exact same clinical benefits. This phenomenon leads to a paradox: How can lesioning and stimulation give the same clinical benefit when the thought of stimulating a cell seems to excite the cell and lesioning the cell destroys it and its output? Recent studies suggest that what may actually be happening is that the stimulation is exciting the target cells, causing a release of neurotransmitters at the terminal ends. This may seem to confuse the matter even further until one thinks of the circuits as interactive with specific frequencies of activity in relation to other circuits. Thus one circuit can be activated an erroneous frequency so the remaining circuits may read this as a null circuit regardless of its activity. This idea may also help explain other apparent paradoxes found in regard to stimulation and lesioning.

Intralaminar centromedian nucleus stimulation has also rendered an inhibitory and a dampening effect on cortical motor movements. It has yielded a facilitatory influence on the processing of language and other higher mental functions (Bhatnagar and Mandybur 2005). This improved performance may have resulted from the activation of the reticularly synchronized response of the cortical mechanism. Stimulation of the subthalamic nucleus has resulted in an improved motor performance in Parkinson patients. This may be related to the reduced inhibitory output of the globus pallidus internal and its facilitatory regulation of cortical motor activity by the theory just explained.

Tardive dyskinesia, commonly seen in patients receiving treatment for psychosis, is one of the complications associated with excessive L-dopa treatment of Parkinson disease. It is characterized by involuntary movements involving facial and lingual muscles, with implications for speech and swallowing. These movements do not vanish even with the discontinuation of the L-dopa treatment. Dyskinesia of facial and lingual movements, similar to that seen in patients with Parkinsonism who have had long-term L-dopa therapy, also can occur in patients who receive neuroleptics (antipsychotic) drugs, such as trifluoperazine, phenothiazines, and haloperidol. The mechanism of action is not well understood; however, it is believed that the drugs block dopaminergic cells, altering the balance between the intrastriatal dopaminergic, cholinergic, and GABAergic systems.

Huntington Chorea

Huntington chorea is another well-understood disease of the BG. George Huntington, an American physician, first

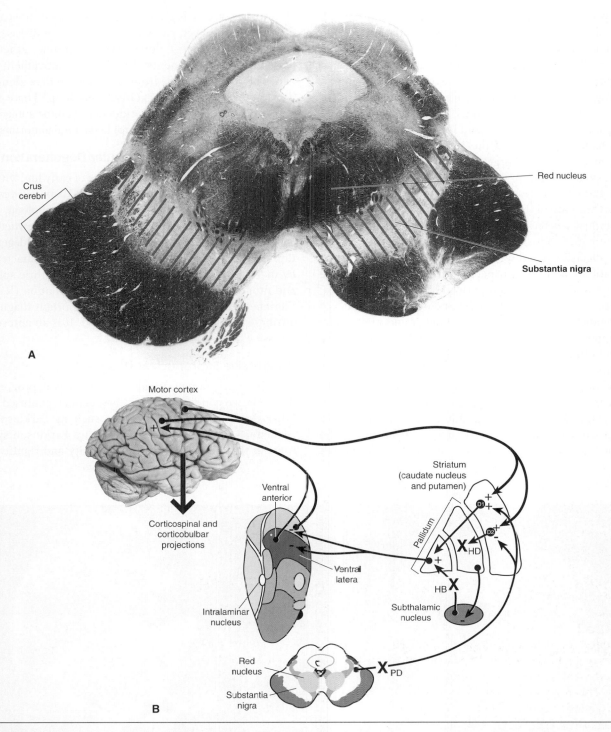

Figure 13-6 A. Schematic illustration of a degenerative lesion in the substantia nigra. B. A schematic illustration of anatomic-chemical disconnectivity involving the pathways underlying Parkinson disease (PD) with two dopaminergic receptors in the striatum: D1(direct) and D2 (indirect). The D1 receptors, that incorporate GABA and substance p neurotransmitters, serve as disinhibitory to the thalamus thus facilitatory to cortical movements; the D2 receptors that use GABA and enkephalin neurotransmitters activate globus pallidus (GPi) that is inhibitory to thalamus and cortical movements. The loss of nigrastriatal projections in PD not only impedes the facilitation of D1 receptors but also disinhibits D2 receptors. This disconnectivity results in reduced (bradykinesic/akinesic) movements. The management (subthalamic stimulation and pallidotomy) for PD improves the movement quality by reducing inhibitory GP output. Interruption (reduction) of subthalamic projections to GPi results in hemiballism. Loss of D2 projections alone to the GPi is known to result in reduced inhibition of the GPi and caues choreic movements that are seen in Huntington chorea.

described it in 1872. Huntington, his father, and his grandfather observed the same symptoms in members of successive generations of the same families. Huntington disease has the following four characteristics: hereditary transmission, adult onset, chorea, and cognitive deficits (dementia). Huntington chorea is inherited as an autosomal dominant disease in which each offspring of an affected parent has a 50% chance of inheriting and developing the disorder (see Chapter 20). Around the 3rd decade, the first signs of the disease appear: forgetfulness, personality changes, and clumsiness in motor movements. The choreiform movements gradually increase. The cognitive deficits lead to the subcortical type of dementia. Speech becomes dysarthric and gradually deteriorates into muteness. The prevalence of Huntington chorea is 5–10/100,000 in the United States, and it affects men and women in equal proportions.

Patients exhibit nonspecific atrophy in the caudate nucleus and prefrontal and parietal lobes. In Huntington chorea, the involvement of the caudate nucleus leads to degeneration of intrinsic striatal cholinergic and striatonigral GABAergic neurons (Fig. 13-7). Enzymes that biosynthesize acetylcholine and GABA also are decreased, contributing to further loss of GABA inhibition of the globus pallidus. In addition, the loss of striatonigral inhibition leads to the disinhibition of dopaminergic cells in the substantia nigra (Fig. 13.6). The nigrostriatal projections primarily inhibit pallidal output to the thalamus, resulting in the choreic movements of Huntington disease. If a patient with

Huntington disease is given L-dopa, the choreic movements get worse. Moreover, patients with Parkinson disease who are given too much L-dopa develop choreic, athetotic, and dystonic movements. Involuntary movements are caused by an imbalance from lesions anywhere along the dopaminergic–cholinergic–GABAergic loop. There is no cure for the condition; haloperidol (a dopamine antagonist) is usually administered to control behavioral abnormalities.

Wilson Disease: Hepatolenticular Degeneration

Wilson disease is a progressive disease of early life, with the onset of clinical manifestations between 10 and 25 years of age. It results from a disorder of copper metabolism, leading to the degeneration of internal brain regions, particularly the basal ganglia, and to cirrhosis (damage to and degeneration of hepatic cells) of the liver. It is clinically characterized by increased muscular rigidity, tremor, dysarthric speech, and progressive dementia. Corneal pigmentation (Kayser-Fleischer ring) is perhaps the most important diagnostic attribute of Wilson disease (Fig. 13-8). It is an autosomal recessive disease (see Chapter 20).

Progressive Supranuclear Palsy

Progressive supranuclear palsy (PSP), a slowly progressive degenerative condition of the CNS, is often confused with other neurodegenerative diseases, such as Parkinson or Alzheimer disease. This disease mimics Parkinson symptoms in that patients have gait difficulty and rigidity, but

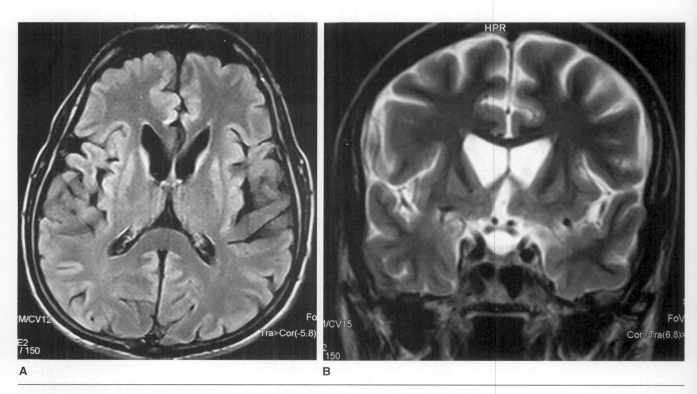

A   **B**

Figure 13-7 T2 axial (A) and coronal (B) MRI studies showing the caudate degeneration and dilated ventricles in a patient with Huntington disease.

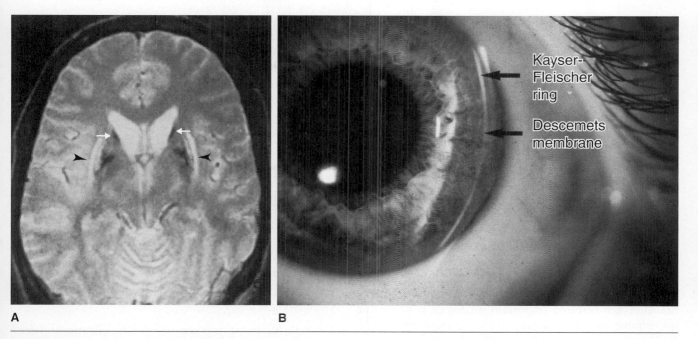

Figure 13-8 A. MRI study showing copper accumulation in the basal ganglia. B. Note the Kayser-Fleischer ring, which is marked by a yellowish discoloration of the Descemet layer.

there is usually no tremor. Unlike Parkinson disease, the neck is often rigid in extension, rather than flexion. The age of onset is 50 years or older. Early clinical symptoms include lack of balance, bradykinesia (decreased spontaneity in movement initiation), impaired gait control, and supranuclear gaze palsy, or loss of voluntary eye movements. This usually begins with impaired downgaze, later upgaze, and late in the course horizontal gaze. The inability to look down, together with the neck extension, makes it hard for the patient to walk down steps. Some patients do not have the extraocular motor palsy until late in the course, which makes diagnosis difficult. The patient often has a eyes-wide-open expression (look of perpetual astonishment). Additional symptoms include facial grimaces, dysarthria, and dysphagia. Speech is marked with imprecise consonants, reduced loudness, vowel prolongation, and increased intersyllabic juncture, regressing high and soft-pitch articulation. In its advanced stage, patients experience dysphagia and become wheelchair bound or bedridden. PSP patients also exhibit personality changes marked with a loss of interest in activities that were liked before and become quiet and socially withdrawn. Some patients develop cognitive impairments (forgetfulness, slow thinking, and inattention) or even dementia.

The underlying cause involves cellular degeneration in the brainstem, including the substantia nigra, which explains why patients with PSP share some of the motor phenomena of Parkinson disease. There is an accumulation of tau protein, a feature also of frontotemporal dementia and Pick disease. At present, there is no known treatment for the disease. PSP patients may show minimal response,

in terms of motor symptoms, to L-dopa (as in Sinemet), the drug that is used to treat Parkinsonism. Botulinum toxin injections have been used to treat the involuntary eyelid closure.

Basal Ganglia and Higher Mental Disorders

Traditionally, the functions of the BG nuclei were implicated exclusively with the refinement of cortically generated motor movement; this view was based on the BG projections to the cortical motor neural circuitry. Recently, however, the consideration of BG connectivity and excitability and the temporal relationship between the neuronal event and function have revealed that BG nuclei have additional roles in emotions, personality, and cognition (Bhatnagar and Mandybur 2006). Research has determined that a substantial amount of the BG connectivity is to the orbital, dorsolateral, and medial prefrontal regions (Brodmann areas 9, 12, 46, and 47) and to the inferior temporal region (Middleton and Strick 2000).

The prefrontal cortex is involved with cognition (planning, organizing, sequencing goal-oriented movements, learning, regulating attention, and solving problems), motivation, emotion, and personality, and the striatum is concerned with cortically mediated higher functions (Paxinos and Mai 2004). The dorsolateral striatum receives projections from the entire frontal cortex, whereas the ventromedial striatum is connected to the orbital (emotional) and medial (motivational) prefrontal lobe and the limbic motor (cingulate) region. Striatal cellular activity has been associated with movement selection and initiation, repetitive and overlearned movements, working memory, and the development of reward-based behavior. Caudate pathology has been associated with an acquired deficit in memory related to delayed tasks (Levy et al. 1997) and sequential movement learning in humans nonhuman primates.

The clinically confirmed presence of cognitive disorders, seen in virtually all patients with Huntington chorea and Wilson disease, and some of those with Parkinson disease, has further provided strong support for the cognitively relevant neural circuitry in the striatum and the reciprocally connected pars reticulata region of the substantia nigra.

Basal Ganglia and Psychiatric Disorders

The BG based movement disorders are also known to have psychiatric concomitants. There is a high incidence of depression in patients with Parkinson disease; similarly, patients with Huntington chorea exhibit a high suicide rate along with obvious personality and mood disorders. Research has revealed important analogies between the neurotransmitter dysfunctions in movement disorders and psychiatric illnesses, such as schizophrenia and depression, and in Tourette syndrome and dopaminergic receptors. Furthermore, a wide range of motor disorders, such as rigidity, dystonias, and tardive dyskinesia, are known to result from the use of neuroleptic medications. Used for behavioral modification and for treating psychiatric conditions, the neuroleptic drugs cause dysfunction of the striatal dopaminergic system by either blocking or changing the sensitivity of dopaminergic receptors, which results in dyskinesias. The presence of the psychiatric condition has a further effect on the effectiveness of the treatment rendered to improve the motor speech quality.

The discovery of the Huntington gene, which is localized to chromosome 4, has revealed how molecular genetics is involved with the mind–body relationship. This gene encodes the protein huntingtin, which gradually accumulates and damages dopaminergic receptors. Identification of the gene has contributed to the development of a genetic test to diagnose Huntington disease prenatally or before symptoms appear.

Summary of Basal Ganglia

The BG nuclei are a series of interconnected anatomic loops that are functionally contiguous with the thalamus and neocortex. The interconnected loops are the sites of reverberating circuits of electrical currents sustaining and modulating motor activity. The subthalamic nuclei and rostral brainstem also tie into the circuit, contributing to its stability. Lesions in one or more components of the system result in dyskinesias of varying types. Ballism is the only dyskinesia known to be produced by a single lesion in the subthalamic nucleus. The rest of the dyskinesias seem to be associated with diffuse lesions in different parts of the system. The neurotransmitter dopamine is deficient in Parkinsonism owing to the degeneration of the substantia nigra dopaminergic cells that project to the striatum.

Dopamine-replacement therapy and surgical intervention have been helpful in relieving Parkinsonian tremors, but neither is a cure. In recent years, chronic electrical stimulation in the thalamus has been found to control some forms of dyskinesia, such as Parkinson disease. Many BG disorders cause significant cognitive and emotional deficits.

CLINICAL CONSIDERATIONS

PATIENT ONE

A 60-year-old woman had suddenly developed partial paralysis (weakness or paresis) in her left leg while sewing. Within 24 hr, the paralytic attack was replaced by involuntary movements in her leg and arm. She was admitted to the hospital. On testing, she exhibited the following signs:

- Wild swinging movements of the left arm and leg that gradually became more intense
- Flaccid muscle tone
- Altered speech quality similar to mild dysarthria

A brain MRI study revealed an infarct in the right subthalamic nucleus. The swinging movements gradually became more intense. Several weeks of conservative therapy did not decrease the movements, so an electrolytic lesion was stereotactically placed in the right subthalamic nucleus, relieving the dyskinesia. She could then walk and eventually feed herself, and there were no complications. Her speech also improved.

Question: How can you relate the infarct of the subthalamic nucleus with the BG mechanism?

Discussion: The subthalamic nucleus renders facilitatory influence on the intrinsically inhibitory globus pallidus. The irritative infarct impaired the smooth flow of facilitating impulses to the globus pallidus and inhibitory BG projections to the motor cortex, which resulted in hemiballism in the limbs contralateral to the lesion site.

PATIENT TWO

A 64-year-old college dean saw his physician after he began having muscle rigidity and mild involuntary movements, primarily in his right hand, and difficulty with articulator precision when speaking. He was easily tired, and the impairment affected his ability to work. Examination revealed the following:

- Tense face without much expression
- Impaired ability to initiate a movement
- Mild pill-rolling tremor in both hands with more tremor in the right hand
- Awkward gait, resembling shuffling

- Mild dysarthria (his words were uttered quickly and lacked precision)
- Slightly stooped posture

A brain MRI study revealed changes bilaterally in the lower brainstem. The attending physician suspected this to be a case of akinesia and tremor associated with the degeneration of neurons in the substantia nigra.

Question: How can you explain these clinical symptoms in light of bilateral degenerative changes in the lower midbrain?

Discussion: This is a case of Parkinson disease, the most commonly known BG disease, which results from a degeneration of the dopaminergic neurons in the substantia nigra. Its symptoms include tremor at rest, cogwheel muscular rigidity, bradykinesia (slowed execution of body movements), akinesia (slow beginning or inability to initiate a movement), shuffling gate, expressionless face, flexed posture, and dysarthria. The muscle rigidity in Parkinson disease is commonly treated with L-dopa, a dopamine-replacement drug.

PATIENT THREE

A 37-year-old teacher began to experience weakness and uncontrollable clumsiness in his movements. He also exhibited dysarthric speech, some confusion, and mild cognitive impairments. This also changed his personality, and he gradually was becoming a recluse. His wife took him to their family doctor, who made the following observations:

- Postural imbalance
- Mild weakness of the upper and lower limbs
- Hypotonia and hyporeflexia
- Choreic movements involving the shoulders, head, and tongue
- Dysarthric speech
- Family history of similar condition; his father and uncle died young with similar symptoms, including dementia

A brain MRI study revealed wider lateral ventricles anteriorly, indicating the degeneration of the caudate head. Some degenerative changes were also noted in the basal region of the prefrontal lobe. The physician suspected this to be a case of a BG condition of dominant inheritance.

Question: What clinical characteristics helped the physician make this diagnosis?

Discussion: This is a case of Huntington chorea, which is characterized by four clinical characteristics: heredity, onset in early adult age, chorea, and cognitive deficits (dementia). Personality changes and mood disorders, including depression, are also present. This neurologic condition, a autosomal dominant disease, is associated with degenerative changes in the corpus striatum (putamen and caudate nucleus) followed by changes in other cortical areas.

PATIENT FOUR

A 35-year-old male unpaid politician became concerned about his gradually worsening speaking ability and shaking movements involving both arms. He consulted a neurologist who noted the following:

- Involuntary arrhythmic movements of the hands
- Rigidity in limb muscles
- Rigidity in both legs with an unsteady gait
- Amnesia for recent events
- Short attention span
- Presence of pigmentation at the sclerocornea junction (Kayser-Fleischer rings
- Unintelligible speech

speech language pathologist (SLP) consultation revealed the following:

- Irregular articulatory breakdown
- Voice stoppages
- Loudness variations
- Prolonged intervals
- Vowel prolongation
- Consonant distortion
- Confused language
- Anomia

A brain MRI study revealed degenerative changes bilaterally in the basal ganglia. Laboratory testing also confirmed cirrhosis (dysfunction) of the liver. The attending neurologist diagnosed it as a case of hepatolenticular degeneration, an autosomal recessive condition of impaired copper metabolism.

Question: How can you relate these speech, language, and motor symptoms to the underlying disease process?

Discussion: This is a case of Wilson disease which is marked by the retention of copper in the body. In normal conditions, the liver releases absorbed copper into the bile, which helps with digestion. The damaged liver in Wilson disease, however, frees copper into the bloodstream, which carries it to different organs in the body, damaging the kidneys, brain, and eyes. Copper accumulation around the cornea (Kayser-Fleischer ring) supports the diagnosis of Wilson disease. Basal ganglia degeneration affects the motor speech processes (hyperkinetic dysarthria) and produces tremor, rigidity, ataxia, and choreic movements. This pathophysiology has implications for language functions and eventually leads to dementia.

SUMMARY

Both the reticular formation and BG play important roles in motor activity. The reticular formation uses integrated sensory and motor input to regulate spinal motor activity and influence muscle tone. The BG, consisting of a series of interconnected anatomic loops, is the site of reverberating circuits of electrical currents that sustain and modulate motor activity. Furthermore, the abnormalities of neurotransmitters in the BG also produce specific dyskinetic conditions, such as Parkinson disease, Huntington chorea, progressive supranuclear palsy, and Wilson disease.

QUIZ QUESTIONS

1. Define the following terms: athetosis, ballism, basal ganglia, chorea, tardive dyskinesia, tremor.

2. Briefly describe the following diseases:

   Huntington chorea
   Parkinson disease
   Wilson disease

3. Match each of the following numbered definitions with its associated lettered statement.

1. wild flinging movements involving one or both sides of the body
2. rhythmic pill-rolling movements of fingers during rest
3. rhythmic, quick, involuntary movements of proximal muscles
4. difficulty in performing voluntary movements and abnormally sustained posture
5. slow twisting movements in the muscles of the upper extremities

   a. athetosis
   b. chorea
   c. ballism
   d. dyskinesia
   e. tremor

TECHNICAL TERMS

acetylcholine
akinesia
athetosis
autosomal dominance
ballism
basal ganglia
bradykinesia
chorea

cogwheel rigidity
decerebrate rigidity
dopamine
GABAergic neurons
reticular formation
tardive dyskinesia
tremor

Motor System 4: Motor Cortex

LEARNING OBJECTIVES

After studying this chapter, students should be able to:

- Discuss the motor roles of the primary motor cortex and surrounding cortical areas

- Outline the anatomic organization of the primary motor cortex

- Describe the functions of the corticospinal and cortico-bulbar pathways

- Discuss the bilateral cortical innervation of speech-related cranial nerve nuclei

- Describe the location of upper motor neurons

- Explain the pathophysiology and signs of upper motor neuron syndrome

- Differentiate between upper motor neuron and lower motor neuron syndromes

- Explain the pathophysiology of spastic hemiplegia

- Discuss the pathophysiology of pseudobulbar palsy and describe its effects on speech muscles

- Explain the physiology of intact emotional responsiveness in pseudobulbar palsy

- Discuss the pathophysiology of alternating hemiplegia and describe its clinical symptoms

U p to this point, motor functions have been discussed in relation to the spinal cord, cerebellum, and basal ganglia. These structures represent motor organizational levels that do not initiate volitional motor movements on their own but instead act on efferent information that originates in the cerebral cortex and/or sensory information derived from various parts of the body and the environment.

The efferent impulses from the **primary motor cortex** (**PMC**) activate spinal motor neurons and induce contraction of specific muscles. The cortical motor projections regulate a series of movements that are complex, discrete, precise, and skilled, such as finger tapping, dancing, running, and

speaking. In addition to activating the lower motor neurons (LMNs) in the brainstem and spinal cord (see Chapter 11), the PMC, in conjunction with afferents from the **premotor, prefrontal, sensory**, and **associational cortices**, participates in the cognitive planning of motor activity. This planning includes the integration of sensory information regarding what and where the object is, calculation of the extent of muscle movements, determination of body parts that must be recruited, and generation of efferent signals for regulating specific muscles. The cerebral motor cortex executes movements with constant and updated feedback to and from the adjacent cortical and subcortical areas.

ANATOMY OF MOTOR CORTEX

The PMC is in the **precentral gyrus** of the frontal lobe (Fig. 14-1; see Fig. 2-5), which is rostral to the **central sulcus**. The PMC (Brodmann area 4) contains large **Betz cells**, which are unique to this cortical area and are important in voluntary motor movement. A low intensity of electric stimulation can evoke motor acts from this cortical area. The organization of the PMC can be represented in terms of the body (**motor homunculus**). The face, speech muscles, and head are shown in the lower third of the motor cortex near the **sylvian fissure**, the arms and trunk are in the upper motor cortical region, and the legs and toes are in the mid-sagittal area (see Fig. 2-6). In comparison, the face and mouth occupy a large cortical area in the motor cortex caudal to the premotor area. The disproportionately large representation of the face and mouth in the human PMC corresponds to the uniqueness of the elaborate apparatus required for speech, an important point for professionals in human behaviors to remember.

The motor neural impulses that travel in the **pyramidal tract** originate from the three cortical regions (Fig. 14-2): PMC, **premotor cortex**, and **primary sensory cortex**. In humans, 25–30% of the pyramidal tract fibers are known to arise from the PMC. Of those, only 2% come from the large Betz cells. The Betz cells are pyramidal cells whose long axons extend to the lower limbs and thus require large cell bodies for metabolic support. There are relatively few large motor cells because humans have a much greater need of the shorter cortical projections to the cranial nerve nuclei

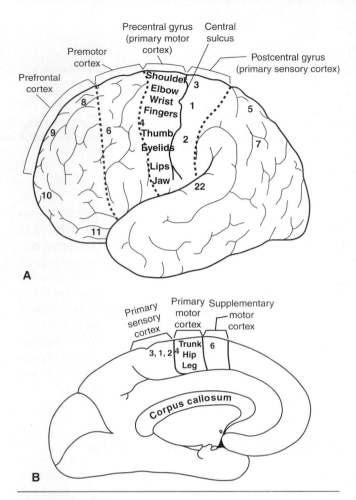

Figure 14-1 The human body in the primary motor cortex and important Brodmann areas on the lateral (**A**) and medial (**B**) brain surfaces.

(**corticobulbar projections**) and upper limb levels in the cord (**corticospinal projections**). Therefore, the small neurons in the motor cortex give rise to the remaining pyramidal fibers. Approximately 30% of the remaining descending motor fibers arise from the premotor cortex (Brodmann area 6), which extends midsagittally within the interhemispheric fissure as the **supplementary motor area** (Fig. 14-1*B*). The remaining 40% of the motor fibers arise from the primary sensory cortex (Brodmann areas 3, 1, 2) in the parietal lobe and the adjacent somatosensory association cortex (Brodmann areas 5 and 7) (Figs. 14-1 and 14-2). Most of the efferents from the cortex project to the contralateral limbs. Substantial bilateral projections, however, are known to exist, particularly from the supplementary cortical area.

The motor cortex circuitry is organized into columns of neurons arranged vertically from the surface into the depth of the cortex. Each single column provides circuitry responsible for directing a group of muscles. Thus the simultaneous and sequential organization of fine movement patterns,

but not the individual muscles, are considered to be organized in the motor cortex. Direct control from the cortex allows higher primates, including humans, to control individual and grouped proximal and distal muscles to perform specific movements.

This cortical motor system is maintained and enhanced by the thalamocortical excitatory loop, which itself is modulated by the intrinsic inhibitory basal ganglia functions and excitatory afferents from the cerebellum (see Chapters 12 and 13). To maintain the precision, accuracy, smoothness, and sequential nature of the motor activity, the motor cortex depends on constant feedback from the adjacent cortical and subcortical regions. The cortical input includes afferents from the premotor cortex (Brodmann area 6), which, with input from the prefrontal cortex (Brodmann areas 8–and 10), is concerned with setting up a motor plan of a skilled movement pattern involving specific limbs. The prefrontal cortex, the site of reasoning, thinking, and planning, receives inputs from the occipital, parietal, and temporal lobes. The **supplementary motor cortex** (Brodmann area 6) regulates planning and implementing the bilateral aspects of a motor pattern. Projections from the somesthetic cortex (Brodmann areas 3, 1, 2) modulate sensory feedback, whereas fibers from the association somesthetic cortex (Brodmann areas 5 and 7) regulate higher-order spatial aspects of the movement plan.

Much highly skilled movement is learned through a background of species-specific, built-in capabilities. The sensory feedback aspects of the sensorimotor cortex and corticospinal projections to the spinal cord contribute to the process of motor learning. Once a skilled movement pattern is well learned, these feedback systems are usually not required unless a deterrent to the movement is encountered.

Lesions of the motor cortex and its descending fibers (**upper motor neuron: UMN**) result in paralysis and slowed movement because they interrupt voluntary and precise motor control, especially of the limb muscles used in fine manipulative skills and the muscles involved in speech and facial expression in the acute stage. However, there can be a gradual return of gross function.

INNERVATION PATTERN

The motor cortex is organized **contralateral** to output and input. The short (corticobulbar) and long (corticospinal) efferent projections from the motor cortex cross the midline to innervate contralateral cranial nerve and spinal output nuclei. Consequently, a lesion of the motor fibers above the **pyramidal decussation** produces clinical signs contralateral to the locus of damage (Fig. 14-3). In the case of a lesion below the pyramidal decussation in the caudal medulla, clinical signs in the spinal UMNs and lower motor neurons (LMNs) are **ipsilateral** to the site of the damage.

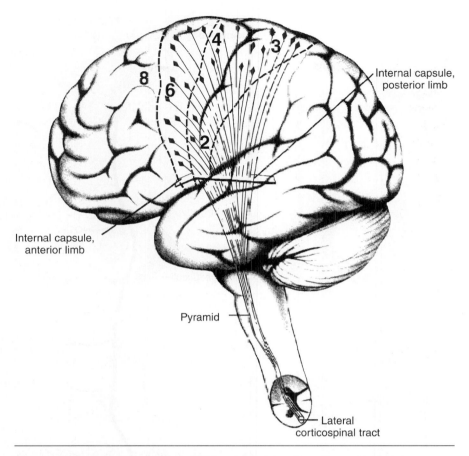

Figure 14-2 The pyramidal tract fibers originating from the sensorimotor cortex: premotor, motor, and sensory cortical areas. *Numbers* refer to Brodmann areas.

CLINICAL TERMS

Common clinical terms associated with cortical motor dysfunctions are paralysis, **UMN syndrome**, **LMN syndrome**, and **spasticity**. Clinical terms related to paralysis (loss of voluntary muscle movement) are **monoplegia**, **hemiplegia**, **triplegia**, and **quadriplegia**. Monoplegia refers to the paralysis of a single limb, hemiplegia is the paralysis of one side of the body involving both upper and lower limbs, paraplegia involves the paralysis of both lower limbs, and quadriplegia refers to the conditions characterized by the paralysis of all four (upper and lower) limbs.

The term UMN is used in reference to the cortical motor neurons and their axons before they synapse on the spinal motor neurons. These are also called pyramidal neurons because their descending axons pass through the pyramids in the medulla. Its damage is associated with specific symptoms of delayed muscle spasticity, increased tone and reflexes, and paralysis. The term LMN is used in reference to the neurons located in the brainstem and spinal cord that directly project to the skeletal muscles. Its damage is associated with symptoms of flaccid paralysis, decreased tone and reflexes, and muscle atrophy. Spasticity refers to increased muscle tone and resistance to passive manipulation of the muscle that is not under voluntary control.

DESCENDING PATHWAYS

Impulses from the motor cortex to the LMNs travel on one of two pathways, either the **corticospinal tract** or the **corticobulbar tract** (Fig. 14-3). The corticospinal tract, which contains merely 30% of the descending motor fibers, mediates voluntary movements of the skeletal muscles through the spinal α-motor neurons (LMNs). The corticobulbar tract, which contains ~ 70% of the remaining motor fibers, controls the facial and associated muscles through activation of cranial nerve nuclei in the brainstem. Virtually all efferent fibers in both tracts cross the midline before synapsing on their respective motor neurons.

Corticospinal Tract

The corticospinal fibers arise from the upper two-thirds of the PMC (precentral gyrus), premotor cortex, and sensory cortex. These fibers travel through the **corona radiata** and then descend, in a compact bundle, through the posterior limb of the **internal capsule** of the forebrain (see Fig. 2-5). Later, they run through the midbrain **pes pedunculi**. These descending fibers separate into several longitudinal but diffuse fascicles as they pass between the masses of neurons in the ventral pons, mingling with the pontine nuclei (Fig. 14-3A). Some fibers terminate in

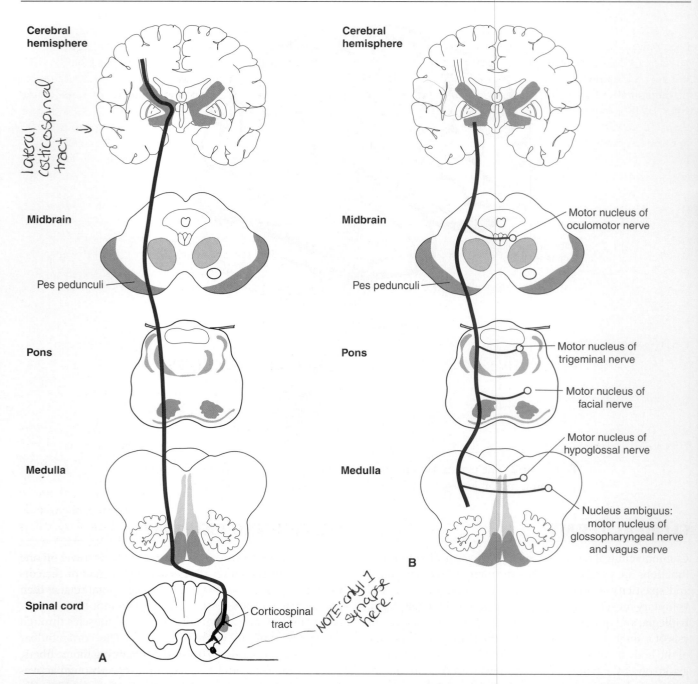

Figure 14-3 Origin and course of the pyramidal fibers. **A.** Corticospinal fibers projecting to the spinal motor nuclei. **B.** Corticobulbar fibers projecting to the motor nuclei of the cranial nerves. Most motor nuclei of the cranial nerves receive motor commands from the contralateral motor cortex; the motor nucleus for the upper face and jaw receives bilateral projections.

the pontine nuclei, while the rest continue to the medulla to form the **pyramids** (source of the term: the pyramidal tract) before crossing at the caudal end of the medulla. After crossing, the motor fibers descend into the **lateral corticospinal tract** of the spinal cord (Figs. 14-2 and 14-3A), named after the location of these fibers in the lateral funiculus of the spinal cord. Through the fibers of the lateral corticospinal tract, the motor cortex participates in digital control of the skeletal muscles of the distal limbs (fingers and toes) required for fine manipulative skills.

An uncrossed smaller fasciculus of motor fibers (**anterior corticospinal tract**) descends into the ventral funiculus of the spinal cord, which eventually crosses the midline before synapsing on the α-motor neurons (see Fig. 11-7). The anterior corticospinal tract fibers control the proximal axial and girdle muscles, which provide the postural platform required for skilled digital movements.

The UMN fibers of the lateral corticospinal tract terminate on the interneurons and α-motor neurons (LMNs) in the spinal anterior gray horns to initiate movements (Box 14-1). Some of the fibers also terminate on γ-motor neurons, providing a means for the motor cortex to modulate the stretch reflex. This ensures an appropriate level of tone in the muscles in which the α-motor neurons are influenced to provide the motor control. Some fibers also synapse on the sensory cells in the dorsal gray horns through which the cortex modulates somesthetic feedback data, which consist largely of messages noting deviations from what the premotor cortex planned and the motor cortex actuated. On its way to the spinal motor neurons, the corticospinal tract also emits multiple collaterals to the basal ganglia, thalamus, brainstem reticular formation, and pontine nuclei. The axonal processes of the LMNs exit at all levels of the spinal cord, terminating in the skeletal muscles.

Corticobulbar Tract

The corticobulbar fibers, similar to the fibers of the corticospinal tract, control skilled and fine movements. However, the corticobulbar fibers exclusively control the skeletal muscles of the head and face through the motor nuclei of the following cranial nerves (CNs): trigeminal (CN V), facial (CN VII), glossopharyngeal (CN IX), vagus (CN X), spinal accessory (CN XI), and hypoglossal (CN XII). The corticobulbar fibers arise from the lower third of the motor cortex and adjacent area and travel through the genua of the internal capsule and pes pedunculi. The corticobulbar projections to the cranial nerve nuclei do not cross the midline at a single point; rather, they do so at multiple points before synapsing on the cranial LMNs (Fig. 14-3*B*).

The corticobulbar projection to some cranial nerves is contralateral, whereas the corticobulbar regulation of some cranial nerve LMNs is bilateral (see Chapter 15). The corticobulbar fibers from the left motor cortex innervate both the left and right motor nuclei of some of the cranial nerves. Similarly, projections from the right motor cortex control the functioning of some cranial nerve nuclei on both sides, which include the nuclei of the trigeminal (CN V), facial (CN VII), vagus (X), and glossopharyngeal (IX) nerves. The pontine gaze center controls the ocular cranial nerves on both sides (see Fig. 15-6).

An important clinical point is that because the muscles of the jaw, larynx, and upper face receive projections from the bilateral motor cortices, a unilateral cortical lesion does not profoundly impair the function of some cranial nerves (facial [CN VII], trigemina [CN V], and vagus [CN X]) and spares mastication, phonation, and speech. The functions of such cranial nerves are severely affected only in the case of a bilateral cortical pathology or after a LMN lesion.

CLINICAL CONCERNS

Differential Involvement of the Arm and Leg After Cerebral Lesion

There is a close clinical relationship between vascular functioning and neuroanatomy. Cerebral injuries mostly affect the contralateral limbs, and the upper limbs are more involved than the lower limbs. This observation is clinically crucial because the lateral cortical surface, with motor representation for the arm and face is served by the **middle cerebral artery**, whereas the medial extension of the motor cortex, with motor representation for the leg and toes, is served by the **anterior cerebral artery**. Because the middle cerebral artery is most commonly involved with cerebral infarction, a greater prevalence of paresis of the arm than leg occurs (see Chapter 17).

Spastic Hemiplegia

Interruptions of the corticospinal fibers result in **spastic hemiplegia**. Lesions of the corticospinal tract at various neuraxial locations usually produce different symptoms concomitant with the hemiplegia. As a result, involvement of the corticobulbar fibers also results in the paralysis of the facial, lingual, palatal, and laryngeal muscles. Because corticospinal fibers cross the midline at the medulla, any lesion involving the pyramidal system in the brainstem above the pyramidal decussation produces clinical symptoms contralateral to the locus of damage. However, in the case of a lesion below the decussation point, the clinical signs from spinal UMNs and LMNs occur ipsilateral to the side of the damage.

Common causes of spastic motor dysfunctions are **cerebrovascular** accidents, **tumors**, and **degenerative diseases** of the nervous system. None of these causes respects the anatomic boundaries; therefore, the clinical pictures

---

BOX 14-1

Rationale for Contralateral Symptoms with Damage to Upper Motor Neurons

The point of crossing for the descending motor fibers has significant implications for contralateral and ipsilateral symptoms. Any pathologic involvement of the motor fibers before the point of decussation results in weakness and paralysis in the body contralateral to the site of lesion; any neuraxial lesion below the point of decussation will produce weakness and paralysis in limbs ipsilateral to the lesion site. The LMN receives only the crossed efferents. Consequently, an involvement of the motor nuclei in the brainstem and spinal cord invariably affects the muscles ipsilateral to the lesion site.

evolving from these conditions are usually mixed and may also implicate extrapyramidal structures.

Typical spastic hemiplegia consists of a flexed upper arm, thumb, and fingers with the neck bent toward the affected side (Fig. 14-4A). While walking, the patient circumvents the affected leg. The clinical symptoms appearing immediately after an acute pyramidal tract lesion include profound weakness and flaccidity, especially in contralateral distal muscles; loss of delicate and manipulative skills; loss of abdominal and **cremasteric reflexes**; positive **Babinski reflex**; and flaccid tone in the affected muscles. Within 1–4 weeks, the muscle tone not only returns but increases and the muscle becomes spastic.

The spasticity is most evident in passive manipulation of the affected limb, as there is a resistance to a passive limb extension. This is mostly present in antigravity muscles such as the proximal flexors in the upper extremity and extensors in the lower extremity. Spasticity is speed dependent, and it is stronger if the affected limb is moved rapidly. Furthermore, it is present only in the muscles that are not under voluntary control. If pressure is persistently applied, the muscle resistance may suddenly disappear. This is called **clasp-knife** spasticity. This is different from the jerky **cogwheel muscle** rigidity seen in patients with Parkinson disease. Extreme levels of hypertonia and the clasp-knife characteristics of the limbs are rarely seen in lesions restricted to the corticobulbar system. Furthermore, corticobulbar damage does not usually produce the same

level of spasticity as that which develops in the distal limbs after a corticospinal tract lesion.

The gradual emergence of spasticity is related to the outgrowth of local stretch afferents, which fill the depopulated synapses on the α-motor neurons after a cortical lesion. This growth may subsequently promote increased afferents on type Ia fibers from the muscle spindles, causing greater activation of the motor neurons. This axonal outgrowth takes considerable time, explaining the span of several weeks that it takes for spasticity to appear.

Pseudobulbar Palsy

Bilateral spastic paralysis of the speech musculature is called pseudobulbar (supranuclear) palsy. This indicates that the lesion is not in the medulla but rather in the motor pathways to the pons and medulla. It results from bilateral involvement of the corticobulbar pathways, which causes a supranuclear paralysis of the cranial nerves. The patient has difficulty controlling facial muscles for delicate and discrete motor control, such as in speech; however, there is little spasticity in facial and neck muscles.

Furthermore, the facial emotional response pattern remains intact. Consequently, when the patient attempts to move the facial muscles, they respond poorly. However, the patient's facial muscles respond strongly to an emotional stimulus, which is not considered under direct control by the cerebral cortex. The pathways activated during a true emotional response are not as fully understood as are the direct pathways that control voluntary actions. The emotional response may involve some limbic afferents. When the cranial nerve motor nuclei are activated through the so-called intact emotional pathways, the facial response is actually exaggerated; when asked to show the teeth or perform a voluntary smile, the patient may assume the appearance of a Greek mask of tragedy, with forceful contraction of the same muscles that otherwise appear to be weak. Often these exaggerated emotional responses are accompanied by excessive laughter, sobbing, or choking, and they may pose a hazard to the patient if he or she is eating.

Alternating Hemiplegia

Lesions at the brainstem level produce **alternating or crossed hemiplegia**, which can result from an obstruction of small brainstem arteries (see Chapter 17). A lesion on one side of the brainstem affects the cranial nerve motor nuclei and/or nerves (motor units) extending to the innervated muscles. The LMN signs are **unilateral** to the side of the lesion. The lesion also interrupts the unilateral corticospinal fibers, which descend to cross the midline in the caudal medulla. A brainstem lesion results in an alternating pattern of symptoms: ipsilateral pharyngeal, facial, and/or ocular palsy symptoms and contralateral hemiplegia (Fig. 14-4B).

Unilateral damage to the motor nucleus of the vagus (CN X, LMN) nerve produces flaccid paralysis of the pharyngeal and/or laryngeal muscles, resulting in a weak and

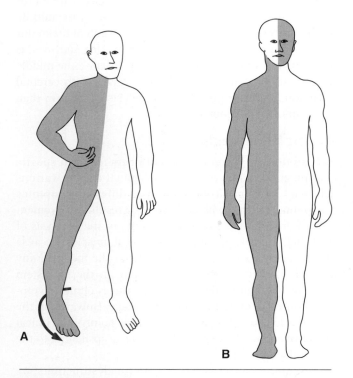

Figure 14-4 A. Right spastic hemiplegia. B. Left alternating hemiplegia, which is characterized by left facial palsy and right-sided hemiplegia and hemianesthesia.

hoarse voice and swallowing difficulty. Unilateral involvement of the motor nucleus of the facial (CN VII; LMN) nerve causes facial asymmetry and affects eating and articulation. Unilateral damage to the motor nucleus of the hypoglossal nerve (CN XII; LMN) produces flaccid paralysis of the intrinsic and extrinsic lingual muscles, resulting in eating and speaking disturbances. If the lesion is large and extends to the lateral brainstem, it also produces contralateral hemianesthesia because of an interruption of the ascending somesthetic fibers. A lesion impairing the LMNs alone produces symptoms of flaccid paralysis, absent reflexes, muscular fibrillation, and eventual atrophy of the involved muscle (Fig. 14-5, Lesion B; see Fig. 11-15).

Upper Motor Neuron Syndrome

Interruption of the descending motor (corticospinal and corticobulbar) tracts have two clinically important components: the UMN (central nuclei and fibers) and the LMN (spinal and cranial nuclei and peripheral fibers). The UMNs relate to the cell bodies in the motor cortex and descending axonal processes before they synapse on the cranial or spinal motor neurons. The LMNs are the cell bodies in the anterior gray column in the spinal cord or cranial motor nuclei in the brainstem (see Chapters 11 and 15). The LMNs provide the output pathway to peripheral functions via their axons and innervate muscle fibers. The difference between the locations of the UMNs and LMNs has important clinical implications (Fig. 14-5, Table 14-1).

Lesions of the corticospinal fibers result in UMN syndrome, which is characterized by immediate flaccid muscle weakness (Fig. 14-5, Lesion A); this is followed by increased muscle tone (spastic hemiplegia) after several weeks. Additional symptoms are a positive Babinski sign, hyperreflexia, and loss of the abdominal and cremasteric reflexes. With the loss of the pyramidal motor system, there is no cortical motor control on limb muscles and the patient loses precise and delicate motor control of the distal limb muscles used in fine manipulative skills, along with the head and neck muscles used for speech and facial expression. However, the paralyzed muscles do not atrophy (degenerate), because with intact LMNs their reflexive functions are preserved.

Flaccid in the beginning, the muscles gradually become spastic because of both pyramidal and extrapyramidal involvement. Spasticity, which includes hyperexcitability of reflex, takes 1–4 weeks to develop. This is largely the result of collateral sprouting (scrambled wiring) of the type Ia (annulospiral) endings to the spinal motor neurons, which fill depopulated or denuded corticospinal synapses. Contralateral spinal reflexes are hyperactive (Table 14-1). The abdominal and cremasteric reflexes are absent, with no muscle contraction in response to stroking the abdomen and inner thigh. A positive Babinski sign is characterized by an extension of the toes in response to stroking the bottom of the foot with a pointed object (Fig. 14-6*B*).

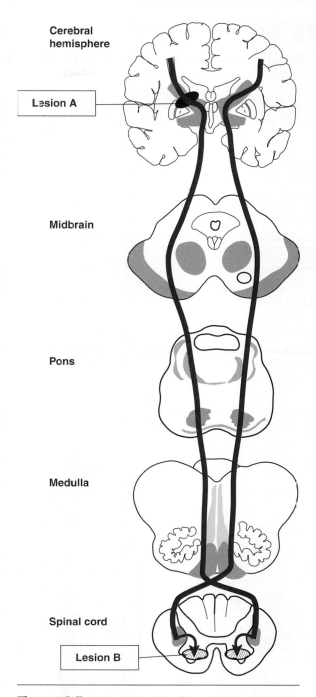

Figure 14-5 Lesion sites implicated in upper and lower motor neuron syndromes. Each site results in a different set of clinical symptoms. Lesion A (upper motor neuron lesion) results in a contralateral hemiplegia (flexed arm and extended leg), increased muscle tone (spastic), hyperactive reflexes, no muscle atrophy, and Babinski sign. Lesion B (lower spinal motor neuron lesion) results in ipsilateral paralysis of specific muscles, absent muscle tone (flaccid), hypoactive or absent reflexes, muscular atrophy, and muscle fasciculations.

Table 14-1

Clinical Characteristics of Upper and Lower Motor Neuron Syndromes

Characteristic	Upper Motor Neuron Syndrome	Lower Motor Neuron Syndrome
Lesion site	Cortical motor neurons and their axons before synapses on spinal/cranial motor nuclei	Spinal/cranial motor neurons and their axons
Paralysis	Paralysis (spastic) or weakness	Paralysis (flaccid) or weakness
Muscle tone	Increased tone	Decreased tone
Muscle atrophy	Not present	Present
Denervation	No twitching or fasciculation	Fibrillations and fasciculations
Reflexes	Hyperreflexia	Hyporeflexia
Abnormal reflexes	Babinski and Hoffman	No abnormal reflexes
Limb involvement	Multiple muscles or limbs (monoplegia, hemiplegia, or quadriplegia)	A single limb or selected muscles

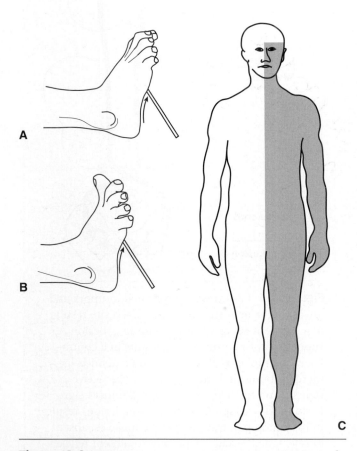

Figure 14-6 Upper motor neuron symptoms. **A.** Normal motor response. **B.** The Babinski sign in adults indicates dysfunctioning of the corticospinal system. **C.** Left hemiplegia.

A positive Babinski sign in a child is not an indication of disorder. Before maturation of the corticospinal system, during the first 5–7 years of development, earlier (or primitive) reflexes are pronounced; these include the protective flexor-withdrawal reflex. As the developing corticospinal system begins to dominate, Babinski and related primitive reflexes disappear. Corticospinal damage removes this domination, and the earlier reflexes, including Babinski, reappear.

There is always some recovery from spastic paralysis, and it may result in varying degrees of flexion in the upper extremity and hyperextension in the lower limbs (Fig. 14-6C). In general, gross motor movements recover, with proximal muscles displaying the greatest recovery.

No treatment is available to alleviate UMN symptoms other than minimizing the damage by reducing cerebral edema and by enhancing the blood supply to the damaged tissue. Future treatment is concerned with finding a way to get UMN axons to grow past the damage and reinnervate former targets, an extremely challenging task. This central nervous system nerve growth factor, when fully understood, would have enormous implications for rehabilitation.

LESION LOCALIZATION

Rule 8: Upper or Lower Motor Neuron Lesion Presenting Symptoms

Increased reflexes and spastic tone in a symptomatic (sensorimotor) limb indicate an UMN lesion. Reduced reflexes and attenuated muscle tone in the same symptomatic limb imply a peripheral or LMN lesion.

Rationale

The UMN regulation of the LMNs via the corticospinal and corticobulbar systems is excitatory. A lesion interrupting the excitatory projections from the UMNs first produces early signs of loss of precise motor control, especially of distal limb muscles, muscle weakness, flaccid tone, and hyporeflexia. However, in several weeks, the hyporeflexia and flaccid tone are replaced by increased reflexes and spasticity, which result from the increased power of the stretch reflexes because of the filling of the denuded corticospinal synapses to the LMNs.

The hyperactive antigravity stretch reflexes and spastic muscle tone take 1–4 weeks to be demonstrated clinically. The LMN cell body provides the only output pathway to peripheral function via its axon, which traverses the ventral root and peripheral nerves to innervate a skeletal muscle, where it makes multiple axon branches to innervate and contract many muscle fibers. This entire single neuron–multiple muscle fiber functional unit is the motor unit. Damage to the LMN cell and/or its axon eliminates the entire function of a motor unit. This both weakens the muscles and reduces tendon reflexes. Additional LMN symptoms are flaccid muscle tone, muscle weakness, and muscle atrophy. These symptoms are seen in neurologic conditions affecting motor units, diseases of the skeletal muscles (e.g., muscular dystrophy), and reduced nerve–muscle transmission (e.g., myasthenia gravis).

Rule 9: Brainstem Lesion
Presenting Symptoms

- Motor and sensory losses of the extremities associated with cranial nerves (facial [VII], ocular [III], lingual [XII], trigeminal [V]) imply a brainstem lesion.
- An altered level of consciousness, cranial nerve impairments (facial paralysis, hearing impairment, nystagmus, dysarthria, dysphagia) on the same side (ipsilaterally), paralysis of the body on the opposite side (alternating or crossed hemiplegia), and hemianesthesia all imply a brainstem lesion.

Rationale

A lesion anywhere in the neuraxis affects the ascending and descending fibers causing sensory loss and paralysis. However, an involvement of cranial nerves suggest a brainstem location of the lesion. In alternating hemiplegia, the involved cranial nerves receive contralateral projections that have already crossed the midline, whereas the descending corticospinal fibers have not yet decussated. Thus brainstem involvement results in crossed or alternating symptoms, whereas hemiplegia involves the body contralateral to the lesion and the cranial nerve signs occur on the side of the brainstem lesion. Furthermore, dysarthria (laryngeal, pharyngeal, facial, or glossal dysfunctions) and dysphagia imply the involvement of cranial nerves and their nuclei, which are present in the brainstem. Disorders

of consciousness can result from either the involvement of the brainstem reticular formation, which is essential for alertness and consciousness, or extensive bilateral cortical destruction or lesions.

CLINICAL CONSIDERATIONS

PATIENT ONE

A 47-year-old woman had a stroke while sleeping. When she awoke, her left arm and leg would not move. She could talk, but her speech was dysarthric (imprecise articulation and weak and breathy voice). She was rushed to the hospital, and on testing, the medical team noted the following:

- Weakness in the left upper and lower limbs (hemiplegia)
- Drooping lower left face
- Distorted smile with the mouth pulled to the normal (right) side
- Intact upper facial functions: intact frowning and eye closing
- Loss of proprioceptive, discriminative, and pain sensation on left side of the body
- Hyperactive deep tendon reflexes, including a positive Babinski sign on the left side.

A brain MRI study revealed an infarct in the posterior region of the right internal capsule.

Question: How can you relate this lesion site with her UMN symptoms?

Discussion: The right internal capsule lesion affected the following structures:

- Damaged corticospinal fibers caused the left spastic hemiplegia.
- Damaged portions of the corticobulbar fibers supplied the motor nucleus of the facial (CN VII) nerve (loss of delicate motor control for left lower facial muscles), hypoglossal (CN XII) nerve (imprecise speech), and vagus (CN X) nerve (weak voice). There was a differential effect of the lesion on the muscles of the larynx, lower face, and tongue. The effect was minimal on phonation because of the bilateral innervation of the nucleus ambiguus, and maximal on articulation because of the unilateral innervation of the facial (CN VII) and hypoglossal (CN X) nuclei (see Chapter 15).
- Interruption in the thalamocortical (medial lemniscus) projections resulted in loss of proprioceptive and discriminative touch on the left half of the body.
- Damage to the thalamocortical projections accounted for the left-sided loss of pain and temperature sensation.

PATIENT TWO

A 61-year-old man had a stroke while confined to a hospital for heart disease. He suddenly felt that he had no control of his left arm and leg and could not move his mouth. He was seen by a physician, who observed the following:

- Weakness in the right half of the face
- Inability to close his right eye and a widened palpebral fissure
- A weak bite on the right side
- No pain and touch sensation in the right half of his face
- Spastic paralysis of the left upper and lower limbs
- Positive left-sided Babinski sign

A brain MRI study revealed a massive infarct in the right ventrolateral pons extending rostrally. He was diagnosed with alternating hemiplegia.

Question: How is it that there was sensorimotor loss of the right face and right masticator muscles and yet left hemiplegia? Can you account for the discrepancy in the clinical features observed?

Discussion: The ventrolateral pontine infarct on the right side affected the following structures:

- Damaged facial (CN VII) nucleus and nerve (LMN syndrome) caused the paralysis of the right half of the patient's face.
- Damaged trigeminal (CN V) motor nucleus (LMN symptom) caused the weakness of the right mastication muscles.
- Damaged chief sensory nucleus and spinal trigeminal nucleus affected pain and touch sensation from the right half of the face.
- Damaged uncrossed corticospinal fibers resulted in paralysis of the left side of the body. These fibers cross the midline at the caudal medulla. A positive Babinski sign implicates an UMN lesion site.

PATIENT THREE

A 55-year-old man had a stroke while sleeping; he woke up and noted that he had no control of his right limbs and did not speak well. He was taken to the emergency room and was seen by a neurologist who noted the following:

- Right hemiplegia: paralysis of the right lower and upper limbs, respectively
- Right hemianesthesia: loss of touch and pain in right lower and upper limbs
- Drooping right lower face
- When smiling the weakened right side of the face moved to the left
- Intact upper right facial functions, such as wrinkling
- Weakened tongue deviating to right
- Dysarthria with imprecise articulation

- Nonfluent, effortful, and halting verbal output containing two- to three-word utterances

A brain MRI study revealed a large infarct in Brodmann area 4, extending to parts of areas 3, 1, 2 and area 44 in the left hemisphere. The patient was seen again 3 weeks later and exhibited the following additional symptoms:

- Hyperactive deep tendon reflexes
- Spasticity in limb muscles
- Positive Babinski sign

Question: How can you relate these symptoms to the cortical lesion evident on MRI?

Discussion: This case may look similar to that of patient one, but patient three has a different lesion site. A cortical lesion had affected the following structures and their functions:

- Damaged corticospinal fibers in Brodmann area 4, caused the right (UMN) spastic hemiplegia.
- Affected corticobulbar fibers supplied the motor nucleus of the facial nerve (loss of motor control for right lower facial muscles) and hypoglossal nerve (imprecise speech), resulting in attenuated cranial nerve functions marked with facial and lingual paralysis and dysarthria. The effect on the upper facial muscles was minimal because they receive bilateral cortical projections (see Chapter 15).
- Partial involvement of the somatosensory cortex resulted in the loss of pain, touch, and temperature.
- The involvement of the Brodmann area 44 (anterior association language cortex) resulted in nonfluent and effortful verbal output.

PATIENT FOUR

A 65-year-old man suffered a stroke while sleeping and woke up to find that he could not use his right limbs and had problems speaking. He was taken to the hospital where the physician noted the following:

- Dysarthric speech subsequent to a left-sided lingual paralysis
- Swallowing difficulty owing to weakness of the pharyngeal muscles
- Loss of pain and temperature on the left side of the face
- Loss of pain and temperature on the right half of the body
- Paralysis of the right limbs
- No sign of aphasia or cognitive impairment

A brain MRI study revealed an infarct in the left brainstem.

Question: What lesion location in the brainstem can account for these symptoms?

Discussion: This is a case of alternating hemiplegia associated with a right medullary lesion that had affected the following brainstem structures:

- Paralysis of the left hypoglossal (CN XII) nerve contributed to the speech unintelligibility.
- Involvement of the pharyngeal branches of the vagus (CN X) nerve resulted in the paralysis of the pharyngeal muscles, contributing to dysphagia.
- Involvement of the descending trigeminal (CN V) nucleus contributed to the facial anesthesia.
- Interruption of the ascending fibers of the lateral spinothalamic tract resulted in the loss of pain and temperature on the right half of the body.
- Involvement of the uncrossed descending motor fibers (pyramidal tract) contributed to the right hemiplegia.

SUMMARY

The several motor cortices control voluntary manipulative and delicate motor movements and initiate motor performance. Descending cortical projections to the motor neurons travel via two pathways, the corticobulbar tract and the corticospinal tract, collectively called the pyramidal tract. These tracts control cranial and spinal motor neurons (LMN), respectively. Activity at the motor cortex is influenced by extensive feedback channels from the cerebellum, brainstem, thalamus, and basal ganglia.

A lesion interrupting the excitatory projections from the motor cortex results in a specific loss of delicate motor control. It also results in signs of muscle weakness, flaccid tone, hyporeflexia, and loss of reflexes. However, in several weeks, the hyporeflexia and flaccid tone are replaced by increased reflexes (hyperreflexia) and spastic tone in muscles.

QUIZ QUESTIONS

1. Define the following terms: alternating hemiplegia, Babinski reflex, homunculus, pyramidal decussation, upper motor neurons.

2. List two clinical characteristics of alternating hemiplegia.

3. Match each of the following conditions with its associated lettered lesion site.
   1. muscle atrophy and flaccidity
   2. loss of stretch reflex and hypotonia
   3. spasticity and hypertonia
   4. fasciculation
   5. positive Babinski sign
   6. ataxia and asynergia
   7. tremor and chorea
   8. hemiplegia

   a. LMN
   b. UMN
   c. cerebellum
   d. basal ganglia

4. List four clinical characteristics of UMN syndrome.

TECHNICAL TERMS

alternating hemiplegia
Babinski reflex
corticobulbar tract
corticospinal tract
cremasteric reflex
homunculus
postcentral gyrus
precentral gyrus

premotor cortex
pyramidal decussation
pyramidal tract
spastic hemiplegia
supplementary motor
  cortex
upper motor neurons

Synopsis of Cranial Nerves

LEARNING OBJECTIVES

After studying this chapter, students should be able to:

- List the cranial nerves by their names and numbers

- Relate the cranial nerve numbers to their names

- Follow the rationale for the functional classification of cranial nerves

- Identify the locations of the attachments of cranial nerves in the brainstem

- Explain the brainstem locations of cranial nerve nuclei

- Discuss the cranial nerve nuclei that receive bilateral or unilateral cortical projections

- Explain the clinical implications of the bilateral or unilateral innervation of motor nerve nuclei

- Discuss the branchial and somatic bases of muscles

- List the muscles derived from various branchial arches

- Identify functional components for each cranial nerve

- Relate cranial nerve nuclei and their projections to specific sensorimotor functions

- Explain idiosyncratic distributional patterns and innervational properties of cranial nerves

- Discuss clinical symptoms associated with disorders of cranial nerves and nuclei

- Describe function-based cranial nerve combinations

- Perform an oral–facial examination in accordance with the pertinent functional components of cranial nerves

- Differentiate between upper and lower motor neuron symptoms of the motor cranial nerves.

The **cranial nerves** (CNs) in humans are the result of an evolutionary modification of a basic organizational pattern of the vertebrate central nervous system (CNS), which consists of ~40 bilaterally symmetrical repeating segments, each with a **dorsal horn** and a **ventral horn**. Each

CNS segment innervates the corresponding head or body region by means of the nerve (dorsal and ventral) roots on each side. The peripheral process of the **ganglion** cells in the **dorsal root** innervates the tissue of the body segment as receptor endings, whereas its central axons travel to the dorsal horns of the corresponding CNS segment. The ventral root, containing efferent axons, innervates the somite-derived skeletal muscles of the body.

Early in evolutionary development, additional (intermediate) roots of efferent fibers between the dorsal and the ventral roots emerged. These are present in only the rostral 15 segments of the CNS, extending from the head to the C5 segment. The efferent axons leaving the **intermediate roots** innervate ancient muscles related to gill opening and closing, including filtering food and absorbing oxygen from the water. In mammals, these gill-related muscles evolved into many of the skeletal muscles of the head and face and are modified for other purposes, such as phonation and speech, the area of most concern to students of human communication. This is the evolutionary basis for the muscles now used for human motor speech and explains the origin of the unique functions of the head and face muscles. The cranial nerves that innervate these include the evolutionary remnants of the intermediate nerve roots as well as the expected ventral and dorsal roots that innervate the segmental skeletal muscles of the head and neck (Box 15-1).

The stable arrangement of afferent (sensory) neurons transmitting to the CNS and efferent (motor) neurons innervating somatic muscles on each side of each spinal segment continues in the brainstem. The peripherally located afferent neurons of the cranial nerves are homologous to the spinal dorsal root ganglia and have names such as semilunar ganglion (trigeminal nerve [CN V]), geniculate ganglion (facial nerve [CN VII]), and the superior and inferior ganglia (vagus nerve [CN X]). The efferent neurons of the cranial nerves, whether related to gill muscles or somite muscles, contain both α- and γ-motor neurons and lie within the nuclei of the brainstem. For example, the gill-related motor nuclei are in the facial nucleus, and the somite-related motor neurons are in the abducens nucleus.

The first 2 cranial nerves (olfactory [CN I] and optic [CN II]) are part of the forebrain; the other 10 cranial nerves are attached to the brainstem (Fig. 15-1). Some cranial

Evolutionary Basis of the Cranial Nerves

The cranial nerves are the result of an evolutionary modification of the basic organizational pattern of the vertebrate CNS. In mammals, the ancient gill-related muscles evolved into many of the skeletal muscles of the head and face and were modified for other purposes, such as swallowing, phonation, and speech. These functions, regulated by cranial nerves, are of concern to students of human communication. This explains not only the differential evolutionary basis for the muscles now used for motor speech but also why the head and face muscles are treated as functionally different.

nerves serve only sensory functions; others serve only motor functions. However, many of the nerves are mixed, serving both sensory and motor functions. Furthermore, cranial nerves have evolved specialized functions, not required at the spinal level, such as vision, audition, gustation, and olfaction. Thus the CNs have a more complex organization than do the spinal nerves.

FUNCTIONAL CLASSIFICATION OF CRANIAL NERVES*

Spinal nerves serve general motor and general sensory functions only, involving both somatic (skeletal) and visceral (internal organ) muscles, and can be classified into four functional components (Table 15-1). Besides serving **general motor** and **general sensory** functions, cranial nerves use special receptors and neurons to provide **special** functions. The general and special functional components of the cranial nerves can be further classified by their innervation (somatic muscles or visceral structures) and type of information (sensory [afferent] or motor [efferent]). The somatic component of the cranial nerves with special functions contains only afferent fibers, whereas the visceral component contains both afferent and efferent fibers (see Chapter 1). Thus there are seven functional types of cranial nerves, discussed in the following sections (Tables 15-2 and 15-3; Box 15-2).

Efferent

General Somatic Efferent

The general somatic efferent (GSE) nuclei innervate the skeletal muscles derived from somites. This functional cat-

egory includes the innervation of the ocular muscles (oculomotor [CN III], trochlear [CN IV], and abducens [CN VI]) and tongue muscles (hypoglossal [CN XII]).

General Visceral Efferent

The general visceral efferent (GVE) nuclei regulate the autonomic innervation of smooth muscles and glands. In the cranial nerves, all these serve **parasympathetic** functions. The GVE nuclei are the source of **preganglionic** parasympathetic fibers and include the **Edinger-Westphal** nucleus (oculomotor [CN III]), **superior salivatory** nucleus (facial [CN VII]), **inferior salivary** nucleus (glossopharyngeal [CN IX]), and **dorsal motor nucleus** (vagus [CN X]). These nerves are responsible for pupillary constriction; gland secretion; and the regulation of the muscles of the heart, trachea, bronchi, esophagus, and lower viscera.

Special Visceral Efferent or Branchial Efferent

The special visceral efferent (SVE), or branchial efferent (BE), nuclei control the muscles of the face, pharynx, larynx, and some neck muscles, which evolve from the branchial arches. This functional component consists of the motor nucleus of the trigeminal nerve (CN V), the motor nucleus of the facial nerve (CN VII), the nucleus ambiguus of the glossopharyngeal nerve (CN IX), the vagus nerve (CN X), and the accessory motor nuclei in the C1–C5 segments. They are related to the spinal accessory nerve (CN XI) and control the muscles of expression, mastication, phonation, deglutition, head turning, and shoulder elevation.

Afferent

General Somatic Afferent

The general somatic afferent (GSA) nuclei mediate somesthetic input, including pain, pressure, temperature, and touch sensations from the skin and somatic muscles in the head, neck, and face. This functional category primarily includes the trigeminal (CN V) sensory nuclei (**chief sensory nucleus** and **spinal descending nucleus**).

General Visceral Afferent

The general visceral afferent (GVA) nuclei serve general sensation, including pain and temperature, from the visceral structures of the pharynx, palate, larynx, aorta, and abdomen. This functional category includes the glossopharyngeal nerve (CN IX) and the vagus nerve (CN X).

Special Somatic Afferent

The special somatic afferent (SSA) nuclei regulate special senses, such as vision (optic [CN II]) and audition and equilibrium (vestibulocochlear [CN VIII]). This functional component includes proprioception and stretch afferents from muscle spindles.

Special Visceral Afferent

Special visceral afferent (SVA) nuclei mediate taste (gustation) and smell (olfaction). This functional component

---

*See Chapter 1 for definitions of the terms used in the functional classification of the CNs.

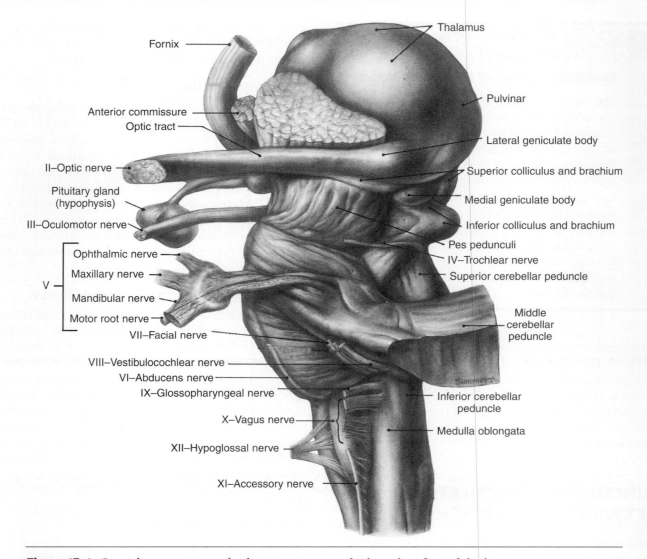

Figure 15-1 Cranial nerve roots and other structures on the lateral surface of the brainstem.

includes the olfactory nerve (CN I), facial nerve (CN VII), glossopharyngeal nerve (CN IX), and vagus nerve (CN X).

BRANCHIAL ORIGIN OF SPEECH-RELATED MUSCLES

The classification of speech and the related muscles of phonation, mastication, deglutition, articulation, head turning, and shoulder elevation as **special visceral efferent** is often confusing for students of communicative disorders because these muscles can be under both voluntary and reflex control and are structurally the same as other skeletal muscles derived from the somites and classified as somatic (Table 15-4; Box 15-3). The muscles related to motor speech processes are classified as SVE because they are derived from the **branchial arches** and gill-related structures of the embryo. To minimize confusion to the stu-

dent, these muscles are also identified as **branchial efferent** in this chapter.

Early in human embryonic development, six branchial arches emerge (Fig. 15-2). The first four arches are well marked, the fifth arch disappears during development, and the sixth arch is present but not obvious. Each branchial arch relates to specific groups of muscles (Table 15-4): the muscles of mastication (trigeminal nerve [CN V]) relate to the **first branchial arch**, the muscles of facial expression (facial nerve [CN VII]) relate to the **second branchial arch**, and the stylopharyngeus muscles (glossopharyngeal nerve [CN IX]) relate to the **third branchial arch**. The remaining pharyngeal muscles (vagus nerve [CN X]) are derived from the **fourth branchial arch**, and the laryngeal muscles (vagus nerve [CN X]) are derived from the **sixth branchial arch**.

The spinal accessory [CN XI] nerve is also a branchial nerve because it is related to a series of unnumbered gill structures that extended down to the C5 segment in mammals. The **lower motor neurons** (LMNs) exiting the

Table 15-1

Functional Components of the Nervous System

General		Special	
Somatic	**Visceral**	**Somatic**	**Visceral**
GSE: controls muscles derived from somites (e.g., skeletal, extraocular, glossal)	GVE: sends preganglionic axons to peripheral parasympathetic ganglia, which regulate autonomic functions of smooth muscles, cardiac muscles, glands	SSE[a]	SVE/BE: controls gill-related muscles of face, pharynx, larynx, and neck (evolved from branchial arches)
GSA: mediates somesthetic input (pain, temperature, touch) from somatic muscles, skin, ligaments, and joints	GVA: mediates sensations of pain, temperature, tissue stretch, and pressure from visceral organs	SSA: conducts special sensory mechanism of vision from retina and audition and equilibrium from inner ear; includes spindle afferents and Golgi tendon organ afferents	SVA: mediates information from specialized receptors related to taste from tongue and pharynx olfaction from nasal mucosa

[a]Special somatic efferent does not exist.

BE, branchial efferent; *GSA*, general somatic afferent; *GSE*, general somatic efferent; *GVA*, general visceral afferent; *GVE*, general visceral efferent; *SSA*, special somatic afferent; *SVA*, special visceral afferent; *SVE*, special visceral efferent.

Table 15-2

Functional Components of the Cranial Nerves

	General				Special[a]		
	Afferent		Efferent		Afferent		Efferent
Nerve	**GSA**	**GVA**	**GSE**	**GVE**	**SVA**	**SSA**	**SVE/BE**
I					+		
II						+	
III			+	+			
IV			+				
V	+						+
VI			+				
VII			+		+		+
VIII						+	
IX		+	−		+		−
X		+	+		+		+
XI							+
XII			+				

[a]Special somatic efferent does not exist.

BE, branchial efferent; *GSA*, general somatic afferent; *GSE*, general somatic efferent; *GVA*, general visceral afferent; *GVE*, general visceral efferent; *SSA*, special somatic afferent; *SVA*, special visceral afferent; *SVE*, special visceral efferent.

Table 15-3

Summary of the Functional Components of the Cranial Nerves

Cranial Nerve (Number)	Classification	Cell Nuclei	Function
Olfactory (I)	SVA	First order: neuroepithelial olfactory cells in nasal mucosa Second order: olfactory bulb	Smell
Optic (II)	SSA	Ganglion cells in retina	Vision
Oculomotor (III)	GSE	Oculomotor nucleus in upper midbrain tegmentum	Eye movements: controls all eye muscles except lateral rectus (CN VI) and superior oblique (CN IV) muscles Regulates eyelid elevation (levator palpebrae superioris)
	GVE	Edinger-Westphal nucleus in midbrain tegmentum Preganglionic parasympathetic projections to ciliary ganglion	Reflexive constriction of pupil and accommodation of lens for near vision
Trochlear (IV)	GSE	Trochlear nucleus in midbrain tegmentum	Eye movements: innervates contralateral superior oblique muscles
Trigeminal (V)	GSA	First order: trigeminal (semilunar) ganglion Second order: primary sensory (pons), descending spinal nucleus (pons, medulla, and upper cervical levels)	Receives pain and touch sensations from skin and muscles in face, orbit, nose, mouth, forehead, teeth, meninges, anterior two-thirds of tongue, external auditory meatus, and external surface of tympanic membrane
		Mesencephalic nucleus (midbrain)	Proprioception from jaw
	SVE/BE	Trigeminal motor nucleus in pons	Innervates muscles of mastication (masseter internal and external pterygoid and temporal), mylohyoid, anterior belly of digastric, tensor velum palatini, and tensor tympani muscles
Abducens (VI)	GSE	Abducens nucleus in tegmentum of pons	Eye movements: innervates ipsilateral lateral rectus muscle
Facial (VII)	GVE	Superior salivatory nucleus: preganglionic parasympathetic to ganglia associated with oral, lacrimal, and nasal glands	Parasympathetic regulation of secretion from nasal, palatal, lacrimal, submaxillary, and sublingual glands and mucous membrane of nasopharynx
	SVA	First order: geniculate ganglion Second order: nucleus solitarius	Mediates gustatory sensation from taste buds in anterior two-thirds of tongue
	SVE/BE	Facial motor complex in lateral pons	Innervates muscles of facial expression and platysma, extrinsic and intrinsic ear muscles, and stapedius muscle

(continued)

Table 15-3

Summary of the Functional Components of the Cranial Nerves (*continued*)

Cranial Nerve (Number)	Classification	Cell Nuclei	Function
Vestibulocochlear (VIII)	SSA	First order: superior and inferior vestibular ganglia Second order: vestibular nuclei in medulla and pons	Maintains equilibrium and head orientation in space
	SSA	First order: spiral ganglion Second order: cochlear nuclei in medulla	Mediates audition
Glossopharyngeal (IX)	GVA	First order: inferior ganglion Second order: nucleus solitarius	Mediates general sensation from palate, posterior third of tongue, oral pharynx, middle ear, eustachian tube (ear ache), and carotid sinus
	GVE	Inferior salivatory nucleus: preganglionic to otic ganglion	Parasympathetic regulation of secretion from parotid gland and oral pharyngeal mucosal glands
	SVA	First order: inferior ganglion Second order: nucleus solitarius	Mediates taste sensation from posterior third of tongue and oral pharynx
	SVE/BE	Nucleus ambiguus	Contributes to swallowing by controlling stylopharyngeus muscle
Vagus (X)	GVA	First order: inferior ganglion Second order: nucleus solitarius	Receives general sensation from pharynx, larynx, thorax, abdomen, carotid body, and aortic body Regulates nausea, oxygen intake, and lung inflation
	GVE	Dorsal motor nucleus: preganglionic parasympathetic innervation	Innervates glands and muscles in heart, blood vessels, trachea, bronchi, esophagus, stomach, and intestine
	SVA	First order: inferior ganglion Second order: nucleus solitarius	Mediates taste sensation from sensory buds in epiglottis and pharynx, and laryngeal pharynx
	SVE/BE	Nucleus ambiguus	Controls muscles of larynx, pharynx, soft palate for phonation, deglutition, and resonance
Spinal accessory (XI)	SVE/BE	Spinal accessory nucleus in C1–C5 ventral horns	Controls head and shoulders by innervating trapezius and sternocleidomastoid muscles
Hypoglossal (XII)	GSE	Hypoglossal nucleus in medulla	Controls tongue movement by regulating intrinsic and most extrinsic muscles

BE, branchial efferent; *GSA*, general somatic afferent; *GSE*, general somatic efferent; *GVA*, general visceral afferent; *GVE*, general visceral efferent; *SSA*, special somatic afferent; *SVA*, special visceral afferent; *SVE*, special visceral efferent.

C1–C5 segments form the spinal accessory nerve and innervate the neck muscles.

CRANIAL NERVES AND THE AUTONOMIC NERVOUS SYSTEM

The cranial nerves also serve autonomic functions. The **parasympathetic efferents** of the **autonomic nervous system** (ANS) exit the CNS from the craniosacral region (cranial brainstem area and spinal segments S2–S4) (see Chapters 2 and 16). Therefore, autonomic components of the cranial nerves have only parasympathetic functions via the innervation of **postganglionic neurons** in the periph-

eral ganglia. These functions, classified as general visceral efferent, are carried out by the preganglionic LMNs in the **Edinger-Westphal nucleus** (oculomotor [CN III]), **superior salivatory nucleus** (facial [CN VII]), **inferior salivatory nucleus** (glossopharyngeal [CN IX]), and the **dorsal vagal nucleus** (vagus [CN X]).

CRANIAL NERVE NUCLEI

Most of the cranial nerve nuclei are in the ventricular floor of the brainstem. Depending on what functions they serve,

Table 15-4

Branchial Arches, Associated Cranial Nerves, and Derived Muscles

Branchial Arch[a]	Cranial Nerve (Number)	Muscles
First (mandibular)	Trigeminal (V)	Of mastication: temporalis, masseter medial, and lateral pterygoid Additional: mylohyoid, anterior belly of digastric, tensor tympani, and tensor veli palatini
Second	Facial (VII)	Of facial expression: buccinator, auricularis, frontalis, platysma, orbicularis oris, and orbicularis oculi Additional: stapedius, stylohyoid, and posterior belly of digastric
Third	Glossopharyngeal (IX)	Stylopharyngeus
Fourth and sixth	Superior laryngeal and recurrent laryngeal branches of vagus (X)	Pharyngeal and laryngeal: cricothyroid, levator veli palatini, constrictors of pharynx, and intrinsic muscles of larynx
Unnumbered gill structures	Spinal accessory nuclei in C1–C5	Sternocleidomastoid and trapezius muscles

[a]The fifth branchial arch is not developed in human embryo.

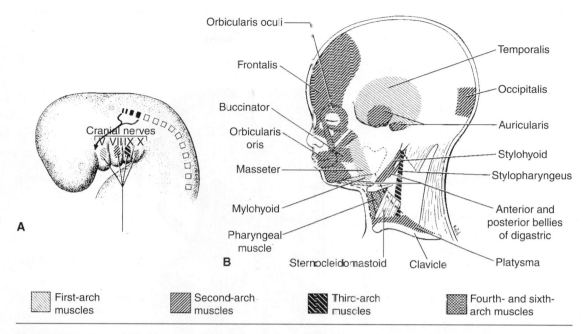

Orbicularis oculi

Frontalis

Buccinator

Orbicularis oris

Masseter

Mylohyoid

Pharyngeal muscle

Cranial nerves
V VII IX X

A

B

Temporalis

Occipitalis

Auricularis

Stylohyoid

Stylopharyngeus

Anterior and posterior bellies of digastric

Platysma

Sternocleidomastoid

Clavicle

First-arch muscles

Second-arch muscles

Third-arch muscles

Fourth- and sixth-arch muscles

Figure 15-2 Lateral view of a 4-week-old embryo. **A.** Arches and the cranial nerves derived from each branchial arch. **B.** Major muscles derived from each arch.

some nuclei are connected to several related nerves. The intramedullary locations of the cranial nerve nuclei are presented in Figures 15-3 and 15-4. Note that the cranial nerves take a fixed path and exit through specific foramina in the skull (Fig. 15-5).

Midbrain

There are three cranial nerve motor nuclei in the adult midbrain tegmentum: Edinger-Westphal nucleus (oculomotor [CN III]), **oculomotor nucleus** (CN III), and **trochlear nucleus** (CN IV). The Edinger-Westphal nucleus contains preganglionic parasympathetic efferents to innervate the **ciliary muscle** and the sphincter (constrictor) fibers of the pupil. The oculomotor nucleus contains the lower motor neurons (LMNs) that control most of the muscles of the eye. The trochlear nucleus contains the LMNs that innervate the superior oblique, one of the muscles of the eye.

Pons

Six major cranial nerve nuclei lie in the pontine tegmentum. There are the three sensory nuclei of the trigeminal nerve (CN V): the **primary sensory** nucleus, **spinal trigeminal** nucleus, and **mesencephalic** nucleus. The first two nuclei join to form the sensory branch of the trigeminal nerve (CN V). The mesencephalic nucleus contains afferents from muscle spindles and regulates the jaw reflex and provides proprioceptive input from the muscles of mastication. Adjacent to the sensory trigeminal complex is the **trigeminal motor nucleus**, which contains LMNs to innervate the muscles of mastication and other associated muscles. Dorsal in the pontine tegmentum is the **abducens**

motor nucleus (CN VI), which contains LMNs to innervate the lateral rectus muscle of the eye. Ventrolateral to the abducens nucleus (CN VI) is the **facial motor nucleus** (CN VII) which contains LMNs to innervate the muscles of facial expressions (Fig. 15-4).

Medulla

There are nine major cranial nerve nuclei in the medulla. The **cochlear** and **vestibular nuclear complexes** (not shown in Fig. 15-4) are lateral to the junction of the pons and medulla (see Chapters 9 and 10). The **nucleus solitarius** serves the sensory function of taste and has gustatory input from the facial nerve (CN VII; intermedius), vagus nerve (CN X), and glossopharyngeal nerve (CN IX). At the rostral medulla is the **salivary nucleus** (shared by the facial [CN VII], glossopharyngeal [CN IX], and vagus [CN X] nerves), a visceral motor nucleus responsible for controlling secretion from various glands. The **dorsal motor nucleus** of the vagus nerve (CN X) controls autonomic motor activity of various visceral organs. Medial to the dorsal motor nucleus is the **hypoglossal nucleus** (CN XII), whose LMNs innervate extrinsic and intrinsic muscles of the tongue. The nucleus solitarius, a visceral sensory nucleus responsible for taste, nausea, heart rate, respiration, and blood pressure, is shared by the facial and glossopharyngeal nerves. Lateral to the nucleus solitarius lies the spinal trigeminal nucleus. The **nucleus ambiguus**, which is between the inferior olivary nucleus and the **spinal trigeminal nucleus**, contains LMNs and controls the movements of the laryngeal and pharyngeal muscles. This nucleus is also shared by the glossopharyngeal (CN IX) and vagus (CN X) nerves. The spinal

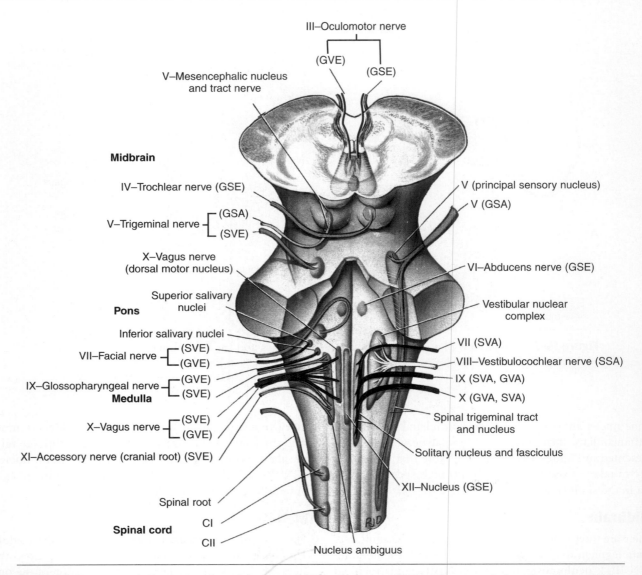

Figure 15-3 Intramedullary cranial nerves, their nuclei of origin, and their functional classifications. *GSA*, general somatic afferent; *GSE*, general somatic efferent; *GVA*, general visceral afferent; *GVE*, general visceral efferent; *SSA*, special somatic afferent; *SVA*, special visceral afferent; *SVE*, special visceral efferent.

accessory nucleus (CN XI), the only cranial nerve nucleus outside the brainstem, is located in the ventral horns of the upper cervical (C1–C5) segments.

PATHWAYS

Motor or Efferent Pathways

The cranial nerve nuclei receive their motor projections from the **corticobulbar fibers** (Fig. 15-6). Corticobulbar fibers arise from the motor cells (**upper motor neurons**; UMNs) in the lower part of the **precentral cortex** (Brodmann area 4) and descend through the internal capsule to synapse on the motor cranial nerve nuclei (LMN) in the brainstem. Before synapsing on the cranial nerve motor nuclei, most corticobulbar fibers cross the midline at different brainstem locations. However, a substantial **bilateral** cortical innervation of the cranial motor nuclei has been reported for the muscles of the face, jaw, larynx, and pharynx.

Cortical damage interrupts the corticobulbar projections, resulting in UMN symptoms of increased deep tendon reflexes and contralateral paralysis (see Chapter 14). The many aberrant corticobulbar fibers in the brainstem provide for safety from damage to cranial nerve motor functions; therefore, cortical lesions generally do not result in profound spasticity and weakness in the cranial muscles. Lesions of the brainstem cranial motor nuclei and their axons (nerves) produce LMN syndrome, which is characterized by **flaccid tone**, muscle paralysis, absent reflexes, fibrillations (single denervated fiber), fasciculation (spon-

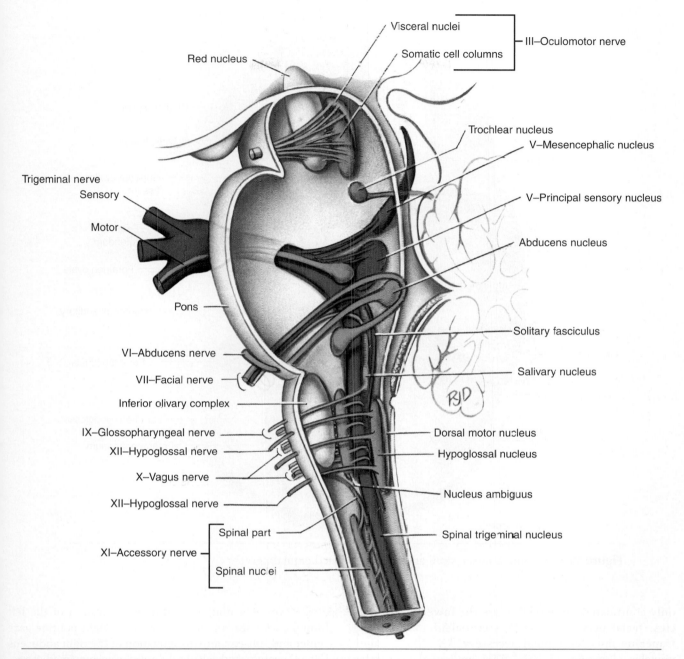

Figure 15-4 Midsagittal view of a hollow brainstem showing the intramedullary nuclei of the cranial nerves. All the cranial nerves and associated nuclei, except the vestibulocochlear nerve, are presented.

taneous firing of motor units), and **atrophy** of the muscles (see Chapters 11 and 14).

Sensory or Afferent Pathways

Most of the sensory pathways of the cranial nerves consist of three-order nuclei and their fibers (Fig. 15-7; see Chapter 7). The cell bodies of the **first-order fibers** are outside the CNS. The **second-order fibers**, with cell bodies in the gray matter of the brainstem, cross the midline and terminate in the thalamus. The **third-order fibers**, with cell bodies in the ventral **posterior medial nucleus** of the thalamus,

project to the sensory cortex in the parietal lobe. Smell, audition, and vision are exceptions to the sensory organization of three-order cells and fibers.

INNERVATION PATTERN

The corticobulbar regulation of several branchial motor nuclei is bilateral (Fig. 15-8; Table 15-5). The nuclei of such cranial nerves receive corticobulbar input from both sides of the motor cortex (Box 15-4). Muscles with

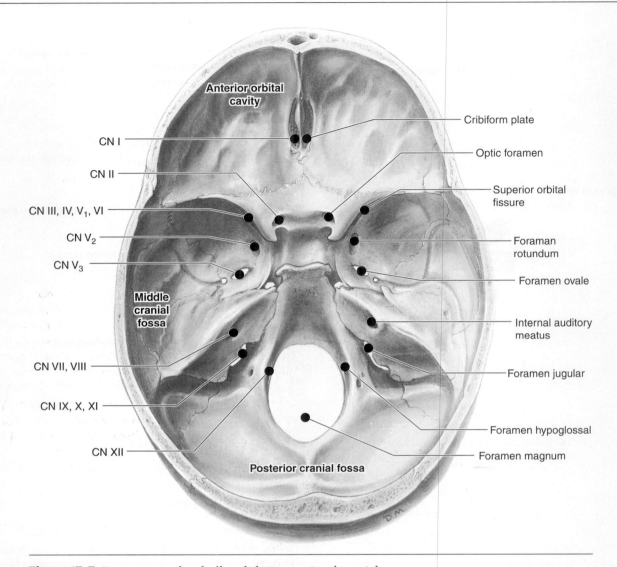

Figure 15-5 Foramina in the skull and their associated cranial nerves.

only contralateral innervation are the **lower facial muscles** (facial nerve [CN VII]), **sternocleidomastoid** and **trapezius muscles** (spinal accessory [CN XI]), **tongue muscles** (hypoglossal [CN XII]), and **ocular muscles** (oculomotor [CN III], trochlear [CN IV], and abducens [CN VI]). Owing to bilateral innervation, a unilateral cortical lesion will not profoundly impair the function of the facial (CN VII; upper face), trigeminal (CN V), vagal (CN X), and glossopharyngeal (CN IX) nerves. The functions of these cranial nerves are severely affected only in the case of bilateral cortical destruction or after a LMN lesion. The presence of many collateral corticobulbar fibers further provides protection from spasticity in the cranial muscles in the case of pyramidal (UMN) lesions.

The pyramidal tract provides minor cortical regulation of eye movement (oculomotor [CN III], trochlear [CN IV], and abducens [CN VI]). For the innervation of ocular muscles, a powerful corticobulbar projection to the **midbrain conjugate gaze** control center coordinates the movement

of the eyes as a unit. For example, activation of the left frontal cortex leads to activation of the right pontine gaze center and subsequently to activation of the right abducens (lateral rectus) and left oculomotor nucleus (medial rectus). This results in contraction of the right lateral rectus and left medial rectus muscles and turns the eyes toward the right.

CRANIAL NERVES AND THEIR SENSORIMOTOR FUNCTIONS

Olfactory Nerve

The olfactory system consists of the afferent neuron in the olfactory mucosal membrane, the olfactory bulb, the olfactory tract, part of the temporal cortex, and a limited region of the inferior fronto-orbital cortex. The cortical olfactory area is located on the basomedial surface of the cerebral hemisphere and includes the **uncus, periamyg-**

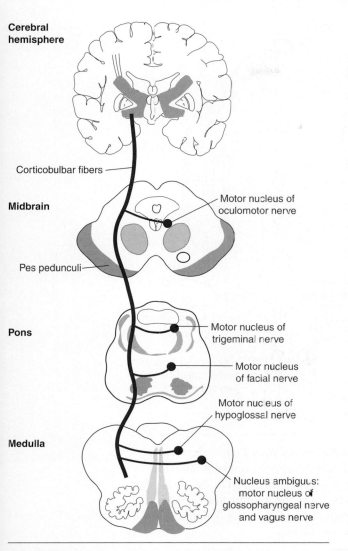

Cerebral hemisphere

Corticobulbar fibers

Midbrain

Motor nucleus of oculomotor nerve

Pes pedunculi

Pons

Motor nucleus of trigeminal nerve

Motor nucleus of facial nerve

Motor nucleus of hypoglossal nerve

Medulla

Nucleus ambiguus: motor nucleus of glossopharyngeal nerve and vagus nerve

Figure 15-6 Corticobulbar fibers projecting to the contralateral motor nuclei of the oculomotor, trigeminal, vagal, and hypoglossal nerves in the brainstem.

daloid nucleus, anterior **hippocampal gyrus**, and parts of the temporal lobe.

Special Visceral Afferent

The SVA begins with neurosensory cells that transduce odor molecules. These are embedded in the olfactory epithelium in the roof of the nasal cavity, which is ~2 cm² (Fig. 15-9A; Table 15-6). Also found in the epithelium are the sensory endings of the trigeminal nerve (CN V), which responds to noxious sensation, such as concentrated ammonia. The unmyelinated axons of the neurosensory (olfactory) neurons group together to form the olfactory nerve (CN I). The olfactory receptor cells are unique: they are the only mammalian neurons that are replaced with new cells in 30–60 days. The unmyelinated olfactory fibers that form the nerve pass through the foramina in the ethmoid cribriform plate, terminating on the **mitral** and other

cells in the olfactory bulbs on the basal surface of the frontal lobe. The axonal projections from the mitral and associated cells form the olfactory tract, which travels caudally to the **olfactory trigone** area and divides into subtracts (Fig. 15-9B).

The olfactory tract divides into three major bundles (striae) of fibers: **intermediate**, **medial**, and **lateral**. The intermediate stria terminates in the trigone area and the **anterior perforated substance** anterior to the **optic chiasm** (Fig. 15-9B). Some medial stria fibers terminate in the **subcallosal area** and are closely associated with the limbic lobe (see Figs. 2-10 and 2-14). Other medial stria fibers cross the midline through the **anterior commissure** and connect with the opposite olfactory bulb. Fibers of the lateral stria, which form the central connections, travel along the anterior perforated substance and terminate in the vicinity of the medial temporal lobe of the (primary) olfactory area, called the **pyriform cortex** because of its pear shape (Fig. 15-9C). This area includes the cortex of the uncus, the amygdaloid nucleus, and the anterior part of the parahippocampal gyrus. The primary cortical region mediates olfactory awareness. Various projections from the primary olfactory cortex to the neocortex and limbic region help integrate smell with the emotional brain and serve many vegetative functions. These extrinsic olfactory connections include projections from the olfactory cortex to the **orbitofrontal cortex** and the **insular cortex**, which plays a role in odor discrimination. Direct olfactory projections to the hypothalamus play an important role in feeding behavior.

Clinical Concerns

At approximately 65 years of age, humans gradually begin to lose acuity of the sense of smell. This is largely caused by ongoing degeneration of olfactory sensory cells. The primary complaint in many such patients with chemosensory disturbance is the loss of taste, which is mostly related to impaired olfaction. A lesion that interrupts the olfactory fibers or the primary olfactory cells causes **anosmia**, a condition in which the ability to smell is partially or fully impaired. Two associated conditions are **hyposmia** and **hyperosmia**. In hyposmia, there is decreased olfactory sensation, whereas in hyperosmia there is an abnormally acute sense of smell. Olfactory loss is also seen in patients with seizure activity involving the uncinate fibers (uncinate fits) in addition to altered consciousness.

Olfactory loss may involve the neural mechanism of olfaction unilaterally or bilaterally. Bilateral lesions drastically restrict olfactory function. Olfactory nerve function is tested by asking the patient to identify various odors, such as coffee, using one nostril at one time.

Optic Nerve

Many anatomists do not consider the optic nerve (CN II) to be a cranial nerve because it, like the olfactory nerve (CN I), is merged with the brain and functions like a CNS tract. The optic system is a brain system because the retina

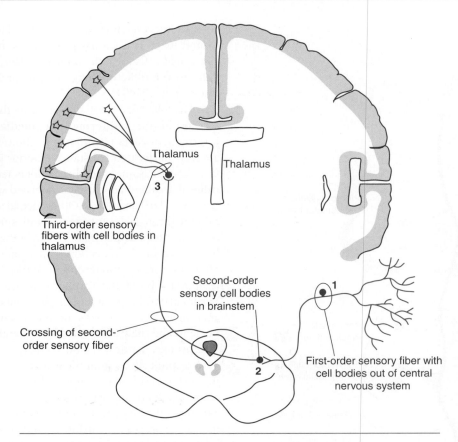

Figure 15-7 Cranial nerve fibers mediating sensation. First-order fibers, with cell bodies external to the central nervous system, transmit information from the periphery to the second-order nuclei in the brainstem. Second-order fibers, with cell bodies in the brainstem, cross the midline and terminate in the thalamus. Third-order fibers, with cell bodies in the thalamus, project to the lower parts of the postcentral gyrus.

is derived from the neural tube. The olfactory system, however, is a sensory system, and its cells are neural crest derivatives. In this book, both are treated as cranial nerves.

Special Somatic Afferent

Light rays entering the eye are bent (refracted) by the curvature of the cornea and lens and converge on rods and cones in the retina (Table 15-7; see Fig. 8-9). The rods populate the peripheral regions of the retina and are sensitive to white light and movement. Rods are capable of considerable adaptation to low-intensity stimulation, such as that needed for night vision. The cones populate mostly the central retinal region (**fovea**), where visual acuity is highest. Cones mediate color vision, which results from the differential sensitivity of the three classes of cones: red, green, and blue. The retina also contains interneurons, which modulate and transform visual input, including bipolar cells and retinal ganglion cells.

The photoreceptor cells transduce light energy into local potentials. These potentials travel to the bipolar cells, which, by means of local potentials and neurotransmitters, affect the excitability of the ganglion, whose axonal processes transmit the action potentials through the optic nerve, optic chiasm, and optic tract. Ganglion cell fibers from the nasal half of the retina cross the midline at the optic chiasm; ganglion cell axons from the temporal retina do not cross through the chiasm. Optic tract fibers, which are formed by the postchiasmatic fibers, travel posteriorly around the pes pedunculi and terminate in the **lateral geniculate body**, the thalamic relay center for vision. Geniculocalcarine projections, also called optic radiations, travel to the visual cortex in the occipital lobe. The visual cortex, in the upper and lower banks of the calcarine fissure, receives projections from both eyes. Because the eyes are separated in space, two views of the visual world are integrated by the visual cortex into a single clear image, with the binocular disparity contributing to the depth perception. In addition to the primary visual cortex in the pole and medial surface of the occipital lobe, other specialized visual cortical areas in the lateral cortex analyze visual information in terms of color, motion, location, depth, and spatial pattern.

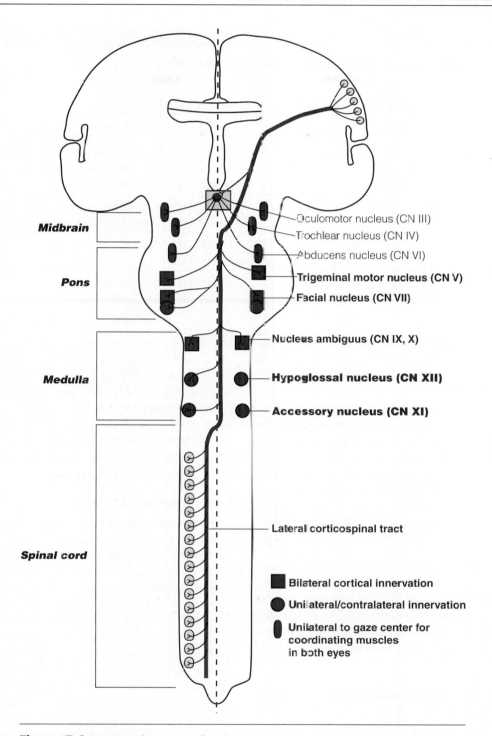

Figure 15-8 Neuronal pattern of unilateral and bilateral innervation of the cranial nerve nuclei.

Clinical Concerns

Injury to any part of the visual pathway results in selected visual field loss. The area and type of loss depend on the site and extent of the lesion. A lesion of the entire optic nerve leads to complete blindness in one eye. Cerebrovascular accidents and neuritis, an inflammation of the optic nerve, are common causes of optic nerve disorders. Common visual field defects are **bitemporal hemianopsia, homonymous** hemianopsia, **homonymous superior quadrantanopia,** and **homonymous inferior quadrantanopia** (see Fig. 8-14).

Visual field loss can be informally tested by having the patient close one eye and fix the other eye on a point straight ahead. The clinician then moves his or her index finger, with arm outstretched, from the periphery to the midline from all directions (left, right, up, and down) and the patient is asked to report the point at which the finger

Table 15-5

Supranuclear Innervation of the Cranial Nerve Motor Nuclei

Cranial Nerve	Associated Function	Innervation Pattern
CN III, IV, and VI	Ocular movements	Contralateral to gaze control
CN V	Mastication	Bilateral (function spared after unilateral lesions)
CN VII	Upper face	Bilateral (spared after unilateral lesions)
	Lower face	Contralateral (face affected after a unilateral lesion)
CN IX and X	Swallowing	Bilateral (transient affection after unilateral lesions)
	Phonation	Bilateral (transient affection after unilateral lesions)
CN XI	Head turning	Contralateral
	Shoulder shrugging	Contralateral
CN XII	Tongue movement	Contralateral

is seen. Any difference in clarity and delay in seeing can be a clue to a visual field defect.

Oculomotor Nerve

All ocular movements are controlled by six extrinsic muscles: **medial rectus**, **lateral rectus**, **superior rectus**, **inferior rectus**, **superior oblique**, and **inferior oblique**. These muscles are controlled by three cranial nerves: the oculomotor (CN III), trochlear (CN IV), and abducens (CN VI), which are interconnected through the **medial longitudinal fasciculus** (**MLF**), a longitudinal fiber bundle in the brainstem (see Chapters 3 and 10). The combined function of these cranial nerves is to track moving objects and maintain visual fixation by regulating conjugate eye movements.

Functional components of the oculomotor nerve consist of the somatic and visceral motor nuclei (Table 15-8). The somatic motor nucleus innervates the extrinsic ocular muscles. The visceral motor (Edinger-Westphal) nucleus provides parasympathetic projections to the constrictor (circular) fibers of the **iris** and **ciliary muscle**, regulating pupil-

lary constriction in response to light and enabling the lens to accommodate for near vision (see Chapter 8). The oculomotor nuclear complex is in the upper tegmentum (**periaqueductal gray**) of the midbrain at the level of the superior colliculus under the **cerebral aqueduct**. The oculomotor fibers travel ventrally through the **midbrain tegmentum**, the **red nucleus**, and **basis pedunculi**, exiting from the ventral surface of the brainstem at the junction of the pons and midbrain (Figs. 15-10, and 15-11).

General Somatic Efferent

The oculomotor nerve (CN III) splits in the orbital cavity to supply the following ocular muscles: superior rectus, medial rectus, inferior rectus, and inferior oblique (Fig. 15-11). In addition, the oculomotor fibers innervate the **levator palpebrae superioris**, the muscle responsible for raising the eyelid and implicated in **ptosis** (upper eyelid paralysis). Each muscle makes an individual contribution to the total eye movement: the superior rectus moves the eyeball upward and inward, the medial rectus adducts the eyeball medially, and the inferior rectus moves the eyeball downward and inward. The inferior oblique and the superior rectus contribute to upward gazing and rotating the eye upward and outward (Table 15-12). These ocular muscles never work alone; they require synergistic participation from all of the muscles of the eye. For example, looking to the left entails contraction of the lateral rectus of the left eye and the medial rectus of the right eye, with simultaneous relaxation of their opposite muscles.

General Visceral Efferent

The Edinger-Westphal nucleus, the visceral oculomotor nucleus, is responsible for the parasympathetic innervation of the intrinsic eye muscles, such as the **iris** and **ciliary muscles** (Figs. 15-10 and 15-12). It supplies the circular (constrictor) fibers of the iris, causing pupillary

BOX 15-4

Bilaterality of Innervation

The cranial nerves are known to have a unique cortical control pattern, in which the nuclei of some cranial nerves receive corticobulbar input from both sides of the motor cortex. This bilaterality of innervation ensures that a unilateral cortical lesion does not profoundly impair the function of some of the cranial nerves. Only bilateral cortical destruction severely affects cranial nerve functioning.

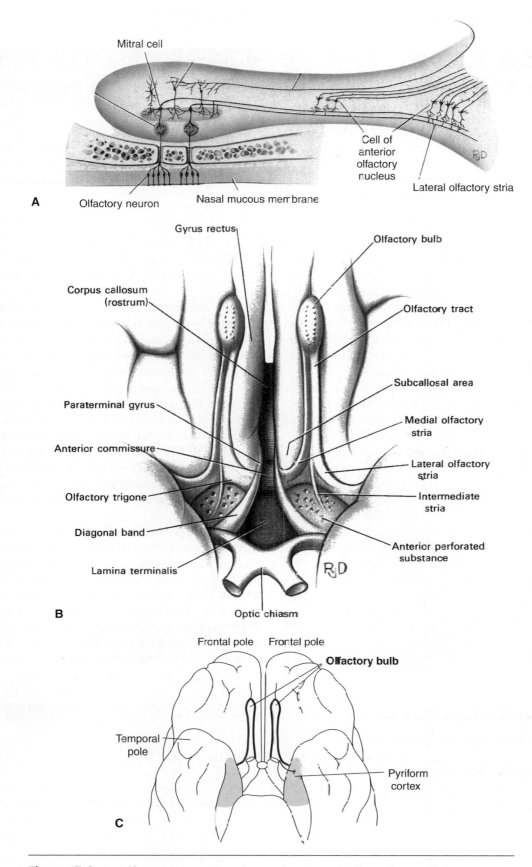

Figure 15-9 A. Olfactory neurons in the nasal mucosa, bulb, and centrally projecting fibers. B. An anatomic view of the olfactory structures on the ventral surface of the frontal lobe from the bulb to the anterior perforated substance. C. Primary olfactory (pyriform) cortex and associated structures on the ventral surface of the frontal and temporal lobes.

Table 15-6

Functional Description of the Olfactory Nerve

Classification	Nuclei	Function
SVA (special visceral afferent)	Neuroepithelial cells in nasal mucosa	Regulates smell

Table 15-7

Functional Description of the Optic Nerve

Classification	Nuclei	Function
SSA (special somatic afferent)	Retinal ganglion cells	Serves vision

constriction in response to light. The light reflex does not involve the visual cortex. The parasympathetic projections of the Edinger-Westphal nucleus to the ciliary muscles regulate the refractive power of the lens by changing its shape during the accommodation reflex for near vision, which requires the participation of the visual cortex, as one has to see something to focus on it. The neuronal circuitry difference between the light and the accommodation reflexes is used to evaluate the extent of CNS damage.

As light shines into an eye, the pupils in both eyes promptly react by constricting. The pupillary light reflex in both eyes is mediated through the Edinger-Westphal nucleus of both sides (Fig. 15-12; Table 15-9; see Fig. 8-9). Visual impulses from the retina travel via the optic tract, passing through the LGB and brachium of the **superior colliculus** to reach the **pretectal area** in the midbrain. The **pretectal nucleus**, anterior to the superior colliculus, projects to both Edinger-Westphal nuclei in the oculomotor complex. The Edinger-Westphal nuclei, which receive crossed and uncrossed projections, send the preganglionic parasympathetic projections along the oculomotor fibers to the ciliary ganglion lateral to the eyeball in the orbit. The postganglionic fibers from the ciliary ganglion supply the constrictor (circular) pupillary fibers of the iris (Fig. 15-12). The pupillary constriction in the illuminated eye is the direct light reflex; that in the contralateral eye is the consensual reflex. In the dark, the

activity of the Edinger-Westphal nucleus is inhibited, and the dilation of the pupils is activated through the sympathetic projections to the dilator (radial) fibers of the iris muscle.

The accommodation reflex refers to adjustments in the shape of the lens to keep a nearing object in focus. As noted earlier, it involves the visual cortex because an organism has to see something to focus on it. This reflex consists of three components: ocular convergence, pupillary constriction, and lens thickening. The reflex is tested by asking the patient to focus on an object moving closer to the eyes. The ability to focus on the nearing object is achieved as the medial rectus muscle contracts for ocular convergence. The ciliary muscle contracts to regulate lens thickening, which narrows the optic globe, releasing tension on the lens capsule and allowing the elastic lens to assume the natural rounded shape that is needed for near vision.

The neural mechanism responsible for the accommodation reflex is slightly different from that of the light reflex because it involves the visual cortex and superior colliculus. Impulses from the retina are relayed to the pretectal nucleus in the midbrain via the visual cortex and superior colliculus. The crossed and uncrossed parasympathetic fibers from the pretectal nucleus reach the ciliary muscle through the Edinger-Westphal nucleus and ciliary ganglion (Fig. 15-12). The lens is connected to the ciliary processes

Table 15-8

Functional Description of Oculomotor Nerve

Classification	Nuclei	Function
GSE (general somatic efferent)	Oculomotor (lower motor neuron) nucleus in midbrain	Responsible for eye movement; regulates the activity of all ocular muscles except superior oblique and lateral rectus; regulates levator palpebrae superioris (lid elevation)
GVE (general visceral efferent)	Edinger-Westphal nucleus in midbrain tegmentum Preganglionic parasympathetic projections to ciliary ganglion	Responsible for reflexive constriction of pupil and lens accommodation for near vision

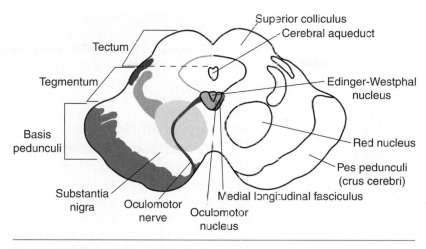

Figure 15-10 Section at the superior colliculus level showing the oculomotor nucleus and its fibers traveling through the midbrain tegmentum.

through the suspensory ligaments. In accommodation, the reflexive contraction of the ciliary muscles pulls the ciliary processes forward, reducing the tension in the suspensory ligaments (zonules of Zinn). Reducing the tension in the suspensory ligaments releases the tension on the lens capsule and allows the elastic lens to assume its natural rounded shape. Consequently, the lens acquires the greater refractive power needed for viewing near objects. The opposite happens during relaxation of the ciliary muscles. As the ciliary muscles relax, they put tension on the suspensory ligaments and lens capsule, causing the lens to flatten and lose its refractive power.

Clinical Concerns

Oculomotor nerve (CN III) pathology results in **external** and **internal ophthalmoplegia**. In external ophthalmo-

plegia, the extrinsic ocular muscles are paralyzed. This results in deviation of the ipsilateral eye to the lateral side (**lateral strabismus**) and **ptosis**, in which the eyelid droops because of paralysis of the levator palpebrae superioris.

In a normal physiologic state, the simultaneous activation of all ocular muscles maintains the eyes slightly deviated to the midline in the horizontal axis. The oculomotor nerve supplies the four extraocular muscles. Impairment of CN III may result in paralysis of those muscles, which causes lateral inferior deviation of the involved eye because of the unopposed action of the intact superior oblique (trochlear [CN V]) and lateral rectus muscles (abducens [CN VI]). A patient with oculomotor paralysis is likely to have difficulty looking up, down, and medially with the affected eye. Failure to direct both eyes toward an object (**strabismus**) in the direction

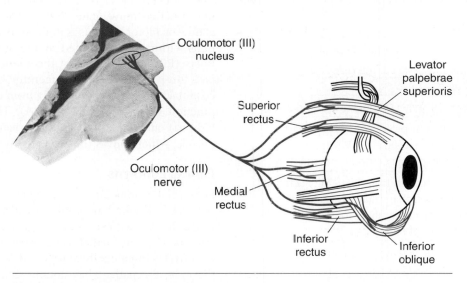

Figure 15-11 Oculomotor nucleus, course of its nerve fibers, and innervated ocular muscles.

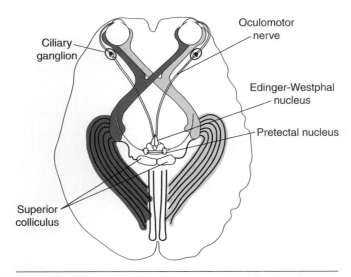

Figure 15-12 Pathway serving the visual reflexes. Retinal-tectal axons (*red*) leave the ipsilateral optic tract to synapse in the pretectal nucleus and related nuclei, which are interconnected through the posterior commissure (*red*). The direct light reflex is pupil constriction to light in the ipsilateral eye, and the consensual light reflex is pupil constriction in the contralateral eye.

opposite to the paralyzed side results in double vision (**diplopia**). A patient with left oculomotor nerve palsy is likely to have double vision when looking either straight or to the right (Fig. 15-13). A patient with ptosis may compensate for the eyelid paralysis by using the frontalis muscle (facial cranial nerve [CN VII]) to raise the eyelid.

Table 15-9

Neuronal Events of the Pupillary Light Reflex

Step	Event
1	Projection of light on retinal photosensors
2	Transmission of visual impulses on optic nerve and tract
3	Activation of pretectal nucleus in midbrain
4	Bilateral efferent projections (via posterior commissure) to Edinger-Westphal (parasympathetic oculomotor) nucleus
5	Efferent projections from bilaterally activated Edinger-Westphal nuclei through oculomotor nerve fibers to bilateral innervation of ciliary ganglion
6	Postganglionic activation of constrictor (circular) fibers of iris
7	Bilateral parasympathetic pupillary constriction

Internal ophthalmoplegia results from the interruption of the parasympathetic fibers to the iris and causes permanent dilation of the pupil (**mydriasis**). This occurs because the fibers of the sphincter muscle become paralyzed, and the sympathetic action on the dilator pupillary muscle fibers is unopposed.

Trochlear Nerve
General Somatic Efferent

The trochlear nerve (CN IV), the second nerve contributing to ocular movement, is the only cranial and motor nerve to exit dorsally from the brainstem (Figs. 15-3 and 15-4). The motor nucleus of the trochlear nerve (CN IV) is in the **periaqueductal gray matter** at the level of the **inferior colliculus** (Figs. 15-3 and 15-14*A*). The trochlear nerve (CN IV) fibers cross the midline in the **anterior medullary velum** and exit dorsally from the brainstem below the inferior colliculus. The nerve fibers enter the orbit with the oculomotor nerve (CN III) and innervate the **superior oblique muscle** (Table 15-10). Contraction of this muscle causes the eye to move downward and laterally (Fig. 15-14*B*).

Clinical Concerns

Damage to the trochlear nerve (CN IV) results in paralysis of the superior oblique muscle, causing difficulty in looking downward and outward. The eye is fixed with an upward medial gaze because the actions of the inferior oblique, superior, and medial recti muscles (oculomotor nerve [CN III]) are unopposed. An attempt to look down and outward results in diplopia because only one eye moves down and out, causing misalignment of the eyes.

Abducens Nerve
General Somatic Efferent

The abducens nerve (CN VI) is the third nerve contributing to ocular movements (Tables 15-11 and 15-12). The abducens motor nucleus is in the dorsal tegmentum of the pons within a loop formed by the facial nerve (CN VII) fibers (Fig. 15-4). Fibers of the abducens nerve (CN VI) pass through the pontine tegmentum and pierce the corticospinal tract, exiting anteriorly from the pontomedullary junction (Figs. 15-4 and 15-15*A*). The abducens nerve (CN VI) enters the orbit and innervates the lateral rectus muscle, which moves the eye laterally (Fig. 15-15*B*).

Clinical Concerns

Because of its long intracranial course, the abducens nerve (CN VI) is highly susceptible to disruption. Its injuries cause the affected eye to turn in medially (**medial strabismus**) because the medial rectus muscle (oculomotor nerve [CN III]) is functionally unopposed. With misalignment of the eyes, the patient has double vision (diplopia) when looking straight or to the affected side (Fig. 15-16). Isolated bilateral damage to the abducens nuclei and nerves results in

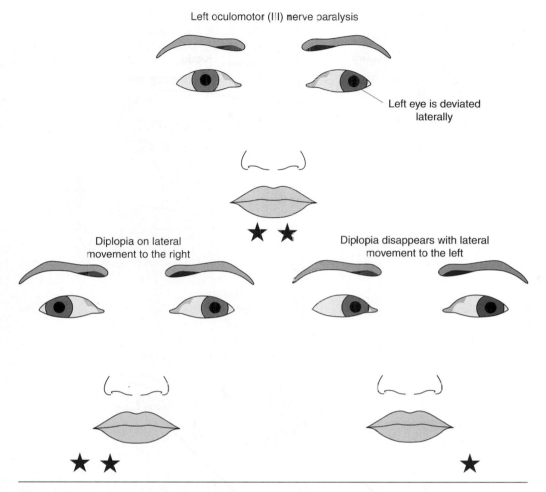

Figure 15-13 Double vision caused by oculomotor nerve paralysis. In left oculomotor paralysis, the eyelid droops (ptosis) and the eye moves laterally, making the eyes disconjugate. As a result, when looking straight ahead (*top*), the patient sees two images. The patient continues to see two images (*bottom left*) when looking to the right because the left paralyzed eye cannot move beyond the midline. However, a left movement of the right eye allows the eyes to conjugate (*bottom right*); hence the diplopia disappears.

medial deviation of both eyes because of unopposed activity of the medial rectus muscles.

The MLF is an important brainstem tract with inputs from the vestibular complex and neck muscles. It projects to the motor nuclei of the ocular cranial nerves: oculomotor (CN III), trochlear (CN IV), and abducens (CN VI) (see Chapter 10). It coordinates the movements of the eye muscles for gaze control and coordinates head position with eye movements. Lesions involving the MLF severely affect gaze control.

Trigeminal Nerve

The trigeminal nerve (CN V) is a functionally mixed nerve. As the principal sensory nerve for the head, face, orbit, and oral cavity, it mediates the sensations of pain, temperature, and discriminative touch (see Chapter 7). It has a small motor component that supplies the mastication (chewing) muscles along with other muscles (Table 15-13). The sensory and motor components together form the reflex arc for the jaw jerk reflex. It also mediates special somatic afferent (kinesthetic and proprioceptive awareness) information, which is responsible for stretch receptor feedback for the masticators.

General Somatic Afferent

The trigeminal nerve (CN V) is responsible for cutaneous (touch, pain, and temperature) and proprioceptive (awareness of posture and muscle movement) sensations from the face, head, oral and nasal cavities, sinuses, teeth, anterior two-thirds of the tongue, anterior half of the pinna, external auditory meatus, and external surface of the tympanic membrane. The sensory function of the trigeminal nerve (CN V) is organized along three neurons (Fig. 7-9): the **semilunar** or **trigeminal ganglion** (first-order nerve cell), **trigeminal complex** (second-order nerve cell), and **ventral posteromedial thalamic**

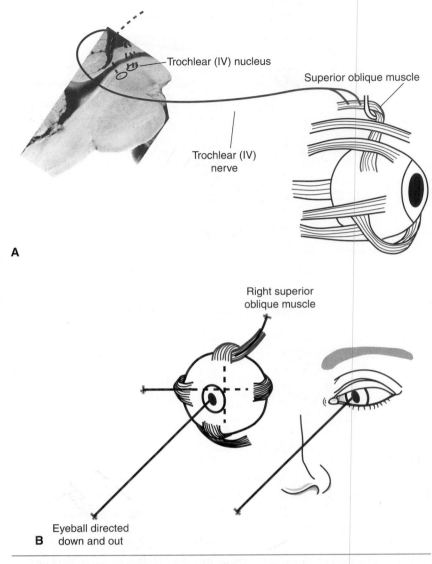

Figure 15-14 A. Trochlear nucleus, intramedullary course of the cranial nerve, and the innervated muscle. B. The functioning of the superior oblique muscle.

nucleus (third-order nerve cell). The trigeminal ganglion is external to the pons.

The trigeminal nuclear complex, consisting of the **chief sensory nucleus, descending spinal nucleus,** and **mesencephalic nucleus,** is in the lateral tegmentum of the pons.

Each of these sensory nuclei mediates different modalities of sensation. The chief sensory nucleus mediates discriminative sensation from the head and face. The descending spinal nucleus is primarily involved with pain and temperature and secondarily with diffuse touch. The descending spinal

Table 15-10
Functional Description of the Trochlear Nerve

Classification	Nuclei	Function
GSE (general somatic efferent)	Trochlear (lower motor neuron) nucleus in midbrain	Responsible for downward and outward eye movement by innervation of the contralateral skeletal muscle (superior oblique)

Table 15-11

Functional Description of the Abducens Nerve

Classification	Nuclei	Function
GSE (general somatic efferent)	Abducens (lower motor neuron) nucleus in tegmentum of pons	Responsible for lateral eye movements (abduction of eyeball) by innervation of skeletal muscle (lateral rectus)

Table 15-12

Cranial Nerves, Innervated Eye Muscles, and Their Functions

Cranial Nerve (Number)	Muscle	Functions
Oculomotor (III)	Inferior oblique	Elevates eyeball upward and outward
	Inferior rectus	Depresses eyeball downward and inward
	Medial rectus	Adducts eyeball medially and inward
	Superior rectus	Elevates eyeball upward and inward
	Levator palpebrae superioris	Elevates upper eyelid
Trochlear (IV)	Superior oblique (contralateral)	Rotates eyeball downward and outward
Abducens (VI)	Lateral rectus	Abducts eyeball laterally and outward

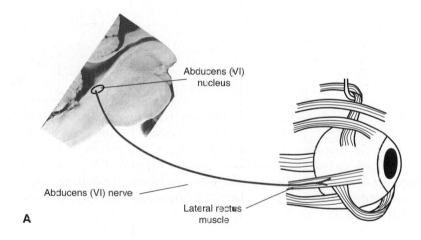

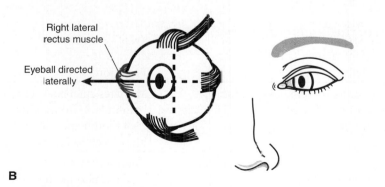

Figure 15-15 A. Abducens nucleus, intramedullary course of the cranial nerve, and the lateral rectus muscle. B. Lateral eye movement as regulated by the lateral rectus muscle.

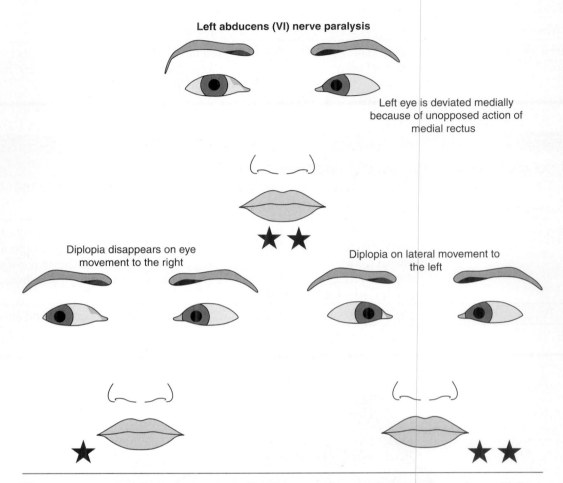

Figure 15-16 Double vision caused by left abducens nerve paralysis. With paralysis of left lateral rectus muscle, the left eye moves medially because of the unopposed action of the medial rectus muscle; thus the eyes become disconjugate. The patient sees two images (diplopia) when looking straight ahead (*top*). The patient has double vision even when looking to the left (*bottom right*) because the in-turned left eye remains disconjugate with the right eye. However, rightward movement of the right eye results in conjugation of the eyes (*bottom left*); thus the diplopia disappears.

Table 15-13

Functional Description of the Trigeminal Nerve

Classification	Nuclei	Function
GSA (general somatic afferent)	First order: trigeminal ganglion Second order: descending spinal nucleus and primary sensory nucleus Mesencephalic nucleus	Mediates cutaneous and proprioceptive sensation from face, front of head, and oral cavity (mucosa of mouth and tongue) Proprioception from jaw muscles
SVE (special visceral efferent)/BE (branchial efferent)	Motor (lower motor neuron) nucleus of trigeminal in pons	Controls jaw movements by innervation of muscles of mastication, tensor veli palatini, tensor tympani, and anterior belly of digastric muscle

nucleus and its tract also receive GSA projections from the facial (CN VII), glossopharyngeal (CN IX), and vagus (CN X) nerves. The mesencephalic nucleus contains the neurons that mediate proprioceptive sensation from the jaw muscles.

The trigeminal nerve has three sensory branches: **ophthalmic**, **maxillary**, and **mandibular** (Fig. 15-17). These nerves project sensory information from the entire face and part of the head to the semilunar ganglion (first-order sensory nucleus). The ophthalmic nerve mediates the sensations of touch, pain, temperature, and proprioception from the skin of the forehead, anterior scalp, vertex, eyeball, upper eyelid, cornea, conjunctivum, anterior and lateral surfaces of the nose, frontal and nasal sinuses, and tentorium cerebelli.

The maxillary nerve mediates sensation from the skin of the temples, posterior portion of the nose, upper cheeks, lower eyelids, and upper lips. Additional innervated oral structures include the upper gum, teeth (molar and premolar), mucosal membrane, and soft and hard palates. The maxillary nerve also receives sensations from the nasal cavity, maxillary sinus, and dura mater in the medial cranial fossa.

The mandibular nerve, the largest of the trigeminal branches, mediates sensations from the skin on the sides of the scalp, the mucosal membrane of the lower gum, the mouth, and the meninges of the anterior and middle cranial fossae. Additional structures innervated by the trigeminal nerve (CN V) include the anterior half of the pinna, external auditory meatus, external surface of the tympanic membrane, and the mucosa of the anterior two-thirds of the tongue.

Special Visceral Efferent/Branchial Efferent

The motor nucleus of the trigeminal nerve (CN V) lies in the midpons, and its fibers exit with the mandibular branch of the nerve (Figs. 15-4 and 15-18). The corticobulbar fibers from both motor cortices, although predominantly from the contralateral motor cortex, supply the trigeminal motor nucleus. The trigeminal motor nucleus controls the muscles

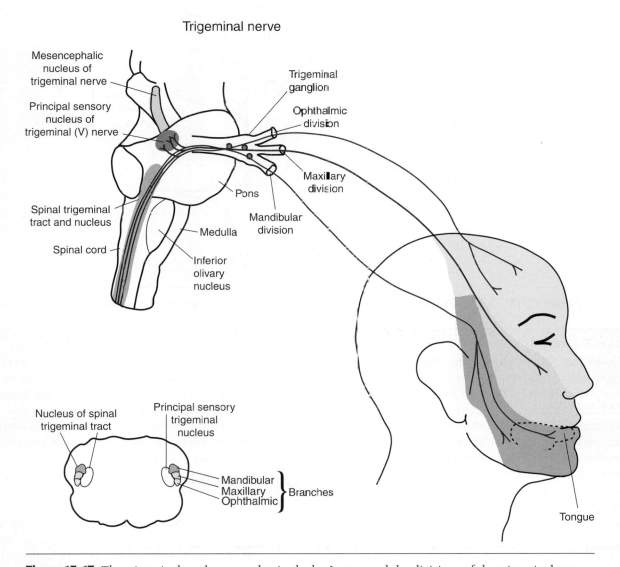

Trigeminal nerve

Figure 15-17 The trigeminal nuclear complex in the brainstem and the divisions of the trigeminal nerve.

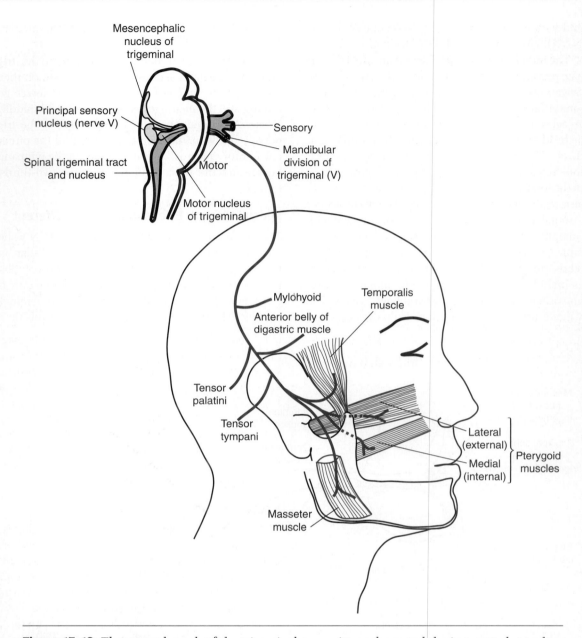

Figure 15-18 The motor branch of the trigeminal nerve, its nucleus, and the innervated muscles.

of mastication, which include the internal and external pterygoid, temporalis, and masseter; these are derived from the first branchial arch (Table 15-14). Other muscles supplied by the trigeminal motor nucleus include the mylohyoid, anterior belly of the digastric, tensor veli palatini (soft palate), and tensor tympani (middle ear). The muscles of mastication (masseter, internal and external pterygoid, and temporalis), working jointly with other muscles, regulate the rotary and lateral motions of the jaw needed for chewing and the up and down motions required for speech. The tensor veli palatini, on contraction, brings the soft palate to one side, which prevents food from entering the nasal pharynx.

The contraction of the tensor tympani muscle has a pulling effect on the malleus in the middle ear; on exposure to very intense sound, the trigeminal nerve (CN V) reflexively contracts the tensor tympani. Believed to be protective, this reflex restricts the movement of the tympanic membrane to prevent damage to the inner ear hair cells from loud sounds. Furthermore, this muscle also contracts to attenuate the internal sensation of sounds generated by the acts of chewing and swallowing.

Clinical Concerns

Sensory

The distribution of the trigeminal branches on the head, face, and oral cavity is well differentiated. Damage to any peripheral branch or branches results in an ipsilateral loss of sensation in the area of distribution for the nerve, which

Table 15-14

Muscles of Mastication and Their Functions

Muscle	Function
Lateral and external pterygoid	Depresses and protrudes mandible toward opposite side; regulates movement side to side
Masseter	Elevates, closes, and slightly protrudes mandible
Medial and internal pterygoid	Elevates and assists in mandible protrusion
Temporalis	Elevates and retracts mandible

includes the face, rostral tongue, teeth and gingiva, and the cavities of the nose, orbit, and mouth. The sneezing and blinking reflexes are also lost because of the interrupted innervation of the nasal mucosa and exterior surface of the eye (Table 15-20). The affected branch of the nerve and the related modality (touch, pain, temperature) of sensation can be determined by clinical testing with various sensory stimuli (cotton and pinprick) and by assessing the sneeze and corneal reflexes.

The most common trigeminal pathology is **trigeminal neuralgia** (pain), or **tic douloureux** (Box 15-5). It is marked by an excruciating chronic pain of unknown cause, usually in the territory of the ophthalmic or mandibular branch. This pain, often described as burning or stabbing, can be elicited by the slightest tactile stimulus in the trigger zones of the trigeminal distribution. The recurrent stabbing pain of trigeminal neuralgia has often been surgically treated by transecting the involved nerve branch or by sectioning the sensory nerve root.

Motor

An injury in the trigeminal motor nucleus or its fibers produces a LMN syndrome characterized by a flaccid paresis

or paralysis of the ipsilateral muscles of mastication. The jaw slightly deviates toward the side of the injury; this deviation is exaggerated on jaw protrusion. Along with this, the muscles twitch and gradually atrophy, and the jaw-jerk reflex is absent. Because the muscles of mastication receive corticobulbar projections from the bilateral motor cortices (Fig. 15-8), any unilateral cortical or corticobulbar (UMN) injury is likely to have only a mild effect on the strength of the masticator muscles. Bilateral cortical (UMN) lesions, however, produce marked paralysis of the masticators bilaterally, and the mandible hangs low, causing structural difficulty in the production of vowels and labial and lingual consonant sounds. The motor strength in patients with masticator palsy is assessed by asking them to bite down on a tongue depressor, move the jaw laterally against resistance, or open the jaw against resistance.

Facial Nerve

The facial nerve (CN VII) is functionally mixed. It is primarily a motor nerve for the facial muscles and the stapedius muscle of the middle ear, but it also contains a small sensory component (Table 15-15). The facial nerve complex supplies the muscles of the face and scalp (facial expression), which are derived from the second branchial arch. It also contains secretory parasympathetic efferents to the lacrimal, sublingual, and submandibular glands and to the secretory glands in the mouth and nasal cavities. The sensory function of the facial nerve (CN VII) involves the mediation of taste sensation from the anterior two-thirds of the tongue and the nasopharynx.

The facial nuclear complex, which is in the lateral caudal pons at the level of the abducens nucleus, consists of three nuclei: facial motor nucleus, superior salivatory nucleus, and nucleus solitarius (Figs. 15-3, 15-4, and 15-19). The facial nerve (CN VII) fibers pass upward lateral to the abducens nerve nucleus, loop over the top of the nucleus at the floor of the fourth ventricle, and descend to exit laterally in the caudal pons (the junction of the pons and medulla). After exiting, the nerve fibers enter the **internal acoustic meatus** along with the vestibulocochlear nerve (CN VIII) (Fig. 15-5). At the end of the meatus is the geniculate ganglion (Fig. 15-19), where the facial nerve (CN VII) fibers separate from the vestibulocochlear nerve,

BOX 15-5

Trigeminal Neuralgia

Trigeminal neuralgia (pain), or tic douloureux, is a common condition associated with trigeminal pathology. It is marked by an excruciating chronic pain of unknown cause, usually in the territory of the ophthalmic or mandibular branch. This pain, often described as burning or stabbing, can be elicited by the slightest tactile stimulus in the trigger zones of the trigeminal distribution. The recurrent stabbing pain of trigeminal neuralgia has often been surgically treated by transecting the involved nerve branch or by sectioning the sensory nerve root.

Table 15-15

Functional Description of the Facial Nerve

Classification	Nuclei	Function
GVE (general visceral efferent)	Superior salivatory nucleus: preganglionic parasympathetic to pterygopalatine, submandibular, and sublingual ganglia associated with glands	Regulates secretions from lacrimal gland and mucosal glands of nasopharynx and salivary secretion from sublingual and submaxillary glands
SVA (special visceral afferent)	First order: geniculate ganglion Second order: nucleus solitarius	Mediates taste sensations from anterior two-thirds mucosa of tongue and palate
SVE (special visceral efferent)/BE (branchial efferent)	Motor (lower motor neuron) nucleus in lateral pons	Innervates muscles of facial expression, scalp muscles, and stapedius muscle of the middle ear

enter the facial canal, and finally emerge from the **stylo-mastoid foramen**. Before exiting the stylomastoid foramen, the nerve diverges to supply the muscles of facial expression and the stapedius muscle in the middle ear.

General Visceral Efferent

The GVE fibers of the facial nerve (CN VII) arise from the superior salivatory nucleus in the brainstem and supply the lacrimal, submandibular, and sublingual glands with visceral efferent impulses. The GVE fibers leave the facial nerve (CN VII) at the geniculate ganglion and carry the preganglionic parasympathetic fibers to the pterygopalatine ganglion and lacrimal nucleus. Postganglionic projections from the lacrimal nucleus and pterygopalatine ganglion are parasympathetic to the lacrimal glands in the eye and the glands in the nose and palate. The lacrimal gland produces tears, and the glands in the palate secrete saliva (Fig. 15-19B).

Some of the GVE fibers continue in the facial nerve (CN VII) and join the **chorda tympani nerve**, a sensory branch of the facial nerve (CN VII) that merges with the lingual branch of the trigeminal nerve (CN V). These GVE fibers transmit impulses to the submaxillary ganglion. The submaxillary ganglion provides the secretory parasympathetic fibers to the sublingual and submandibular glands, which regulate the secretions from the mucous membrane in the mouth and pharynx (Fig. 15-19B).

Special Visceral Afferent

The sensory root of CN VII carries gustatory sensation from the taste buds in the anterior two-thirds of the tongue. These taste-carrying afferent fibers travel along the lingual nerve of the mandibular branch of the trigeminal nerve (CN V) and join the chorda tympani nerve. The fibers of the chorda tympani merge with the facial motor fibers toward the end of the facial canal in the middle ear. The sensory fibers with the first-order nerve cells in the geniculate ganglion enter the brainstem and terminate in the tractus and nucleus solitarius (Fig. 15-19), which sends this taste sensation to the sensory cortex through the **ventral posterior medial nucleus** of the thalamus.

Special Visceral Efferent/Branchial Efferent

The SVE/BE functional component of the facial nerve innervates all the muscles of facial expression. Fibers from the facial nucleus move toward the floor of the fourth ventricle in the pontine tegmentum and make a U-turn over the abducens nucleus (Figs. 15-3 and 15-4). The facial nerve (CN VII) fibers travel downward and exit from the lateral portion of the caudal pons (Fig. 15-19). After exiting, the nerve divides into the temporal, zygomatic, buccal, mandibular, and cervical branches to innervate the muscles of facial expression (depressor anguli oris, depressor labii inferioris, levator anguli oris, mentalis, orbicularis oculi, orbicularis oris, platysma, risorius, buccinator, and zygomaticus), which are jointly responsible for kissing, blowing, speaking, smiling, frowning, grimacing, raising the eyebrows, and exhibiting emotional expressions such as happiness, apathy, and sorrow (Table 15-16).

The buccinator muscle in particular contributes to swallowing by compressing the cheeks to prevent food accumulation in the buccal (facial) sulci. The fibers of these facial branches also innervate the extrinsic muscles of the ear, middle ear stapedius muscle, stylohyoid muscle, and posterior belly of the digastric muscle.

Clinical Information

The facial nerve (CN VII) fibers are responsible for different sensorimotor functions and thus take different routes to their destinations. The site of a given lesion determines which clinical signs emerge in the facial muscles. For example, an injury near the pons and surrounding area is likely to affect all three functions of the facial nerve (CN VII), resulting in paralysis of the ipsilateral facial muscles, excessive secretion from the glands, and loss of taste from the

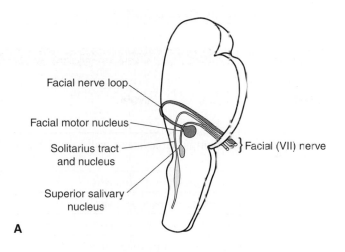

A

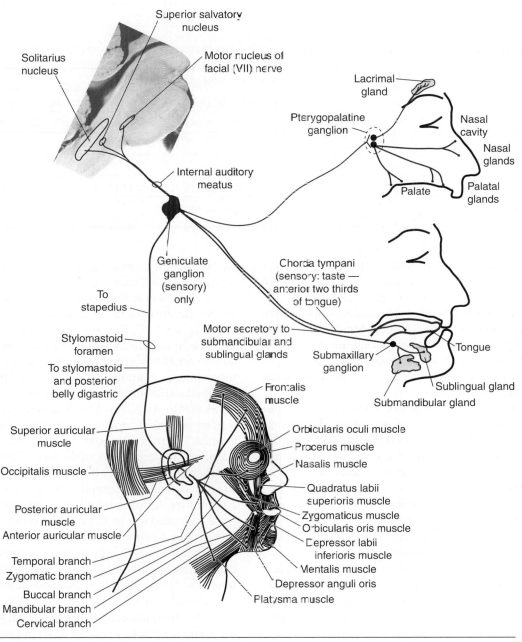

B

Figure 15-19 A. The facial nuclear complex in the brainstem. B. Sensorimotor branches of the facial nerve, and innervated structures (glands, oral pharynx, and muscles).

Table 15-16

Muscles of Facial Expression

Muscle	Function
Buccinator	Presses cheeks against teeth and forms stable lateral wall to oral cavity; prevents accumulation of food
Corrugator	Draws eyebrows together during expression of suffering
Depressor anguli oris	Draws mouth down and to the side in grimace and smile
Depressor labii inferioris	Draws corners of lips downward
Frontalis	Raises eyebrows and contributes to wrinkling of forehead.
Levator anguli oris	Draws corner of lips and raises angle of mouth
Levator labii superioris	Lifts angle of upper lip and turns it outward
Mentalis	Raises, protrudes, and wrinkles lower lip
Orbicularis oculi	Surrounds orbit; contributes to eye closing
Orbicularis oris	Contributes to closing lips, pressing lips against teeth, and shaping lips for speech
Platysma	Pulls lower lip and corner of mouth downward; draws neck skin up; contributes to smiling
Risorius	Retracts corners of mouth
Superioris alaeque nasi	Elevates and protrudes upper lip
Zygomaticus major	Functions as a sling with depressor anguli oris; draws angle of mouth up and to side
Zygomaticus minor	Raises upper lip, contributing to a broad smile

anterior two-thirds of the tongue (Fig. 15-19). An injury in the facial nerve (CN VII) fibers at or beyond the stylomastoid foramen, where its fibers separate, is likely to result in paralysis of the ipsilateral half of the facial muscles, sparing glandular secretion and taste sensation. Similarly, an injury to the chorda tympany fibers before they merge with the facial motor root affects only taste sensation from the anterior two-thirds of the tongue and secretion from sublingual and submandibular glands.

Involvement of the GVE fibers to the pterygopalatine ganglion causes secretory dysfunctions of the glands in the eye and palate. Interruption of the efferents to the middle ear causes paralysis of the stapedius muscle (working jointly with the tensor tympani); impaired control of stapedius results in **hyperacusia**, a condition in which normal sounds seem very loud. The stapedius muscle, when functioning properly, reflexively dampens the ear drum and constricts ossicular movements, a reflex function that protects the delicate organ of Corti from extreme movement.

The corticobulbar fibers differentially innervate the upper and lower face muscles (Figs. 15-8 and 15-20; Box 15-6). The motor nucleus that controls the lower half of the face receives projections from the **contralateral** motor cortex alone. However, the facial nucleus innervating the upper facial muscles (frontalis and orbicularis) receives corticobulbar projections from both motor cortices (**bilateral innervation**). This scheme of motor innervation

has significant clinical implications for UMN (supranuclear) and LMN (internuclear) syndromes.

A dysfunction in the unilateral motor cortex (UMN) affects the muscles in the contralateral lower half of the face (Fig. 15-20A). The upper facial muscles are spared in the case of a contralateral cortical lesion. The patient is able to wrinkle the forehead and close the eye, because these muscles continue to receive partial projections from the **ipsilateral motor cortex**. Complete destruction of either the facial nucleus (LMN), which involves the nuclear regions for both the upper and the lower face, or a bilateral cortical lesion is necessary to cause paralysis of all the upper and lower muscles in the face (Fig. 15-20B); it produces disastrous effects on the articulation of labial and labiodental sounds. Bilateral corticobulbar (UMN) lesions, also known as pseudobulbar palsy, produces bilateral facial palsy and results in profound impairments of motor speech (see Chapter 14). Patients lose delicate and discrete motor control, and muscles become paralyzed. In bilateral facial paralysis, the lips may be parted at rest and remain so during a smile and/or speech attempts.

A condition commonly associated with facial nerve (CN VII) dysfunctioning is **Bell palsy**, an LMN syndrome. It is characterized by a sudden onset of paralysis of all ipsilateral upper and lower facial muscles (Fig. 15-20B). The muscles of the lower face sag, the fold around the lip and nose (nasolabial fold) flattens, and the palpebral fissure

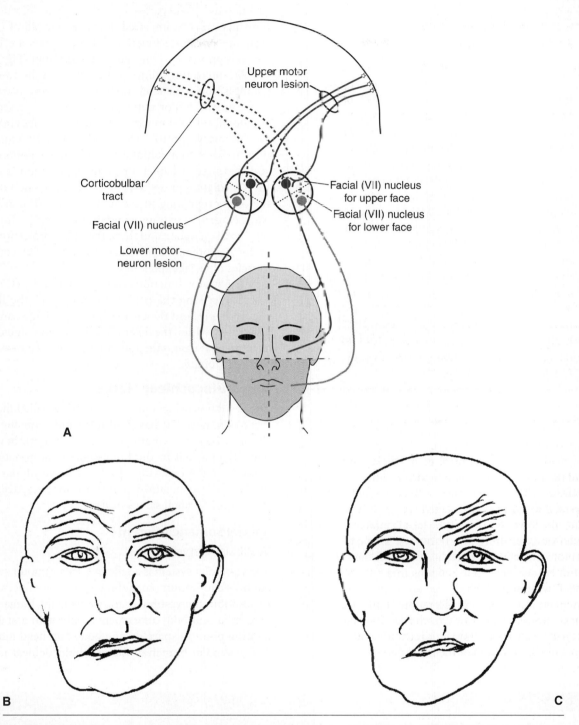

Figure 15-20 A. Distribution of the facial nerve fibers carrying unilateral and bilateral projections from the cortex. The upper portion of the face receives bilateral cortical projections, and the lower half of the face receives efferent commands from the contralateral motor cortex only. This differential neuronal organization for the facial muscles accounts for different patterns of facial paralysis after upper and lower motor neuron lesions. B. In upper motor neuron syndrome, the patient exhibits only lower facial palsy (loss of the nasolabial fold and sagging of the lower mouth) and has preserved strength in the frontalis and ocular muscles. C. In lower motor neuron syndrome (Bell palsy), the entire side of the face is paralyzed.

BOX 15-6

Facial Innervation

The cortical control of the facial muscles is somewhat atypical. The motor nucleus that controls the lower half of the face receives projections from the contralateral motor cortex alone, whereas the facial motor nucleus innervating the upper facial muscles (frontalis and orbicularis) receives corticobulbar projections from both motor cortices (bilateral innervation). This scheme of motor innervation has differential clinical implications for UMN (supranuclear) and LMN (internuclear) syndromes. A unilateral motor cortex lesion (UMN) affects only the muscles in the contralateral lower face, and the patient is able to wrinkle the forehead and close the eye, because these muscles continue to receive partial projections from the ipsilateral motor cortex. Bilateral corticobulbar (UMN) lesions produces bilateral facial palsy and results in profound impairments of facial function and motor speech.

widens. On the side of the lesion, the patient is unable to wrinkle the forehead, close the eye, show the teeth, or purse the lips. With no motor control of the facial muscles, the corner of the mouth droops and food and saliva accumulate in the affected side of the mouth. The paralyzed side of the face is pulled toward the unaffected side. While the person is smiling, the lower portion of the face is pulled toward the unaffected side, resulting in a transverse shape of the lips. Furthermore, the corneal reflex is absent on the side of the lesion, but corneal sensation remains intact (Table 15-20). Additional symptoms include impairments of sublingual and submandibular salivary secretion, hyperacusis, and loss of taste from the anterior two-thirds of the tongue.

Bell palsy may result from a degenerative inflammatory injury or from an infection of the facial nerve (CN VII) after its exit from the brainstem. Depending on the site of the lesion, sensory and parasympathetic (gland secretions) functions may also be impaired. For example, all of the motor, secretory, and taste functions of the nerves are lost if the lesion is proximal to the geniculate ganglion (Fig. 15-19).

An interesting clinical observation in the case of facial paralysis from a bilateral supranuclear lesion (pseudobulbar palsy) in the motor cortex (UMN) is the preservation of emotional expression while the facial muscles are paralyzed for voluntary control. The paralyzed facial muscles continue to respond involuntarily to genuine emotional stimuli and states (see Chapter 14). One explanation is that pathways mediating preserved emotional expression differ from the ones originating in the motor cortex. Emotional pathways consist of extrapyramidal integrated prefrontal, limbic, basal ganglia, and hypothalamic projections to the brainstem premotor reticular generator that controls the muscles of facial expression.

The motor functions of the facial nerve (CN VII) are tested by asking the patient to smile, part the lips, show the teeth, puff out the cheeks, pucker the lips, and express emotions, while the examiner looks for signs of facial asymmetry. Sugar, salt, and vinegar are used to assess taste from the tongue.

Vestibulocochlear Nerve

The vestibulocochlear nerve (CN VIII) is called the vestibuloacoustic nerve. It has vestibular and acoustic branches (Table 15-17; see Chapters 9 and 10). Both branches are laterally attached to the brainstem at the junction of the medulla and pons (Fig. 15-1). The vestibular division mediates head position (equilibrium) in space, whereas the acoustic branch serves hearing.

Special Somatic Afferent

Vestibular Nerve

The vestibular system is a reflexive sensorimotor system that controls equilibrium, including regulation of neck position. In addition, the vestibular apparatus helps humans coordinate head and body movements and retain a stable visual fixation point in space during body and head movements. The vestibular branch of the vestibulocochlear nerve (CN

Table 15-17

Functional Description of the Vestibulocochlear Nerve

Classification	Nuclei	Function
SSA (special somatic afferent)	First order: superior and inferior vestibular ganglia Second order: vestibular nuclei in caudal pons	Maintains equilibrium and head orientation in space
SSA (special somatic afferent)	First order: spiral ganglia Second order: cochlear nuclei in caudal pons	Mediates audition

VIII) originates from the **vestibular** (superior and inferior) **ganglia** equivalent of the **dorsal root ganglia** (DRG) neurons in the internal auditory meatus. The distal fibers of the vestibular ganglia innervate the hair cells in the cristae of the semicircular canals, saccule, and utricle. Their proximal axons make up the vestibular nerve and project impulses from the hair cells to the vestibular complex in the floor of the medulla's fourth ventricle (see Fig. 10-4). The vestibular nuclei send ascending projections to the flocculonodular lobe of the cerebellum, reticular formation, MLF, and motor nuclei of other cranial and spinal nerves (see Chapter 10). The descending projections from the vestibular nuclei to the spinal cord coordinate the limbs for standing balance. The importance of the vestibular system becomes evident in patients whose body equilibrium is impaired by vestibular dysfunctioning, as in **Ménière disease** or because of a **vestibulocochlear schwannoma**.

Auditory Nerve

The acoustic fibers of the vestibulocochlear nerve (CN VIII), which serve hearing, originate in the spiral ganglia (equivalent to DRG neuron); the peripheral processes of the cells in the spiral ganglia innervate the hair cells in the organ of Corti in the inner ear. The proximal axons of the spiral ganglion, the primary cell bodies of the auditory nerve, mediate auditory impulses to the cochlear nuclei in the rostrolateral medulla (see Fig. 9-6). Some of the auditory fibers from the cochlear nuclei ascend ipsilaterally, whereas several others cross the midline through the **trapezoid bodies**. Most of the crossed auditory fibers terminate in the **superior olivary nucleus**, although some bypass it and ascend to the midbrain.

Besides transmitting the information, the function of the superior olivary nucleus is to compare the timing of the auditory signals received from the two ears, which provides the basis for the judging the sound source direction. The projections from the superior olivary nucleus form the **lateral lemniscus**, which ascends to the inferior colliculus of the midbrain. The fibers from the inferior colliculus travel through the brachium of the **inferior colliculus** to the **medial geniculate body** of the thalamus. The auditory fibers from the thalamus pass posterior to the internal capsule, then project to the primary auditory cortex in the temporal lobe. The auditory nerve has two important characteristics: its crossed and uncrossed fibers result in bilateral projections to the cortex and throughout its projections to the brain, a spatial tonotopic representation in tract fibers of various frequencies is discretely maintained.

Clinical Concerns

Injuries to the vestibulocochlear nerve are associated with disturbances of equilibrium and audition. Symptoms of vestibular nerve dysfunctioning are impaired equilibrium, vertigo or dizziness (the sensation of moving around in space), and nystagmus (rhythmic movement of the eye in which the eye moves slowly away from the center and then returns rapidly).

There are two types of hearing impairment: **conductive and sensorineural**. The exact nature of a hearing impairment depends on the site of the lesion. Damage to the peripheral mechanism involving the tympanic membrane and/or middle ear ossicles results in conductive hearing loss, which may not be very disabling. Damage to the **labyrinthine systems** (organ of Corti), spiral ganglia, cochlear nerve, and cochlear nuclei results in sensorineural impairment, which can be disabling. For example, if the cochlear nerve is damaged, hearing impairment in the affected ear may be permanent and profound. However, in the case of a brainstem lesion (central auditory pathways), impairment is only partial because of the bilaterality of auditory projections to the cortex. An important symptom of sensorineural hearing loss is tinnitus, a sensation of ringing, buzzing, or other noises in the absence of any external sounds (see Chapters 9 and 10).

Glossopharyngeal Nerve

The glossopharyngeal nerve (CN IX) and vagus nerve (CN X) share similar anatomy and functions, although they follow different peripheral pathways. The glossopharyngeal nerve serves both sensory and motor functions (Table 15-18). The sensorimotor nucleus complex of the nerve consists of the inferior salivatory nucleus, **nucleus ambiguus**, and **nucleus solitarius** (Figs. 15-21 and 15-22); the latter two nuclei are shared with the vagus nerve (CN X). After exiting laterally from the medulla posterior to the inferior olivary nucleus, the nerve fibers leave the skull through the **jugular foramen** (Fig. 15-5; see Figs. 2-49 and 2-50). At the opening of the foramen are two DRG of the glossopharyngeal nerve (CN IX): superior and inferior ganglion. The superior ganglion contains stretch afferent cell bodies innervating stylopharyngeus muscle spindles; the inferior ganglion contains GVA (cutaneous) and SVA (taste) DRG cell bodies of CN IX.

General Visceral Afferent

GVA fibers, which are primarily concerned with the initiation of reflexes, mediate the touch, pain, tension, and temperature sensations from intraoral visceral structures including the upper pharynx, tonsils, eustachian tube, middle ear cavity, soft palate, and mucosa of the posterior third of the tongue. With the primary sensory cell bodies in the inferior ganglion near the jugular foramina, the central processes from the inferior ganglion project to the nucleus solitarius in the medulla (Fig. 15-22). This sensory information later travels to the **ventral posterior medial nucleus** of the thalamus via the **ventral secondary ascending trigeminal tract** and subsequently to the sensory cortex in the rostral parietal lobe (see Chapter 7).

The GVA fibers also receive inputs from the carotid body (chemoreceptors) and middle ear. The carotid body

Table 15-18

Functional Description of the Glossopharyngeal Nerve

Classification	Nuclei	Function
GVA (general visceral afferent)	First order: inferior ganglion Second order: nucleus solitarius	Mediates gag and respiratory reflexes by regulating visceral sensation (pain and pressure) from oral pharynx mucosa, soft palate, palatal arch, posterior third of tongue mucosa, eustachian tube, middle ear cavity, and carotid sinus
GVE (general visceral efferent)	Inferior salivatory nucleus with preganglionic parasympathetic projections	Regulates salivatory secretion from parotid gland and mucous secretion from oral pharynx
SVA (special visceral afferent)	First order: inferior ganglion Second order: nucleus solitarius	Transmits taste sensation from posterior third of tongue, oral pharynx, and epiglottis
SVE (special visceral efferent)/BE (branchial efferent)	Nucleus ambiguus (lower motor neuron)	Contributes to swallowing reflex by activating stylopharyngeus and upper pharyngeal constrictor fibers

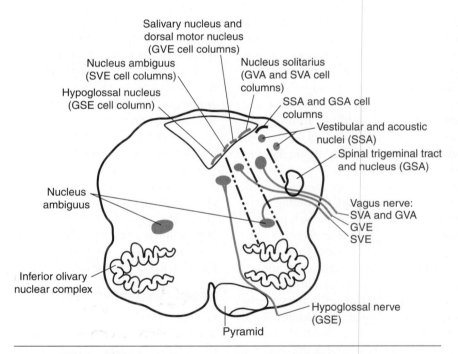

Figure 15-21 Cross-section of the medulla showing the locations of the nuclei: hypoglossal nucleus (general somatic efferent [*GSE*]), nucleus ambiguus (special visceral efferent [*SVE*]/branchial efferent [BE]), salivary nucleus and dorsal motor nucleus (general visceral efferent [*GVE*]), nucleus solitarius (general visceral afferent [*GVA*] and special visceral afferent [*SVA*]), vestibular and acoustic nuclei (special somatic afferent [*SSA*]), and trigeminal nucleus (general somatic afferent [*GSA*]). Many of these nuclei are shared by the glossopharyngeal and vagus nerves.

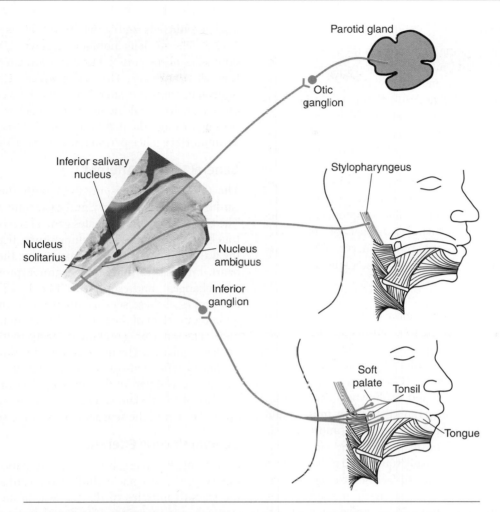

Figure 15-22 The glossopharyngeal nerve, its nuclear complex, and its projections to the brainstem.

chemoreceptors respond to changes in the carbon dioxide and oxygen content of the circulating blood and reflexively control the rate of respiration through modulation of the reticular respiratory center (see Chapter 16). The carotid sinus baroreceptors respond to increased blood pressure and reflexively control the flow of blood by dilating peripheral blood vessels. GVA afferents also mediate pain from the middle ear, which is often seen in the case of infection.

General Visceral Efferent

The GVE system is concerned with the autonomic control of visceral body organs including glands and cardiac muscles. The inferior salivatory nucleus mediates parasympathetic projections to the parotid gland. The preganglionic parasympathetic fibers from the inferior salivary nucleus supply the otic ganglion, which regulates secretion from the parotid gland in the oral cavity (Fig. 15-22).

Special Visceral Afferent

The SVA fibers mediate taste information from taste buds in the posterior third of the tongue and scattered throughout the oral pharynx. The sensory processes, with their primary cell bodies in the inferior ganglion, send projections to the medulla where they travel in the tractus solitarius, later terminating in the rostral nucleus solitarius (Fig. 15-22). Fibers from the nucleus solitarius proceed in the medial lemniscus to the ventral posterior nucleus of the thalamus and then to the tongue area in the primary sensory cortex.

Special Visceral Efferent/Branchial Efferent

The SVE/BE projections of the glossopharyngeal nerve contribute to swallowing by innervating the stylopharyngeus, a branchial or special visceral muscle derived from the third branchial arch (Fig. 15-2). The BE fibers of the glossopharyngeal nerve (CN IX) originate in the rostral region of the nucleus ambiguus, a column of motor nuclei also shared by the vagus cranial nerve (CN X). The nucleus ambiguus, dorsolateral to the inferior olivary nucleus (Fig. 15-21), receives UMN input from both sides of the motor cortex (corticobulbar tracts), with contralateral input being somewhat stronger. The fibers from the nucleus ambiguus exit the lateral medulla, supplying the ipsilateral stylopharyngeus muscle (Fig. 15-22).

Clinical Concerns

Because of the overlapping of nuclei and their proximity to other cranial nerves and nuclei, a lesion selectively affecting the glossopharyngeal nerve (CN IX) or its nuclei is rare. Nevertheless, a discrete lesion results in partial paresis of the unilateral stylopharyngeal muscle, impairing ipsilateral pharyngeal elevation in deglutition. An additional symptom is loss of general and taste sensation from the ipsilateral posterior third of the tongue. Impaired cutaneous sensation from the posterior tongue causes loss of the gag reflex. Furthermore, poor control of the parotid gland leads to excessive oral secretion. The symptoms are particularly pronounced after bilateral damage of the nerve. Dysfunctions of the glossopharyngeal nerve (CN IX) are usually assessed with the functions of the vagus nerve.

Vagus Nerve

The vagus nerve (CN X), with a more extensive distribution than any other cranial nerve, is 90% sensory and 10% motor (Table 15-19). From the perspective of students and professionals in communicative disorders, by far the most important function of the vagus nerve (CN X) is its control of the muscles used for phonation and swallowing (deglutition). The vagus nerve (CN X) innervates the cardiac muscles and smooth muscles of the esophagus, stomach, and intestine, and the branchial muscles of the pharynx and larynx. This nerve mediates sensations of pain, touch, and pressure from mucosa of the pharynx, inferior surface of the epiglottis, the trachea, bronchi, esophagus, and stomach. It also mediates general somesthetic (pain) input (GSA) and stretch afferent feedback (SSA) from the pharyngeal and laryngeal muscles.

The vagal nuclear complex is in the ventricular floor of the medulla oblongata. It consists of the dorsal motor nucleus, nucleus ambiguus, and nucleus solitarius (Fig. 15-21). The nucleus ambiguus receives UMN input from both sides of the cortex, but the contralateral projection is somewhat stronger. The vagus nerve (CN X) exits the brainstem from the lateral medulla between the inferior olivary nucleus and the inferior cerebellar peduncle; after passing through the jugular foramen, it distributes its sensorimotor branches peripherally (Figs. 15-1 and 15-5).

General Visceral Afferent

The GVA sensation is involved with the regulation of cardiovascular, respiratory, and gastrointestinal functions. The GVA component mediates general sensation, including touch, pain, tension, and temperature, from receptors in the walls of the viscera: pharynx, larynx, thorax, abdomen, heart, bronchi, carotid sinus (baroreceptors; detect pressure changes), and esophagus (Fig. 15-23). The primary cell bodies of these sensory fibers are in the inferior ganglion (equivalent of the DRG), which is in the jugular foramen. The inferior ganglion projects to the tractus and nucleus solitarius. The nucleus solitarius projects into many medullary reflex networks and through the medial lemniscus to a special part of the ventral posterior medial (VPM) nucleus of the thalamus and then to the parietal superior opercular part of the sensory cortex in the sylvian sulcus.

General Visceral Efferent

As part of the ANS, the GVE fibers parasympathetically innervate the viscera, including the cardiac muscles and the smooth muscles of the trachea, bronchi, esophagus, stomach, and intestines. The dorsal motor nucleus, which is laterally in the ventricular floor, receives afferents from the hypothalamus, brainstem reflex network, and solitary tract. The long fibers leaving the dorsal motor nucleus send

---

Table 15-19		
Functional Description of the Vagus Nerve		
Classification	Nuclei	Function
GVA (general visceral afferent)	First order: inferior ganglion Second order: nucleus solitarius	Receives general sensation from muscles of pharynx, larynx, thorax, carotid body, and abdomen Regulates nausea, oxygen intake, and lung inflation (respiratory reflex)
GVE (general visceral efferent)	Dorsal motor nucleus with preganglionic projections to visceral plexuses	Innervates glands, cardiac muscles, and muscles of heart, trachea, bronchi, esophagus, stomach, and intestine
SVA (special visceral afferent)	First order: inferior ganglion Second order: nucleus solitarius	Mediates taste sensation from mucosa of posterior pharynx, larynx, and epiglottis
SVE (special visceral efferent)/BE (branchial efferent)	Nucleus ambiguus (lower motor neuron)	Controls muscles of larynx, pharynx, and soft palate for phonation, swallowing, resonance, and for opening respiratory pathway

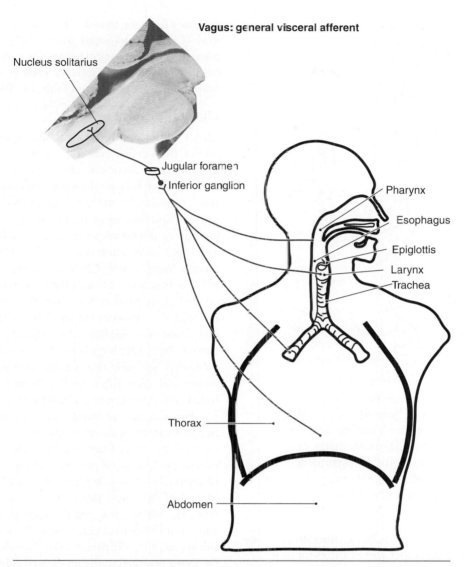

Vagus: general visceral afferent

Nucleus solitarius

Jugular foramen

Inferior ganglion

Pharynx

Esophagus

Epiglottis

Larynx

Trachea

Thorax

Abdomen

Figure 15-23 The nucleus solitarius with its general visceral afferent fibers, which mediate the general sensation from the muscles of the pharynx, larynx, thorax, and abdomen.

preganglionic projections to distal ganglia in the walls of the alimentary canal and digestive organs, including the trachea, bronchi, heart, esophagus, stomach, and intestines. The short postganglionic fibers regulate the functions of these structures (Fig. 15-24). The parasympathetic autonomic innervation of the rectum, bladder, and genitals is supplied via the S2–S4 spinal segments (see Chapter 16).

Special Visceral Afferent

The SVA fibers mediate taste sensation from the pharyngeal area. The sensory fibers from the base of the tongue, epiglottis, larynx, and pharynx have their cell bodies in the inferior ganglion (equivalent to the DRG); they project to the tractus and nucleus solitarius in the medulla oblongata (Fig. 15-25). The fibers from the nucleus solitarius ascend in the medial lemniscus to the VPM nucleus of the thala-

mus, from which fibers project to the sensory cortex in the parietal lobe. The primary (inferior ganglia) and secondary (solitarius) nuclei are shared by the glossopharyngeal nerve (CN IX) while serving similar SVA and GVA functions.

Special Visceral Efferent/Branchial Efferent

SVE/BE projections of the vagus nerve (CN X) innervate muscles that are important to students of communicative disorders: those of the larynx, pharynx, and the upper part of the esophagus (Fig. 15-26). These motor fibers of CN X originate from the posterior two-thirds of the nucleus ambiguus (one-third of the nucleus is related to the glossopharyngeal [CN IX]), which is known to receive corticobulbar projections from both sides of the cortex. The efferent fibers supply the branchial muscles of the pharynx, the muscles of the soft palate (except for the tensor palatini, which

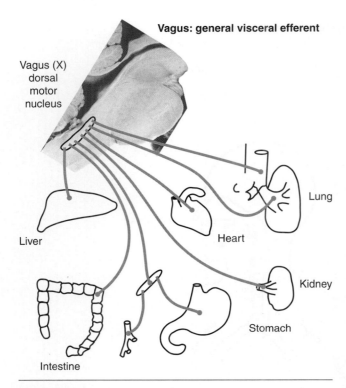

Vagus: general visceral efferent

Vagus (X) dorsal motor nucleus

Liver

Heart

Lung

Kidney

Stomach

Intestine

Figure 15-24 The dorsal motor nucleus of the vagus nerve in the medulla and its general visceral efferent nuclei projections to the smooth muscle fibers of the heart, trachea, bronchi, esophagus, stomach, and intestine. *Red lines,* preganglionic parasympathetic fibers, which innervate the postganglionic cells in the small ganglion near the target structures.

is served by the trigeminal nerve [CN V]), the intrinsic muscles of the larynx, and the upper area of the esophagus.

The pharyngeal branch of the nerve supplies the three constrictor muscles (superior, middle, and inferior) of the pharynx and all soft palate muscles (palatoglossus and levator palati), except for the tensor palatini (trigeminal nerve [CN V]). The superior laryngeal branch of the vagus divides into internal and external laryngeal branches. The external branch of the superior laryngeal nerve controls the cricothyroid muscle, an internal laryngeal muscle. The internal branch is sensory to the mucous membrane as far down as the vocal cords and adjacent area.

The recurrent laryngeal branch of the vagus (CN X) takes different routes on the two sides. It curves around the subclavian artery before emerging on the right side but curves around the aortic arch on the left side. The recurrent laryngeal nerve fibers innervate the intrinsic muscles of the larynx and epiglottis and, therefore, play an important role in phonation (Fig. 15-26). While these branches provide motor control to the larynx, some of its fibers are responsible for sensory innervation of the mucous membrane inferior to the vocal cords.

The nucleus ambiguus also receives afferent projections from the tractus solitarius, which contains stretch afferent

feedback from the muscles innervated by the glossopharyngeal (CN IX) and vagus nerves (stretch reflexes). These afferent and efferent projections form the reticular neuronal circuitry that enables reflexes such as gagging, coughing, vomiting, and swallowing (Table 15-20).

Clinical Concerns

The medulla oblongata, the site of many reticular networks, vital reflex centers, and several cranial nuclei, is an important anatomic structure. Reflexes required for survival—such as swallowing, gagging, coughing, sneezing, vomiting, breathing, and cardiac rate—require the normal functioning of output nuclei (e.g., from nucleus ambiguus, dorsal vagus nucleus, and hypoglossal nuclei) and input association nuclei (especially the nucleus solitarius). Vagus nerve (CN X) fibers participate in almost all of these functions. Most of the networks that organize and control these vital reflexes involve many regions of the reticular formation in the medulla, with hierarchical control from the higher CNS. Consequently, medullary lesions, especially large ones that damage both sides of the medullary reticular area, can damage aspects of these networks and their input and/or output nuclei, often with lethal consequences (see Chapter 16).

For students of communicative disorders, the functions of the nucleus ambiguus are essential. A unilateral lesion of the nerve fibers and/or nucleus ambiguus is likely to result in ipsilateral paresis or paralysis of the soft palate, pharynx, and larynx. Injuries specifically to the pharyngeal branch of the vagus nerve (CN X) cause paralysis of the pharynx and the soft palate, leading to swallowing difficulty. With unilateral paralysis of the levator muscle of the soft palate, the soft palate lowers on the affected side, and the uvula is pulled to the unaffected side (Fig. 15-27). With bilateral soft palate paralysis, despite symmetry, the soft palate hangs lower than its normal curvature (Fig. 15-27). Recurrent laryngeal nerve disorders lead to paralysis of the vocal folds. Unilateral LMN paralysis of the vocal folds causes breathy voice, diplophonia, and hoarseness but only minimally affects the ability to phonate. Vocal cord paralysis may also cause choking and pulmonary aspiration. Bilateral injury to the recurrent laryngeal nerve, however, produces inspiratory stridor and aphonia. It can also be life-threatening if the paralyzed vocal cords impair air flow.

Unilateral central (UMN) lesions in the brainstem involving the corticobulbar fibers cause harsh voice quality. However, such lesions do not produce severe phonatory and swallowing symptoms because the nucleus ambiguus receives UMN input from both sides of the cortex (Fig. 15-8). Bilateral central (UMN) lesions will produce profound phonatory and swallowing problems.

With vagus nerve injuries, many autonomic functions and visceral reflexes, such as coronary circulation, heart rate, and relaxation and contraction of tracheal and bronchial muscles, are impaired. Altered autonomic reflexes include

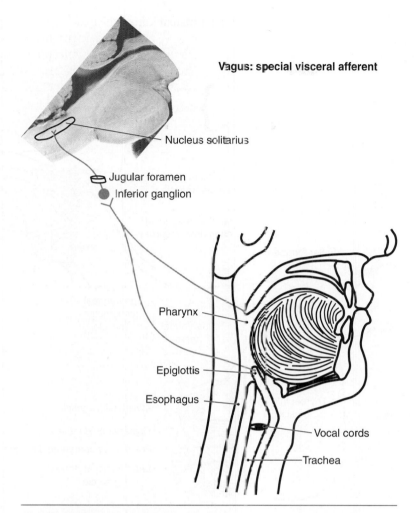

Vagus: special visceral afferent

Nucleus solitarius

Jugular foramen

Inferior ganglion

Pharynx

Epiglottis

Esophagus

Vocal cords

Trachea

Figure 15-25 The nucleus solitarius and special visceral fibers from the muscles of the larynx, pharynx, epiglottis, and palate.

vomiting, coughing, sneezing, sucking, hiccupping, and yawning. Damage to the sensory nuclear complex of CN X leads to anesthesia of the larynx, pharynx, and associated structures and to loss of taste sensation from the pharyngeal and epiglottic areas. Because the glossopharyngeal nerve (CN IX), vagus nerve (CN X), and spinal accessory nerve (CN XI) all pass through the jugular foramen, peripheral lesions involving the vagus nerve alone are uncommon. Loss of vagus nerve functions are tested by visual examination of the soft palate and pharyngeal cavity and assessment of quality in phonatory and swallowing tasks.

Spinal Accessory Nerve
Special Visceral Efferent/Branchial Efferent

The spinal accessory nerve (CN XI) is a branchiomeric motor nerve that receives projections primarily from the contralateral motor cortex (Table 15-21). The corticospinal projections transmit nerve impulses through the spinal roots of the nerve. As mentioned earlier, the remnants of gill-related muscles continue to C1–C5. These fibers are

classified as a cranial nerve, even though they originate from the spinal cord. The efferents from the LMNs in the ventral horns in C1–C5 fuse longitudinally to enter the cranial cavity through the foramen magnum and leave the cranium via the jugular foramen (Figs. 15-1 and 15-3). They follow the vagus nerve (CN X), and the efferent fibers innervate two neck muscles: the trapezius and sternocleidomastoid (Fig. 15-28). The trapezius muscle tilts the head back and to the side and contributes to shrugging. The sternocleidomastoid muscle pulls the mastoid process as well as clavicle closer together on one side, rotating the head and jaw to the opposite side.

Clinical Concerns

The trapezius and sternocleidomastoid, combined with other adjacent neck muscles, contribute to tilt, forward and backward extension, and lateral rotation of the head. Accessory nerve dysfunctions affect the ability to control head movements. Accessory nerve function is tested by asking the patients to turn the head and raise the shoul-

Vagus: special visceral efferent

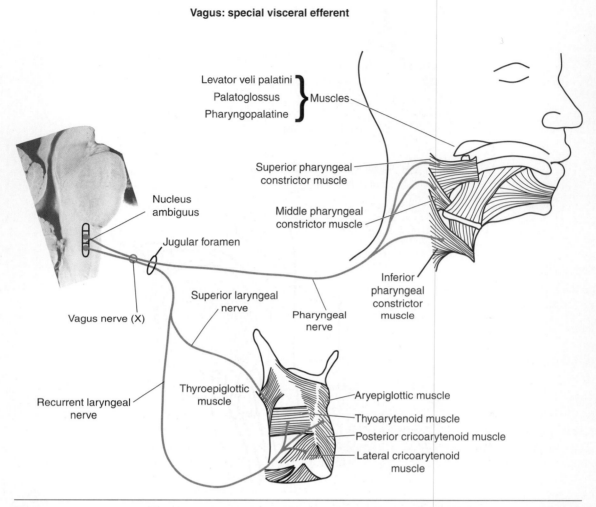

Figure 15-26 The vagus nucleus ambiguus with its special visceral efferent fiber/branchial efferent projections to the branchial muscles of the larynx and pharynx.

der against an opposing force provided by the clinician (Fig. 15-29). An interruption of the nerve supply to the trapezius muscle results in a dropped shoulder that cannot be raised. Damage to the sternocleidomastoid restricts head turning to the side away from the lesion. Paralysis of these muscles may also indirectly affect speech resonance.

Hypoglossal Nerve
General Somatic Efferent

The hypoglossal nerve (CN XII) is a motor nerve (Table 15-22). The nerve fibers originate from the hypoglossal nucleus in the ventricular floor of the fourth ventricle

Table 15-20

Common Cranial Nerve–Mediated Reflexes

Reflexes	Reflexive Activity	Initiating Stimulus
Pupillary	Pupillary constriction (CN III efferent fibers)	Shining light in eye (CN II afferent fibers)
Corneal	Eye blink (CN VII efferent fibers)	Touching cornea (CN V afferent fibers)
Gag	Involuntary effort to vomit (CN X efferent fibers)	Pharyngeal touch (CN IX and X afferent fibers)
Sneeze	Involuntary contraction of muscles of expiration (CN X efferent fibers)	Nasal mucous membrane irritation (CN III afferent fibers)

CN, cranial nerve.

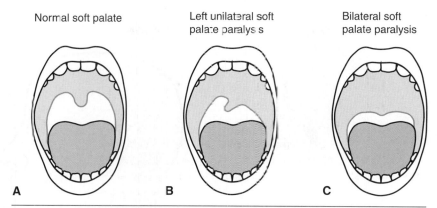

Normal soft palate   Left unilateral soft palate paralysis   Bilateral soft palate paralysis

A   B   C

Figure 15-27 A. The normal soft palate. B. Paralysis of the left soft palate and pharyngeal wall from a lower motor neuron lesion. Sagging of the left pharyngeal wall and palatal arch moves the uvula to the right, away from the side of the lesion. The muscles involved in this paralysis include the levator veli palatini, palatoglossal, and palatopharyngeus. C. In bilateral soft palate paralysis, the palatal arch remains symmetrical, although its curvature hangs lower than normal. Complete vagus nerve interruption causes many additional problems involving the muscles of the pharynx, palate, and larynx.

close to the midline in the medulla (Figs. 15-1 and 15-3). The hypoglossal nucleus receives its direct corticobulbar input from the contralateral motor cortex (Fig. 15-8). The efferent fibers from the hypoglossal nucleus travel anteriorly, pass through the medullary substance medial to the inferior olivary nucleus, and exit lateral to the pyramidal tract (Fig. 15-21).

The hypoglossal nerve (CN XII), which controls tongue movement, innervates all ipsilateral intrinsic and most extrinsic (genioglossal, styloglossus, and hyoglossus) tongue muscles except the palatoglossal, which is controlled by the vagus nerve (CN X) (Fig. 15-30; Table 15-23). The afferent projections from the nucleus solitarius and trigeminal sensory nuclei are functionally linked with efferent hypoglossal fibers. This forms the neuronal circuitry for eating, sucking, and chewing reflexes.

Clinical Concerns

Unilateral damage to the hypoglossal nucleus or interruption of nerve projections in the distributions of the nerve results in LMN symptoms. Consequently, when the ipsilateral half of the tongue is paralyzed, it becomes flaccid

and wrinkled. With no voluntary control or reflexes, the paralyzed half of the tongue eventually atrophies, which is characterized by loss of contour and corrugation of the edge. This weakness and muscle atrophy contribute to dysarthria and chewing difficulty, in which the patient has problems with formation and control of the bolus that is essential for normal swallowing. On palpation, the affected side of the tongue appears flaccid (soft) and wrinkled. On protrusion, the tongue deviates to the side of the lesion because of the unopposed protrusion of the normal half of the tongue (Fig. 15-31A). Bilateral LMN damage to the nucleus or nerve is likely to cause severe difficulty in swallowing, eating, and speaking (Fig. 15-31B).

After a unilateral supranuclear lesion, the loss of UMN influence on the contralateral hypoglossal nucleus results in significant loss of skill in using the contralateral half of the tongue during articulation and eating. However, the presence of some aberrant corticobulbar fibers may somewhat limit the effect of the loss. The affected and weakened tongue in such a case moves away from the side of the affected hemisphere with a supranuclear (UMN) lesion. The hypoglossal nerve is tested by asking the patient to protrude,

Table 15-21		
Functional Description of the Spinal Accessory Nerve		
Classification	Nuclei	Function
SVE (special visceral) efferent)/BE (branchial efferent)	Spinal accessory nucleus in C1–C5 ventral horns of spinal cord	Controls head position by controlling trapezius and sternocleidomastoid muscles

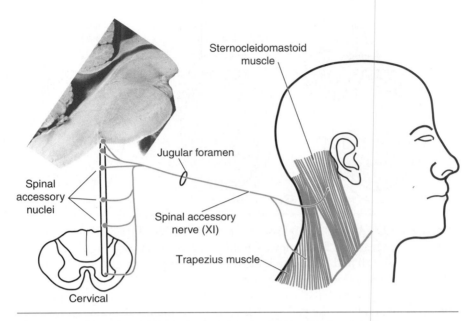

Figure 15-28 Origin of the spinal and cranial fibers of the spinal accessory nerve and distribution to the muscles in the neck.

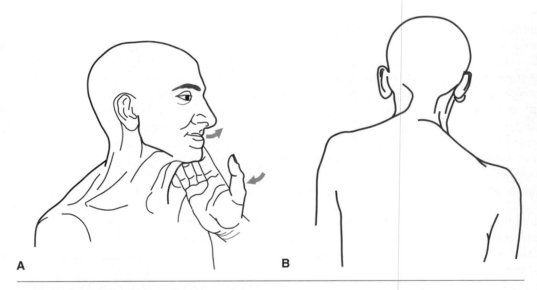

A   **B**

Figure 15-29 Paralysis of the spinal accessory nerve. **A.** The sternocleidomastoid muscle pulls the mastoid process and clavicle closer together on one side, rotating the head and jaw to the opposite side. Paralysis of the sternocleidomastoid muscle restricts movement of the jaw and neck, thus limiting the head movement opposite the side of damage. **B.** With paralysis of the trapezius muscle, the ipsilateral shoulder sags because of the loss of the normal contour between the neck and shoulder.

Table 15-22

Functional Description of the Hypoglossal Nerve

Classification	Nuclei	Function
GSE (general somatic efferent)	Hypoglossal nucleus (lower motor neuron) in medulla	Controls motor movements of tongue by regulating intrinsic and extrinsic glossal muscles

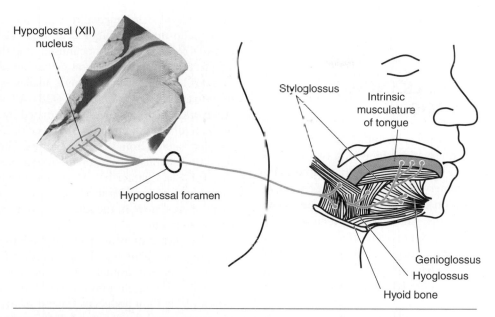

Figure 15-30 The hypoglossal nucleus in the medulla, the intramedullary course of the nerve, and the distribution of the nerve fibers to the glossal muscles.

Table 15-23

Muscles of the Tongue

Muscle	Function
Extrinsic muscles	
Genioglossus (CN XII)	Raises hyoid bone and protrudes and retracts tongue
Hyoglossus (CN XII)	Retracts tongue and lowers its side
Palatoglossus (CN X)	Narrows fauces and elevates back of tongue
Styloglossus (CN XII)	Retracts and elevates tongue
Intrinsic muscles	
Superior longitudinal	Shortens and curls tip of tongue upward
Inferior longitudinal	Shortens and curls tip of tongue downward
Transverse	Elongates and narrows and raises sides of tongue
Verticalis	Flattens and broadens tongue

CN, cranial nerve.

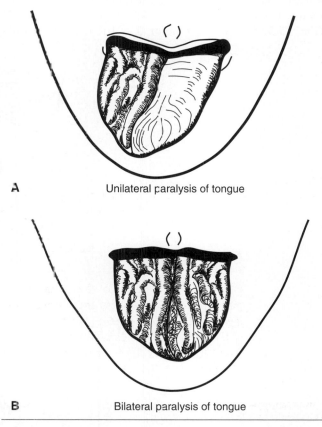

A — Unilateral paralysis of tongue

B — Bilateral paralysis of tongue

Figure 15-31 Paralysis of the right half of the tongue. A. The loss of bulk is evident; and on protrusion, the tongue deviates to the side of weakness. B. Bilateral palsy of the tongue is characterized by general atrophy.

retract, raise, and move the tongue laterally and by examining the quality of lingual and dental sounds.

FUNCTION-BASED CRANIAL NERVE COMBINATIONS

There are two important aspects of cranial nerve functions. The first is multiple innervation, in which two or more cranial nerves innervate the same anatomic structure. For example, several cranial nerves combine to serve eye movement, sensory innervation of the tongue, and soft palatal and pharyngeal movements. The second is that some cranial motor (branchial) nuclei nerves receive corticobulbar projections from both motor cortices, although the contralateral projection is somewhat stronger. This has significant clinical implications for preserved motor speech functions after a unilateral lesion.

Motor Control of Eye Muscles

The ocular movements of each eye are controlled by six muscles that are regulated by three cranial nerves: oculomotor (CN III), trochlear (CN IV), and abducens (CN VI) (Fig. 15-32A). The oculomotor (CN III) nerve innervates four ocular muscles: medial rectus, inferior rectus, superior rectus, and inferior oblique. The trochlear (CN IV) nerve controls the superior oblique muscle, and the abducens (CN VI) nerve regulates the lateral rectus muscle. Each of these muscles, combined with others, makes specific contributions to eye movements (Fig. 15-32B). All of the ocular muscles work together and are coordinated by the gaze centers in the midbrain and pons, which receive coordinated corticobulbar signals from the motor cortex. The motor nuclei of these three cranial nerves are interconnected by the fibers of the MLF (see Chapter 10). This brainstem tract ensures that the activity of muscles in the two eyes is coordinated and that the eyes move in the same direction concurrently with head movement.

The midbrain **conjugate gaze control center** coordinates the movement of both eyes together. For example, activation of the left frontal cortex (premotor area) leads to activation of the right pontine gaze center and then to activation of the right abducens (lateral rectus) and left oculomotor nucleus (medial rectus). This results in contraction of the right lateral rectus and left medial rectus muscles to ensure a smooth turn of both eyes toward the right. The activation of the right frontal cortex (premotor area) would lead to activation of the left pontine gaze and cause the contraction of the left lateral rectus and right medial rectus muscle.

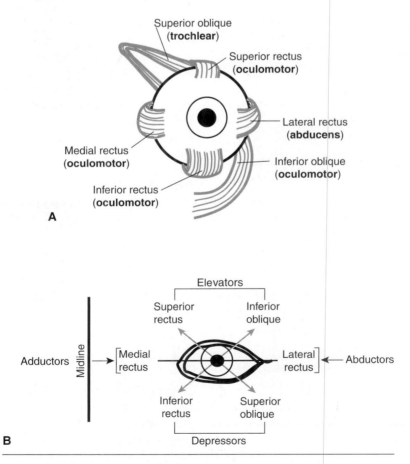

Figure 15-32 A. Muscles of the left eye and the cranial nerves responsible for their innervation. B. Group actions of the ocular muscles of the left eye.

Sensory Nerve Supply to Tongue

The tongue displays a distinctive pattern in which three cranial nerves innervate general (cutaneous) and special (taste) sensations from its anterior and posterior regions (Fig. 15-33). The general sensations of pain, touch, and proprioception from the anterior two-thirds of the tongue are carried in the lingual branch of the trigeminal nerve (CN V). General sensations from the posterior third of the tongue are relayed by the glossopharyngeal nerve (CN IX) branches (Table 15-24).

Two cranial nerves also participate in the mediation of the special sensation of taste from the tongue. Special sensation of taste from the anterior two-thirds of the tongue is carried by the chorda tympani, a branch of the facial nerve (CN VII) complex. Taste sensation from the posterior third of the tongue is carried by the fibers of the glossopharyngeal nerve (CN IX).

Motor Nerve Supply to the Soft Palate and Pharynx

The soft palate and tube-shaped pharyngeal cavity are important in swallowing and speech resonance. The soft palate seals the nasopharynx to prevent the entrance of food during swallowing. It also regulates speech nasality. The circular constrictor (superior, middle, and inferior) muscles of the pharynx perform squeezing actions on the bolus, and vertical muscles (stylopharyngeus, palatopharyngeus, and salpingopharyngeus) elevate the larynx during swallowing. The motor innervation of the muscles of the soft palate and pharyngeal cavity is supplied by the pharyngeal branches of the vagus nerve (CN X), except for the tensor veli palatini (trigeminal [CN V]) and stylopharyngeus (glossopharyngeal [CN IX]). (Fig. 15-34).

Sensory Innervation of the Soft Palate and Pharynx

The glossopharyngeal nerve (CN IX) and vagus nerve (CN X) are responsible for general sensation from the pharynx,

a visceral structure. The vagus alone carries the general sensation from the larynx, another visceral structure. However, a branch of the facial nerve (CN VII) complex (pterygopalatine nerve) mediates general sensation (GVA) and taste (SVA) from the nasopharynx and soft palate.

CLINICAL CONCERNS

Upper and Lower Motor Neuron Syndromes

Lesions involving the UMNs and LMNs affect the function of buccofacial muscles differently. Interruption in corticobulbar projections from the motor cortex to the cranial nerve motor nuclei on the opposite side results in UMN syndrome, which is characterized by a loss of discrete and delicate motor control, muscle weakness, and brisk reflexes. The substantial number of collateral corticobulbar fibers probably provides safety from damage in the brainstem for cranial nerve functions. This explains why damage to the pyramidal fibers after they have separated from the major pyramidal tract does not result in any more than a minimal spasticity in cranial muscles. Furthermore, most buccofacial muscles that receive corticobulbar projections from both sides of the cortex may not be severely impaired by a unilateral UMN lesion.

Bilateral involvement of UMN (pseudobulbar palsy), which profoundly affects cranial muscle function and motor speech, is characterized by hypertonia and loss of discrete motor control, again with little or no spasticity in the cranial muscles. LMN lesions affect the motor cranial nuclei (final common pathways) and their projections and produce the LMN symptoms, which include flaccid paralysis, absent or reduced reflexes, muscular fibrillations and twitching, and muscle atrophy.

The muscular twitching results from spontaneous firing of an α-LMN cell body or its axons, resulting in an entire motor unit firing at the same time. It is caused by irritation, infection, or hyperexcitability of the LMN cell body. If the LMN cell body dies, the innervating terminals (neuromuscular junctions) degenerate, and fasciculation ceases.

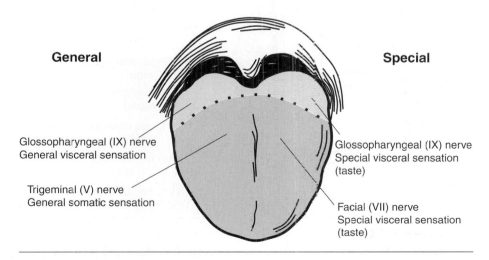

Figure 15-33 General and special sensory innervation of tongue.

Table 15-24

Sensory Innervation of the Tongue

Cranial Nerves (Number)	General Sensation (GSA)	General Visceral (GVA)	Taste Sensation (SVA)	Tongue Region
Lingual branch of trigeminal nerve (V)	+			Anterior two-thirds of tongue
Glossopharyngeal nerve (IX)			+	Taste buds in mucosa of posterior third of tongue
Chorda tympani of facial nerve (VII)			+	Taste buds in mucosa of anterior two-thirds of tongue
Glossopharyngeal nerve (IX)		+		Posterior third of tongue

GSA, general somatic afferent; *GVA,* general visceral afferent; *SVA,* special visceral afferent.

When deprived of efferent impulses (reflexive or voluntary) from the LMN cell body, the muscle fibers eventually atrophy and degenerate. LMN lesions greatly affect the functioning of the buccofacial, glossal, laryngeal, and neck muscles.

UMN signs are contralateral to the locus of damage, whereas LMN signs are ipsilateral to the damage of the cell body or axon in the brainstem. An exception to this rule is the trochlear nerve (CN IV), which innervates the superior oblique muscle. Damage to its nucleus results in a contralateral LMN syndrome, and the nerve involvement results in ipsilateral signs.

COMMON CRANIAL NERVE SYNDROMES

Cranial nerve nuclei are packed in a small area of the brainstem (Fig. 15-3; Table 15-25). Their compact location and close proximity to both crossed and uncrossed ascending and descending fibers makes them susceptible to even small brainstem lesions. The selective cranial nerve involvement has resulted in a few established neurologic syndromes: **Weber, Millard-Gubler, locked-in, medial medullary,** and **Wallenberg.** Most of these syndromes involve motor speech functions.

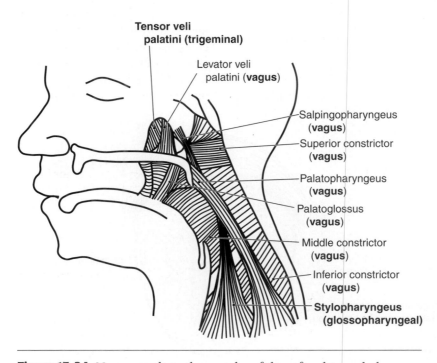

Figure 15-34 Nerve supply to the muscles of the soft palate and pharynx.

Table 15-25

Brainstem Cranial Nerve Syndromes

Syndrome	Affected Structures	Clinical Symptoms
Weber syndrome (midbrain lesion)	Corticospinal fibers Oculomotor nerve (CN III)	Contralateral hemiplegia Ipsilateral ocular paralysis (lateral strabismus) Dilated pupil
Millard-Gubler syndrome (lower pons)	Corticospinal fibers Abducens nerve (CN VI)	Contralateral hemiplegia Ipsilateral ocular impairment (medial strabismus)
Locked-in syndrome (bilateral basal pons)	Bilateral corticospinal fibers	Paralysis of all voluntary movements (quadriplegia) Preserved vertical eye movements Intact sensation
Wallenberg syndrome (lateral medulla)	Nucleus of trigeminal spinal tract Nucleus ambiguus Spinal lemniscus (spinothalamic fibers)	Loss of pain sensation from ipsilateral face and contralateral side of body Dysarthric speech marked by paralysis of muscles of pharynx, larynx, and soft palate
Medial medullary syndrome	Pyramidal fibers Medial lemniscus Hypoglossal nerve (CN XII)	Contralateral hemiplegia Contralateral loss of pressure and vibration (medial lemniscus) Dysarthria owing to ipsilateral lingual paralysis

Weber Syndrome (Midbrain Lesion)

Weber syndrome is associated with a ventral medial midbrain lesion which affects the oculomotor nerve (CN III) along with descending corticospinal (pes peduncle) fibers (Fig. 15-35). It is marked with contralateral hemiplegia (with interruption of the descending motor fibers) and ipsilateral ocular paralysis (with the involvement of the oculomotor [CN III] nerve fibers). With the paralysis of all the muscles except the lateral rectus (abducens [CN V] nerve) and superior oblique (trochlear [CN IV] nerve), the patient displays ptosis (impaired ability to raise eye),

pupil dilation (parasympathetic CN III paralysis), and lateral deviation of the ipsilateral eye (secondary to the unopposed activity of the lateral rectus muscle). An extended lesion may also affect the red nucleus, which causes incoordination and tremor of the opposite arm.

Millard-Gubler Syndrome (Pons)

In Millard-Gubler syndrome, a lower caudal pontine lesion affects the abducens nerve (CN VI) and the descending motor fibers in the basal pons (Fig. 15-36A). This pontine lesion results in alternating symptoms, which are marked

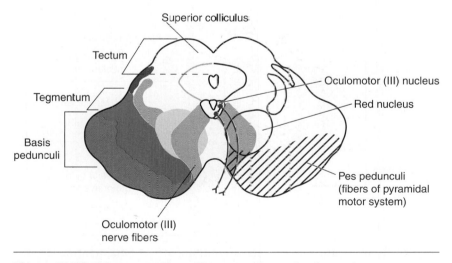

Figure 15-35 A lesion in the midbrain involving the descending corticospinal fibers and the oculomotor nerve.

by contralateral hemiplegia and ipsilateral paralysis of the lateral rectus muscle (abducens nerve [CN VI]), resulting in medial strabismus. The eye deviates medially because of the unopposed activity of the medial rectus muscle (oculomotor nerve [CN III]) and affects horizontal gaze. An extended lesion can also affect the adjacent facial nerve (CN VII) fibers, which may lead to ipsilateral facial palsy, resulting in motor speech symptoms. This syndrome is usually associated with the occlusion of the pontine branches of the basilar artery.

Locked-In Syndrome (Basal Pons)

Locked-in syndrome is associated with a bilateral pontine lesion, which interrupts all the descending fibers (Fig. 15-36B). It is clinically characterized by quadriplegia (paralysis of all voluntary movements) and loss of all motor speech functions. Only vertical eye movement (oculomotor nerve [CN III]) is preserved, which the patient can use for communicating. The patient remains fully awake, can feel somatosensation, and is able to hear and understand what others say. This clinical condition is commonly seen in patients with traumatic brain injury and is often misinterpreted as coma, which has implications for the type and quality of treatment.

Wallenberg Syndrome (Lateral Medulla)

Wallenberg syndrome is caused by a lateral medullary lesion and is associated with the occlusion of the branches of the vertebral or posterior inferior cerebellar arteries, which affects the trigeminal spinal tract: nucleus, nucleus ambiguus, and spinothalamic fibers from the contralateral half of the body (Fig. 15-37A). It causes a dissociated loss of sensation secondary to the levels of fiber crossings. The syndrome is marked by the loss of pain sensation from the ipsilateral face (trigeminal nerve [CN V]) and the contralateral side of the body (spinothalamic tract fibers). The involvement of the nucleus ambiguus (vagus [CN X] and glossopharyngeal nerves [CN IX]) limits the movements of the pharynx, larynx, and soft palate. When the medial lemniscus fibers are spared, touch sensation in the affected area is preserved (see Chapter 7).

Medial Medullary Syndrome

Medial medullary syndrome, caused by a medial medullary infarct as a result of involvement of the anterior spinal artery branches or the medullary branches of the vertebral artery, includes the descending pyramidal fibers, medial lemniscus, and hypoglossal nerve (CN XII) fibers (Fig. 15-37B). This infarct results in contralateral hemiplegia (pyramidal tract

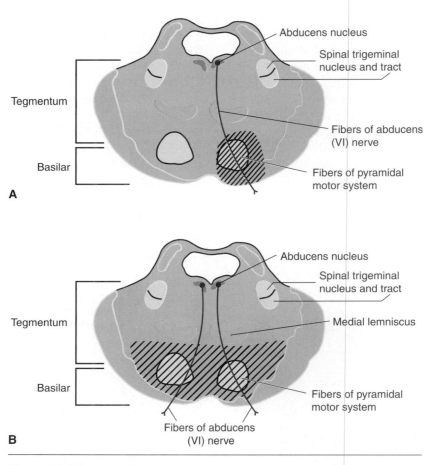

Figure 15-36 Pontine cranial nerve syndromes. **A.** A basal pontine lesion involving the descending corticospinal fibers and the abducens nerve fibers. **B.** A bilateral pontine lesion associated with locked-in syndrome.

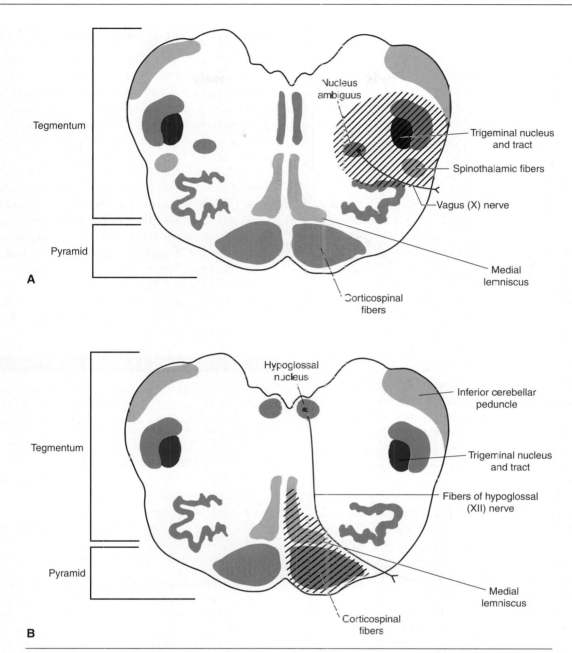

Figure 15-37 A. A lesion producing lateral medullary syndrome. B. A lesion producing medial medullary syndrome.

fibers), contralateral loss of pressure and vibration (medial lemniscus), and ipsilateral lingual paralysis (hypoglossal nerve), which has speech-related implications.

CLINICAL CONSIDERATIONS

PATIENT ONE

A 60-year-old man had several lacunar strokes (deep cortical infarcts) bilaterally in the region of the internal capsule and basal ganglia, as demonstrated on MRI

studies. The bilateral UMN lesions to the corticobulbar fibers affected multiple cranial nerves and caused sensorimotor dysfunctions in the extremities. Neurologic examination revealed the following abnormalities:

- Mild cognitive decline (impaired short-term memory)
- Stiff gait with slow, short steps
- Hyperactive muscle stretch reflexes and bilateral Babinski signs
- Impaired control of the facial muscles, with inability to show his teeth, pucker his lips, or wrinkle his forehead
- Exaggerated facial movement when he laughed

- Difficulty controlling excessive laughter and sobbing
- Difficulty protruding the tongue
- Difficulty chewing and swallowing; food accumulating in his mouth
- Failure of the soft palate to rise on phonation

Question: What cranial nerves control the muscles of facial expression, mastication, and deglutition? Can you account for this clinical picture based on lesions affecting those nerves?

Discussion: The functions of facial movement are mediated by the facial nerve (CN VII), and mastication is mediated by the trigeminal nerve (CN V). Deglutition involves the pharyngeal plexus of the glossopharyngeal nerve (CN IX) and vagus nerve (CN X), and the tongue is controlled by the hypoglossal nerve (CN XII). In this case, the lacunar lesions impaired voluntary control of the connected muscles by injuring the corticobulbar pathways from the cortex to the nuclei of those nerves. This is known as a UMN lesion. This clinical condition, also called pseudobulbar palsy, is associated with bilateral cortical lesions. The term *pseudobulbar* implies that the problem is not in the medulla and does not affect the LMNs; rather it involves the bilateral corticobulbar pathways to the brainstem. Another term used to refer to a UMN lesion is supranuclear paralysis (injury above or rostral to the cranial nerve motor nuclei of the brainstem) owing to bilateral involvement of corticobulbar or corticonuclear pathways.

When the patient attempts to move his facial muscles, the muscles respond poorly, but they respond strongly to an emotional stimulus, which is not under direct control of the cerebral cortex through the corticobulbar pathways that have been damaged. The pathways that are functional during an emotional response are not as well understood as are the direct pathways controlling voluntary actions. The pathways involved with emotions are known to escape injury from lacunar strokes and cortical lesions in typical locations. When the cranial nerve nuclei are activated through the indirect and spared pathway known to mediate emotions, the facial response is actually exaggerated; the patient's face may assume an expressive mask, with forceful contraction of the muscles that otherwise appeared to be weak when he was asked to show his teeth or perform a voluntary smile. An emotional smile, in contrast, resulted in an exaggerated emotional expression accompanied by sobbing. It is important to avoid emotional stimulation when the patient is eating to minimize the risk of aspirating food or saliva.

Slow gait with hyperactive muscle stretch reflexes (deep tendon reflexes) and extensor plantar responses (Babinski signs) imply UMN symptoms. This means that the nerves of the LMNs directly supplying the muscles have not been damaged, but the descending corticospinal motor pathways from the brain have been damaged. The resulting spastic weakness with impaired voluntary control but uninhibited reflex activity (the hyperactive knee-jerk and ankle reflexes, for example) is characteristic of UMN syndrome (see Chapter 14).

The reason the reflex activities of laughing and crying are not just intact but are actually overactive or exaggerated in pseudobulbar palsy has the same basis for why hyperactive muscle stretch reflexes are observed. The reflexes are normally modulated, or somewhat inhibited, by the activity in the intact corticonuclear or corticospinal pathways (corticonuclear or corticobulbar for the display of emotion in the face; corticospinal for the stretch reflexes in the limbs). When that inhibition is removed as the result of a lesion, the responses are uncontrolled, or hyperactive. The signs of cognitive impairment in this patient resulted from multiple cortical infarcts.

PATIENT TWO

A 63-year-old man had a stroke while sleeping and woke up in confusion and panic. He was taken to the emergency room where the examining physician noticed the following:

- Complete left-side facial paralysis
- Inability to move his left eye laterally (the eye was adducted medially)
- Hearing loss in the left ear
- Absence of pain and touch sensation on the left side of the face
- Some weakness in jaw movement

A brain MRI study revealed a small stroke in the left superior tegmentum of the pons that affected the LMN nuclei of the following nerves: facial (CN VII), abducens (CN VI), and trigeminal (CN V). The lesion also extended laterally, affecting the cochlear nuclei within the substance of the brainstem.

Question: How can you account for these cranial nerve–related sensorimotor symptoms on the left side and no paralysis in the muscles of the extremities?

Discussion: The pontine tegmental lesion affected four cranial nerves (abducens [CN VI], trigeminal [CN V], facial [CN VII], and vestibulocochlear [CN VIII]), which caused adduction of the left eye (impaired abducens function), analgesia and anesthesia on the left face (trigeminal [CN V] interruption), paresis in the jaw (trigeminal [CN V] motor nerve involvement), left facial paralysis (facial [CN VII]), and hearing loss (vestibulocochlear [CN VIII]). The typical location of the lesion did not affect the descending corticospinal fibers, so limb motor functions were spared.

PATIENT THREE

A 60-year-old man developed gradually worsening ringing in his left ear; he also noticed decreased hearing in that ear. He began to hold the telephone to his right ear instead of the left. Shortly before consulting his physician, he began to walk with a stiffly extended right leg, tending to scrape the toe of the right foot. He was also somewhat clumsy with his right hand. Examination by the physician revealed the following abnormal signs:

- Mild right-sided weakness of the hand and lower limb
- Increased muscle stretch reflexes (deep tendon reflexes) and Babinski sign on the right
- Tendency to stagger and fall to the left while walking (a sign of cerebellar or vestibular injury)
- Decreased sensitivity to temperature and pinprick on the left side of the face
- Normal light touch sensation
- Absence of left corneal reflex
- Mild left-sided weakness when wrinkling his forehead, forcibly closing his eye, and retracting the corner of his mouth
- Loss of hearing in left ear, with lateralization of the tuning fork to the right ear on the Weber test and severely diminished air–bone conduction on the left

A brain MRI study revealed an egg-shaped mass in the left cerebellopontine angle that was expanding the internal auditory meatus of the temporal bone, compressing the left cerebellar hemisphere from below, and indenting the pons and upper medulla on the left side.

Question: Can you account for the cranial nerve symptoms based on the tumor mass at the cerebellopontine angle? Can the location of the mass account for the spastic (UMN) weakness of the right side of the body (the side opposite the lesion) and the tendency to fall to the left side (ipsilateral to the lesion)? How does cranial nerve injury explain the sensory findings on the face and facial weakness? Does the hearing loss indicate disease of the middle ear or of the statoacoustic vestibulocochlear (CN VIII) nerve? If it is nerve injury, would you expect any other abnormality of function of the vestibulocochlear nerve?

Discussion: UMN signs produced by a lesion anywhere above the decussation of the pyramids in the caudal medulla manifest on the opposite side of the body. Therefore, a mass at the level of the pons and rostral medulla on the left can account for right-sided hemiparesis. Cerebellar signs of unsteadiness appear on the same side as the lesion, and injury to the left cerebellar hemisphere accounts for falling to the left, the side of the lesion. Therefore, a single site of lesion can account for both of these clinical abnormalities. The decreased sensation on the face can be explained by partial injury to the

trigeminal (CN V) nerve on the left, with pain perception more affected than perception of touch. It may also be explained by injury to the sensory pathway for pain and temperature inside the brainstem on the left, because fibers mediating pain and temperature sensation (known as the descending or spinal tract of the trigeminal nerve) enter the brainstem at the midpons as part of the trigeminal nerve (CN V), then descend through the caudal pons and medulla as far as the high cervical spinal cord before synapsing and sending second-order sensory neurons across the midline to ascend to the thalamus on the right. The fibers mediating touch do not follow this descending course. They synapse, and the second-order axons cross at the level of entry in the midpons.

Absence of the corneal reflex can be explained by the loss of pain sensation on the cornea. The weakness of eye closure is also relevant to loss of the reflex, but without the sensory loss, some response of eye closure to touching the cornea with a wisp of cotton is likely, and the patient would feel the irritation of the stimulus.

The weakness of the face affects all components. When there is UMN facial weakness, the functions of forehead muscles are usually intact because they are controlled by both ipsilateral and contralateral descending motor pathways. Therefore, in this case, the weakness appears to be of the LMN variety (involvement of the nerve itself). This is consistent with the mass on the left at the level of the lateral recess of the medulla, where the facial and vestibulocochlear nerves enter the brainstem. The loss of hearing is the sensorineural type, affecting both air and bone conduction. Therefore, it is likely to originate in the nerve and is not consistent with middle ear disease, in which bone conduction is preserved.

The slow development of symptoms is consistent with benign tumor. Usually, a tumor in the cerebellopontine angle develops on the vestibular division of the vestibulocochlear nerve (CN VIII) from nerve sheath cells. The tumor is often called an **acoustic neuroma**, but better names for it are schwannoma (or Schwann cell tumor) and neurolemma. It is necessary to remove a schwannoma surgically to prevent further compression of vital structures of the medulla. Because the tumor tends to surround the facial nerve (CN VII) but not destroy it, facial weakness, if present, is usually mild before surgery. It may not be possible to preserve the nerve during the operation, however, because it is engulfed in tumor, and the face may be paralyzed postoperatively. Similarly, hearing is usually not restored; and because the tumor most often develops on the vestibular division of the nerve, caloric testing (irrigating the ear canal with warm or cold water) gives no response—that is, there is no vertigo or nystagmus when the test is performed on the damaged side. This is true before the operation as well, if the test is performed during the diagnostic workup.

PATIENT FOUR

A 60-year-old priest was taken to the emergency room for sensorimotor problems that developed abruptly while speaking to the members of his church during a Sunday mass. The attending physician noted the following:

- Unintelligible speech because of dysarthria
- Hypernasality with lowered left palate
- Dysphagia
- Sensation loss on the left side of the face
- Difficulty balancing, with falling to the left
- Left-sided facial paralysis
- Weakness in the right leg and arm

A brain MRI study revealed an infarct in the left caudal lateral ventral pons and medulla.

Question: Can you account for the symptoms of the left face and the paralysis of the right half of the body?

Discussion: A left pontine-medullary lesion resulted in alternating symptoms:

- The effects on the facial nerve (CN VII) and trigeminal nerve (CN V) fibers, along with the rootlets of the vagus nerve (CN X), were facial motor disturbance, loss of sensation from the face, palatal paralysis, and swallowing difficulty.
- Involvement of the vestibular nuclei resulted in the equilibrium problem.
- Interruption of the long descending pyramidal (corticospinal) fibers above the point of decussation produced paralysis in the right arm and leg.

PATIENT FIVE

A 39-year-old woman suffered a stroke while sleeping. When she woke, she was unable to speak and control her right limbs (arm and leg). She was taken to the emergency room where the examining neurologist noted the following:

- Adducted (drawn toward the median plane) left eye with inability to move it laterally
- Paralysis of the left face with drooling from the left of mouth
- Slowly uttered unintelligible speech marked by slurred articulation, imprecise consonants, and vowel prolongation
- Weakened tongue deviating to the left
- Loss of pain sensation on the entire left face
- Profoundly impaired hearing in the right ear
- Right hemiplegia
- Loss of pain and temperature on right half of the body

A speech language pathologist (SLP) consultation revealed:

- Poorly articulated, breathy, and aphonic speech, affecting its intelligibility

- Swallowing difficulty
- No sign of aphasia or cognitive impairment

An MRI study revealed a large infarct in the right rostral medulla.

Question: How can you explain the symptoms in relation to the right medullary lesion?

Discussion: This is a case of alternating hemiplegia in which a medullary lesion resulted in cranial nerve (LMN) symptoms on the ipsilateral side and hemiplegia (UMN) and hemianesthesia on the body contralateral to the lesion site. The lesion not only affected the cranial nerve projections but also interrupted long ascending and descending fibers:

- The ocular adduction (impaired ability to the move eye laterally) implies paralysis of the lateral rectus muscle subsequent to abducens nerve (CN VI) involvement; this nerve exists medially from the pontomedullary junction.
- Facial paralysis and subsequent drooling of saliva resulted from the involvement of the facial nerve (CN VII), which exits laterally at the pontomedullary junction.
- The decreased pain and temperature sensation on the face was the result of interrupted fibers of the trigeminal nerve, which exits from the pontine tegmentum.
- Hypoglossal nerve (CN XII) involvement resulted in the paralysis of the right half of the tongue. Hearing impairment (sensorineural type) indicated the involvement of the vestibulocochlear nerve (CN VIII), which is located lateral to the facial nerve at the pontomedullary junction. The presence of right hemiplegia and anesthesia resulted from the interruption of long ascending and descending projection fibers.

PATIENT SIX

A 50-year-old woman with a complaint of excruciating facial pain gradually was disinclined to speak and began communicating with gestures. She was diagnosed with possible depression and was taken to a neurologist who noted the following:

- Malnourished body habitus
- No limb or facial paralysis
- No sensory loss on either side of her face or body
- Excruciating episodic pain involving the face any time the patient touched the inner upper lip with the tongue tip
- No evidence of language or cognitive impairment

A brain MRI study revealed no abnormality. The attending neurologist concluded it to be a case of cranial nerve dysfunction associated with a trigger zone on the upper lip.

Question: What reasons can you give for this patient's disinclination to speak and for her facial pain?

Discussion: This is a clear case of trigeminal neuralgia, which is characterized by episodes of intense (sudden and stabbing) pain. The cause of neuralgia is not fully known. However, inflammation of the trigeminal ganglion and pressure caused by an arterial loop against the trigeminal nerve (CN V) are commonly implicated. The pain was initiated by touching a trigger zone, which for this patient was in the upper lip area. This evoked pain that caused her to refrain from speaking and eating.

PATIENT SEVEN

A 55-year-old SLP professor woke up in the middle of the night to use the bathroom; she was shocked to see asymmetry in her face. She first thought that her husband had played a trick by placing a special (fun house) mirror in the bathroom. She was taken to the emergency room where the attending neurologist noted the following:

- The mouth on right was lower with dripping saliva
- No motor control on her entire right face
- Inability to close her right eye.
- Speech was slow, slurred and unintelligible
- No sign of aphasia or amnesia
- No hemiplegia or hemianesthesia

A brain MRI study revealed no abnormality.

Question: How can you explain these selected facial symptoms?

Discussion: This unilateral facial palsy is a case of Bell palsy, which could be caused by an idiopathic involvement of the facial nerve (CN VII). With no other sensorimotor (hemiplegia or hemianesthesia) symptoms and no higher mental functions (aphasia and amnesia), this is a case of focal pathology, most likely a viral infection, one of the most common causes of facial palsy. In this case, the inability to close the eye has serious implications, because a constantly exposed cornea leads to dryness and, if untreated, can lead to corneal ulceration and eye damage.

PATIENT EIGHT

A 52-year-old woman, diagnosed with a brainstem (medullary) stroke, was seen by a consulting SLP who noted the following:

- Moderately unintelligible speech marked with slurred articulation, articulatory breakdown, hypernasality, impaired phonation, and intermittent breathiness
- Inability to protrude the tongue
- Difficulty with swallowing
- No other sensorimotor impairment
- No sign of language or cognitive disorder

The attending SLP suspected the involvement of several cranial nerves.

Question: How can you explain these symptoms and relate them to a brainstem stroke?

Discussion: The motor nuclei for the vagus (CN X), hypoglossal (CN XII), and glossopharyngeal (CN IX) nerves are located in the upper medial medulla. A localized medullary stroke had selectively affected the nucleus ambiguus, which is shared by the glossopharyngeal (CN IX) and vagus nerve (CN X) (altered phonation and dysphagia). This also affected the hypoglossal nucleus, which resulted in lingual paralysis and further contributed to the dysarthria.

SUMMARY

The human cranial nerves are the result of evolutionary modifications to a basic vertebrate pattern of CNS organization, constructed of ~40 bilaterally symmetrical repeating segments. During development, the first 2 nerves (olfactory [CN I] and optic [CN II]) became elaborated as the forebrain and involve the thalamus before reaching the cortex. The remaining 10 cranial nerves originate from the brainstem and innervate the muscles of the head, neck, face, larynx, tongue, and pharynx. These muscles serve speech, resonance, swallowing, facial expression, chewing, and phonation. Besides serving special senses such as vision, audition, smell, and taste, the cranial nerves regulate autonomic secretive functions of glands in the oral, nasal, and orbital cavities.

Some cranial nerves mediate only sensation, whereas others exclusively serve motor functions. However, most nerves have both sensory and motor functions. Some cranial nerves serve only a single functional component, whereas others contain fibers to serve two or more functional components. Several motor cranial nuclei receive corticobulbar projections from both sides of the motor cortex. This bilaterality of projection has important clinical implications for the motor speech processes.

QUIZ QUESTIONS

1. Define the following terms: anosmia, diplopia, ophthalmoplegia, pseudobulbar palsy.

2. Match each of the following numbered classifications with its associated lettered statement.

1. GSA	a.	pain and temperature
2. GSE	b.	vision and audition
3. SSA	c.	eye movements
4. SVA	d.	speech, phonation, and swallowing
5. SVE/BE	e.	taste and smell
6. GVA	f.	organ content
7. GVE	g.	autonomic activities

3. Match each of the numbered branchial arches with its lettered motor cranial nerve.

   1. first
   2. second
   3. third
   4. fourth and sixth

   a. glossopharyngeal nerve
   b. vagus nerve
   c. facial nerve
   d. trigeminal nerve

4. A 45-year-old woman experiences decreased hearing in the right ear, the entire right side of her face is paralyzed, and she has no reflex to touch in the cornea of the right eye. What cranial nerves are suspected to be damaged?

5. Some clinical symptoms demonstrated by a stroke patient were left ptosis, pupil unresponsiveness to light with dilated left pupil, and laterally deviated left eye. Discuss what cranial nerve is involved.

6. Define the following clinical conditions: trigeminal neuralgia and Bell palsy.

TECHNICAL TERMS

accommodation
atrophy
Bell palsy
branchial arch
ciliary muscle
cranial nerves
cutaneous
diplopia
flaccid
hypotonia
iris

light reflex
lower motor neuron
neuralgia
ophthalmoplegia
paralysis
postganglionic neuron
preganglionic neuron
somatic
strabismus
upper motor neuron
visceral muscles

Axial-Limbic Brain: Autonomic Nervous System, Limbic System, Hypothalamus, and Reticular Formation

LEARNING OBJECTIVES

After studying this chapter, students should be able to:

- Describe the structural organization of the autonomic nervous system

- Discuss the functions of the sympathetic and para-sympathetic systems

- Explain the central neural mechanism that controls the autonomic nervous system

- Describe the anatomic organization of the limbic system

- Discuss the functions of the cingulate gyrus, amygdala, septum, and hippocampus

- Describe the anatomic organization of the hypothalamus

- Discuss the autonomic and endocrinic functions of the hypothalamus

- Describe the functions of common hormones

- Explain the anatomic organization of the reticular formation

- Discuss the important functions of the reticular formation, including cortical arousal, attention, swallowing, and respiration

The autonomic nervous system (ANS), limbic lobe, hypothalamus, and reticular formation are functionally and anatomically integrated and are identified as the limbic–axial brain. As early-developing parts of the brain, these structures control basic physiologic functions and behaviors at the unconscious level. Together, the four components of the limbic–axial brain control all visceral and somatic activities vital to sustaining body functions. The ANS regulates the functions of the heart, lungs, and blood vessels as well as the organs of the digestive, reproductive, and urogenital systems. As a transitional structure, the limbic lobe (central unit of the limbic system) connects the thinking (neocortical) brain to the nonthinking and older (subcortical) axial brain and regulates drives, moods, motivation, and visceral activities that relate to the emotional aspects of sensorimotor behaviors and learning.

The hypothalamus, a visceral–somatic and metabolic control system, is functionally related to the limbic system, controls activity of the ANS, and influences behaviors including copulation, defecation, urination, alimentation, and aggression. In addition, the hypothalamus contains centers that control respiration, blood pressure, pulse rate, temperature, electrolyte balance, fluid balance, food intake, metabolism, diurnal (repeating daily) rhythms, and endocrine production. Furthermore, it contributes to the internal emotional state of well-being and pleasure.

The brainstem reticular formation influences brain activity by regulating the alerting mechanism. As the integrator of the sensory and motor mechanisms, the reticular formation participates in generation of well-coordinated motor functions, such as speech, eye–body coordinated movements, swallowing, and respiration. It also regulates blood pressure, rate, respiration, vomiting, and sleep and awake states.

All four components of the limbic–axial brain are connected by a system of complex fiber bundles. Only the basic anatomy of these related systems and their important functions are discussed in this chapter.

AUTONOMIC NERVOUS SYSTEM

The ANS involuntarily regulates visceral body functions by controlling the cardiac muscles, smooth muscles, and glands. This brings together all vital body functions, including the cardiovascular, pulmonary, digestive, urinary, and reproductive systems, maintaining body homeostasis. The ANS is integrated tightly with automatic and volitional sensorimotor behaviors.

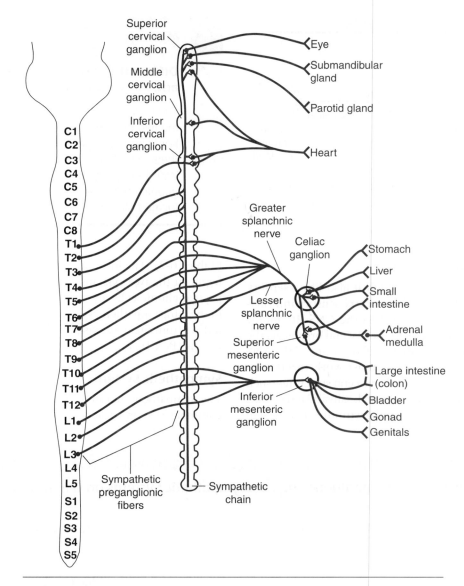

Figure 16-2 The sympathetic autonomic nervous system.

in the **intermediolateral gray matter** between the sensory and motor columns in the thoracic and upper lumbar segments of the spinal cord (Fig. 16-2). These cell bodies give rise to preganglionic efferent fibers. Efferent fibers of the preganglionic cells leave through the ventral spinal roots of the **thoracic** and **lumbar** segments and travel through the **white communicating ramus** of each spinal nerve (Fig. 16-3). They are white because most of the fibers are myelinated. These fibers terminate on the postganglionic neurons in the sympathetic chain or on other postganglionic sympathetic neurons in the abdomen around the aorta. The postganglionic neurons in the sympathetic chain are also known as the **paravertebral ganglia**, and the postganglionic sympathetic neurons close to the large abdominal arteries are called **prevertebral ganglia**. The prevertebral ganglia surround the visceral branches of the aorta and include the **coeliac, superior mesenteric,** and **inferior mesenteric**

ganglia. The sympathetic ganglionic chain extends from the base of the skull to the coccyx along the anterolateral area of the vertebral column.

The cervical portion of the sympathetic trunk contains three ganglia that are formed by a fusion of the original eight segmental ganglia: **superior, middle,** and **inferior cervical** (Fig. 16-2). The cervical sympathetic ganglia innervate the smooth muscles and glands in the head and upper limbs. Postganglionic fibers from the 11 thoracic ganglia innervate the heart, lungs, and thoracic and abdominal viscera. Postganglionic fibers from the lumbar ganglia are distributed via the spinal nerves and innervate the upper abdominal viscera, intestines, bladder, and genitals. Some of the unmyelinated sympathetic postganglionic fibers rejoin the spinal nerves via the gray communicating ramus (Fig. 16-3). They travel with the spinal nerves and separate from them before innervating blood vessels, smooth muscles, and sweat glands.

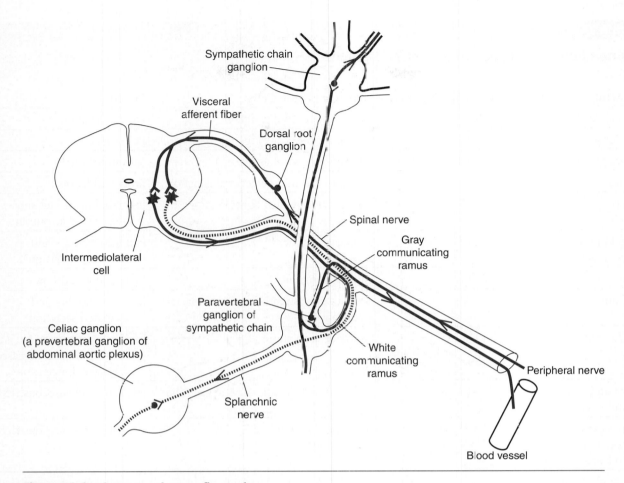

Figure 16-3 The sympathetic reflex arch.

The sympathetic system mobilizes metabolic energy for expenditure. This is common in stressful situations and emergencies in which a person's heart rate accelerates, arterial pressure rises, blood sugar level increases, and blood flow diverts from the visceral structures to the skeletal muscles (Table 16-3).

Parasympathetic System

The parasympathetic system preserves or restores metabolic energy. This system is also known as the **craniosacral system** because the cell bodies giving rise to preganglionic fibers are in the brainstem and sacral region of the spinal cord. The parasympathetic efferent fibers innervate the visceral structures in the head, neck, thorax, much of the abdominal cavity, and pelvic organs (Fig. 16-4; Table 16-4). The cranial section of the parasympathetic system includes the following cranial nerves (CNs): oculomotor (CN III), facial (CN VII), glossopharyngeal (CN IX), and vagus (CN X). The Edinger-Westphal nucleus, the visceral component of the oculomotor complex in the midbrain (see Chapter 15), sends preganglionic fibers to the postganglionic neurons in the ciliary ganglion. The postganglionic fibers from the ciliary ganglion innervate the sphincter of the iris and smooth muscle of the ciliary body. The facial preganglionic parasympathetic fibers supply the pterygopalatine and sub-

mandibular ganglia; the postganglionic fibers innervate the lacrimal glands and their blood vessels as well as the mucous membrane glands. Postganglionic fibers of the facial cranial nerve also innervate the submandibular and sublingual salivary glands and the mucous membranes in the floor of the mouth. Postganglionic fibers from the otic ganglion of the glossopharyngeal nerve activate the parotid gland.

The largest source of preganglionic parasympathetic fibers is from the vagus nerve (CN X), which supplies practically all of the thoracic and abdominal viscera except for the pelvis. The vagus nerve (CN X) supplies the parasympathetic ganglia in the heart, bronchial musculature, stomach, large and small intestines, liver, pancreas, and kidneys. In the intestinal system, short postganglionic fibers terminate in the smooth muscle and glands and serve motor and secretory functions. The sacral parasympathetic postganglionic fibers supply the urinary bladder, colon, rectum, accessory reproductive organs, and intestinal viscera not innervated by the vagus nerve (CN X).

The parasympathetic system dominates during periods of relaxation because it reduces the activity of various organs and conserves metabolic energy. Common parasympathetic activities include decreasing heart rate, lowering blood pressure, constricting pupils, and increasing digestion.

Table 16-3

Sympathetic Innervation of the Visceral Organs

Structure	Preganglionic Cells	Postganglionic Cells	Function
Eyelid cartilage	C8–T2	Superior cervical ganglion	Eyelid elevation
Iris muscle	C8–T2	Superior cervical ganglion	Pupil dilation
Saliva gland	C8–T2	Superior cervical ganglion	Salivation (thick)
Lungs	T1–T5	Stellate and middle cervical ganglion	Bronchodilation
Heart	T1–T5	Stellate and middle cervical ganglion	Increased heart rate and greater cardiac output
Small intestine (stomach)	T6–T10	Celiac ganglion	Reduced motility and decreased secretion
Liver	T6–T10	Celiac ganglion	Increased blood flow
Column	T8–L2	Mesenteric (superior and inferior) ganglion	Reduced motility and decreased secretion
Bladder and ureter	T11–L12	Inferior mesenteric	Inhibition of ureter contraction and increased internal sphincter tone
Neck and heart glands and vessels	C8–T3	Superior and middle cervical ganglion	Sweating and vasoconstriction
Upper extremity and upper chest glands and vessels	C8–T5	Stellate ganglion and T2–T5 paravertebral ganglion	Sweating and vasoconstriction
Lower chest and abdominal glands and vessels	T6–L2	T6–L2 paravertebral ganglion	Sweating and vasoconstriction
Lower extremity gland and vessels	T10–L2	L1–S4 paravertebral ganglion	Sweating and vasoconstriction

Visceral Afferent System

Sensory fibers from the thoracic, abdominal, and pelvic viscera travel through sympathetic nerves, ultimately reaching the sympathetic chain. They enter the T1–L2 region of the cord via the white communicating rami. From there they ascend into the dorsal lemniscus and anterolateral systems. The visceral afferent fibers of the vagus nerve (CN X), which has cell bodies in the inferior (nodose) ganglion, are distributed peripherally in the heart, lungs, and other viscera. Fibers from the bladder, rectum, and accessory genital organs travel through the splanchnic nerves and enter the spinal cord through the S2–S4 nerves.

Afferent visceral fibers are important for visceral and viscerosomatic reflexes mediated through the spinal cord, brainstem, and hypothalamus. For example, sacral visceral afferents from stretch receptors of the urinary bladder control the bladder reflex and sensations that occur with bladder distension. The nucleus of the solitary tract in the medulla receives stimuli from the walls of the digestive tract, respiratory tract, and heart as well as its vascular trunks. These projections mediate respiratory and cardiovascular reflexes regulated by the medulla and hypothalamus.

Most autonomic sensory reactions remain subconscious but cause visceral pain, distress, nausea, hunger, and other less well-localized visceral sensations. A constant stream of visceral impulses allows for the general feeling of either internal well-being or malaise. Almost all visceral abdominal pain is projected in the sympathetic system. Intense visceral pain from internal organs often is felt on the skin in an area supplied by the somatic fibers arising from the same cord segment; this is known as referred pain (see Chapter 7).

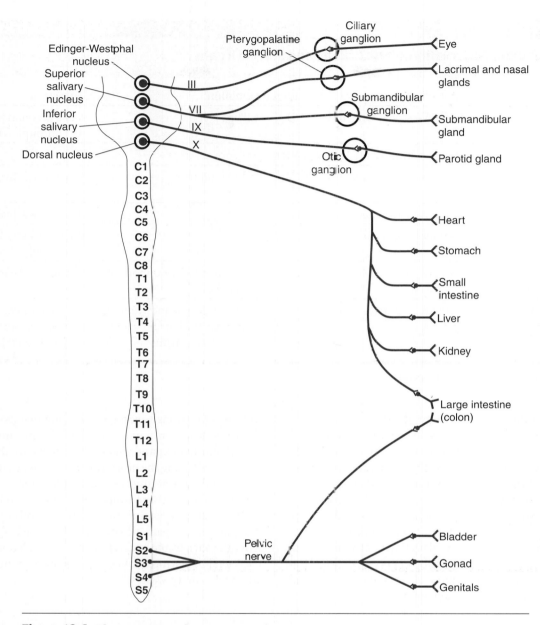

Figure 16-4 The parasympathetic autonomic nervous system.

Neurotransmitters

Acetylcholine is the main neurotransmitter for the preganglionic and postganglionic fibers of the parasympathetic system and for the preganglionic fibers of the sympathetic system. The postganglionic sympathetic nerves secrete norepinephrine as a transmitter (Table 16-5).

Central Autonomic Pathways

The **hypothalamus** centrally controls the ANS. The hypothalamic regulation of the ANS is mediated in part by a series of synaptic relays from the neocortex, limbic system, diencephalon, brainstem, and spinal cord. Activation of the anterior hypothalamus stimulates the parasympathetic system, whereas activation of the posterolateral hypothalamus stimulates the sympathetic system. Hypothalamic impulses are transmitted to the midbrain via a descending component of the **medial forebrain bundle**, the **mamillotegmental tract**, and through other descending projections. Continuing from the midbrain, hypothalamic impulses are relayed caudally through synaptic relays in the brainstem reticular formation, which in turn conveys the impulses to visceral motor nuclei of the brainstem and spinal cord.

Clinical Concerns

Interruptions of the autonomic regulation of visceral functions are characterized by impaired control of blood pressure,

Table 16-4

Parasympathetic Innervation of the Cranial and Sacral Organs

Structure	CNS Cell Body	Ganglion	Function
Ciliary and pupillary muscles	Edinger-Westphal nucleus (CN III)	Ciliary	Lens accommodation and pupil constriction
Lacrimal gland	Superior salivatory nucleus (CN VII)	Sphenopalatine	Tears
Submandibular and sublingual glands	Superior salivatory nucleus (CN VII)	Submandibular	Excessive saliva (thin)
Parotid gland	Inferior salivatory nucleus (CN IX)	Otic	Excessive saliva (thin)
Small intestine	Dorsal motor nucleus (CN X)	None	Increased secretion and mobility
Heart	Ambiguus nucleus (CN X)	Intracardiac and pulmonary ganglia	Decreased heart rate
Column, rectum, and genitals	Intermediate spinal gray nuclei (S2–S4)	Vesicular ganglia in myenteric plexus of colon and ganglia in walls of organs	Contraction of bladder, colon, rectum, and penile erection

CN, cranial nerve; *CNS*, central nervous system.

respiration, cardiovascular activity, gland secretion, sexual activity, bladder incontinence, and urinary retention. In the case of disturbance in the sympathetic system, unopposed parasympathetic control of visceral structures results in symptoms indicating the restoration of metabolic energy in activities, such as decreased heart rate, lowered blood pressure, constriction of the pupils, and increased digestion. The reverse is true in cases of parasympathetic disturbance in which unopposed activity of the sympathetic system results in expenditure of metabolic energy (e.g., acceleration of the heart rate, elevation of arterial pressure, and increased blood flow to the skeletal muscles) (Tables 16-3 and 16-4).

Summary of the Autonomic Nervous System

The ANS regulates visceral functions and maintains homeostasis by regulating vital body systems, including the cardiovascular, pulmonary, digestive, urinary, and reproductive systems. The ANS uses its sympathetic and parasympathetic systems—functionally antagonistic components—to render opposite effects on organ activities. For instance, sympathetic neurons expand metabolic energy by dilating the pupils, accelerating the heartbeat, inhibiting intestinal movements, and contracting the rectal sphincters. Conversely, the parasympathetic neurons constrict the pupils, slow the heart, increase peristaltic movement, and relax the sphincters. The parasympathetic system is concerned with anabolic activities, such as the restoration and conservation of energy. The sacral parasympathetics activate the excretion of intestinal and urinary wastes.

LIMBIC SYSTEM

The limbic system (visceral brain) refers to closely related functional structures of the limbic lobe, diencephalon, septum, and midbrain. The limbic lobe includes the **subcallosal gyrus**, **cingulate gyrus**, **isthmus**, **parahippocampal gyrus**, **hippocampus**, **olfactory cortex**, **uncus**, and **amygdala** (Figs. 16-5 and 16-6). The **septal area**, located at the rostral diencephalon, forms the septo-hypothalamus-midbrain continuum. It is essential for completing the limbic system's bidirectional circuitry, connecting the limbic lobe to the hypothalamus, thalamus, and midbrain. The **fornix**, a large C-shaped bundle of bidirectional fibers, serves as the main circuitry connecting the limbic lobe to the diencephalon and visceral centers of the hypothalamus.

The limbic system regulates emotion, motivation, learning, and memory. Limbic projections to the forebrain con-

Table 16-5

Sympathetic and Parasympathetic Neurotransmitters

Structure	Sympathetic	Parasympathetic
Preganglionic cells	Acetylcholine	Acetylcholine
Postganglionic cells	Norepinephrine	Acetylcholine

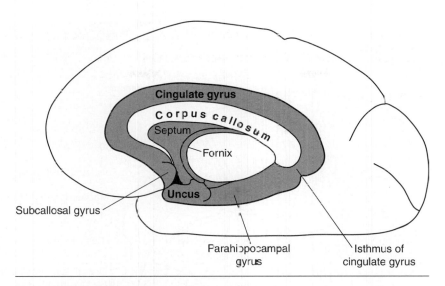

Figure 16-5 Midsagittal view showing the limbic structures.

tribute to emotions and provide motivation for behaviors that are fundamental to survival (feeding, mating, aggression, and flight). With connections to prefrontal lobe and hippocampus, the limbic structures also participate in memory and learning. Most understanding of limbic behaviors and their impairments, such as **Klüver-Bucy syndrome**, is based primarily on animal experiments. Humans with dementias, carbon monoxide poisoning, and temporal lobe seizures may exhibit the behavior found in animals with impaired limbic systems.

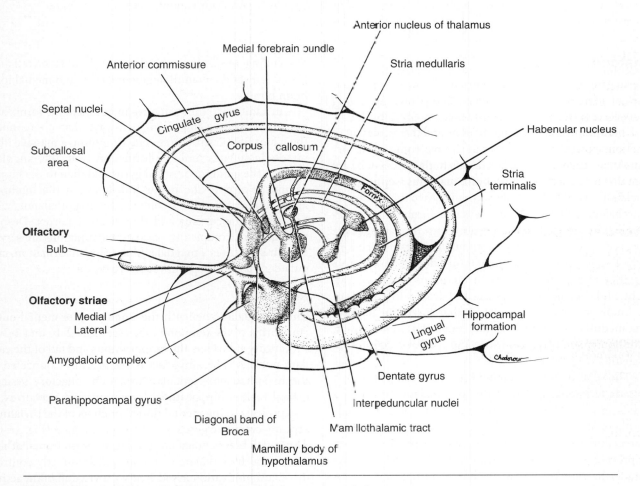

Figure 16-6 Medial view of the major limbic structures and their connections.

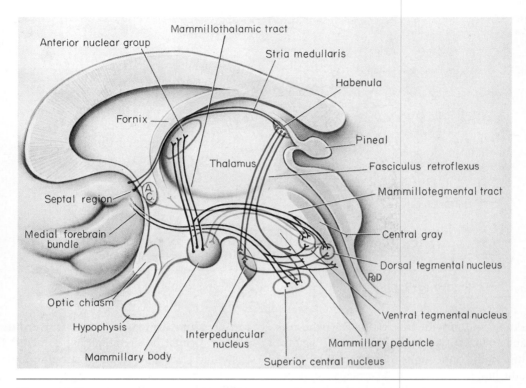

Figure 16-7 The major limbic pathways: medial forebrain bundle, mamillothalamic tract, mamillotegmental tract, and stria medullaris. *A.C.*, Anterior Commissure.

Anatomic Structures

The key limbic structures are connected by an extensive network of afferent and efferent fibers. These interconnecting fibers account for the limbic influence on virtually all cortical, brainstem, and visceral functions and the regulation of emotions and motivation. Not all limbic connections are completely understood. Major inputs to the limbic lobe are from the **neocortex**, **olfactory bulb**, **thalamus**, **septum**, and reticular formation. The limbic output goes to the neocortex, hypothalamus, thalamus, and reticular formation. Projections to the prefrontal lobe in the neocortex regulate affective aspects of emotion, such as moods and feelings. Projections to the hypothalamus and reticular formation regulate ANS activities and motor aspects of emotions, such as fear, flight, and sex. Major ascending and descending tracts of the limbic system include the **medial forebrain bundle**, **stria medullaris**, **stria terminalis**, **mamillothalamic tract**, **mamillotegmental tract**, fornix, and **medial longitudinal fasciculus** (Fig. 16-7).

The septum is connected with the amygdala through the stria terminalis and with the hypothalamic mamillary bodies through the fornix and ascending and descending fibers of the medial forebrain bundle (Fig. 16-6). The stria medullaris forms the limbic–thalamic pathway, which reciprocally connects the septum with the thalamus. The mamillothalamic tract mediates limbic outputs to the neocortex via the **anterior nucleus** of the thalamus. The limbic descending projections travel to the brainstem reticular formation via the mamillotegmental tract and medial forebrain bundle.

In addition to the structures mentioned, the fornix and cingulum are two important pathways that interconnect the major limbic structures. The cingulum, a massive fiber bundle, circulates limbic information from the cingulate gyrus to the parahippocampal gyrus and then to the hippocampus. Forming the major link between the forebrain and midbrain, the fornix connects the hypothalamus with both the hippocampus and the olfactory cortex. Despite this anatomic complexity, basic limbic functions are served by four structures: amygdala, hippocampal formation, cingulate gyrus, and septum (Table 16-6).

Amygdala

The amygdala is beneath the uncus in the medial anterior cortex of the temporal lobe (see Figs. 2-16 and 3-30). Posteriorly, it borders the hippocampus and tail of the caudate nucleus. The amygdala is reciprocally connected to the hypothalamus, reticular formation, olfactory system, orbital region, hippocampal formation, and neocortex. It also projects to the **medial dorsal nucleus** of the thalamus, septum, cingulate gyrus, and prefrontal region (Fig. 16-6). Along with bidirectional projections to the prefrontal orbital cortex and hypothalamus, the amygdala directly controls drive and motivation associated with visceral brain activities and the accompanying internal feelings.

Table 16-6

Limbic Structures and Their Functions

Structure	Afferents	Efferents	Functions
Amygdala	Hypothalamus, reticular formation, olfactory system, orbital region, hippocampal formation, and neocortex limbic cortex	Thalamus, septum, cingulate, hypothalamus, and prefrontal cortex	Aggression, mating, stress-mediated responses, memory, feeding, and drinking
Hippocampus	Neocortex, limbic cortex, olfactory area, hypothalamus, and septal area	Amygdala, septum, hypothalamus, and thalamus	Memory and learning
Septal nuclei	Hippocampus, amygdala, and hypothalamus	Hippocampus, amygdala, and hypothalamus	Hormonal secretion, behavioral reaction, and memory facilitation
Cingulate gyrus	Hypothalamic mamillary bodies and anterior thalamic nucleus	Hypothalamic mamillary bodies and anterior thalamic nucleus	Anxiety and altered behavior (panic and compulsion)

Stimulation-based investigations of amygdaloid function in animals suggest that its activation with high-threshold stimulation can produce all the behaviors that are elicited from the hypothalamus—for example, defecation, micturition, pupillary dilation, hair erection, pituitary hormone secretion, blood pressure and heart rate changes, and gastrointestinal motility and secretion. Other behaviors are associated with sexual activities: erection, copulatory movements, ejaculation, ovulation, uterine activity, and premature labor. Rage, escape, punishment, and fear also are associated with the amygdala. Stimulation of the amygdala results in motor activities such as head movements, circling, dystonic movements, licking, chewing, swallowing, and vomiting. Combined stimulation of the amygdala and hypothalamus facilitates the rage reaction, and amygdala stimulation may increase or decrease hypothalamic-induced rage.

Bilateral ablation of the amygdala and surrounding temporal tissues is associated with Klüver-Bucy syndrome, which is characterized by indiscriminate eating, oral exploration, fearlessness, loss of aggression, psychic blindness, and inappropriate hypersexuality. Complex partial seizures, which emanate from the amygdala and surrounding temporal lobe structures, are characterized by automatic aggressive behavior, memory impairment, and automatisms (impaired ability to monitor behavior and realize subsequent consequences) (see Chapter 20).

Hippocampus

The hippocampus is in the ventromedial temporal lobe beneath the **hippocampal gyrus**. It forms the ventromedial wall of the lateral ventricle temporal (inferior) horn (see Fig. 3-30). The principal sources of afferents to the hippo-campus are the polysensory association cortical areas. Impulses to the hippocampus travel via the parahippocampal and occipitotemporal gyri (Fig. 16-6). The hippocampus also receives projections from the septum, hypothalamus, and midbrain via the medial forebrain and fornix fiber bundles. Primary efferents from the hippocampus are to the amygdala, septum, and hypothalamus. Hippocampal stimulation and ablation implicate endocrine and autonomic functions that are generated in the hypothalamus. However, the hippocampus is best known for its involvement with memory and learning.

In the early 1950s, drastic anterograde memory deficits were noted to have occurred after radical bilateral ablations of the hippocampal formation that extended posteriorly in the region of the caudal parahippocampal and fusiform (occipitotemporal) gyri. Patients could not remember their experiences from one moment to the next. A hippocampal lesion was associated with severe anterograde amnesia with preserved retrograde memories. In other words, patients lost newly acquired data but retained memory of events that preceded the lesion. Clinical and experimental findings suggest that the anterograde memory deficit may be the result of the interruption of reverberating cortical circuits that connect the polysensory association cortices with the parahippocampal and fusiform gyri.

Cingulate Gyrus

Located above the corpus callosum, the cingulate gyrus receives projections from the hypothalamic mamillary bodies by way of the mamillothalamic tract and the anterior thalamic nucleus (Figs. 16-5 and 16-6; see Fig. 2-10 and Chapter 6). The cingulate gyrus projects to the hypothalamic mamillary bodies via the fornix fibers that arise in

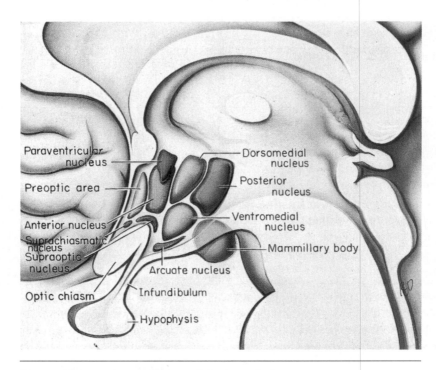

Figure 16-8 Midsagittal view of the hypothalamic nuclei.

the entorhinal cortex (part of the hippocampus and uncus forming the lateral olfactory area). Clinically, this limbic circuit has been associated with anxiety and obsessive–compulsive behaviors.

Septum

The septum consists of two parts. Dorsally, it consists of a midline fibrous sheet attached to the corpus callosum (Figs. 16-5 and 16-6; see Fig. 2-11). Ventrally, it consists of a collection of nuclei. In conjunction with the diencephalon and brainstem and a major component of the axial brain, the septum forms the septo-hypothalamus-midbrain continuum. The fornix provides a vital portal entry connecting the limbic lobe to the diencephalon and brainstem. It is also involved actively in processing autonomic, visceral, endocrine, sensorimotor, reproductive, neurotransmitter, emotional, and motivational functions.

Clinical Concerns

Clinical symptoms that appear after limbic system lesions involve emotions and motivation. They are characterized by uninhibited instinctual behavior, altered sexual behavior, excessive fear, aggression, and disturbances in circadian rhythm. Limbic dysfunctions also have substantial implications for memory and learning (Table 16-6).

Summary of the Limbic System

Anatomically, limbic structures form the inner brain neural circuitry that connects the cortex to the diencephalon and midbrain structures. Functionally, they regulate all visceral, endocrine, and sensorimotor functions. With rich interconnections, the limbic system forms the neural mechanism responsible for motivational drive and emotions.

HYPOTHALAMUS

Consisting of only 4 g of gray matter and occupying a small area in the anterior region of the diencephalon beneath the thalamus, the hypothalamus has an importance that greatly exceeds its size. Interconnected with the forebrain, brainstem, and spinal cord, the hypothalamus is the central structure for controlling autonomic and visceral behaviors, such as vasodilation, body homeostasis (internal body environment), anger, reproduction, hunger, and thirst. With its projections to the limbic lobe, it provides the substrates for regulating motivation and emotions. The neurosecretory cells of the hypothalamus regulate the production and circulation of hormones by the pituitary gland.

Anatomic Structures

The hypothalamus is exposed fully on the medial surface of the brain and is located symmetrically along the lateral walls of the third ventricle (see Figs. 2-11 and 2-12). Dorsally delineated by the hypothalamic sulcus, the hypothalamus extends from the optic chiasm to the posterior border of the mamillary bodies. The anterior commissure identifies its rostral limit, whereas caudally it extends to the central gray matter in the midbrain tegmentum. The internal capsule marks the lateral limit of the hypothalamus.

On the midsagittal surface, the hypothalamus is divided into the **anterior, tuberal**, and **posterior regions** (Fig. 16-8). The anterior hypothalamus is above the optic chiasm. The tuberal region is enclosed by the optic chiasm, optic tract,

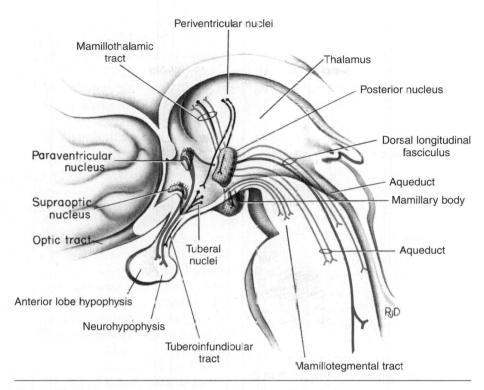

Figure 16-9 The major hypothalamic primarily efferent pathways.

and mamillary bodies. The posterior hypothalamic region includes the mamillary bodies and the nuclei above them. The principal hypothalamic nuclei are **preoptic, supraoptic, ventromedial, dorsomedial, paraventricular, anterior, posterior,** and **mamillary body** (Fig. 16-8).

The **infundibulum,** is the stalk of the **pituitary gland;** it comes from the floor of the third ventricle. As the transitional structure between the CNS and peripheral endocrine system, the infundibulum is the interface between the brain and pituitary gland. The median eminence (**tuber cinereum**) is just caudal to the infundibulum. Above this tuberal level are the ventromedial and dorsomedial hypothalamic nuclei.

The hypothalamus is connected to the cerebral cortex, thalamus, and midbrain with extensive afferent and efferent fiber tracts. Afferents to the hypothalamus come primarily from the limbic region of the forebrain, brainstem, and spinal cord. The bidirectional connections of the hypothalamus to the brainstem and spinal cord regulate visceral and autonomic functions. Its interconnections to the limbic lobe account for motivational drive and emotions (Fig. 16-7). The major fiber bundles that interconnect the hypothalamus with other neuraxial structures are the medial forebrain bundle, stria terminalis, fornix, and mamillothalamic, mamillotegmental, and dorsal longitudinal fasciculi (Figs. 16-7 and 16-9).

Afferents

The medial forebrain bundle regulates the forebrain input to the hypothalamus and is the major bidirectional tract formed by the cells in the olfactory region, septum, and amygdala. This pathway mediates information basic to the emotional drives. Other important input for emotional drives comes from the amygdala, which is connected to the hypothalamus via the stria terminalis (Fig. 16-6). The fornix, a large bidirectional pathway, curves around the thalamus and connects to the hypothalamic mamillary bodies with the hippocampus via the septum. The bidirectional fibers of the mamillothalamic tract connect the mamillary bodies to the anterior nucleus of the thalamus, which projects to the cingulate gyrus of the limbic lobe (Fig. 16-7). The brainstem and reticular input to the hypothalamus enter by way of the mamillary bodies, dorsal longitudinal fasciculus, and medial forebrain bundle (Figs. 16-7 and 16-9).

Efferents

Efferents of the hypothalamus project to the forebrain limbic structures (septum, hippocampal formation, and amygdala). Projections also reach the brainstem reticular region, which includes the periaqueductal gray matter, by way of bidirectional fibers in the tracts described under afferents. The efferent hypothalamic projections to the limbic lobe travel via the septum to the hippocampus and by way of the mamillothalamic tract to the cingulate gyrus (Fig. 16-9). The mamillothalamic fibers connect the hypothalamus to the anterior thalamic nucleus (see Chapter 6), which in turn connects to the cingulate gyrus, another limbic structure. Hypothalamic projections to the amygdaloid nucleus travel primarily via the stria terminalis and hypothalamus-amygdaloid fibers. The multisynaptic outputs travel through the fibers of the dorsal longitudinal tract to the sympathetic and parasympathetic preganglionic cranial and spinal cells. Because of this, the hypothalamus controls the autonomic system and regulates eating and drinking.

Additional projections to the lower brainstem and spinal preganglionic autonomic nuclei come from the reticular formation, which in turn receives hypothalamic input via fibers of the mamillotegmental tract (Fig. 16-9). Other important neural projections of the hypothalamus travel to the posterior pituitary gland. Hypothalamic neuronal influence on the anterior pituitary gland controls the secretion of gonadotropic, adrenocorticotropic, and thyrotropic hormones.

Hypothalamic Functions

Most understanding of hypothalamic functions is based on the electrical stimulation of the hypothalamus and/or observations of impaired functions after lesions induced in the hypothalamus of animals. In addition to regulating autonomic (sympathetic and parasympathetic) functions, the hypothalamus has specific centers for controlling eating, drinking, reproduction, aggression, and biologic body rhythms. The hypothalamus also contributes to blood electrolyte balance and temperature control. Most important, it controls endocrine-monitored behaviors through the secretion of hormones. Only a few hypothalamic functions are discussed here.

Autonomic Innervation

The posterior hypothalamic region controls activity of the sympathetic nervous system, which regulates activities such as pupil dilation, piloerection, somatic hyperactivity, inhibition of the gut and bladder, increased heart rate, blood pressure, and respiration. Electrical stimulation of this region activates thoracolumbar outflow, which increases metabolic and somatic activities typical of emotional stress and aggression. The control center for the parasympathetic system is in the anterior and medial hypothalamic regions, which on activation increase vagal and sacral autonomic responses, such as reduced heart rate, peripheral vasodilation, and increased tone and motility of the alimentary and bladder walls.

Body Temperature Regulation

Body temperature regulation involves the balanced coordination of the sympathetic and parasympathetic nervous systems. Neurons in the anterior hypothalamus are sensitive to increases in blood temperature. They react to an increase in temperature by dissipating excess heat through sweating (a sympathetic activity) and by inhibiting the sympathetic system, causing cutaneous blood vessels to dilate. The posterior hypothalamus, however, preserves heat by inhibiting the sympathetic system in constricting cutaneous vessels and stopping sweat secretion. This is accompanied by shivering (a somatic activity) and decreased visceral activity.

An anterior hypothalamic lesion impairs the heat dissipation mechanism and results in **hyperthermia**, whereas a posterior hypothalamic lesion impairs the pathways responsible for both heat conservation and dissipation, resulting in a **poikilothermic state** in which body temperature is governed by environmental temperature.

Water Intake Regulation

Adequate water input and output, essential for normal body activity, is regulated by vasopressin, an antidiuretic hormone. Synthesized in the supraoptic nucleus of the anterior hypothalamus, vasopressin is released into the bloodstream per physiologic circumstances by way of the posterior pituitary gland. Vasopressin production is controlled by blood osmotic pressure and hydration. A rise in blood osmotic pressure or a reduction in circulating vascular volume increases vasopressin production, causing fluid retention. A dehydrated state activates the supraoptic hypothalamic vasopressin system. Vasopressin is resynthesized and stored in the posterior pituitary gland after water balance is re-established.

Activation of the anterior hypothalamus causes increased water intake. In fact, the anterior hypothalamus regulates both food and water intake. Small lesions in the lateral hypothalamus cause adipsia (a lack of desire to drink), and large lesions cause both **adipsia** and **aphagia** (inability to eat). A lesion in the supraoptic nucleus results in increased water intake (polydipsia) and increased urine output (polyuria), a condition clinically known as diabetes insipidus.

Feeding

The feeding (phagic) center is in the lateral hypothalamus. A lesion in this area causes anorexia, a decreased desire to eat. The ventromedial nucleus of the hypothalamus is the site of a satiety center. Lesions of the ventromedial nucleus of the hypothalamus cause hyperphagia, obesity, and aggressive behavior.

Punishment

The periventricular hypothalamus regulates feelings like fear, terror, and the desire to flee, which are engendered by challenging situations. These structures extend posteriorly to the central gray matter surrounding the cerebral aqueduct or aqueduct of Sylvius in the midbrain. Prolonged stimulation in these areas may cause death. By varying the electrical parameters, stimulation of the ventromedial hypothalamus may elicit fear, rage, and aggression. Stimulation of the more rostral midline preoptic area elicits the fear and anxiety that are associated with escape. In generating these behaviors, the cerebral cortex, in conjunction with various environmental inputs, must recruit somatic and hypothalamic visceral systems. Together they control the expression of pleasure or displeasure associated with the behavior.

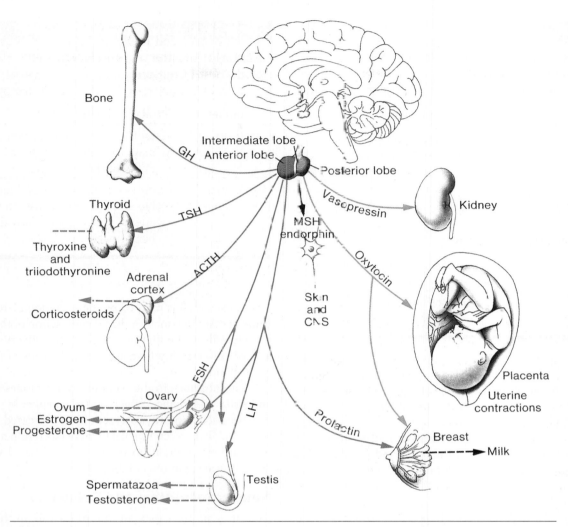

Figure 16-10 Commonly secreted pituitary hormones in the adenohypophysis and neuro-hypophysis. Hormones of the anterior pituitary gland, or adenohypophysis, are growth hormone (*GH*), thyrotropin, adrenocorticotropic hormone (*ACTH*), gonadotropin, and prolactin. The posterior pituitary lobe, or neurohypophysis, contains vasopressin and oxytocin. Secreted by cells in the supraoptic and paraventricular hypothalamic nuclei, these hormones regulate kidney function (vasopressin) and glands of the breasts (oxytocin). *CNS*, central nervous system; *FSH*, follicle-stimulating hormone; *LH*, luteinizing hormone; *MSH*, melanocyte-stimulating hormone; *TSH*, thyroid-stimulating hormone.

Hypothalamic Regulation of the Pituitary Gland (Hypophysis)

Nicknamed the master gland, the pituitary gland forms the central endocrine system and works with the nervous system to maintain body homeostasis. The pituitary gland controls the functioning of other glands and tissues in the body by secreting hormones and chemical messengers. The pituitary gland consists of a large anterior lobe (adenohypophysis) and small posterior lobe (neurohypophysis) (Fig. 16-9).

The release of hormones produced in the neurosecretory hypothalamic cells stimulates the adenohypophysis to secrete the following hormones: **growth hormone, thyro-** tropin, adrenocorticotropin, gonadotropin, and prolactin. The releasing hormones are transported into the anterior lobe of the pituitary gland through the hypothalamic hypophyseal portal (blood) circulation (Fig. 16-10; Table 16-7).

Thyrotropic hormones stimulate and regulate thyroid gland hormone secretion. Adrenocorticotropin regulates steroid secretion by the adrenal cortex. Gonadotropin (follicle-stimulating hormone) stimulates production of ova and sperm. Prolactin (lactogenic hormone), in conjunction with other hormones, stimulates and maintains milk secretion by the mamillary glands. Growth hormones stimulate and maintain the growth of bones and muscles. Hyposecretion and hypersecretion of growth hormones are related

Table 16-7

Anterior Pituitary Gland Hormones and Their Functions

Hormones	Primary Function
Growth hormone	Controls general body growth.
Thyroid-stimulating hormone (thyrotropic)	Controls thyroid hormone secretions
Adrenocorticotropic hormone	Controls secretion of adrenal cortex hormones
Gonadotropic hormone	Initiates sperm production in males; promotes development of ova in females
Prolactin	Promotes milk secretion by mamillary glands

Table 16-8

Posterior Pituitary Gland Hormones and Their Functions

Hormones	Primary Function
Oxytocin	Stimulates uterine contraction and mamillary gland alveoli, causing milk secretion
Vasopressin	Decreases urine volume and raises blood pressure by constricting arterial lumen, particularly during hemorrhage

to dwarfism and gigantism. These growth hormones also regulate the rate of protein synthesis, fat burning, and conversion of glycogen into blood glucose.

Two peptide hormones, vasopressin and oxytocin, are released from the posterior pituitary gland (Table 16-8). Vasopressin is synthesized predominantly in the supraoptic nucleus, whereas oxytocin is synthesized in the paraventricular nucleus of the hypothalamus. They are both transported axonally to the posterior hypophysis, where they are stored and then released into the bloodstream. Vasopressin is an antidiuretic hormone that increases water reabsorption in the kidney and is used to raise blood pressure in states of hypotension. Lesions of the posterior lobe cause diabetes

insipidus, which is marked by the excretion of 10–15 L of urine per day. Oxytocin-induced contraction of the smooth muscle cells of the uterus assists in the delivery of a baby and in milk ejection by contracting the cells of the mammary gland.

An imbalance in the secretion of hormones results in endocrine disturbance, which is marked either by decreased hormone secretion (hyposecretion) or increased hormone secretion (hypersecretion). The hypersecretion and hyposecretion of common hormones are associated with specific clinical symptoms (Table 16-9).

Neurotransmitters and Behaviors

Neurotransmitters play an important role in the regulation of behaviors mediated by the hypothalamus. The interaction of vasopressin with noradrenergic synapses influences memory consolidation. Norepinephrine released in the hypothalamus may block visceral drives, such as eating,

Table 16-9

Disorders Associated with Hormone Disturbances

Hormone	Disturbance	Condition
Growth hormone	Hyposecretion	Dwarfism
	Hypersecretion	Gigantism
Thyrotropic hormone	Hyposecretion	In infancy, results in low metabolism, low body development, and mental retardation; in adults, causes lethargy, excessive sleeping, and slow mental activity
	Hypersecretion	Increased metabolic rate increases hunger and food intake
Adrenocorticotropic hormone	Hyposecretion	Impaired synthesis of glucose and loss of sodium in urine
	Hypersecretion	Decreased immune response and excessive fat deposits
Gonadotropic hormone		Impaired sexual functions
Vasopressin		Water imbalance

drinking, and sexual behavior. This suggests that while norepinephrine activates the neocortex it inhibits the competing visceral drives. Excessive production of norepinephrine causes manic psychosis, whereas insufficient production of it causes depression. Stimulation of dopamine projections to the hypothalamic area enhances eating and fighting drives. A bilateral hypothalamic lesion that impairs the dopaminergic systems reduces these drives.

Clinical Concerns

Clinical symptoms that commonly result from hypothalamic dysfunction are characterized by disturbances of food intake, water balance, libido, menstruation, and temperature control. Also, pituitary hormone changes can affect body growth, the ability to reproduce, and milk secretion.

Summary of the Hypothalamus

The hypothalamus is the central structure for controlling autonomic and visceral behaviors. It is the central generator of motivational and emotional–motor behaviors and controls visceral functions, such as vasodilation, body homeostasis (internal body environment), reproduction, hunger, and water and food intake. Its neurosecretory cells regulate pituitary gland hormone production and release.

RETICULAR FORMATION

The reticular formation (RF) consists of a group of neurons that are interconnected by a complex web of parallel and serial running neuronal circuits. Composing most of the brainstem (medulla, pons, and midbrain), it is also functionally wired to nuclei in the thalamus and spinal cord (see Fig. 2-23). With their central location, the neuronal circuits of the RF converge or diverge to inhibit, facilitate, modify, and regulate all cortical functions and further integrate all sensorimotor stimuli with internally generated thoughts, emotions, and cognition. It also is responsible for maintaining the homeostatic state of the brain, which is essential for regulating visceral, sensorimotor and neuroendocrine activities such as sleep, blood pressure, posture, and movement. The RF also regulates emotions, mood, and cognition. Furthermore, it energizes the **reticular activating system** (RAS), which controls arousal and consciousness. A single lesion of the RAS can produce complex illnesses and altered states of arousal or permanent unconsciousness, such as coma, stupor, insomnia, headaches, depression, tremors, aggression, and forgetfulness. Descending reticular fibers regulate the quality of motor movement and muscle tone. They also inhibit sensory inputs at the spinal level. Finally, for students of communicative disorders, two important functions of the RF are its regulation of respiration and swallowing.

Anatomic Structures

The reticular circuitry is characterized by a web of multiple parallel and serial running circuits that can diverge or converge. This organization of circuitry allows for reticular cells to influence over 25,000–30,000 neurons in the brainstem. This architectural property also enables the reticular cells, first, to amplify a weak impulse and, second, to disseminate the amplified signal to thousands of other nuclei. The RF can concentrate impulses from thousands of neurons to a single neuronal circuit. It can also channel and screen information and respond to the amount of information rather than to the details.

The reticular cells are arranged longitudinally in transverse modules and project to overlapping dendrites, which generally lack dendritic shafts. The dendritic processes look like radiating spokes of a wheel. Each dendrite shaft receives input from different combinations of axons throughout the neuraxis. The axons, the efferent component of the reticular cells, are long (**Golgi type I**) and tend to bifurcate and project in opposite directions to distant structures. Projections run caudally to the spinal cord and rostrally throughout the brainstem, diencephalon, limbic structures, basal ganglia, and cortex.

The brainstem reticular cells are arranged in three broad longitudinal columns: **median**, **medial**, and **lateral** (see Fig. 13-1). The median reticular cell column contains the midline nucleus raphe, which forms a continuous cellular column in the brainstem and consists of regions that provide projections to the brain and spinal cord. The medial cell column consists of a central group of reticular nuclei, including the gigantocellular reticular nucleus, whereas the lateral cell column contains small- to intermediate-size nuclei.

Afferents

Overlapping afferents, some of which are inhibitory and others facilitatory, converge on a given reticular neuron. Reticular afferents consist of collaterals from the ascending and descending spinal tracts (pain, proprioception, tactile, temperature, and vibration), cranial nerve nuclei, cerebellum, midbrain, thalamus, subthalamus, hypothalamus, striatum, limbic lobe, and various cortical areas.

Efferents

Through its direct and indirect projections, the RF influences all nervous system functions. It sends projections to somatic and autonomic nuclei in general, autonomic and somatic motor nuclei of cranial nerves in the brainstem, and interneuronal pools in the spinal cord. Direct and indirect reticular projections also travel to the cerebellum, red nucleus, substantia nigra, midbrain tectum, subthalamic nuclei, thalamus, hypothalamus, and limbic lobe (septum, hippocampus, amygdala, and cingulate gyrus).

Functional Considerations

Within the diffuse reticular core of nuclei in the brainstem, specific nuclear cell aggregates form closed-loop circuits and serve as the reticular centers for regulating various sensori-motor, visceral, and cortical activating functions. Reticular centers may combine to form reticular networks that help regulate complex sensorimotor and visceral behaviors, such as eating, swallowing, vomiting, coughing, sneezing, copulation, and fighting.

Examining all of the unifying functions of the RF is beyond the scope of this chapter. However, to provide a simpler way to describe these functions, the reticular functions have been divided into three types: cortical arousal, sensorimotor elaboration, and visceral integrated activity.

Regulation of Cortical Arousal

The activation and regulation of cortical arousal are perhaps the best known functions of the RF. The serotonergic, cholinergic, and catecholaminergic cells of the ascending RAS and their projections from the brainstem to the neocortex and limbic structures collectively contribute to cortical arousal (Box 16-3). The RAS is indiscriminate to variations between sensory input and its modality; rather it responds best to stimulus intensity and novelty.

Clinically, cortical electrical activity is the best indicator of cortical arousal and brain functions. Various patterns of the brain's electrical activity are known to relate to different mental states of arousal. For example, if a person is relaxed with closed eyes, the usual electrical activity observed is the α-rhythm (see Chapter 20). Opening the eyes or exposing the individual to other sensory stimuli causes the α-rhythm to change to a high-frequency, low-amplitude (electroencephalographic [EEG] activation) wave pattern. This electrical activity reflects changes in the arousal or alertness of the cerebral cortex and is related to functions of the reticular system.

Terms that are related to clinically altered consciousness or awareness are *drowsiness* (impaired awareness associated with sleep), *stupor* (impaired consciousness in which the patient can be transiently aroused by stimulation), and *coma* (a state of profound unconsciousness). All these levels of altered consciousness are exhibited by patients with brain damage, and each affects the patients' ability to use language and cognition.

BOX 16-3

Reticular Serotonin and Depression

Low levels of serotonin in the brain are associated with mental illness, such as depression and obsessive–compulsive disorder. Selective serotonin reuptake inhibiting drugs, such as Prozac, Celexa, Zoloft, and Paxil are used to increase serotonin by preventing its cellular reuptake.

Sleep is related to the state of arousal and consciousness and is involved directly with the functioning of the RAS. In general, there are two sleeping states: deep sleep, or non-rapid-eye movement (NREM) and paradoxical, or rapid-eye movement (REM) sleep. NREM sleep has several substages, representing progressively deeper states of unconsciousness and characterized by slower and higher-amplitude EEG patterns. EEG recordings of deep sleep are characterized by slow-frequency waves of large amplitude from which one can recover with full restoration of awareness and cognitive functions.

Deep sleep is interrupted periodically by REM sleep, in which the individual is as physically relaxed as in deep sleep but displays the EEG pattern characteristic of being awake. This is associated with the dream state. REM sleep also is characterized by variations in heart rate, blood pressure, and respiration. Being awake is accompanied by a low-voltage and fast-frequency desynchronized wave form. Electrical stimulation of the RF can change EEG patterns of deep sleep to the pattern of wakefulness, indicating that the RASm may regulate levels of cortical arousal and wakefulness.

The median raphe nucleus (serotonergic) and locus ceruleus (noradrenergic) are two important reticular neurotransmitter nuclei concerned with sleep (see Fig. 13-1B); their alternating actions trigger NREM and REM sleep. The median raphe nucleus generates the high-amplitude, slow waves of deep sleep. A lesion of the raphe nucleus causes constant wakefulness or insomnia. Conversely, the nucleus locus ceruleus generates REM sleep. If the locus ceruleus is damaged, REM does not occur.

Most coma or altered consciousness-causing lesions are at the midbrain, hypothalamic, and thalamic junctions. The lesion can result from traumatic injury, vascular occlusion, tumors, or encephalitis. Impairment of the brainstem RF may be a major causative factor, especially at the midbrain level. Arousal, a state of awareness or wakefulness, is also related to attention, the central-most attribute of cognition, besides memory, that regulates the operation of higher mental functions allows focusing on a particular modality-specific stimulus, and is an a essential skill for new learning.

Central to the neural circuitry of arousal and its integration with attention are the diffuse cortical projections of the medial reticular formation (MRF) by way of thalamic nuclei, such as intralaminar centromedianum and reticular thalamicium. Documenting the driving force of this mechanism, Moruzi and Magoun (1963) noted that centromedianus stimulation with afferents from the MRF induced a global cortical activation, exemplifying the electroencephalic pattern of one being fully awake and alert. The reticular activation not only tunes the physiology for cognitive functions but also promotes learning by facilitating information flow to the brain and by opening the neuronal gates.

Stimulation of the centromedianus nucleus with an externally applied current has been found to enhance the processing of virtually each language function in neurologically impaired patients. This performance enhancement was measured in terms of response latencies and reduced number of errors (Bhatnagar and Mandybur 2007). The neuronal circuitry interacts with the prefrontal lobe to drive intentional–attentional mechanisms, which allow focusing on selective modality processing in the tactile, visual, or auditory mode. Reactive attention, on the other hand, involves simple environmental (visual, auditory, and painful) stimuli that initiate bodily reactions such as removing oneself from the path of danger or recognizing a friendly face. Behavior triggered by visual recognition involves the participation of the parietal association cortex.

Regulation of Sensory Functions

The reticulospinal projections also modulate the quantity and quality of sensory information and employ a gating mechanism that screens information at both the spinal and thalamic levels. The brainstem collateral terminals of the primary sensory fibers are under direct reticular influence. The RF affects sensory impulse transmission in presynaptic and postsynaptic terminals.

Reticular nuclei send input to brain structures that process specialized and general sensory input, such as the cochlear and vestibular nuclei, tectal and pretectal structures, geniculate nuclei, and thalamic nuclei. These direct reticular projections influence information processing by either accentuating or attenuating the sensory (audition, vision, olfaction, pain, temperature, and tactile) stimuli. There is a reticular pain-monitoring and -control system at the midbrain level and posterior diencephalic RF, especially in the tegmental and periaqueductal regions.

Integrated Motor Functions

Integrated motor functions include unconscious activities that are vital to survival and are controlled by the brainstem reticular nuclei. The RF uses convergent multimodal input and diffuse divergent output to control the vital centers of the brainstem that regulate cardiac activity, respiration, and swallowing. The reticular modulation of the lower motor neuron (LMN) and resultant altered muscle tone are discussed in Chapter 13.

Cardiovascular Activity

The reticular nuclei regulating vasomotor functions of the heart extend from the rostral medulla to the midpons. These nuclei receive extensive projections from peripheral receptors and are in part controlled by the hypothalamus. They project information via fibers of the vagus nerve (CN X). Stimulation of the lateral reticular pressor center increases heart rate and causes vasoconstriction. However, stimulation of the depressor center in the lower medulla decreases heart rate and causes vasodilation. Most spinal nerves and some cranial nerves, when stimulated, raise arterial pressure by exciting the pressor region and inhibiting the depressor region. Lesions of the medullary center for cardiovascular control can cause cardiac irregularities and blood pressure changes, both of which are life-threatening.

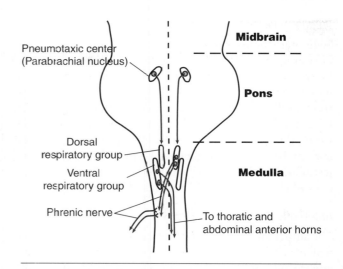

Figure 16-11 Autonomic (pontine and medullary) respiratory centers.

Respiration

Though the primary function of respiration is to maintain the proper level of oxygen in body tissue and remove carbon dioxide through the regulated cycles of inhalation and exhalation, respiration is the most basic process underlying speech. Changes in the concentration of any of these constituents render an immediate effect on the respiratory activity. For example, the concentration of carbon dioxide, which is detected by chemoreceptors located in the carotid and aortic bodies, can stimulate the respiratory center through inspiratory and expiratory signals to the respiratory muscles.

The primary muscles of respiration are the diaphragm, **internal** and **external intercostals**, and **abdominal** muscles. The contraction of the diaphragm and external intercostal muscles increases the intrathoracic volume and decreases the pleural cavity pressure, thus prompting the inspirational phase, in which air is forced into the pleural cavity according to Boyle law. Expiration is a passive process controlled by the elasticity of the lungs and the walls of the abdomen and chest. However, forced expiration, as during coughing and defecating, requires muscle contraction from the abdominals and internal intercostals.

Neural Control of Respiration

The neural control of respiration is not as clear as generally depicted. The regulation of breathing involves two controls: **voluntary** and **autonomic**. The nuclei forming the **voluntary respiratory control center** are in the motor cortex. The **autonomic brainstem respiratory center** consists of several groups of scattered neurons in the RF; it is divided further into two distinct centers: **pontine pneumotaxic center** and **medullary respiratory center**. The medullary respiratory center is further divided into the **dorsal respiratory group** and **ventral respiratory group** of neurons (Fig. 16-11). A lesion in the pontomedullary respiratory center causes asphyxia and, eventually, death if artificial respiration is not administered.

Voluntary Respiration Control

Temporary increases and decreases in the rate and depth of breathing owing to different motor activities are regulated by the voluntary respiratory center. This center is in the motor cortex. Projections from the motor cortex descend through the internal capsule (diencephalon), pes peduncle (midbrain), and pyramidal fibers (medulla) before innervating the spinal motor neurons in the cervical, thoracic, and lumbar regions of the spinal cord. The neuronal projections from the cervical and thoracic regions of the cord control the activity of the muscles of respiration.

Automatic Respiration Control

The autonomic center of the brainstem, containing the pacemaker cells, includes the pneumotaxic center of the pons and dorsal and ventral respiratory nuclei of the medulla (Fig. 16-11). The function of the pontine pneumotaxic center is to limit the duration of the inspiration phase in the lungs. Based on physical activity and bodily needs, the strong signals from the pneumotaxic center temporarily shorten the filling phase of the lungs. However, weaker signals from this center lengthen the inspirational phase, resulting in excessive filling of the lungs. By limiting the duration of inspiration, the pneumotaxic center also regulates the duration of expiration; it controls respiratory depth and rate by constant inhibition of the medullary respiratory centers. In normal physiologic conditions, the activity of the pontine pneumotaxic center, in conjunction with vagal afferents from the brachial stretch receptors, inhibits strong inspiratory activity (Box 16-4).

The dorsal medullary respiratory center contains reticular nuclei, including the **nucleus** of the **tractus solitarius**, which is responsive to afferents from the carotid and aortic chemoreceptors through the vagus (CN X) and glossopharyngeal (CN IX). These signals, along with the sensory information from the lungs, help control respiratory activity. The fibers descending from the dorsal medullary respiratory neurons cross to activate the anterior horn LMNs of the cervical region of the cord. Efferent projections from C3–C5 (predominantly from C4) form the phrenic nerve, which causes contraction of the diaphragm, the main muscle of respiration (see Chapter 2). Contraction of the

---

BOX 16-4

Important Role of the Brainstem in Respiratory Function

Acting as a pacemaker, the brainstem respiratory centers regulate the depth, rhythm, and duration of breathing. Thus brainstem lesions, commonly seen in traumatic brain injuries, can cause respiratory dysfunctioning. Furthermore, vagus nerve (CN X) dysfunction, anesthetic drugs, and barbiturates can depress the activity of the respiratory pacemaker cells, causing apnea.

---

diaphragm increases the intrathoracic volume, beginning the cycle of inspiration. The dorsal respiratory area is known to regulate respiratory rhythm.

Next to the dorsal respiratory group of nuclei is the ventral group of respiratory nuclei, which is inactive during the normal respiratory cycle. It becomes active when high levels of pulmonary ventilation are required. Projections from the ventral medullary respiratory nuclei cross the midline to activate the contralateral thoracic motor nuclei; their projections regulate the activity of the spinal intercostal and abdominal muscles. Both the dorsal and ventral respiratory nuclei of the medulla contain the mechanism responsible for controlling the rhythmic activity of the respiratory muscles.

Muscles of Respiration

The most important function of the spinal cord for motor speech is its control of the muscles that regulate respiration, a patterned cycle of inhalation and exhalation that not only is vital for survival but also contributes to loudness, an important motor speech process (Table 16-10).

Respiration involves about 15 muscles, the four major groups of which are the diaphragm, abdominals, external intercostals, and internal intercostals. The sternocleidomastoid and scalenus are also important accessory muscles. The motor nuclei from the anterior horns of the C3–C5

Table 16-10

Motor Innervation of the Muscles of Respiration

Spinal Roots	Muscles	Functions
C3–C5, mainly C4	Diaphragm	Increases intrathoracic volume for inspiration
T1–T12	External intercostals	Increases intrathoracic volume by raising ribs for inspiration
T1–T12	Internal intercostals	Decreases intrathoracic volume by depressing ribs for expiration
T6–T12	Abdominal muscles	Increases intrathoracic pressure for expiration

(with predominance from C4 through the phrenic nerve) innervate the diaphragm. The efferents to the internal and external intercostals exit from T1–T12. The abdominal muscles receive efferents from the motor nuclei of T6–T12. The diaphragm and external intercostals are the primary muscles of inspiration, whereas the abdominal and internal intercostals participate in forced expiration (Table 16-10).

During the inspiratory phase, contraction of the diaphragm and external intercostals increases the intrathoracic volume, which lowers the pressure within the lungs and thoracic cavity. The reduced intrathoracic pressure forces air into the lungs through the trachea. Exhalation is initiated by an increase in intra-abdominal pressure and a decrease in intrathoracic volume caused by the abdominal and internal intercostal muscles. In quiet inspiration, the diaphragm and external intercostals actively participate, whereas quiet exhalation does not require active muscular activity because the elastic recoil of the lungs restores intrathoracic volume to the resting level. However, forced inspiration (during exercise) and expiration (while blowing out a candle or coughing) requires active muscle contraction.

These facts are clinically important because spinal lesions involving motor nuclei at different levels differentially affect respiration (Box 16-5). For example, a patient with a complete spinal lesion above C3 has complete paralysis of all respiratory muscles and is likely to lose the ability to breathe spontaneously. Such a patient requires artificial respiration/tracheostomy for survival. Patients with a spinal injury below C4 and above T12 have varying degrees of paralysis of all primary respiratory muscles except the diaphragm. With basic control over the diaphragm, such a patient may continue to inhale and quietly exhale because of the elastic recoil of lungs. With full control of diaphragm, inspiration is not a problem; however, with reduced or impaired control over the abdominal and internal intercostal muscles, such a patient would not be able to undertake the forced exhalation needed for coughing, bowel movements, and blowing. In the case of any lesion below T12, the patient's control of respiratory muscles is likely to remain intact.

Swallowing

The physiology of deglutition, or swallowing, has recently become an important clinical issue in communicative disorders because many clinicians are now diagnosing and managing disorders of this mechanism. As with respiration, the reticular nuclei regulate the act of swallowing by integrating the functions of the following cranial nerves: trigeminal (CN V), facial (CN VII), glossopharyngeal (CN IX), vagus (CN X), and hypoglossal (CN XII). Swallowing is a reflexive action instigated by the sensory and motor components of these cranial nerves along with reticular participation.

Swallowing has two stages: **voluntary** and **involuntary**. The voluntary stage consists of masticating a bolus and moving it into the pharyngeal cavity. The involuntary or reflexive stage is the passage of the bolus through the pharynx and esophagus. The voluntary stage covers the act of chewing, bolus formation, and bolus movement in the oral cavity. It ends as the upward and backward motion of the tongue forces the bolus against the palate. As the bolus presses against the palate to enter the pharynx, the involuntary stage begins through sensory projections from the posterior palate to the reticular swallowing center in the lower pons and upper medulla.

The reticular swallowing center directs projections to the adjacent respiratory center and subsequently to the nuclei of trigeminal (CN V), facial (CN VII), glossopharyngeal (CN IX), vagus (CN X), and hypoglossal (CN XII) nerves, which initiate a series of reflexive motor actions to ensure proper breathing management while the bolus passes through the pharynx. Major reflexive actions include the upward movement of the palate to close the nasopharynx, backward and downward movement of the epiglottis to seal off the glottis, raising of the larynx to close the airway, and enlarging the esophageal opening to allow entrance of the bolus. As the bolus passes the pharyngeal phase, the reticular respiratory center regulates the reopening of the respiratory passageway.

Brainstem lesions interrupting the afferent and efferent projections of the RF also alter the integrity of the swallowing reflex and cause aspiration. Common disturbances of swallowing seen in neurogenic patients are poor mastication, delayed swallowing reflex, reduced peristalsis of the bolus through the pharynx, and aspiration.

Vomiting

The reticular nuclei that regulate vomiting are in the medulla. They receive inputs from the oropharynx and gastrointestinal tract. Noxious impulses mediating irritations of the intestinal tract and oropharynx initiate reflexive vomiting. Projections from the vomiting center in the medulla descend through the fibers of the glossopharyngeal nerve (CN IX) and vagus nerve (CN X) and coordinate the

---

BOX 16-5

Clinical Implications of Spinal Lesions Affecting the Muscles of Respiration

A complete spinal transection above C3 causes a complete paralysis of all respiratory muscles; patients with such a lesion lose the ability to breathe spontaneously and immediately require artificial respiration/tracheostomy for survival. Patients with a spinal injury below C4 but above T12 exhibit varying degrees of paralysis of all respiratory muscles except the diaphragm. With basic control over the diaphragm, the individual can inhale and quietly exhale because of the elastic recoil of lungs but cannot undertake activity related to forced expiration.

contraction of the abdominal, diaphragmatic, and inter-costal muscles. The oropharyngeal musculature, which facilitates vomiting, works with all of these muscles.

Coughing

Afferents mediating irritation from laryngeal and tracheal lining tissues initiate the coughing reflex via vagus nerve (CN X) and solitary tract nuclei. As with the vomiting reflex, the diaphragm, abdominal, and intercostal muscles are involved; however, they contract alternately, not simultaneously.

Autonomic Functions

The RF contributes to the autonomic system through its reticulobulbar and reticulospinal fiber projections. Input to the reticular autonomic regulatory system comes from limbic and diencephalic structures of the forebrain, which include the orbitofrontal cortex, cingulate gyrus, amygdala, hippocampus, hypothalamus, and the medial, anterior, and dorsal groups of the thalamic nuclei. Reticular projections regulate hypothalamic centers specializing in endocrine production and release, temperature, food and fluid intake, sexual activity, diurnal body rhythms, blood electrolyte balance, visceral and autonomic functions, emotional states, and learning.

Biologic Rhythms

A self-regulated internal clock, a characteristic of all living systems, determines the turnover rates of macromolecules, annual seasonal variations, and daily environmental changes in the body. Biologic rhythms govern reproductive cycles and development, division, and death of cells. Many rhythms depend on an intact hypothalamus with its multiple connections, including those from the RF. The RF is also indirectly involved in neural control of the pineal gland, a structure that participates in regulating circadian rhythms (repetitive cycles or biorhythm).

Self-Awareness

Deep cellular layers of the superior colliculus receive multimodal inputs that outline the space around the body. This input stems from overlapping visual, auditory, and somatic stimuli, representing various temporal and spatial reference points surrounding the body. These stimuli form a three-dimensional body image in the midbrain RF. The RF projects this image to nonspecific and specific thalamic nuclei and thus enables humans to have conscious self-awareness. The thalamus in turn relays information to the neocortex for further in-depth analysis.

Head and Eye Movement

The RF regulates the rotation of the head and eyes. Through fibers of the medial longitudinal fasciculus, the RF mediates impulses connecting various participating cranial and cervical muscles that control head and eye movements

(see Chapter 10). Their integrated activity is responsible for head and body movements, such as circling in one direction.

Reticular Neurotransmitters

The RF uses a variety of neurotransmitters to communicate with the brain, spinal cord, and neighboring reticular regions. These neurotransmitters are synthesized by a specialized population of cells (see Chapter 5). A monoamine imbalance can generate somatic and psychic symptoms such as excitement, agitation, depression, anxiety, and insomnia. For example, an overabundance of norepinephrine can lead to the somatic symptoms of speech disfluency, rapid heart rate, increased blood pressure, dry mouth, and cessation of intestinal peristalsis; whereas low levels of serotonin are associated with depression and anxiety.

Serotonin

Electrical discharge firing rates of serotonin and noradrenergic neurons fluctuate with sleep and wakefulness. Therefore, they participate in the general activity level of the CNS. Serotonin is thought to be concerned with overall levels of arousal and slow-wave sleep as well as severe depression (Box 16-3). In the treatment of depression, antidepressant drugs appear to enhance the concentration of serotonin at the synapse by reducing its uptake. Serotonin is also an important contributor to the descending pain control system.

Norepinephrine

The **locus ceruleus** is the major noradrenergic reticular nucleus. Noradrenergic projections have a profound influence on brain function and are known to regulate brain tone by inhibiting background activity, thus enhancing the signal-to-noise ratio in the brain. Behaviorally, the locus ceruleus contributes to the generation of REM sleep (see Chapter 20). Along with other noradrenergic neurons, the locus ceruleus is also thought to mediate attention and vigilance. Depression can be treated with drugs that enhance the transmission of norepinephrine at the synapse.

Dopamine

Degeneration of dopamine-producing cells has been associated with Parkinsonism, a motor disorder consisting of a shaking palsy, akinesia, a masked face, drooling, and a shuffling gait (see Chapter 13). Dopamine projections to the cortex and limbic structures seem to influence cognitive functions and motivation. Cocaine and amphetamine, drugs that enhance the action of dopamine, induce syndromes resembling paranoid schizophrenia. Drugs of substance abuse cause dopamine release in the nucleus accumbens, suggesting that this mesolimbic projection may be associated with a sense of pleasure. Thorazine and related drugs used in the treatment of schizophrenia block dopamine receptors, which suggests that the mesolimbic and mesocortical dopaminergic systems may be involved in this psychotic disorder.

Enkephalins

Enkephalins in the RF contribute to pain suppression. As a subgroup of the endorphin opiates, they are primarily present in the PNS. They form local neuronal circuits found in the gastrointestinal system, which respond to opiates by reducing gastrointestinal motility. Abdominal pain (colic) often responds best to opiates.

Substance P

Substance P has a slow and long-lasting inhibitory effect on neuronal firing. It attenuates pain and is present in the RF and spinal dorsal root ganglia. Fibers of the opiate-like enkephalin cells form axoaxonic synapses with substance P fibers. This connectivity is thought to control the pain that may occur with movement disorders, such as Parkinson disease.

γ-Aminobutyric Acid

γ-Aminobutyric acid (GABA), the most prevalent inhibitory transmitter, dominates in local circuit neurons. It is produced from the decarboxylation of glutamate. GABA serves as the inhibitory neurotransmitter from the Purkinje cells to the deep cerebellar nuclei, from the striatum to the globus pallidus and substantia nigra, and from the globus pallidus and substantia nigra to the thalamus.

Tranquilizers, such as diazepam (Valium), bind to GABA receptors and increase the effects of the transmitter released at GABA synapses. Abnormal movements, as seen in Huntington chorea, are caused by the loss of GABA neurons in the caudate and putamen. This elevates the ratio of dopamine to acetylcholine, producing abnormal movements. However, a reduced ratio of dopamine to acetylcholine causes the abnormal motor movements of Parkinsonism.

Clinical Concerns

Clinical symptoms that may occur after lesions of the RF are irregularities in sleep, blood pressure, pulse rate, respiration, vigilance, and states of consciousness. Motor dysfunctions may include tremors and altered muscle tone, ranging from hypertonic rigidity to flaccidity. Speech and swallowing disorders may occur after lesions in the caudal brainstem RF.

Summary of the Reticular Formation

A diffuse core of nuclei in the brainstem, the RF serves as a fine-tuner of cortical functions. With extensive dendrites and axons, it regulates sensorimotor, visceral, and cognitive functions. An important function of the RF is to regulate cortical arousal, which is measured by various patterns of brain electrical activity. It also regulates functions such as sleep and awake states.

CLINICAL CONSIDERATIONS

PATIENT ONE

A 55-year-old schoolteacher consulted his physician for what he thought was a strange feeling of nervousness and embarrassment. This was marked by bladder incontinence. Other sensorimotor functions were normal. A spinal MRI study revealed a tumor in the sacral region of the spinal cord.

Question: How does a sacral lesion cause bladder incontinence?

Discussion: With the tumor compressing the sacral cord, all afferent and efferent impulses of the spinal reflex to the bladder were interrupted. Bladder control was lost and the bladder became flaccid. Once the bladder was full, the urine dripped out gradually.

PATIENT TWO

A 45-year-old unpaid politician consulted his physician about asymmetrical pupil sizes. On examination, he exhibited right pupil constriction (meiosis). Additional signs included ptosis of the right upper eyelid and an inability to perspire on the forehead. The attending physician suspected Horner syndrome, an autonomic nervous system impairment, and a spinal MRI study confirmed an infarct in the right cervical sympathetic chain.

Question: How does a cervical sympathetic chain lesion cause these symptoms?

Discussion: Horner syndrome results from a lesion of the sympathetic pathways to the eye and forehead. Clinical characteristics are miotic (constricted) pupil, ptosis of the upper eyelid, and inability to sweat on the forehead. Pupil constriction (meiosis) is regulated by parasympathetic impulses, whereas pupil dilation (mydriasis) is controlled by sympathetic impulses. Sympathetic impulses originate in the ipsilateral hypothalamus and descend to the motor neurons in the T1–T2 segments. Preganglionic neuron projections travel to the superior sympathetic cervical ganglion, which projects to the smooth dilator muscle of the iris. Damage to the superior cervical ganglia affected the sympathetic projections, resulting in unopposed actions of the parasympathetic system. This caused the pupil constriction and contributed to the inability to sweat.

PATIENT THREE

A 25-year-old woman was very slim and had a history of poor appetite, weight loss, and episodes of high fever. She had lost interest in sex and her menses were irregular. She drank large quantities of water but considered her behavior to be normal. Her physician suspected it to be a case of anorexia subsequent to a lower diencephalic lesion.

Question: How can a lower diencephalic lesion cause these symptoms?

Discussion: Hypothalamic damage usually causes an imbalance in food and water intake and temperature control as well as a decrease in sexual drive. Weight loss is seen commonly in patients with anorexia. A vasopressin (antidiuretic hormone) deficiency causes excessive thirst and accompanying increased urinary output. Alterations in gonadotropic hormones lead to changes in the cycle of menses. Furthermore, hypothalamic damage causes a disturbance in temperature control.

PATIENT FOUR

A 35-year-old man had a history of temporal lobe seizures. During his seizure attacks, he would become very violent, throwing objects at people. He frequently harmed his wife and abused his children. Strangely, he retained no memory of his actions.

Question: How did seizure activity in the temporal (limbic) lobe affect memory?

Discussion: Abnormal electric discharges of the temporal lobe stimulated the hippocampus and amygdala, resulting in automatic behaviors for which there was loss of conscious control. The involvement of association cortices during his seizures impaired his memory.

PATIENT FIVE

A 25-year-old automobile salesperson was in a head-on car collision in which his forehead slammed against the dashboard. He was unconscious for a week. When he recovered, he had no memory of the accident or the events preceding it. According to his wife, he became a different person after regaining consciousness. He lost energy and had no ambition. Physically, his actions were slow. With faulty reasoning, he could not think abstractly or make decisions. He also lost interest in grooming and hygiene.

Question: How can the loss of consciousness, memory loss, and personality changes in this patient can be accounted for?

Discussion: The laceration and concussion of the prefrontal lobe account for his personality changes and cognitive deficits. The temporarily impaired functioning of the brainstem reticular formation was related to his loss of consciousness.

PATIENT SIX

On his first day of work at a hospital, a rookie speech language pathologist (SLP) met a neurologist who informally began discussing a 20-year-old traumatic brain injury (TBI) patient whom she had seen that morning. The patient had no apparent cognitive or communicative problems but presented with an excessive perspiration, irregular sleep–wake cycle, and altered sexual behavior with no libido. His speech was a little slurred as he spoke with a mouth full of saliva. "This is a classical case of a lesion in the lower diencephalon," she stated before rushing off to a call.

Question: How can you explain these symptoms?

Discussion: It is a hypothalamic syndrome. The hypothalamus serves autonomic, visceral, and endocrine functions, including sexual drive, appetite, sleep–wake cycle, and body heat production. Impaired ANS control of the oral glands resulted in excessive saliva secretion.

PATIENT SEVEN

A 19-year-old man with TBI caused by a car accident was referred for a speech-language-cognitive assessment. The attending SLP noted the following:

- Mild retrograde amnesia
- Profound anterograde amnesia
- Agitated behavior
- Uninhibited expression of sexuality
- Inappropriate and vulgar language

Question: How can you relate these symptoms to the associated damaged structure?

Discussion: Functionally related and adjacently located structures of the limbic lobes are involved with the reported behavioral symptoms of agitation and aggression (limbic lobe) and memory impairment (hippocampal formation).

SUMMARY

The ANS, limbic lobe, hypothalamus, and RF are functionally integrated structures with nebulous anatomic borders. Working together, they influence the vital automatic and unconscious bodily functions that are indispensable for reproduction and survival. The system's interwoven cellular networks modulate visceral, somatic, autonomic, endocrine, alimentary, vascular, respiratory, and sexual behaviors. Each of these systems is represented by specialized overlapping cellular networks that extend throughout the septum, hypothalamus, and brainstem RF.

By using sympathetic and parasympathetic projections, the autonomic nervous system (ANS) controls visceral functions, regulating body homeostasis and the functioning of the cardiovascular, pulmonary, digestive, urinary, and reproductive systems. The integrated activity of the limbic system regulates the emotional and motivational aspects of behavior fundamental to survival, such as feeding, mating, aggression, and flight.

The hypothalamus, as the central regulator of the ANS and endocrine functions, controls visceral functions, including vasodilation, body homeostasis, reproduction, hunger, and the intake of water and food. The neurosecretory cells of the hypothalamus regulate pituitary gland hormone production and endocrine body functions.

By integrating stimuli with internally generated thoughts, feelings, and emotions, the RF regulates the homeostatic state of the brain essential for controlling sleep and vigilance. It also controls metabolic, respiratory, visceral, sensorimotor, neuroendocrine, emotional, and cognitive activities. A single lesion of the reticular system may generate complex illnesses characterized by a variety of symptoms, including insomnia, headaches, depression, tremors, aggression, and forgetfulness.

QUIZ QUESTIONS

1. Define the following terms: adipsia, amnesia, aphagia, asphyxia, hippocampus, postganglionic, preganglionic

2. Define the functions of the sympathetic and parasympathetic systems of the ANS.

3. Describe the functions of the limbic system and name its major structures.

4. Which anatomic structure(s) regulate(s) water intake, food intake, and body temperature?

5. Which structure is responsible for regulating cortical arousal, cardiovascular activity, respiration, swallowing, vomiting, and coughing?

TECHNICAL TERMS

acetylcholine
adenohypophysis
adipsia
akinesia
α-rhythm
amnesia
amygdala
aphagia
asphyxia
catecholaminergic
cholinergic
cingulate gyrus
colic
diurnal
Edinger-Westphal nucleus
gonadotropic
hippocampus
insomnia
Klüver-Bucy syndrome
noradrenergic synapses

parasympathetic system
peristalsis
polydipsia
polyuria
portal system
postganglionic
preganglionic neuron
preoptic
raphe nucleus
serotonergic
subcallosal gyrus
supraoptic
sympathetic
tegmentum
tremors
uncus
vasodilation
vasopressin
visceral
viscerosomatic

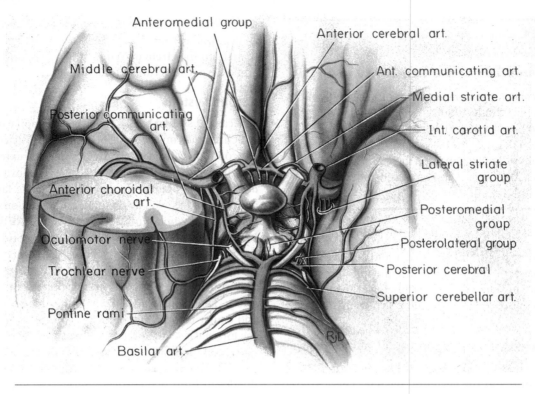

Figure 17-2 Cerebral arterial structure at base of brain depicting large and small arteries.

Vertebral Basilar System

Two **vertebral arteries** arise from the **subclavian arteries** and ascend through the bony foramen of the **upper cervical vertebrae.** They enter the **posterior cranial fossa** of the skull through the **foramen magnum** and continue along the ventrolateral surface of the medulla oblongata (Fig. 2-31). At the level of the caudal pons, both vertebral arteries merge to form a single **basilar artery** that courses upward along the pontine midline, eventually joining the circle of Willis (Figs. 17-1 and 17-2).

Before terminating in the circle of Willis, the vertebral basilar arteries give rise to numerous small branches that supply blood to the spinal cord, medulla, pons, midbrain, and cerebellum (Tables 17-1 and 17-2). Each vertebral artery gives rise to three major arteries: **posterior spinal, anterior spinal** (Fig. 17-6), and **posterior inferior cerebellar** (Figs. 17-1 and 17-2). Some of the branches of the descending posterior spinal artery also supply the dorsal medulla, while the remaining travel caudally to supply the dorsal third of the spinal cord. The dorsal medullary column with nuclei (**nucleus Gracilis** and **nucleus Cuneatus**) and their fibers mediates sensation. Consequently, circulatory disorders in the posterior spinal artery cause medullary symptoms and a loss of epicritic sensation in half of the body.

The anterior spinal artery from each vertebral artery merges and descends along the midline. Some of its branches supply the lower median medulla, which contains the

pyramidal fibers, pyramidal decussation, and **medial lemniscus** fibers (Figs. 3-7 and 3-9). The remaining branches supply the ventral two-thirds of the spinal cord. Interruption of the vascular flow of the anterior spinal artery affects motor fibers and causes hemiplegia as well as protopathic (pain and

Table 17-1

Arteries of the Brainstem, Cerebellum, and Spinal Cord

Structures	Arteries
Midbrain	Posterior cerebral artery
Pons	Basilar artery Anterior inferior cerebellar artery
Medulla	Posterior spinal artery Anterior spinal artery Basilar artery
Cerebellum	Posterior inferior cerebellar artery Anterior inferior cerebellar artery Superior cerebellar artery
Spinal cord	Posterior spinal artery (posterior third of cord) Anterior spinal artery (anterior two-thirds of cord)

Table 17-2

Signs of Vertebral Basilar Involvement

Area Supplied	Structures Affected	Signs of Involvement
Vertebral arteries: medulla (pyramid, medial lemniscus, and CN IX–CN XII), cerebellum (posterior inferior cerebellar arteries), and choroid plexus of fourth ventricle	Pyramidal tract	Contralateral hemiplegia
	Trigeminal tract and nucleus	Loss of discriminative touch, temperature and pain sensation from ipsilateral face
	Lateral spinothalamic tract	Loss of pain and temperature sensation from contralateral trunk and limb
	Cerebellum	Ipsilateral ataxia
	CN VIII: vestibular portion	Vertigo, nystagmus, and vomiting
	CN IX, CN X, and CN XII (pharynx, palate, glottis, and tongue)	Dysphagia and dysarthria
Basilar artery: lateral pons, cerebellum (anterior inferior cerebellar and superior cerebellar arteries), and CNs (V, VII, VIII, and X)	Pyramidal tract	Hemiplegia
	Cerebellum	Ataxia
	CN V	Loss of facial sensation
	CN VII and nucleus	Facial paralysis
	CN VIII and nucleus	Deafness, nystagmus, and vertigo
	CN X	Vomiting

CN, cranial nerve.

temperation) hemisensory loss. Occlusion of the anterior spinal artery branches that supply the medulla results in **alternating hemiplegia**, which is associated with ipsilateral paralysis of the face and tongue as well as contralateral paralysis of the extremities. In alternating hemiplegia, the lesion is above the pyramidal decussation in the medulla. This syndrome is discussed in detail in Chapter 14.

Each *posterior inferior cerebellar artery* supplies the ipsilateral posteroinferior cerebellum, which plays a significant role in the coordination of rapid movements. Immediately after its formation, the basilar artery gives rise to **anterior inferior cerebellar arteries**, which proceed downward and laterally to serve the anterior and lateral surfaces of the cerebellum. At the pontine level, the basilar artery gives rise to many rami bilaterally that supply the pontine structures (Fig. 17-2). One of the most important basilar as well as anterior inferior cerebellar artery branch is the **labyrinthine (internal auditory) artery** (Fig. 17-1). This branch delivers blood to the cochlea and vestibular apparatus in the inner ear.

Immediately before the basilar artery joins the circle of Willis and forms the **posterior cerebral artery (PCA)**, it gives rise to the **superior cerebellar arteries** at the level of the midbrain. These arteries supply the anterior and dorsal surfaces of the cerebellum, and their branches anastomose (connecting blood vessels) with the other cerebellar arteries. Pathology implicating the cerebellar arteries may result in motor incoordination, impaired balance, and dysarthric speech.

Circle of Willis

The wreath-shaped circle of Willis is at the ventral surface of the brain, and it connects the carotid arterial system with the vertebrobasilar system (Figs. 17-1*B* and 17-2). The circle of Willis consists of the **anterior** and **posterior communicating arteries** and the proximal portions of the anterior cerebral (ACA), middle cerebral (MCA), and posterior cerebral (PCA) arteries. The ACAs are rostrally interconnected via the anterior communicating artery. The posterior communicating arteries connect the internal carotid arteries with the basilar artery. The circle of Willis is an important anastomotic point that serves to equalize the vascular blood supply to both sides of the brain. However, because of usual pressure equalization in both arterial systems, very little blood normally flows through the communicating arteries to the left and right sides of the circle.

Two types of arteries, **cortical** and **central**, arise from the circle of Willis. The cortical branches are large arteries that primarily supply the external brain structures (Table 17-3) and give rise to branches to anastomose with other cortical arteries. The central (penetrating) branches are small arteries that penetrate the ventral surface of the brain to supply the internal and subcortical brain structures.

Cortical Arteries

Anterior Cerebral Artery

After arising from the bifurcation of the internal cerebral artery at the circle of Willis, the ACA travels rostrally in the interhemispheric fissure along the midsagittal surface of the

Table 17-3

Vascular Supply to the Brain Surface and Lobes

Brain Area	Artery
Frontal lobe	
Lateral surface	Middle cerebral artery
Medial surface	Anterior cerebral artery
Inferior surface	Middle and anterior cerebral arteries
Parietal lobe	
Lateral surface	Middle cerebral artery
Medial surface	Anterior cerebral artery
Occipital lobe	
Lateral and medial surfaces	Posterior cerebral artery
Temporal lobe	
Lateral surface	Middle cerebral artery
Medial surface	Jointly by middle cerebral, posterior cerebral, posterior communicating, and anterior choroidal arteries
Inferior surface	Posterior cerebral artery

brain. It follows the genu of the corpus callosum and continues posteriorly along the dorsal surface of the corpus callosum (Fig. 17-3). Its main branches are the **orbital**, **frontopolar**, **callosomarginal**, and **pericallosal** arteries, which supply the orbital and medial cortical surfaces of the frontal and parietal lobes. In the posterior medial cortical area, the branches of the ACA anastomose with branches of the PCA. Many terminal branches of the ACA cross over to the lateral cortical surface and develop anastomosing continuity with the branches of the MCA in the **watershed zone**, where the distribution of major cerebral arteries overlaps.

The interruption of blood circulation in the ACA usually results in paralysis of the legs and feet because of decreased blood supply to the midsagittal extension of the motor cortex (Table 17-4; Figs. 2-6 and 14-1). The vascular impairments of this artery may also lead to many prefrontal lobe symptoms, which include disorders of thinking, reasoning, abstracting, self-monitoring, and planning. Additional impairments include decreased spontaneity, motor inaction, impaired judgment, reduced concentration, and impaired executive function.

Middle Cerebral Artery

The MCA, the largest of the cortical arteries, is the direct continuation of the internal carotid artery. After leaving the circle of Willis, it runs laterally and emerges through the sylvian fissure on the lateral brain surface. On the lateral surface, it divides into the temporal (anterior and posterior),

frontal (rolandic and prerolandic), and parietal (anterior, posterior, and angular) artery branches (Fig. 17-4, A and B). The MCA branches supply blood to the entire lateral surface of the brain, which includes the sites for speech, language, and a large part of sensorimotor areas. The important areas are the somatosensory cortex in the postcentral gyrus, motor cortex in the precentral gyrus, Broca area in the premotor region, prefrontal cortex, primary auditory cortex in the transverse Heschl gyrus on the superior surface of the first temporal gyrus, Wernicke area in the superior posterior temporal lobe, and angular and supramarginal gyri in the inferior parietal lobe.

While passing through the lateral sulcus, the MCA gives off **lateral** and **medial lenticulostriate** branches that supply the basal ganglia and diencephalon (Fig. 17-5). The medial lenticulostriate artery supplies blood to the globus pallidus, the posterior internal capsule, and medial ventral area of the thalamus. The lateral lenticulostriate artery supplies the entire pulvinar and caudate nucleus except for its anterior portion, which is served by the ACA.

Impaired vascular circulation of the MCA results in contralateral hemiplegia (motor disorder) and impaired sensory functions that include discriminative and diffuse touch, position sense, and pain and temperature (Table 17-4). Other symptoms, depending on the lesion side, are aphasia, constructional apraxia, temporospatial deficits, homonymous hemianopia, and reading as well as writing deficits. Lenticulostriate artery damage results in involuntary motor movements and sensorimotor symptoms.

Posterior Cerebral Artery

The basilar artery bifurcates to form two posterior cerebral arteries (PCA). With a potential anastomotic flow from the posterior communicating artery, each PCA curves laterally and caudally along the inferior brain surface to supply blood to the anterior and inferior temporal lobe; it covers important structures, such as the uncus, inferior temporal gyri, and inferior and medial occipital lobe, including the primary visual cortex in the calcarine region. The end branches of the artery also cross over to the lateral surface and anastomose in the watershed region with the terminal branches of the MCA.

Occlusion of the PCA results in homonymous hemianopsia. Occlusion of the basilar artery, which provides blood to both PCA, results in total blindness as well as numerous pontine and cerebellar symptoms (Table 17-4). Bilateral involvement of the occipital lobe is associated with cortical blindness where the patient cannot see but can detect light.

Central Arteries

The central arteries are the branches that arise either from the proximal portions of the cortical arteries or from the circle of Willis and penetrate the inferior surface of the brain (Fig. 17-2). These supply blood to the following subcortical structures: thalamus, hypothalamus, caudate nucleus, putamen, globus pallidus, basal ganglia, internal capsule,

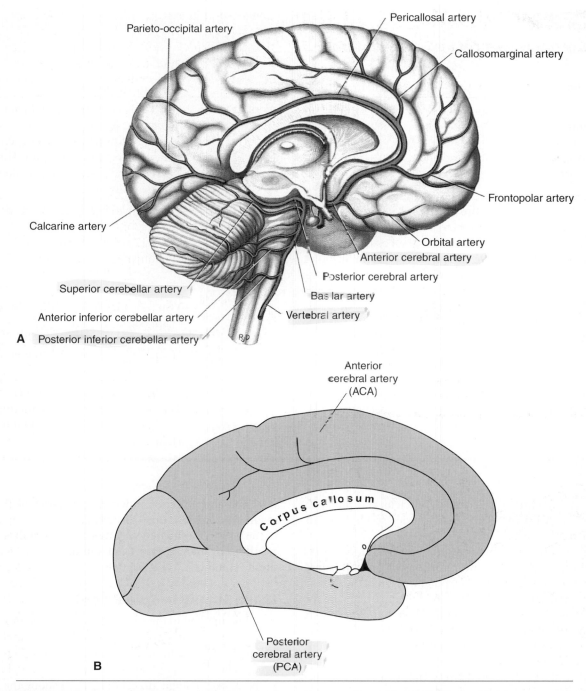

Figure 17-3 A. Anterior and posterior cerebral arteries together with cerebellar and brainstem arteries on midsagittal brain surface. B. Diagram of the midsagittal territory covered by the anterior cerebral and posterior cerebral arteries.

choroid plexus, and others (Table 17-5). One important aspect of the circulation by central arteries is the marked overlapping of blood supply as the branches distribute to the subcortical areas. The overlapping blood supply facilitates the development of anastomotic channels in response to occlusive or ischemic vascular problems. Important central arteries are the **anteromedial, medial striate, anterior choroidal, posterior choroidal, posteromedial,** and **posterolateral** (Fig. 17-2).

The anteromedial arteries arise from the anterior communicating and anterior cerebral arteries and penetrate the **anterior perforated area** to supply the hypothalamus and suprachiasmatic regions of the brain. Involvement of these arterial twigs results in disorders of the **autonomic nervous system (ANS)** and hypothalamus. The medial striate arteries arise from the ACA and supply blood to parts of the caudate nucleus, putamen, and anterior limb of the internal capsule. The lenticulostriate branches of the MCA supply

Table 17-4

Signs of Involvement of the Cortical Arteries

Area Supplied	Structures Affected	Signs of Involvement
Anterior cerebral artery: medial aspect of frontal lobe, anterior 80% of corpus callosum, and partial supply to basal ganglia (caudate head and putamen)	Sensory and motor cortices (medial surface) Prefrontal cortex	Loss of somatic sensory and paralysis of opposite leg and foot Mental impairments: lack of spontaneity, easy distraction, problem-solving deficit, indecisiveness, and altered personality
Middle cerebral artery: entire lateral surface of cerebral hemisphere (including sensorimotor area, premotor area, language cortex, and associational cortex), inferior frontal lobe, basal ganglia (body and head of caudate, lateral globus pallidus, and putamen), and internal capsule	Precentral gyrus Postcentral gyrus Visual radiation fibers in temporoparietal lobes Dominant hemisphere Nondominant hemisphere Prefrontal lobe Internal capsule: lateral striate arteries	Contralateral hemiplegia with spared leg and foot Contralateral hemianesthesia Homonymous hemianopsia Aphasia Visual–spatial deficit and constructional apraxia Cognitive impairments Hemiplegia and hemianesthesia without aphasia
Posterior cerebral artery: medial surface of occipital lobe and inferior surface of occipital and temporal lobes	Calcarine cortex Thalamus Upper midbrain Subthalamic nucleus	Contralateral homonymous hemianopsia Thalamic syndrome: low pain threshold Coma and cranial nerve symptoms Hemiballism

the remaining parts of the caudate nucleus and putamen. Circulatory disturbances in these arteries result in motor movement disorders.

The anterior choroidal artery supplies blood to the choroid plexus, hippocampus, portions of the globus pallidus, posterior internal capsule, putamen, tail of the caudate nucleus, and lateral geniculate body. Signs of its occlusion consist of contralateral hemiplegia, hemianesthesia, involuntary movements, and memory disturbances. Circulatory involvement of the hippocampus results in memory impairment.

The posterior choroidal artery (not shown) originates from the PCA and supplies blood to the choroid plexus of the third ventricle, tectum, and pineal gland. The posteromedial arteries supply blood to parts of the thalamus, red nucleus, substantia nigra, medial portion of the cerebral peduncle, subthalamic nucleus, midbrain reticular formation, and superior cerebellar peduncle. Occlusion of these arteries results in multiple problems. Damage to the red nucleus leads to contralateral ataxia; damage to the substantia nigra leads to involuntary movements; damage to the subthalamic nucleus leads to hemiballism; and most importantly, damage to the midbrain reticular formation results in a coma.

The posterolateral arteries penetrate the inferior surface of the brain to supply blood to the parts of the lateral thalamus and the posterior pulvinar. Occlusion of this artery results in somatosensory disturbances in the opposite half of the body. Threshold to various sensory stimuli is lowered, resulting in intense pain from stimuli that would usually not be painful.

Blood Supply to Spinal Cord

Blood is supplied to the spinal cord by two major longitudinal arteries, the anterior and posterior spinal arteries, both of which originate from the vertebral arteries (Figs. 7-1 and 17-6). The anterior spinal artery from each vertebral artery joins to form a single descending artery along the midline, giving rise to branches on the left and right to serve the anterior two-thirds of the spinal cord, which contain sensorimotor fibers and motor neurons. Interruption in the vascular flow of the anterior spinal artery affects sensory and motor fibers and causes hemiplegia and protopathic hemisensory loss.

The posterior spinal arteries descend on the dorsal surface of the cord and supply the dorsal spinal area (Fig. 17-6), which contains the dorsal lemniscal fibers and dorsal gray column. Circulatory disorders in the posterior spinal artery result in a loss of epicritic sensation.

The vascular supply to the spinal cord is augmented further by the segmental radicular arteries; these arteries

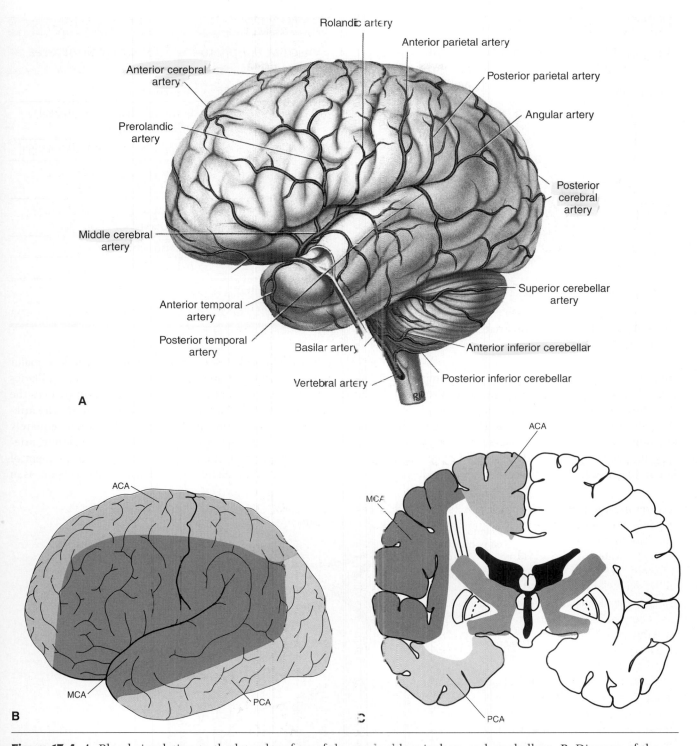

Figure 17-4 A. Blood circulation to the lateral surface of the cerebral hemisphere and cerebellum. B. Diagram of the lateral cortical surface marking the territories of three cortical arteries. C. Coronal illustration of the territories of three cortical arteries. ACA, anterior cerebral artery; MCA, middle cerebral artery; PCA, posterior cerebral artery.

descend from the aorta and enter the spinal column through the intervertebral foramina along with the spinal nerves. Each of the radicular of spinal arteries supplies blood to about six spinal segments, except the great radicular **artery of Adamkiewicz**. At the lower thoracic and upper lumbar level, one of the radicular arteries enlarges to form the

artery of Adamkiewicz; this supplies most of the caudal third of the cord.

Collateral Circulation

Collateral circulation refers to the alternative supply to a given structure after it has lost its primary arterial blood

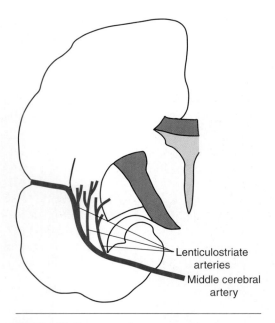

Figure 17-5 Lenticulostriate arteries.

Table 17-5

Vascular Supply to the Subcortical Structures

Structure	Artery
Thalamus	Posteromedial, posterolateral, and choroidal
Hypothalamus	Anteromedial and posteromedial
Caudate nucleus	Anterolateral, medial striate, and lenticulostriate
Putamen	Lenticulostriate, medial striate, and anterior choroidal
Globus pallidus	Anterior choroidal
Subthalamus	Posteromedial
Red nucleus and substantia nigra	Posteromedial

supply (Box 17-2). Collateral circulation is important in the natural recovery process of damaged brain structures. There are many potential channels for alternative blood circulation; however, not all are effective. The variability in **arterial anatomy** and the **degree of vascular pathology** are two factors that contribute to the development of collateral circulation. In general, better collateral circulation develops if an

artery is blocked closer to the main arterial trunk or major branches. Obstruction of the terminal arteries or capillaries after they have penetrated deep into the brain reduces the capabilities of developing collateral circulation. The arterial system from one hemisphere can never adequately perfuse the other hemisphere. A gradually developing arterial insufficiency facilitates the maximum development of compensatory circulation. A sudden arterial occlusion, as in

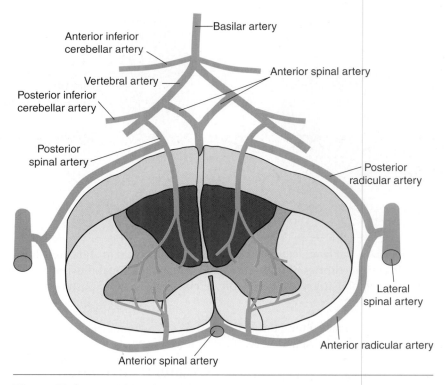

Figure 17-6 Spinal blood distribution through posterior and anterior spinal arteries and its augmentation by the radiculospinal arteries.

surface, which is highly probable in the case of reduced blood volume through any one of the three cortical arteries. The watershed zone constitutes the terminal distribution of blood supply to a given area in relation to its source.

Vascular Pathology

Vascular diseases of the brain are the most frequent causes of neurological deficits and adult disabilities in the United States and are ranked as the third most common cause of death after cancer and heart disease. Vascular interruption deprives the brain tissues of life-sustaining oxygen. Without oxygen, the brain cells die (infarction). **Cerebrovascular accidents** (CVA/Stroke) are characterized by sudden development of focal neurological deficits, which fall into three common types: **occlusive vascular pathology** (**thrombosis** or **embolism**), **hemorrhage** (bleeding from ruptured vessels), and **arteriovenous malformations** (AVM) (Table 17-6); these largely involve arteries.

Occlusive Vascular Pathology

Atherosclerosis, which consists of hardened arterial walls, is the primary cause of local arterial occlusion. Atherosclerosis is a slow process in which various lipids, blood platelets, calcium deposits, fatty particles, and other undissolved substances in the blood gradually accumulate along the inner walls of blood vessels and cause narrowing of the arterial lumen. An **atheroma** takes years to form. The adherence of lipids and platelets usually occurs at an ulcerated or injured site, commonly a point of bifurcation. Increased blood coagulability can contribute to an occlusive disease.

Since a narrowed or blocked arterial lumen (channel) decreases or stops blood flow, the brain suffers from ischemia (insufficient blood supply). A **transient ischemic attack** (**TIA**) is a temporary interruption of blood circulation to the brain. This is caused by mechanisms that interfere with blood supply to the brain, such as occlusive carotid disease, emboli from the heart, or proximal part of an artery,

The Point of Anastomosis

A natural interconnection between two blood vessels (anastomosis) forms the mechanism of the collateral vascular circulation, which, if functional, provides an alternate source of vascularization in the case of vascular insufficiency. In general, a slowly developing arterial insufficiency facilitates the maximum development of compensatory circulation. This collateral vascularization is associated with the natural recovery of functions after stroke. Serving to equalize the vascular blood supply to both sides of the brain, the circle of Willis serves as an important anastomotic point for the revascularization.

stroke, usually does not lead to the development of a substantial source of alternate circulation.

There are four potential points of collateral circulation within one hemisphere or across both. First, the anterior communicating artery connects the two anterior cerebral arteries. Second, the vertebral basilar system feeds through the posterior communicating artery if the internal carotid artery blood flow is insufficient. Similarly, the posterior communicating arteries may draw from the internal carotid artery and feed into the posterior cerebral arteries if the vertebral basilar arterial system is occluded. Third, although infrequent, thromboembolic involvement of the internal carotid artery can trigger retrograde blood flow from the external carotid artery through the ophthalmic artery branches in the eye. Fourth, the terminal branches of all three cortical (anterior, middle, and posterior cerebral) arteries may anastomose in the **watershed zone** on the lateral brain

---

Table 17-6

Principal Types of Stroke

Type	Location	Time of Occurrence	Warning Signs
Thrombosis	Occlusion at atherosclerotic lesion	During sleep and periods of low physical activity	Transient ischemic attacks, headaches, and seizures
Embolism	Occlusion of smaller artery by displaced clot moving peripherally	When awake and active	None; possible headaches and seizures
Hemorrhage	Rupture of arterial wall or aneurysm	Anytime, usually during awake hours	None
Arteriovenous malformation bleed	Twisted arteriovenous malformation	Bleed anytime, usually during awake hours	Recurrent headaches

and infrequently spasms of arterial muscles. The exact symptoms depend on the brain area affected. A patient with TIA may have several of the following suddenly emerging symptoms: **focal weakness**, **double vision**, **headache**, **paresthesia**, **hemianesthesia**, **dysarthria**, and **dizziness**. These may last from a few minutes to an hour. If these symptoms last longer, it is a full stroke.

The transient symptoms of a TIA are clinically significant, since their presence indicates that a larger stroke may be in progress (Table 17-7). Not all strokes are preceded by a TIA; only about one-third of individuals with TIA later have a major stroke. Administration of blood-thinning medication at this stage may prevent a major CVA. In arteriosclerosis, the heart initially compensates for the reduced blood flow by pumping blood with greater force. However, this compensatory pumping may lead to **high blood pressure** (**hypertension**). Once the atherosclerotic process has begun (Fig. 17-7A), it interrupts the blood supply by forming either an embolus (Fig. 17-7B) or a thrombus (Fig. 17-7C).

Comprising 25% of the CVAs, embolism is blockage in a distal artery with a narrow lumen. An embolus is a clot that breaks free from a thrombus and enters the bloodstream, eventually blocking a small end artery.

Table 17-7
Warning Signs of Stroke
Sudden onset of numbness or weakness on one side of body
Suddenly emerged difficulty in speaking and understanding others
Sudden difficulty in seeing with one or both eyes; double vision
Sudden loss of balance and dizziness
Headache with no cause

Cerebral emboli produce rapid development of neurological signs that mostly do not progress. Embolic strokes usually occur during a period of activity and often affect young people.

Accounting for 65% of the CVAs, thrombosis is a local buildup of fatty substances and blood platelets in a cerebral vessel that is caused by an atherosclerotic plaque; the buildup mostly occurs at sites of arterial bifurcation or at

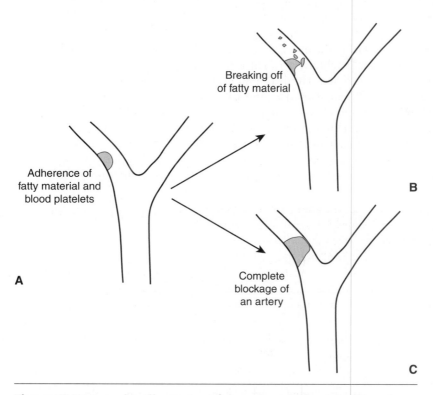

Breaking off of fatty material

Adherence of fatty material and blood platelets

Complete blockage of an artery

A

B

C

Figure 17-7 A graphic illustration of thromboembolism. **A.** Thromboembolism forms in vascular system. **B.** Embolus is a detached part of thrombosis, which occludes a smaller vessel at a distance from the original site. **C.** Thrombosis completely blocks a blood vessel by local accumulation of undissolved substances, including globules of fat, clumps of bacteria, and blood platelets.

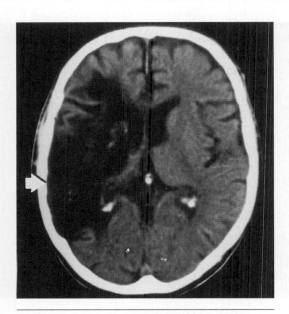

Figure 17-8 Large right middle cerebral artery infarct (*arrow*) on an axial CT image.

sites subjected to injury and inflammation. The presence of plaque causes the degeneration of the vessel wall, and damage to the endothelial layer attracts fibrin and blood platelets to the site. The thrombosis grows slowly; it can take several years before the arterial lumen closes. A thrombosis becomes symptomatic only in the mid and late years (Fig. 17-7). By then, the arterial lumen mostly is blocked. Most thrombotic strokes occur during sleep or a period of inactivity. Patients, unaware of their deficits, awaken to find themselves paralyzed. The reason a thrombotic stroke tends to occur during sleep is that the lower blood pressure during inactivity allows vessels to narrow or close (Fig. 17-8). One warning sign of a thrombotic stroke is TIA (occurring in 30% of patients who later develop stroke).

Hemorrhage

Accounting for 10% of CVAs, hemorrhagic strokes are associated with sudden onset of neurological symptoms and may cause coma and stupor that may progress with time. Hemorrhagic strokes result from bleeding of ruptured blood vessels. They occur when a weakened arterial wall ruptures under the pressure of constant blood flow. Hemorrhages can occur anywhere in the arterial system; however, the lenticulostriate arteries that supply the thalamus and basal ganglia are the most common sites (Fig. 17-5). The major types of hemorrhagic strokes are **lacunar strokes, intracerebral hemorrhage, subdural hematoma,** and **subarachnoid hemorrhage.** Lacunar strokes and intracerebral hemorrhage are traditionally considered strokes, while subdural hematoma is subsequent to trauma and arachnoid hemorrhage results form a rupture of an aneurysm as well as **arteriovenus malformation.**

Lacunar strokes involve small arteries of the basal ganglia and thalamus. They occur abruptly or in spurts over

days. They are commonly found in individuals with idiopathic hypertension. Intracerebral hemorrhages are space-occupying lesions involving the rupturing of an intracranial artery. Blood released from the ruptured artery, if not surgically drained, accumulates to form a hematoma, which encroaches on vital cortical centers. Intracerebral hemorrhages usually occur during an active or awake state. The full extent of deficit is seldom present at the outset but develops over several hours.

In subdural hematoma, which can result from a traumatic injury, a blood vessel ruptures in the arachnoid tissue beneath the dura mater. The accumulated blood, if not surgically drained, will expand and compress the soft underlying brain tissues, causing irreversible brain damage. Another potential site for hemorrhage is the subarachnoid space, which usually develops after physical exertion. Subarachnoid hemorrhage is commonly seen with the bleeding of an AVM or aneurysm.

An **aneurysm**, a vascular condition associated with hemorrhage, is a local balloon-like dilation of an artery (Fig. 17-9). It usually occurs at points of bifurcation of major cerebral arteries. The outpouchings of an aneurysm are due to either weakness in the vessel wall or congenital arterial defect. An aneurysm causes neurological symptoms in two ways: (*a*) the mass effect of arterial dilation can compress the surrounding structures and (*b*) the aneurysm can no longer withstand the blood flow pressure, and it ruptures, releasing blood into the brain or onto its surface.

Arteriovenous Malformations

Arteriovenous malformations are congenital or fetal conditions in which tangled dilated arteries and veins become connected in a local area (Fig. 17-10), thus with capillaries, the blood bypasses cortical tissue and is drained back to the heart. With age, they may become large and are susceptible to hemorrhage because of their thin walls. These malformations often cause seizures and recurrent headaches (mimicking migraines). Depending on the location of the malformations, they can also cause language impairments, motor speech problems, visual disorders, sensory loss, and hemiplegia.

SELECTIVE VULNERABILITY TO ANOXIA

Since the brain receives its energy supply entirely from the oxidative **metabolism** of glucose supplied by the blood, a reduction in the vascular supply in stroke results in sudden onset of neurological symptoms because of **anoxia** in the brain cells. However, the nerve cells in various regions of the brain are differentially vulnerable to anoxia. The general rule seems to be that the brain cells that are inherently active at all times because of constant sensory input are the most susceptible to anoxia. This perhaps accounts for the high vulnerability of the cerebral cortex, cerebellum (Purkinje cells), and the cells of the hippocampus. The con-

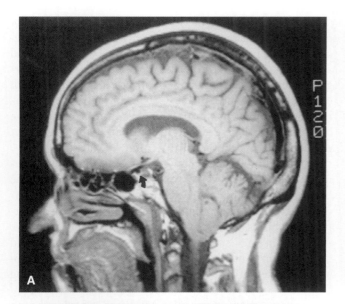

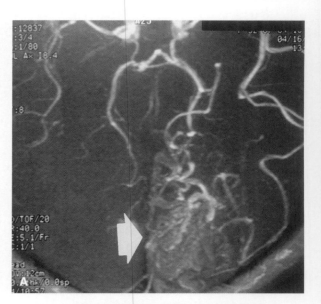

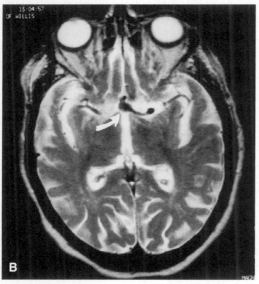

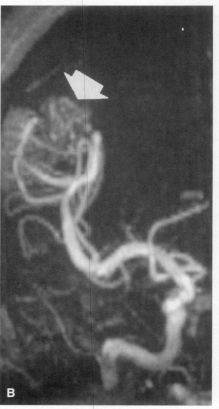

Figure 17-9 A. Sagittal T1-weighted MRI of aneurysm (*curved arrow*) of the internal carotid artery. B. T2-weighted axial MRI of an anterior communicating artery aneurysm (*curved arrow*).

Figure 17-10 A. Axial MRI of a left occipital AVM (*arrow*) in the branches of the left PCA. B. Reconstructed MRI of the right cerebral artery AVM.

stant state of inherent sensorimotor activity also makes the parietal, frontal, and occipital lobes, along with the anterior and dorsomedial thalamus, highly susceptible to anoxia.

RISK FACTORS

There are two types of risk factors for stroke: modifiable and nonmodifiable (Table 17-8). Medical conditions and lifestyle related issues can be controlled either medically or by changing living habits; these include hypertension, heart disease, diabetes mellitus, and high cholesterol. Lifestyle related modifiable risk factors are smoking, obesity, and physical inactivity. Advancing age, gender, hereditary predisposition, and ethnic composition are the risks that cannot be treated. Untreated hypertension can damage the arterial walls so that they become sites of atherosclerotic plaques. High blood pressure is the single most common risk factor for strokes, and controlling hypertension contributes to a significant decline in the incidence of stroke.

Table 17-8

Modifiable and Nonmodifiable Risk Factors for Stroke

Modifiable	Nonmodifiable
Medical	Age
Hypertension	Gender
Hypercholesterolemia	Ethnicity
Hyperlipidemia	Heredity
Carotid artery disease	
Diabetes	
Lifestyle	
Physical inactivity	
Oral contraceptive use	
Cigarette smoking	
Obesity	

Heart disease is another frequent cause of the embolic stroke, as clots leaving the heart can block brain arteries. Persons with **coronary heart disease (CAD)**, who experience symptoms such as heart attack and chest pain, are at twice as much risk of having a stroke as the general population. Diabetic mellitus, another cause of stroke, is known to accelerate the development of atherosclerosis. Also, high cholesterol levels cause buildups on arterial walls, narrowing their passageways and leading to heart attack and stroke (Box 17-3). Lifestyle related habits, such as smoking, substantially increases risk for coronary artery disease (CAD); quitting smoking alone can lower the risk for CVA by 50–70% within 5 years (American Heart Association).

VENOUS SINUS SYSTEM

Veins and sinuses collect deoxygenated blood and transport it back to the heart and lungs for reoxygenation. Drainage of the blood first begins at the capillary level, where the intraparenchymal capillaries unite to form small veins that are called venules. Venules collect the blood from capillaries and transfer it to the network of large veins. Veins drain the surface as well as deep brain structures and empty blood into the sinuses. The sinuses, which consist of large spaces between the periosteal and meningeal layers of dura mater, are in the cranium (Fig. 2-43).

Dural Sinuses

The dural sinuses form a network of cavities in and around the brain (Figs. 2-43 and 17-11). The **superior sagittal sinus** runs along the dorsomedial line on the vertex in the falx cerebri, receiving blood from the superior cerebral veins and **cerebrospinal fluid (CSF)** drained through the arachnoid villi. The **inferior sagittal sinus** runs in the inferior margin of the falx cerebri over the dorsal edge of the corpus callosum. Posteriorly, it joins the straight (rectus) sinus, which runs posteriorly and empties into the sinus confluence. The paired transverse sinuses arise from the confluence of sinuses, which course laterally, rostrally, then down and forward to form the internal jugular vein. The **cavernous sinus**, a large, irregular network of smaller veins, is around the pituitary gland. The cavernous sinus drains into the transverse sinuses through the petrosal sinuses. The sinuses siphon off all the collected blood and shunt the cerebrovascular fluid to the **internal jugular veins** through which blood returns to the heart.

Cerebral Veins

Veins collect the circulating blood from the cortical and subcortical areas and empty it into the sinus network. There are two types of cerebral veins, superficial and deep. The superficial cerebral veins collect circulated blood from the neocortex and subcortical white matter and drain it into the superior sagittal sinus (Fig. 17-12). The large, superficial veins include the **superior, inferior,** and **superficial middle cerebral veins**. The superior cerebral veins collect blood from the middle surface and the vertex and drain it into the superior sagittal sinus. The inferior cerebral veins drain the basal surface of the brain and empty blood into the **cavernous, petrosal,** and **transverse** sinuses. The superficial middle cerebral veins collect blood from the lateral brain surface and drain it into the cavernous sinus.

The deep cerebral veins include numerous smaller veins such as the internal cerebral, basal, choroidal, and thalamostriate. They all drain blood from the subcortical structures, including the striatum, thalamus, choroid plexus, and hippocampus, and empty into the **great cerebral vein of Galen**. The great vein opens to the **straight sinus**.

Veins of the Spinal Cord

The venous drainage system of the spinal cord is similar to the arterial network. The anterior and posterior spinal veins are joined by the anterior radicular veins. The spinal venous system also communicates with internal and external venous plexuses adjacent to the spinal dural sac and vertebral column.

REGULATION OF CEREBRAL BLOOD FLOW

The vascular circulatory system is a closed system in which the blood movement requires a constant pressure. To a large extent, arterial response and regulation of blood flow are adjusted autonomically depending on the brain's metabolic needs. Additional factors that regulate the blood flow are reflexive contraction and expansion of arterial walls, CO_2 blood level, and blood pressure changes. These maintain a constant blood flow with mean arterial pressure in range of 60–140 mm Hg. On average, for normal functioning the

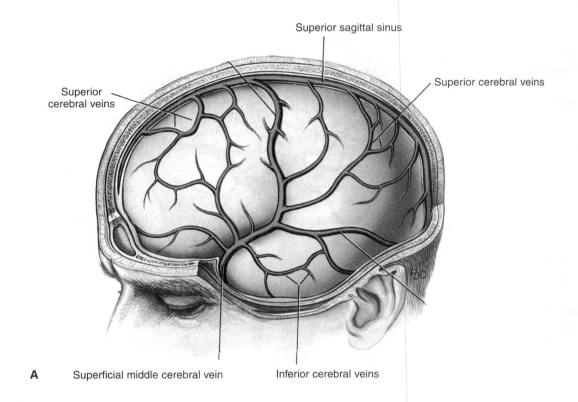

A   Superficial middle cerebral vein   Inferior cerebral veins

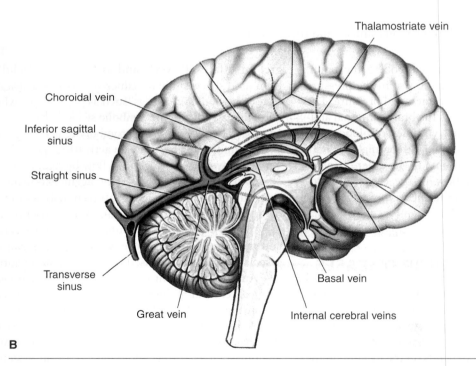

B

Figure 17-12 Superficial and deep veins. A. Large veins on the lateral surface include branches of superior cerebral and inferior cerebral veins and superficial middle cerebral veins. B. Midsagittal view of internal cerebral veins.

Table 17-9

Blood Flow for Brain Functioning

Flow (mL/100 g brain tissue/min)	Levels of Brain Functioning
45–55	Normal level of brain function
20–45	Lower efficiency of brain function
15–20	Impaired or loss of brain function
Consistently <15	Loss of function owing to tissue damage

stroke, which accounts for over 83% of reported cases of stroke.

In the case of a hemorrhagic condition, medically optimal treatment is the reduction of elevated blood pressure. Medical management of an aneurysm, a common site of hemorrhagic stroke, entails reducing blood pressure to prevent bleeding; clipping is used surgically to obliterate the neck of the aneurysm, thus disabling it. Aneurysms also are treated without opening the skull through coiling, which involves placing a platinum coil in the aneurysm. This coil causes a blood clot to form, sealing off the aneurysm.

BLOOD–BRAIN BARRIER

The **blood-brain barrier** (BBB) is an important clinical concept. It restricts movement of specific substances, such as infectious microorganisms, from the bloodstream to the brain tissue and extracellular fluid, which is similar to CSF. The BBB applies only to the CNS because in brain capillaries, unlike the muscle capillaries, endothelial cells form a continuous interior lining membrane. These cellular elements are joined tightly and there are no adjacent intracellular pores or fenestrations. The endothelial cell membrane in the CNS is surrounded further by the end feet of astrocytes outside the capillary wall (Fig. 17-13). Both of these add to the selective membrane permeability, restricting the flow of certain substances in the blood to the extracellular space and restricting flow from the choroidal capillaries to the CSF.

Information regarding which substances cross the BBB is important in the administration of medicine. Although it keeps harmful microorganisms out of the brain, the BBB also keeps many helpful antibodies out, making the treatment of many cerebral infections difficult.

Some disease states in the brain disrupt the BBB by enabling some normally excluded substances to enter into the cerebrospinal and cellular interstitial fluids. Meningitis and brain tumors are two conditions that alter the BBB and allow toxic substances to enter the brain. In brain tumors,

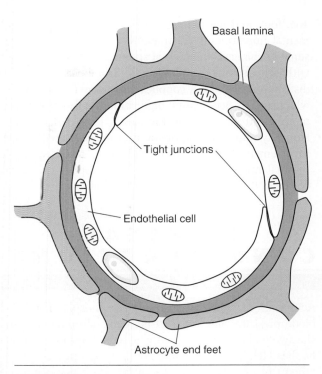

Figure 17-13 Structural properties that contribute to the blood-brain barrier.

new proliferating capillaries are known to have intracellular pores, which affect the capillary permeability. This has some diagnostic significance because radioactive amino acids can exit through pores into the brain, allowing localization of the tumor.

LESION LOCALIZATION–RULE 10: VASCULAR SYSTEM DISORDER

Presenting Symptoms and Rationale

- Sudden development of **contralateral hemiplegia of the lower face, arm, and upper extremity, more than the leg,** with accompanying sensory loss results from occlusion of the MCA, which may be caused by either thrombosis or embolism. The symptoms discussed under rule 1 (see Chapter 2) also may appear. An abrupt onset of symptoms usually indicates vascular pathology, while gradual progression of symptoms indicates a mass lesion. The regions of the motor cortex involved with the representation of different body parts are served by two arteries, the MCA and ACA. The MCA supplies the area of motor control for the face, hand, and upper extremity, while the ACA serves the motor area for the leg (Figs. 14-1 and 17-4). Involvement of the somatomotor cortex and corticospinal fibers accounts for the contralateral paralysis of the upper face, trunk, and upper extremity. Involvement of somatosensory cortex and thalamocortical fibers results in hemianesthesia for the trunk, face, and upper extremity.

- **Toe, foot, and leg paralysis** as well as sensory loss and mental impairments (distractibility, indecisiveness, personality changes, and lack of spontaneity) are associated with ischemia due to embolism or thrombosis in the ACA distribution. The ACA supplies the medial frontal cortex, which serves personality, higher mental functions, and motor control for the leg (Figs. 14-1, 17-3, and 17-4).
- **Homonymous hemianopsia** is associated with PCA involvement. Low pain threshold also is seen because of the thalamic involvement. The PCA supplies the visual cortex in the occipital lobe and the thalamus (Fig. 17-3).

CLINICAL CONSIDERATIONS

PATIENT ONE

A 55-year-old woman was admitted to a hospital for high blood pressure. She had a stroke while sleeping. When she awoke, her right hand and leg would not move, and her head felt heavy. She could not find appropriate words to explain the loss of motor control. She was examined by a neurologist and at his recommendation, a speech language pathologist. They observed the following:

- Right hemiplegia with intact sensation for touch, pain, and temperature
- Moderate difficulty finding words
- Limited verbal output
- Impaired verbal repetition
- Impaired reading and writing
- Near-normal auditory comprehension

Within a few days, her speech improved, but it still was sparse and consisted of only a few words. She used many gestures and pointed with her left arm. Failure to communicate frustrated her, and she was depressed. The brain MRI revealed a large infarct in the left frontal lobe anterior to the central sulcus that involved the anterior language cortex and a large part of the motor cortex.

Question: How can you relate the manifestations of aphasia with the site of infarct?

Discussion: A stroke involving the anterior branches of the MCA affected the motor cortex and Broca area (Brodmann areas 44 and 45).

PATIENT TWO

A 65-year-old right-handed businessman was admitted to a hospital after sudden development of confusion. Initially, the man did not speak much except some jargon and stereotyped expressions. After 3 weeks of care and recovery, he exhibited the following:

- Severe receptive aphasia
- Fluent and copious verbal output

- Severe anomia marked with many (related and unrelated) paraphasic errors and perseverations
- Excessive usage of general pronouns
- Semantically empty speech
- Limited repetition
- Severe difficulty in understanding others
- Moderate alexia
- Poor writing
- Intact somatosensory and motor functions
- Right visual field defect

The brain MRI revealed an infarct in the posterior left superior temporal gyrus and parts of the inferior parietal lobe.

Question: How can you relate the manifestations of receptive aphasia with the temporoparietal site of infarct?

Discussion: A stroke in the posterior branches of the MCA affected the temporal cortex, including the classical Wernicke area (Brodmann area 22), which impaired comprehension and expression in this patient. The temporal lesion also affected the geniculocalcarine visual radiation fibers. Intact sensorimotor function was related to the spared ascending branches of the MCA.

PATIENT THREE

A 59-year-old woman woke up blind in the right eye. She was taken to a hospital, where the attending physician noted the following:

- A history of elevated blood pressure
- No history of trauma
- No previous episode of TIA
- Right homonymous hemianopia

With selective visual symptoms, a vascular cause was suspected. However, computed tomography (CT) of the head produced normal findings. Since the patient's visual difficulty persisted, a repeat CT of the head, undertaken after 3 days, showed an infarct in the left occipital lobe.

Question: How can you account for these symptoms on the basis of your understanding of the vascular supply and the functional organization in the brain?

Discussion: The stroke involving the left occipital lobe accounts for the focal symptom of right homonymous hemianopsia. The sudden emergence of the symptom implies a vascular cause (gradual appearance of the symptoms indicates a tumor). The stroke affected the PCA, which supplies blood to the visual cortex in the occipital lobe (Figs. 17-3 and 17-4). The infarct was visualized only on a repeat CT because it takes nearly 36 hours for infarcts to show on CT.

PATIENT FOUR

A 60 year-old priest was taken to an emergency room for sensorimotor problems that developed abruptly while he was getting ready to go to church to speak for a Sunday service. The attending physician noted the following:

- Unintelligible speech because of dysarthria
- Hypernasality (with lowered left palate)
- Dysphagia
- Sensation loss on the left side of the face
- Difficulty balancing with falling to the left
- Left-sided complete facial paralysis
- Weakness in the right leg and arm

The brain MRI revealed an infarct in the left caudal lateral–ventral pons extending to the medulla.

Question: How can you account for these symptoms of the left face and paralysis of the right half of the body? Can these symptoms be related to the involvement of the blood supply to the pontomedullary area? If so, how?

Discussion: Small lateral arterial branches of the basilar artery supply the pons and part of the medulla. The lateral medulla, which contains sensorimotor fibers, is supplied by the posterior inferior cerebellar artery, a branch of the vertebral artery.

A pontomedullary stroke involving the branches of the vestibular artery affected the trigeminal (CN V), facial (CN VII), and vestibuloacoustic (CN VIII) nerves, as well as rootlets of the vagus (CN X) nerve. Effects on the facial (CN VII) and trigeminal (CN V) nerve fibers along with the rootlets of the vagus (CN X) nerve resulted in facial motor weakness, loss of sensation from the face, palatal paralysis, and swallowing difficulty. The involvement of vestibular nuclei resulted in impaired equilibrium with a tendency to fall to the left. The interruption of the descending pyramidal (corticospinal) fibers above the point of decussation produced right (contralateral) paralysis in the right arm and leg. The implicated cranial nerve fibers already had crossed, so there was left (ipsilateral) facial paralysis. This clinical picture is called alternating or crossed hemiplegia, which is a classical lateral medullary syndrome (see Chapters 14 and 15).

PATIENT FIVE

A 55-year-old man suffered a stroke while sleeping. He woke up with a headache and was perspiring. In the morning, he appeared confused, could not walk, and had difficulty talking. He was taken to the ER where he presented with the following:

- Paralysis of the right-side of the body
- Loss of pain and temperature loss on the right side of the body
- Lower facial palsy
- Paralysis of the right tongue

- Unintelligible speech marked with distorted consonants, slow rate of speech, hypernasality, aphonic and breathy voice
- Impaired swallow marked with premature swallow, and poor bolus control
- Intact ability to wrinkle forehead
- No aphasic or cognitive impairments

The brain MRI revealed an infarct of the left internal capsule, caudate, and Putamen.

Question: How can you explain these symptoms subsequent to a subcortical stroke?

Discussion: Vascular involvement of the lenticulostriate on the left affected the long sensory and motor projections fibers, which had resulted in right-sided paralysis and hemianesthesia. The involvement of the corticobulbar system also affected the cranial motor nuclei of facial (CN VII), hypoglossal (CN XII), and vagus (CN X) nerves, which had contributed to his dysarthria and speech unintelligibility. He could control the upper face, because it receives projections from both motor cortices.

PATIENT SIX

A 75-year-old right-handed man, who was diagnosed with stroke and aphasia, was seen by a SLP, who noted the following:

- Fluently spoken and well-articulated speech
- Speech consisting of a meaningless strings of words
- Poor repetitions
- Impaired comprehension for both spoken and written language
- Moderate anomia.
- Optimistic attitudes

An MRA revealed a large infarct lesion in the left temporal parietal cortex involving Brodmann areas 39, 49, and 22.

Question: How can you identify the aphasia type and account for its association with the lesion site?

Discussion: This neurolinguistic symptomatology (fluently articulated but asemantic verbal output with anomia and impaired comprehension for both spoken and written language as well as euphoria) is indicative of Wernicke aphasia, This aphasia type is associated with damage to the posterior superior temporal region (Brodmann area 22) and the inferior parietal lobule (Brodmann areas 39 and 40) in the dominant hemisphere. This infarct resulted in Wernicke type aphasia.

SUMMARY

The CNS depends on an adequate and uninterrupted supply of blood and oxygen. The heart pumps oxygenated blood to the CNS through two arterial systems, vertebro-basilar and the carotid. Both of these arterial systems ascend and join the arterial circle of Willis at the base of the brain. Three cortical branches and numerous penetrating subcortical branches arise from the circle of Willis and supply blood to the brain. After perfusion, the deoxygenated blood is collected by veins and drained into the sinus system responsible for transmitting the collected blood and cerebrospinal fluid back to the heart for reprocessing.

QUIZ QUESTIONS

1. Define the following terms: anastomosis, aneurysm, arteriovenous malformations, blood–brain barrier, collateral circulation, embolism, hemorrhage, thrombosis, transient ischemic attack.

2. Discuss the relative length of time that brain cells can sustain blood deprivation.

3. List three clinical symptoms that are associated with the involvement of the anterior cerebral artery.

4. List three clinical symptoms that are associated with the involvement of the middle cerebral artery.

5. Discuss two symptoms that might follow after the involvement of the posterior cerebral artery.

TECHNICAL TERMS

anastomoses
aneurysm
arteriosclerosis
arteriovenous
  malformations
atheroma
atherosclerosis
autoregulation
blood–brain barrier
carotid vascular system
cerebrovascular accident

circle of Willis
collateral circulation
embolism
hemorrhage
ischemia
metabolism
paresthesia
sinus
thrombosis
vasodilating
watershed infarction

Survey of the Ventricles and Cerebrospinal Fluid

LEARNING OBJECTIVES

After studying this chapter, students should be able to:

- Discuss the functions of cerebrospinal fluid

- Describe the mechanism of cerebrospinal fluid production

- Outline the circulation of cerebrospinal fluid

- Discuss the circulatory disorders of cerebrospinal fluid

- Discuss the treatment of hydrocephalus

- Explain the diagnostic significance of cerebrospinal fluid

Cerebrospinal fluid (CSF) is a clear, colorless fluid. It is produced by the **choroid plexus** in the ventricular system and circulates from the **ventricles** to the **subarachnoid space** around the CNS. By forming a mechanical cushion around the CNS, the CSF protects the brain and spinal cord from sudden and violent body movements. The buoyancy effect of the floating CSF in the subarachnoid space reduces the brain's weight by more than 95%. Thus a brain weighing 1300–1400 g in the air weighs only 60–70 g when floating in CSF. This buoyancy effect is an important aspect of the protective mechanism. As an active transport mechanism, CSF, with the vascular system, may also participate in the removal of harmful substances and waste resulting from cellular metabolic activities. CSF also is known to regulate extracellular environments.

CHOROID PLEXUS

Extending from the ventricular surface into the ventricular cavity, the **choroid plexus** is formed by an extensive network of infolded **vascular capillaries**, which are surrounded by the **vascular pia mater** (tela choroidea) and connective tissue. This also receives a layer of **epithelium** from the **ependymal lining** of the inner ventricular surface. The choroid plexus, with a minutely folded surface, is a fenestrated structure with tight junctions around its apical regions. The pores or fenestrations are formed by epithelial cells.

The tight junctions between adjacent cells contribute to the barrier for the exchange of solutes between the blood and CSF. The choroid plexus is located primarily in the center of the **lateral** and **fourth ventricles**; its largest formation is around the **collateral trigone** region of the lateral ventricles (Fig. 18-1). No choroid plexus is present in the small opening of the **cerebral aqueduct of Sylvius** or in the **anterior** or **posterior horns**.

CSF is produced by the choroid plexus. The average total volume of CSF present in the human is 120–140 mL. The human brain produces ~ 0.35 mL of CSF every minute, totaling 500 mL/day through passive diffusion from blood. CSF is normally replaced three times within 24 hr and is secreted through the modified **capillary–pia membranous network**. In general, CSF is a filtered form of blood. It resembles blood plasma but differs from blood in its molecular composition—for example, CSF contains less protein and less than half the glucose found in blood and has virtually no white or red blood cells. Diseases of the CNS can change the constituent composition of CSF, an alteration that has diagnostic importance for identifying pathologic changes that occur in the brain and spinal cord.

CEREBROSPINAL FLUID CIRCULATION

CSF circulates in the ventricles and the subarachnoid space. There are four ventricles in the brain (Fig. 18-1): two **lateral ventricles** (one in each hemisphere), the **third ventricle** (in the diencephalon), and the **fourth ventricle** (in the brainstem). CSF flows from both lateral ventricles in the cerebral hemispheres to the third ventricle via the **interventricular (Monro) foramen**. The third ventricle is located vertically between the two **thalami**, and its fluid flows to the fourth ventricle through the **cerebral aqueduct**. From the fourth ventricle, CSF enters the subarachnoid space through three apertures: two lateral **foramina of Luschka** and one mediodorsal **foramen of Magendie** (Fig. 18-1).

The subarachnoid space wraps around the entire CNS between the arachnoid membrane and pia mater. The subarachnoid space varies from region to region: it is narrow over the gyri and wide over the fissures. The arachnoid, which rests under the dura mater, is separated from the dura by a potential **subdural space**, whereas the

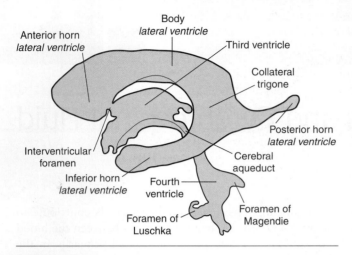

Figure 18-1 Lateral view of the ventricles.

pia mater closely adheres to the cortical surface. **Arachnoid trabeculae** extend from the arachnoid to the pia mater and contribute to the maintenance of the subarachnoid space (Fig. 2-46).

The subarachnoid space houses many **cisterns** that serve as large pockets of CSF. The important cisterns are the **cerebellomedullary**, **superior**, **interpeduncular**, **chiasmatic**, **pontine**, and **lumbar**. Located between the medulla and cerebellum, the cerebellomedullary cistern receives fluid from the fourth ventricle. The interpeduncular cistern is the large pocket of fluid ventral to the midbrain. The chiasmatic cistern lies in front of the optic chiasm, and the pontine cistern is in front of the pons. The lumbar cistern extends from L2 to S2 and contains fibers of the cauda equina nerve roots and filum terminale (Fig. 18-2; see Fig. 2-48).

Once in the subarachnoid space, CSF flows up toward the convexity of the brain or down toward the spinal cord. Some CSF infiltrates the depths of the cerebral cortex along the blood vessels that penetrate the brain. This area around the penetrating blood vessels is the **perivascular space**, the site for possible diffusion of metabolic solutes from the CSF into the extracellular fluid. The diffusion of metabolites has important implications for medical treatment.

ABSORPTION OF THE CEREBROSPINAL FLUID

CSF is absorbed through the **arachnoid granulations**, which are one-way openings. These tufted structures are dorsal along both sides of the **superior sagittal sinus** (see Fig. 2-46B). The arachnoid granulations protrude into the

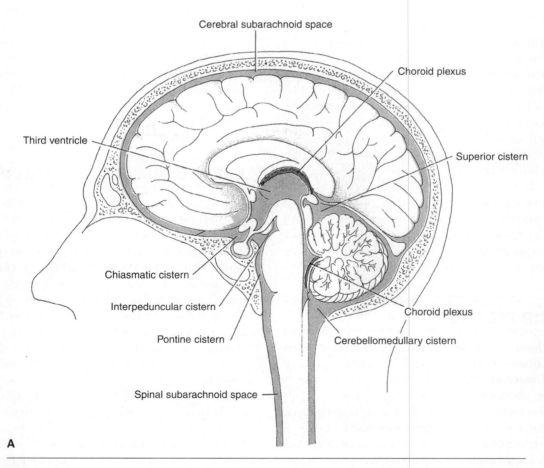

Figure 18-2 A. The subarachnoid space (*shaded*) and major subarachnoid cisterns. (*Continued*)

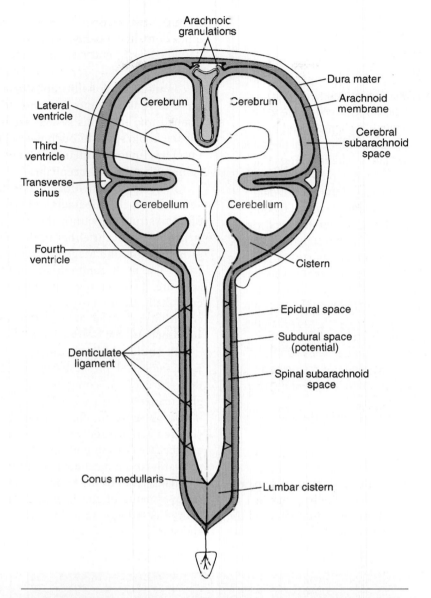

Figure 18-2 (*Continued*) B. The brain and spinal cord showing the locations of the subarachnoid spaces.

dural sinus and empty CSF into the superior sagittal sinus, which also receives venous blood.

CLINICAL CONCERNS

The draining of CSF from the subarachnoid space is a pressure-sensitive process. Emptying CSF into the superior sagittal sinus requires a pressure differential between the subarachnoid space and venous–sinus system. A pressure difference of 30–60 millimeters of mercury (mm Hg) regulates normal CSF drainage through the **arachnoid villi**. If for any reason this pressure differential alters and the sinus pressure exceeds the ventricular pressure, the one-way openings of the arachnoid villi close, ending the draining and subsequently elevating **intracranial pressure**.

The rate of CSF production, however, is independent of its absorption and interventricular pressure. CSF continues to be produced even after an interruption in its drainage into the **sinus system**. A dissociation between production and absorption rates of CSF results in **hydrocephalus** (Box 18-1), a condition to which three factors contribute: the increased production of CSF, blocking of the draining passage through which CSF reaches the subarachnoid space, and impaired absorption of CSF. Choroidal tumors have also been implicated in hydrocephalus. Regardless of the underlying cause, in hydrocephalus, an excessive amount of CSF increases pressure in the brain. Sustained pressure causes enlargement of the ventricles and damage to the surrounding vital cortical tissues (Fig. 18-3). If hydrocephalus begins in infancy, the increased CSF pressure also enlarges the cranial vault.

BOX 18-1

Hydrocephalus

Hydrocephalus is a condition marked by an excessive accumulation of CSF within the ventricular cavity in the brain. It is characterized by dilated ventricles, increased intracranial pressure, and an enlarged cranium in children. The adult skull does not increase in size; rather the ventricles enlarge at the expense of the surrounding cortical tissues. This condition is caused by an obstruction in the flow of CSF from the ventricles to the site of its absorption in the superior sagittal sinus, a structure of the dural meninges at the top of the skull between the cerebral hemispheres. Clinically it is marked by abnormal behavioral symptoms, such as slow thinking and decreased responsiveness, lethargy, and progressing stupor. Untreated hydrocephalus can lead to unconsciousness and coma. Hydrocephalus can be treated surgically by diverting CSF to the peritoneal cavity in the abdomen, the pleural space, or the atrium of the heart.

Circulatory Disorders

Obstruction in the movement of CSF flow or its impaired absorption causes hydrocephalus, which is marked by enlarged ventricles subsequent to the accumulation of the CSF. There are two primary (**communicating** and **obstruc**-tive) and two secondary (**normal pressure** and **ex vacuo**) types of hydrocephalus.

Primary

In communicating hydrocephalus, the problem is impairment of drainage into the sinus. CSF is not adequately drained into the sinus system even though it reaches the subarachnoid space through the foramina of Magendie and Luschka. Tumor or inflammation of the brain often causes communicating hydrocephalus.

In obstructive hydrocephalus, the CSF flow from the ventricles to the subarachnoid space is blocked because of an obstruction within the ventricular cavity. The obstruction can occur either in the ventricular system itself or in Luschka and Magendie foramina in the fourth ventricle. The most common site of blockage is the narrow aperture of the cerebral aqueduct in the midbrain. A mesencephalic tumor also can cause the hydrocephalus by contributing to the stenosis (narrowing) of the cerebral aqueduct.

Regardless of the hydrocephalic type, the final result is the same: CSF pressure rises in the ventricles. It enlarges the ventricles and compresses the surrounding white and gray matters (Fig. 18-3), affecting vital cortical functions, including sensorimotor and higher mental functions. In children with hydrocephalia, the head becomes pyramidal, and the face is disproportionately small with the eyes turned outward. In the most advanced cases of hydrocephalus, a coronal section of the brain reveals nothing but two large compartments of the lateral ventricles, and the cortical mantle is reduced to a thin layer between the ventricles and skull.

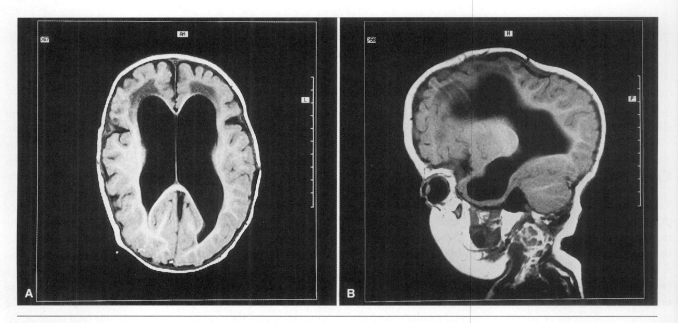

Figure 18-3 MRI studies of the enlarged lateral ventricles in a child with hydrocephaly. A. Transaxial view. B. Sagittal view.

Secondary

Ventricular dilation can also occur subsequent to other brain pathologies, such as brain atrophy (hydrocephalus ex vacua), traumatic injuries, and **meningitis** (normal pressure hydrocephalus). Both of these conditions are commonly encountered in the elderly population by students in human behavior.

Although not a true hydrocephalic condition, hydrocephalus ex vacuo causes a generalized cortical atrophy. With the atrophy of the gray and white matter, the ventricular space is larger but without any increase in CSF pressure. It may take years to develop this condition; symptoms may relate to generalized atrophy of the brain.

Commonly seen among elderly individuals, normal pressure hydrocephalus can result from meningitis, subarachnoid hemorrhage, and/or trauma. The ventricular space is enlarged, though CSF pressure fluctuates from time to time. Common problems seen in patients with normal pressure hydrocephalus are frequent urination, impaired gait, and dementia

Treatment

Hydrocephalus no longer has to be fatal. If diagnosed early, it can be treated surgically. Treatment involves diverting the blocked ventricular CSF to another body cavity for absorption. A thin rubbery tube is inserted surgically into the enlarged ventricular cavity and is used to divert CSF flow to the peritoneal cavity in the abdomen, pleural space, or right atrium of the heart. Usually, the tube has a valve system to help regulate the pressure inside the skull, preventing complete collapse of the brain. This is called a shunt. Draining into the peritoneal cavity is the most common procedure because it is the easiest and safest. Other locations also can effectively absorb CSF, but they require more extensive surgery and/or have a higher failure rate.

Diagnostic Significance of Cerebrospinal Fluid

Changes in the pressure and composition of CSF have diagnostic significance. CSF pressure is measured by **lumbar puncture**. A needle is inserted into the lumbar subarachnoid space between the L4 and L5 vertebrae because spinal penetration at this point does not injure any nerve fibers (see Fig. 2-48). Once CSF starts flowing, the needle hub is attached to a manometer or other pressure-sensitive device. Normal CSF pressure in an adult is 80–150 mm Hg. Ventricular pressure also can be measured by inserting a catheter into the lateral ventricles. A pressure level higher than normal suggests a pathologic process and can occur in response to increased amounts of CSF, brain swelling, and brain tumors.

Spinal puncture also is used to administer anesthesia in the lower spinal region. A fluid anesthetic, such as lidocaine, is injected into the spinal subarachnoid space to suppress pain and other sensations from the lower body up to the level of the spinal injection. The anesthesia prevents nerve impulses from being conducted through the spinal nerves.

Brain pathology also alters the composition of CSF. Consequently, chemical analysis of it may provide important diagnostic information. For example, acute bacterial meningitis, viral infection, or cerebral infarction increases the number of white blood cells. Elevated protein content in the CSF suggests a block in the subarachnoid space by a compressive lesion. Blood pigments in the CSF may indicate an intracranial hemorrhage.

CLINICAL CONSIDERATIONS

PATIENT ONE

A 25-year-old female graduate student had not been feeling well for 3 months. She reported suffering from severe headaches, lethargy, slow thinking, headache, forgetfulness, and frequent attacks of nausea. She was seen by a neurologist who noted that a brain MRI study revealed a tumor that was blocking her cerebral aqueduct.

Question: How can you relate these symptoms with the blocked CSF system and underlying diseased condition?

Discussion: This is a case of an obstructive (noncommunicating) type of hydrocephalus because the CSF did not have access to the subarachnoid space. The symptoms reported by the student are typical of hydrocephalus.

PATIENT TWO

A 65-year-old retired speech language pathology (SLP) professor who had been experiencing memory problems and difficulty in walking straight was examined by a neurologist who noted the following:

- Unsteady gait marked with wavering and tendency to fall
- Frequent need for urination
- Indifferent personality
- SLP consultation revealed
  - Normal comprehension
  - Well-articulated speech
  - Short-term memory problem
  - Difficulty in learning new information
  - Presence of incoherence in spontaneous discourse
  - Impaired pragmatics marked with loss of topic maintenance and turn taking
  - Mild naming difficulty marked with circumlocutions
  - Inattention and reduced verbal spontaneity

The brain MRI revealed large ventricles but the spinal tap examination revealed normal CSF pressure. Nuclear brain scan involving the injection of radioactive substance revealed altered CSF circulation and its absorption from the brain with a notable reflux of CSF into the ventricles. The neurologist diagnosed it to be a typical old-age circulatory problem.

Question: How can you explain these prefrontal cognitive symptoms in a patient with enlarged ventricles in spite of normal CSF pressure?

Discussion: This is a typical case of normal pressure hydrocephalus, which is characterized by urinary incontinence, unsteady gait, impaired equilibrium, and impaired cognition. The prefrontal symptoms result from a pressure to the prefrontal cortex. Meningitis, subarachnoid hemorrhage, and/or trauma are the common causes of this condition. Impaired gait pattern is marked by wide-based stance and walking.

SUMMARY

CSF, which the choroid plexus produces, circulates from the ventricles to the subarachnoid space. Along with the meningeal membranes, CSF protects the brain and spinal cord. Its other function is to regulate extracellular environments. It collects harmful substances and waste products that result from cellular metabolic activities. Inadequate drainage of the CSF results in excessive accumulation of CSF followed by increased intracranial pressure and hydrocephalus. Hydro-

cephalus can be treated by surgically implanting a shunt. However, if not adequately treated, the increased intracranial pressure that accompanies hydrocephalus enlarges the ventricular cavity and causes irreparable brain damage.

QUIZ QUESTIONS

1. Define the following terms: arachnoid granulations, cerebral spinal fluid, choroid plexus, hydrocephalus, lumbar puncture.

2. List four types of hydrocephalus.

3. What is the spinal site used for lumbar puncture? Explain why.

4. List the ventricles and their foramen.

TECHNICAL TERMS

arachnoid granulations	meningitis
cerebrospinal fluid	peritoneal cavity
choroid plexus	spinal anesthesia
ependymal cells	subarachnoid space
hydrocephalus	sinus system
intracranial pressure	ventricles
lumbar puncture	

Cerebral Cortex: Higher Mental Functions*

LEARNING OBJECTIVES

After studying this chapter, students should be able to:

- Describe the functional importance of the primary and associational cortical areas

- Discuss major cortical functions

- Describe the relationship between cerebral dominance and handedness

- Describe the neurologic diagnosis of behavioral deficits

- List the major types of aphasia and describe their linguistic characteristics

- Discuss the neurology of apraxias

- Discuss the neurology of reading and writing

- Describe the neurology of motor speech

- Discuss the neurology of cognition in reference to dementia and traumatic brain injuries

- Provide a clinical discussion of dementia

Chapters 1–18 focus on the structural organization of the nervous system and the sensorimotor functions that are organized bilaterally in the brain. The true uniqueness of the human brain, however, lies in the higher mental functions, such as reasoning, memory, language, speech, calculations, praxis, recognition of objects (gnosis), and the asymmetrical organization of these functions in the cerebral hemispheres. Cerebral dominance, or the specialization of one cerebral hemisphere in specific functions, relates to the unique cytoarchitectural organization of the brain.

The cerebral cortex is a massive, convoluted structure, which is the site of higher mental functions. The cortex makes up an area of about 2.5 ft^2 and contains as many as 14 billion neurons. The brain is divided into four primary **lobes: frontal, parietal, temporal,** and **occipital.** Each lobe has a relatively constant cortical anatomy, which is divided by sulci or fissures into discrete gyri (see Figs. 2-4 and 2-5).

METHODS OF STUDY

Neurology is the study of diseases that affect the nervous system. Classically, neurology depended on observations of behavior gathered during the medical examination of stroke patients, then laboriously correlated with brain lesions seen at autopsy.

Currently, brain imaging modalities permit the simultaneous visualization of brain structure and examination of associated behavior. **Computed tomography (CT), magnetic resonance imaging (MRI), positron emission tomography (PET),** and **single photon emission computed tomography (SPECT)** are commonly used neuroimaging methods (see Chapter 20). The functional brain imaging techniques of functional MRI (fMRI), PET, and SPECT can also be used to study cognitive functions in normal human subjects. The examiner can see which brain areas activate during specific activities, and networks of interrelated brain regions can be delineated. Our knowledge of brain structure and function has advanced much more rapidly since the introduction of these imaging techniques.

Another area of advancement in brain localization is electrical stimulation. The electroencephalogram is an electrical study of neuronal firing patterns in the brain. Computer-assisted techniques such as brain electrical activity mapping increase the anatomic accuracy of the electroencephalogram but are still less precise in anatomic localization than are CT and MRI. Electrical stimulation of the awake patient, used as a guide for excision of epileptic foci in the brain, has further delineated areas of the brain that are important for language and speech (Bhatnagar et al. 2000; Ojemann et al. 1989). Most recently, transcranial magnetic stimulation has been used to activate brain regions noninvasively.

FUNCTIONAL LOCALIZATION IN THE BRAIN

Clinical data obtained from imaging studies such as MRI, PET and SPECT and from patients undergoing surgical ablation of brain structures for epilepsy or brain tumor have helped reveal the functional regional anatomy of the brain in terms of the four major lobes and their cortical gyri. These gyri, or parts of them, operate as modules dedicated to specific cognitive or behavioral functions. The modules act somewhat like the brain centers that 19th-century physicians described, but they are organized not as individual centers but as parts of interacting networks, interconnecting modules in different regions or lobes of the brain. The cortical modules also connect with subcortical centers, such as the basal ganglia and other deep brain structures. The emerging understanding of the major functions of the four lobes of each hemisphere of the brain is summarized briefly here.

In general, the cortex of the brain is divided into primary motor areas, primary sensory areas (for vision, hearing, touch, smell, and possibly taste), and association areas. The association cortex is divided into unimodal association cortices, such as the **visual** and **auditory association cortices**, and heteromodal association cortices. The heteromodal cortical areas include the parietal cortex, a sensory association area for interaction between the senses, and the frontal cortex, which provides the executive function for the entire brain. *Executive function* refers to the processes that decide which of the many incoming sensory stimuli should receive attention and in what order and what responses or motor outputs should be activated and in which order. These heteromodal association cortices represent the areas of largest expansion of the brain from apes to humans, and they are critically important in making possible the extraordinary cognitive and behavioral capabilities that our species, *Homo sapiens,* has attained.

Frontal Lobe

The posterior limit of the frontal lobe, on the lateral surface of the brain, is the precentral gyrus, which contains motor cells of the primary motor cortex (Brodmann area 4). This cortical strip carries a map of the contralateral side of the body (homunculus), with cells programmed to produce contractions of specific muscles or specific movements (see Fig. 2-6). The motor homunculus has its face and lips in the most inferior part of the gyrus, just above the sylvian fissure; the hand and arm are above that and the leg and foot extend over the superior part of the gyrus and continue downward on the medial aspect of the hemisphere. Stimulation of cells in the motor cortex produces specific movements of contralateral parts of the body. The large size of the cortical representation of the thumb, fingers, and hand compared to the arm reflects the importance of fine finger movements. Similarly, the large space reserved for the mouth and lips indicates the importance of speech.

Anterior to the primary motor cortex is the **premotor cortex**, which is involved in the initiation and planning of skilled motor movements. Just anterior to the face area of the motor strip is the cortical Broca area (Brodmann area 44),

thought to program patterned movements of the vocal apparatus to produce phonemes and words. Brodmann area 8, in the superior frontal lobe, is involved in movement of the eyes and head to the contralateral side. The supplementary motor cortex is on the medial side of the hemisphere anterior to the leg area of the primary motor cortex. Stimulation of this area produces complex postures or patterned movements. Lesions in this area also disrupt the initiation of speech.

Another function of the dorsolateral frontal lobe, the frontal heteromodal association cortex of the brain, is critically related to executive functions, as described earlier (Goldman-Rakic 1996). The dorsolateral frontal lobe is also important for working memory, also termed immediate memory or attention span.

Functions of the **prefrontal cortex** anterior to the premotor area and the orbitofrontal cortex are quite complex and are incompletely understood. Lesions of the frontal cortex may produce disinhibition of speech and other behaviors, known as the **frontal lobe syndrome**. Patients with lesions of the orbitofrontal cortex may have normal intelligence and memory, but families may state that the individuals have totally changed personality; examples of such personality changes are short temper, irritability, poor impulse control, sociopathic (antisocial) personality, and a general tendency to act out. Blumer and Benson (1975) refer to this behavior as **pseudopsychopathic**, in that it resembles the behavior of a sociopathic personality.

Such syndromes are frequently seen after frontal head injuries. The lateral frontal convexities also are involved in the initiation of behavior. Bilateral lesions of this area tend to produce a reduction or cessation of behavior, often referred to as **akinetic mutism** or **abulia**. Patients may sit and stare passively, not speaking, or may responding only in a whisper or after a delay. This type of frontal lobe syndrome is called **pseudodepressed**. In general, frontal lobe syndromes resemble psychiatric disorders because they involve profound alterations of behavior and personality, yet the basic cognitive functions, such as memory, language, visuospatial functioning, elementary motor, and sensory functions are intact.

On the medial surface of the frontal lobe lies the cingulum, or cingulate gyrus. This gyrus is a part of the **limbic system**, or **Papez circuit**, of projections from the hippocampus via the septum and fornix to the mamillary bodies and then to the anterior thalamic nuclei. Projections then go to the cingulate gyrus and back to the hippocampus. This circuit is important for memory and for elementary limbic functions, such as motivation and drive (see Chapter 16). The cingulate gyrus is also important for the experience of pain.

Parietal Lobe

The parietal lobe consists of a superior and inferior parietal lobule. The anterior part of the parietal lobe contains

Brodmann areas 3, 1, 2, which are devoted to sensory function. In the inferior parietal lobule are Brodmann areas 39 and 40, the angular and supramarginal gyri. The inferior parietal lobule in the left hemisphere is tied to language function, especially reading and naming; to calculations and arithmetic; and to telling left from right. This region is the second part of the heteromodal association cortex, along with the dorsolateral frontal lobe. The parietal association cortex may be thought of as a center for the association of information from different sensory modalities, such as vision, hearing, and touch.

Gerstmann (1930) associated four deficits with lesions of the left inferior parietal lobule: agraphia, acalculia, right–left confusion, and finger agnosia (loss of the ability to know which finger is which). The inferior parietal lobule in the right hemisphere is involved with the body schema. Right inferior parietal lobe lesions produce neglect of the left side of the body. The superior parts of the parietal cortex are devoted to visuospatial and constructional functions and higher-level cortical sensory functions, such as stereognosis (recognition of palpated shapes) and graphesthesia (ability to recognize letters or numbers drawn on the skin).

Lesions of the right parietal lobe produce important neurobehavioral deficits, including left-side neglect, denial of the presence of a motor deficit (**anosognosia**), and dressing **apraxia** (inability to place garments correctly in relation to body parts). Other spatial and topographical dysfunctions associated with right parietal lobe lesions are difficulty finding one's way around and an inability to draw or read a map. Constructional tasks, such as copying figures, drawing a clock or house, and bisecting a line, may reveal difficulty with spatial relationships or neglect of the left side of space. Although speech and language are relatively well preserved in patients with right parietal lesions, the emotional intonation of speech may be lacking, as may the ability to comprehend emotional tone in the speech of others. These patients often fail to grasp sarcasm or humor. They also may fail to respect the proper turn-taking of a normal conversation, or they respond to questions asked of the patient in the next bed.

Some researchers consider this aspect of language the pragmatics of communication, as opposed to semantics (meanings) or syntax (grammar). Such deficits mean, in effect, that the patient may understand what is said, but not how it is said; in other words, he or she understands only the literal meaning of the words and not the emotional, humorous, ironic, or sarcastic meanings that result from the tone in which the words are spoken. Such paralinguistic disorders are disabling to patients in the social world and affect communication even when speech and language functions are preserved. Emotional indifference often characterizes the mood of these patients; they may be undisturbed by left-sided paralysis or by the impending loss of ability to work. These right hemisphere deficits, expressed over time, change the personality of affected individuals.

Families often have more difficulty accepting a change in personality after a stroke or brain injury than they do in accepting handicaps, such as the inability to speak or understand language, seen after left hemisphere injuries.

Temporal Lobe

The superior temporal gyrus of each hemisphere contains the primary auditory cortex (Brodmann areas 41 and 42), which lies buried within the sylvian fissure. Lesions of the primary auditory cortex on both sides cause cortical deafness. Such patients are rarely totally deaf and often hear some pure tones. In some patients, bilateral superior temporal damage results in **pure word deafness** (inability to understand spoken words, with preserved pure tone hearing and recognition of nonverbal sounds). Another bitemporal syndrome is auditory agnosia, or the inability to recognize nonverbal sounds.

The left superior temporal gyrus contains Wernicke area, which is critical to the comprehension of spoken language. There may be a language comprehension area in the inferior temporal gyrus and adjacent fusiform gyrus, as identified by electrical stimulation (the basal temporal language area; BTLA). It is interesting that surgical ablation of this area usually does not cause lasting **aphasia**. Therefore, the BTLA may be part of a network involved in understanding language but may not be a necessary component to the functioning of the language comprehension system.

The right temporal lobe is a silent, or noneloquent, area of the brain because surgical resection of this area produces only very subtle deficits. Appreciation of rhythm and musical qualities may be affected by right temporal lesions, along with deficits in nonverbal memory. In general, the medial temporal areas, such as the hippocampus, together with their connections to the thalamus, septal area, and cingulate gyri of the medial frontal lobes, are most clearly related to memory. Bilateral lesions produce lasting loss of new learning and recent memory. Unilateral left medial temporal lesions produce disorders of verbal memory, whereas unilateral right temporal lesions produce nonverbal memory loss. Acute lesions of the right temporal lobe, as in strokes, also may cause confusion or delirium.

Occipital Lobe

The most posterior, medial poles of the occipital lobes are the primary visual cortices (Brodmann area 17). Damage to this cortex on one side produces a contralateral hemianopic visual field defect in both eyes. Damage to both sides may produce cortical blindness. Some patients with cortical blindness are unaware of their blindness and confabulate descriptions of objects and scenes they claim to see (Anton syndrome). Adjacent occipital areas (Brodmann areas 18 and 19) are called the visual association cortex and are thought to contribute to complex visual analysis. Lesions of these areas on both sides produce a complex visual syndrome called visual **agnosia**.

DISORDERS OF CORTICAL FUNCTIONS

Cerebral Dominance and Functional Specialization

Since Broca's observations in 1861, it has been known that in most humans the left hemisphere is at least relatively dominant for language. Virtually 99% of right-handed people and most left-handed people have left hemisphere dominance for language. Handedness has some correlation to cerebral dominance, so left-handed individuals are more likely than right-handed people to have right hemisphere language dominance. However, most left-handers still become aphasic if the left hemisphere is damaged, and only a few become aphasic if the right hemisphere is damaged. Some left-handed individuals appear to have mixed dominance, such as having speech expression in the left hemisphere and comprehension in the right hemisphere.

The right hemisphere, often called the minor hemisphere, serves many nonlanguage functions. As discussed with reference to the parietal lobes, right hemisphere functions include visuospatial and constructional tasks, knowledge of maps and topography, dressing, emotional feeling and processing, production of emotional intonation of speech, and music appreciation.

Cerebral dominance may have structural correlates. Geschwind and Levitsky (1968) reported that right-handed people have a longer **planum temporale** in the left hemisphere than in the right (see Fig. 9-10). Similar asymmetries have been described in newborn infants and in illiterate people, suggesting that these anatomic asymmetries are genetically programmed, not acquired through use. Cerebral asymmetries also have been reaffirmed using CT and MRI studies. The relationship of such asymmetries to language dominance, as determined by the Wada test, is being currently investigated.

Speech and Language Disorders

Speech and language disorders have long held great interest for students of the nervous system. First, the ability to communicate verbally sets humans apart from other animal species. Second, language disorders were the first behavioral or cognitive impairments to be correlated with disease processes involving specific areas of the brain; ever since, they have served as an important source of knowledge about the correlation of brain structure with behavior.

Motor Speech Disorders

Motor speech disorders consist of abnormal speech articulation in the absence of any language disorder. Abnormal motor speech control, or **dysarthria**, can involve abnormal strength or place of articulation, abnormal timing or speed of articulatory movement, or abnormal voicing. Dysarthric patients can comprehend both spoken and written language, and their speech output, if comprehensible, can be tran-scribed into normal language. Darley et al. (1975), in a comprehensive study of dysarthric speech at the Mayo Clinic, divide these neurogenic dysarthrias into six types: **flaccid**, **spastic**, **ataxic**, **hypokinetic**, **hyperkinetic**, and **mixed**.

Flaccid dysarthria results from lesions of the bulbar muscles, neuromuscular junction, cranial nerves, and anterior horn cells of the brainstem nuclei and is characterized by hypernasal, breathy speech with imprecisely articulated consonants. Spastic dysarthria is seen in patients with bilateral lesions of the motor cortex or corticobulbar tracts. Speech characteristics involve harsh, strain-and-strangle speech, with a slow speaking rate, low pitch, and imprecisely articulated consonants. A variant of spastic dysarthria is unilateral upper motor neuron (UMN) dysarthria, resulting from a unilateral lesion, such as a stroke. The same characteristics pertain but are less severe.

Ataxic dysarthria, seen in cerebellar disorders, involves irregular cadence or prosody of speech with long pauses and sudden explosions of sound, abnormal and sometimes excessively equal stress on specific syllables, and imprecisely articulated consonants. This pattern is sometimes called scanning speech. Some patients simply speak in a very slow pattern, similar to an exaggerated regional drawl. Hypokinetic dysarthria, classically seen in Parkinson disease, is associated with decreased and monotonous loudness and pitch, occasional rushes of syllables, occasional pauses, and some imprecisely articulated consonants. Hyperkinetic dysarthria, seen in chorea and related movement disorders, including Huntington chorea, is characterized by variable rate, excessive variation in loudness and timing, and distorted vowels. In dystonia, this form of dysarthria can also involve harsh strain-and-strangle speech, with imprecisely articulated consonants.

Mixed dysarthria can involve combinations of any of the other five types. Common examples include **amyotrophic lateral sclerosis** (ALS), in which spastic and flaccid elements co-exist, and **multiple sclerosis**, in which spastic and ataxic characteristics predominate. In practice, there is considerable overlap among the categories of dysarthria.

Apraxia of Speech

Apraxia of speech is difficult to separate from aphasia. Speech apraxia entails abnormal articulation of sequences of phonemes, usually with inconsistent error patterns from one attempt to the next, in contrast to the consistent misarticulations of the dysarthrias. Apraxia of speech is an inability to program sequences of sounds, especially consonants. Consonants are more often substituted than distorted. Apraxia of speech is most obvious with polysyllabic words. Difficulty with initial consonants is common, and speech takes on a hesitant, groping quality. A patient may attempt to say a word like *catastrophe* five times and produce five different errors or may achieve the correct pronunciation once or twice. Apraxia of speech is only rarely seen without aphasia. More commonly, apraxia of speech is part of an aphasic deficit, particularly Broca aphasia.

Aphasia

Aphasia is an acquired disorder of language processing secondary to brain disease (Alexander and Benson 1992). This definition excludes developmental or congenital language problems (dysphasia), motor speech or articulation disorders (dysarthria, dysphonia, and pure apraxia of speech), and impaired thought processes (dementia and psychosis).

Broca Aphasia

The French physician Paul Broca first described Broca aphasia in 1861. It is characterized by nonfluent, often halting, dysarthric, and ungrammatical speech in which meaning is conveyed largely by information-carrying items, such as nouns and verbs, leaving out the minor structural words (Table 19-1). Naming is also deficient, but the patient can often pronounce the first letter or phoneme (tip-of-the-tongue phenomenon). Auditory comprehension often seems relatively normal, although deficits may occur in comprehension of multistep commands or in sentences with complex grammatical structure.

Those with Broca aphasia tend to have difficulty comprehending complex syntax, just as they have difficulty producing such syntax. For example, a person with Broca aphasia might have difficulty with a sentence such as "The book Bill gave to Betty was thick." The patient might understand that a book was given but cannot specify who gave and who received the book. Deficits in comprehension can virtually always be detected on standard language batteries. Repetition in Broca aphasia is usually halting and reduced in fluency. Reading is often more strongly affected than auditory comprehension.

Patients exhibit writing deficits, not only because most of these individuals have right hemiparesis (paralysis of right arm and leg), forcing them to write with their nondominant left hand, but because of the damage to the left frontal lobe. Patients with Broca aphasia have awkward handwriting and spell poorly; many cannot write even single words or short phrases. If forced to use their nondominant hand because of a fracture of the right arm or writer's cramp, patients learn to write quite successfully.

Lesions of Broca aphasia involve the left frontal region. Broca identified the area as the posterior part of the inferior frontal gyrus, although both of his patients had much more extensive lesions. Mohr et al. (1978) found that patients with lesions in or near Broca's area exhibit an excellent recovery within weeks, whereas patients with lasting expressive deficits, such as Broca's original patients, have more extensive lesions involving most of the frontal and parietal lobes. Patients with lasting nonfluent aphasia also have damage to subcortical structures, particularly the subcallosal fasciculus and periventricular white matter (Naeser et al. 1989).

Aphemia, a variant of Broca aphasia, is a rare syndrome of muteness or nonfluent speech with good language comprehension and preserved writing. Because there is very little true language disturbance, aphemia may not be a true aphasia; it has been equated with the equally rare syndrome of pure apraxia of speech.

Wernicke Aphasia

Carl Wernicke described an aphasia syndrome in 1874. In contrast to those with Broca aphasia, patients with Wernicke aphasia speak fluently and effortlessly, although their meaning is obscured by the paucity of meaningful nouns and verbs, overabundance of stock phrases and idioms, and the presence of numerous verbal paraphasic errors (Table 19-1). Neologisms are usually present in severe cases, making the speech jargon. In milder cases, many paraphasic substitutions and idioms take the sentences in directions not intended by the speaker. Naming in Wernicke aphasia is paraphasic, often with bizarre substitutions. Auditory comprehension may be so severely impaired that the patient cannot answer simple yes-or-no questions. Repetition is also paraphasic, and reading comprehension usually mirrors the poor language comprehension seen in auditory testing. In some cases, either auditory comprehension or reading may be less affected than the other

---

Table 19-1					
Language Features of Common Types of Aphasia					
Feature	Broca	Wernicke	Global	Conduction	Anomia
Spontaneous speech	Nonfluent	Fluent and paraphasic	Nonfluent	Fluent	Fluent with pauses
Naming	Impaired	Paraphasic	Poor	Variable	Most impaired
Comprehension	Mildly impaired	Poor	Poor	Intact	Intact
Repetition	Impaired	Impaired	Impaired	Impaired	Intact
Reading	May be impaired	Impaired	Poor	May be intact	Intact
Writing	Impaired	Impaired	Poor	May be intact	Intact

(Kirshner et al. 1989), and this spared language modality can be used to communicate with the patient.

Writing is also abnormal in Wernicke aphasia. Unlike patients with Broca, most of those with Wernicke aphasia have no hemiparesis, and they can grip a pen and write without difficulty. The content of the writing, however, shows the same abnormality as the speech and is characterized by abnormal spelling patterns. Thus writing samples may be a good way to detect mild Wernicke aphasia, as in patients with slowly developing syndromes related to brain tumors.

Lesions associated with Wernicke aphasia generally involve the posterior two-thirds of the left superior temporal gyrus, although in some cases they extend into other parts of the temporal lobe and into the inferior parietal lobule. Lesions that damage most of the traditional Wernicke area are especially well correlated with lasting impairments of comprehension, whereas those involving primarily the inferior parietal lobule may be more associated with reading and writing disorders. As patients with Wernicke aphasia recover, their deficits often evolve into the milder syndromes of conduction or anomic aphasia.

A variant of Wernicke aphasia is pure word deafness, selective loss of auditory comprehension and repetition with preserved naming, reading, and writing. Many patients have mildly paraphasic speech. The syndrome classically results from bilateral temporal lobe lesions, which disconnect the auditory cortices from Wernicke area. Cases resembling pure word deafness have been reported with unilateral, left temporal lobe lesions.

Global Aphasia

Global aphasia may be thought of as the sum of the deficits of Broca and Wernicke aphasias (Table 19-1). Patients with global aphasia are nonfluent or mute, and they exhibit impaired comprehension. All elements of language—speech, naming, comprehension, repetition, reading, and writing—are severely impaired. Syndromes of less severe but equally generalized impairments of language are called **mixed aphasia**. Lesions associated with global aphasia involve much of the left middle cerebral artery territory of the frontal, temporal, and parietal lobes. Large lesions of the subcortical white matter and basal ganglia result in a similar syndrome. As the patient with global aphasia recovers, the deficit profile often evolves toward Broca aphasia.

Conduction Aphasia

Although conduction aphasia occurs in < 10% of aphasia cases, it demonstrates important lessons about language. In this syndrome, repetition is the most severely affected language modality (Table 19-1). Spontaneous speech is fluent, often with many literal paraphasic errors. The patient is aware of these errors and makes efforts at self-correction. Naming is variable, but auditory comprehension is usually normal. The patient understands well but cannot repeat what was said. Reading aloud may show similar deficits to repetition, as may writing to dictation.

Wernicke originally postulated a lesion disconnecting the auditory word association area (Wernicke area) in the left temporal lobe from Broca area in the left frontal lobe. Two general locations of lesion have been reported in conduction aphasia: the left superior temporal region, with incomplete damage to Wernicke area, and the inferior parietal lobule, especially the supramarginal gyrus. Benson et al. (1973) and Damasio (1980) noted that patients with conduction aphasia secondary to parietal lobe lesions often have associated limb apraxia, whereas those with temporal lobe lesions do not. The supramarginal gyrus area may be important to the generation of phonemes in response to repetition or naming (Demonet et al. 1992; Hickok and Poeppel 2000). An alternative explanation for conduction aphasia is a short-term memory deficit specific to auditory verbal material (Shallice and Warrington 1977).

Anomic Aphasia

Also called amnesic or amnestic aphasia, anomic aphasia refers to syndromes in which naming is the most severe deficit. The patient speaks fluently, with some word-finding pauses and circumlocutions. Repetition, auditory comprehension, reading, and writing are intact. Many patients show no other abnormalities on neurologic examination. The lesions producing anomic aphasia are more variable than those underlying the other aphasic syndromes discussed thus far. Some authors have emphasized lesions of the angular gyrus, although lesions there often produce other deficits, including alexia, constructional impairment, and the four elements of Gerstmann syndrome.

Anomic aphasia also is seen in conditions without clearly localized lesions, as in confusional states and dementing disorders, such as **Alzheimer disease** (**AD**). An aphasia test battery given to a patient with early AD will often give a score consistent with anomic aphasia. According to some sources, left frontal lobe lesions disproportionally affect naming of actions (verbs), whereas left temporal lesions are more associated with the misnaming of objects (nouns).

Transcortical Aphasias

The next three aphasic syndromes discussed here are transcortical aphasias; the responsible lesions affect not the primary language cortex or the circuit from Wernicke to Broca area but rather other areas of the brain that project to the language cortex. Specific lesions are quite variable, including cortical damage in the frontal, temporal, and parietal areas and subcortical white matter. Table 19-2 lists key features of the three transcortical aphasia syndromes.

In **transcortical motor aphasia**, the patient speaks little, much as in Broca aphasia. In response to questions, the patient may either remain mute or may give a one- or two-word answer, often in a whisper or after a delay. As in Broca aphasia, the patient utters the most important, meaningful words of a sentence, often communicating adequately. Unlike the patient with Broca aphasia, however, a patient with transcortical motor aphasia can repeat

Table 19-2

Language Features of Transcortical Aphasias

Feature	Isolation	Transcortical Motor	Transcortical Sensory
Speech	Nonfluent and echolalic	Nonfluent	Fluent and echolalic
Naming	Impaired	Impaired	Impaired
Comprehension	Impaired	Intact	Impaired
Repetition	Intact	Intact	Intact
Reading	Impaired	May be spared	Impaired
Writing	Impaired	Impaired	Impaired

normally. Auditory comprehension tends to be preserved, whereas naming, reading, and writing are more variable. Lesions associated with this syndrome usually are in the left frontal lobe, anterior to, superior to, or beneath Broca area. The most common location is the frontal cortex within the territory of the left anterior cerebral artery.

Transcortical sensory aphasia is a Wernicke-like syndrome in which speech is fluent but paraphasic and auditory comprehension is severely impaired. Unlike the patient with Wernicke aphasia, however, the patient with transcortical sensory aphasia can repeat phrases and sentences without difficulty. Naming is typically paraphasic, and reading comprehension and writing are impaired, similar to Wernicke aphasia. Lesions of the left posterior temporo-occipital lobe have been described, and the syndrome also occurs in patients with AD, though more so in moderate stages of the disease.

The final transcortical aphasic syndrome is **mixed transcortical aphasia** (syndrome of the isolation of the speech area). This syndrome is the transcortical equivalent of global aphasia. The patient cannot speak fluently, comprehend spoken language, follow commands, name objects, read, or write. It is surprising, however, that these patients can repeat fluently, and some are even echolalic. A patient reported by Geschwind et al. (1968) could even learn lyrics of new songs popular only after her illness, indicating that some memory storage of words was possible.

Isolation syndrome is an extreme form of transcortical aphasia in which the perisylvian language cortex is intact but not connected to other cortical areas necessary for propositional speech or comprehension. It usually indicates extensive cortical damage to both cerebral hemispheres, sparing the perisylvian cortex, as in watershed infarctions seen in states of hypotension, hypoxia, carbon monoxide poisoning, or bilateral carotid artery occlusion.

Subcortical Aphasias

Subcortical aphasias are defined by the lesion localization rather than by the characteristics of the aphasia. Although aphasia usually reflects dysfunction of the language cortex,

subcortical lesions can disrupt connections to the language cortex. The most common subcortical aphasia syndrome, often called the **anterior subcortical aphasia syndrome**, is seen in patients with lesions involving the head of the caudate nucleus, anterior limb of the internal capsule, and anterior putamen. Speech is usually dysarthric and nonfluent, with mild deficits of repetition and comprehension. Lesions of the dominant thalamus produce fluent aphasia with paraphasic errors but with relatively spared auditory comprehension. Thalamic aphasia also can involve a dichotomy between relatively intact speech when the patient is awake and paraphasic speech when the patient is drowsy. The thalamus may play a role in activating the language cortex; thus thalamic lesions may result in putting the language areas to sleep. Subcortical lesions also can involve the temporal isthmus, cutting off connections to Wernicke area and producing severe disturbance of comprehension. Delineation of the precise neuroanatomy of the subcortical aphasia syndromes is an active area of research.

Alexias: Neurology of Reading

Disordered reading and writing are important aspects of most aphasia syndromes. In some syndromes, however, reading and writing are affected out of proportion to the deficits in spoken language and auditory comprehension. French physician Joseph J. Déjérine delineated the two classical alexia syndromes, with and without agraphia, more than 100 years ago.

Alexia with Agraphia

Alexia with agraphia is acquired illiteracy: the patient becomes unable to read or write (Table 19-3). Although spoken language is relatively intact, most patients have a fluent paraphasic speech pattern. Auditory comprehension and naming are often impaired to some degree. The syndrome results from lesions in the left inferior parietal lobule, including the supramarginal and angular gyri. As such, the syndrome overlaps with Wernicke aphasia, and some cases may evolve as a stage in the recovery of acute Wernicke aphasia.

Table 19-3

Language Features of Alexias

Feature	Alexia with Agraphia	Pure Alexia
Spontaneous speech	Mildly paraphasic	Intact
Naming	Often impaired	Normal except for colors
Comprehension	May be mildly impaired	Intact
Repetition	Intact	Intact
Reading	Poor	Poor; letter reading may be spared
Writing	Poor	Intact

Alexia Without Agraphia

Pure alexia without agraphia (pure alexia or word blindness) can be thought of as a linguistic blindfold in which the inability to read is an isolated deficit (Table 19-3). These patients have normal spontaneous speech, repetition, and auditory comprehension; in fact, most patients can comprehend words spelled aloud, indicating that their spelling is not disturbed. There is often some naming difficulty, particularly for colors. Writing is intact, and one of the most intriguing aspects of the syndrome is that a patient may write a phrase or sentence but shortly afterward may be unable to read it. The inability to read is often complete at first, then improves so that the patient can spell out words letter by letter. Most of these patients have reduced short-term memory and right hemianopsia.

The lesion is almost always a stroke in the territory of the left posterior cerebral artery, which supplies the medial occipital and medial temporal lobes and the splenium of the corpus callosum. Déjérine's explanation was that the left occipital lesion caused right hemianopsia, and the lesion of the corpus callosum prevented visual information from being transmitted from the intact right occipital lobe to the left hemisphere language centers. Thus the patient can see in the left visual field but cannot decode written language. This model of the pure alexia syndrome is a good example of a disconnection syndrome.

Aphasic Alexia

Aphasic alexia occurs in association with aphasic disturbances. Benson (1977) uses the term **third alexia** to characterize the reading disorder of Broca aphasia. In this classification, the first and second alexias are the classical syndromes of alexia with and without agraphia. Benson notes that most patients with Broca aphasia have more difficulty with reading than with auditory comprehension.

Neurolinguists have developed a different classification of reading disorders based on mechanisms of the disorder itself rather than on the pattern of associated language disorders or location of the responsible lesions. **Deep dyslexia**

implies a defect in the basic reading process or the conversion of printed graphemes to spoken phonemes. The characteristics of the reading disorder in deep dyslexia include the inability to read nonwords, semantic and visual errors in reading words (*boat* for *schooner* or *perform* for *perfume*), and marked effects of word class and word image ability on reading performance. Nouns and verbs generally are read better than adjectives, adverbs, and prepositions; likewise, concrete nouns, which have referents that can be visualized, are more likely to be read correctly than abstract nouns. These patients appear to read more by direct recognition of familiar words (access of the semantic system directly from orthography, or spelling) than by conversion of the grapheme into a phoneme, and then processing it into the semantic system. Most deep dyslexic patients have large left hemisphere lesions and significant aphasia of mixed or Broca type.

A second alexia syndrome is **phonologic dyslexia**, which is similar to deep dyslexia except that the reading of single content words may be nearly normal and semantic errors are rare. Reading of nonwords is difficult, as in deep dyslexia. In this syndrome, patients may be able to read aloud not only by recognition of the words' meanings but also by a process of conversion of words to phonemes (lexical–phonologic route). However, conversion of individual graphemes to phonemes is still defective.

Another seemingly opposite type of dyslexia is **surface dyslexia**. This syndrome occurs in patients who can read phonetically by grapheme-to-phoneme conversion but cannot recognize words directly. In this syndrome, words of irregular spelling, such as *yacht* or *colonel*, are particularly difficult to read. Surface dyslexia is a rare syndrome that has been reported in patients with anterior left hemisphere lesions and in primary progressive aphasia.

A fourth neurolinguistic alexia syndrome, **letter-by-letter reading**, is synonymous with the syndrome of pure alexia without agraphia discussed earlier, in which patients have recovered enough reading ability to read letters and to spell words aloud letter by letter.

Agraphia: Neurology of Writing

Writing, a basic element of language, often is disrupted in aphasic syndromes. The classical syndrome of **pure agraphia** affects patients with minimal or no aphasic deficits other than the inability to write. Pure agraphia is a rare syndrome. The diagnosis of pure agraphia requires that the failure to write not be explainable by simple motor deficit (hemiparesis), apraxia (discussed later), or visuospatial difficulties. Lesions of pure agraphia are usually found in the left superior frontal region, although left parietal lesions have been reported to cause pure agraphia as well.

Agraphia is divided into phonologic and lexical types, corresponding to the process of writing by producing a whole word from the semantic meaning (lexical pathway) or by production of the phoneme and then derivation of the corresponding graphemes (phonologic pathway). A patient with phonologic agraphia can write common words from dictation but cannot write dictated nonword phonemes. Such a patient's spontaneous writing contains semantic errors or words of similar meaning but dissimilar spelling to the target word. There is also a preference for concrete over abstract nouns as well as both nouns and verbs over prepositions, adjectives, and adverbs. Phonologic agraphia thus bears a close resemblance to the pattern of deep dyslexia, but the two deficits do not necessarily affect the same patient.

In the other type of agraphia, **lexical agraphia**, the patient can write nonwords from dictation but cannot write irregularly spelled words and is confused by words of the same sound but different spelling (homophones). The clinical syndromes of phonologic and lexical agraphia are still in an investigational stage in terms of correlations with lesion localizations, other aphasia phenomena, and practical use in rehabilitative therapy.

Apraxias: Neurology of Learned Movement

Apraxia is a disorder of learned motor acts not caused by paralysis, incoordination, sensory deficit, or lack of understanding of the desired movement. In practical terms, apraxia is an inability to carry out skilled motor acts to command when it can be demonstrated that the patient understands the command and can perform the same motor act in a different context (Geschwind 1975; Kirshner 1992). Liepmann (1920), a German physician, described three types of apraxia: **ideomotor**, **ideational**, and **limb kinetic**.

It is important to differentiate several diverse motor phenomena that are commonly confused with the principal varieties of apraxia. These are constructional, dressing, oculomotor, and gait apraxia. **Constructional apraxia**, which is characterized by visuospatial difficulties, is associated with right hemispheric lesions. These patients may be unable to construct or copy a drawing of simple items (e.g., a clock or house). In most instances, this deficit is related to neglect of the left side of space or failure to appreciate the spatial relations of items, not to a motor planning deficit. In **dressing apraxia**, which is associated with right hemisphere lesions, the patients have difficulty with the spatial perception of a garment in relation to the body, and the difficulty is not a true motor apraxic deficit. **Oculomotor apraxia** refers to a difficulty with voluntary direction of the eyes in gaze and is associated with damage to the brainstem mechanism for control of eye movements. **Gait apraxia** refers to an inability to walk that is not clearly explained by primary motor weakness, ataxia, or sensory loss. There is no easy way to demonstrate that the same sequential actions can be performed normally in a different context; therefore, it is unclear whether this gait disorder is a true apraxia. Perhaps even more problematic is apraxia of speech (discussed earlier). Whether apraxia of speech is a true apraxia is debated by aphasiologists.

Ideomotor Apraxia

Ideomotor apraxia refers to the failure to carry out a motor act in response to a verbal command when the patient understands the command and has the motor capacity to perform the same motor act under a different context. By Liepmann's (1920) model, the idea of the movement, decoded in Wernicke area, is disconnected from its execution in the premotor cortex of the frontal lobe. Ideomotor apraxia often accompanies aphasia in patients with left hemisphere lesions (Geschwind 1975). In published series, only a small percentage of patients with ideomotor apraxia have right-sided lesions. A high percentage of patients with aphasia and left hemisphere lesions have ideomotor apraxia, whereas a much smaller percentage of nonaphasic patients with left hemisphere lesions demonstrate such apraxia (DeRenzi et al. 1980). Patients with ideomotor aphasia typically fail to carry out the test act to verbal command and perform only slightly better in imitation of the examiner; however, they carry out the act almost normally if given the actual object.

According to the anatomic model of Liepmann (1920), later modified by Geschwind (1975), a lesion in the left temporal lobe, which also causes aphasia, prevents information regarding the desired act from reaching the left premotor area. Thus ideomotor apraxia may be part of the deficit in Wernicke aphasia, but the impairment of comprehension makes it questionable whether the patient has understood the command.

In conduction aphasia and Broca aphasia, there may be associated ideomotor apraxia that interferes with the carrying out of commands with limbs on either side of the body. Such apraxic deficits may create the mistaken impression that the patient has a comprehension deficit; asking the patient yes or no questions or simple pointing commands can be used to establish normal comprehension. Finally, lesions of the corpus callosum can prevent motor information from reaching the right hemisphere motor area. This callosal apraxia affects movement of the left limbs only. The existence of callosal apraxia implies that the left hemisphere is dominant not only for speech but also for learned motor acts, because the right hemisphere cannot program the skilled movement independently.

This association of aphasia and apraxia may reflect the underlying symbolic nature of both speech and gestural expression, or it may simply reflect the anatomic contiguity of centers for speech–language function and those for learned motor acts. The association between apraxia and aphasia explains why most aphasia patients cannot learn complex linguistic gestural systems, such as American Sign Language.

Ideational Apraxia

Ideational apraxia is an even more complex phenomenon than ideomotor apraxia. Heilman proposes the term *conceptual apraxia* as a similar form of apraxia. There are two competing definitions of ideational apraxia. First, some authors use it to mean apraxia for real objects. Ochipa et al. (1989) describe a patient who could name objects but not demonstrate their uses, as if he had lost the concepts of their purposes (apraxia for tool use). The second definition of ideational apraxia is loss of the ability to carry out a multistep activity, although each individual step may be performed appropriately. For example, a patient may not be able to fill, light, and smoke a pipe or assemble a coffee percolator and make coffee. This type of apraxia may reflect a motor planning difficulty, as seen in frontal lobe lesions. It also may simply be a more sensitive test for apraxia than single motor commands. However defined, ideational apraxia also is associated with left hemisphere lesions, more often temporoparietal lesions associated with severe aphasia. Both ideomotor and ideational apraxia occur in AD.

Limb-Kinetic Apraxia

The third of Liepmann's types of apraxia is limb-kinetic apraxia, a deficit of fine motor acts involving only one limb. Patients with mild pyramidal tract lesions may not be weak in gross limb movements but may have difficulty with rapid or fine movements of the fingers. Such apraxia may be a sign of a partial corticospinal tract lesion with mild weakness. Heilman et al. (2000) refer to this type of apraxia as a loss of deftness. A left hemisphere lesion may be associated with limb-kinetic apraxia of both hands, whereas a right hemisphere usually is associated with limb-kinetic apraxia of the left hand only.

Agnosias: Neurology of Recognition

Agnosias are disorders of recognition. Most affect a single sensory system (visual, auditory, or tactile agnosia), whereas others involve selected classes of items within a modality (prosopagnosia, or agnosia for faces). In each case, the patient must be shown to have normal primary sensory perception, normal ability to name the item once it is recognized, and no general cognitive deterioration or dementia. For example, a patient with visual agnosia may fail to recognize a key ring by sight but is able to identify and name it from the sound of the keys jingling or from the feel of the keys in his or her hand. Each sensory modality carries a somewhat arbitrary division between primary sensory

cortical deficits and agnosia. Most agnosias require bilateral cortical lesions, cutting off input from the sensory modality to the left hemisphere language centers.

In the visual system, bilateral occipital lesions may cause cortical blindness. More partial lesions, however, may permit primary visual perception of the elements of an object or picture, such that the patient can even draw lines or angles representing the item but cannot identify the item. Shown a bicycle, the patient may report two circles and identify it as eyeglasses. Prosopagnosia, or failure to identify faces, is a subtype of visual agnosia in which patients cannot recognize family members or friends, though they can describe features, such as hair color, a mustache or beard, or accessories (e.g., hats or glasses). Frequently, the prosopagnostic patient identifies the person by voice or gait pattern. Oliver Sacks (1998) described prosopagnosia, or perhaps a more profound visual agnosia, in *The Man Who Mistook His Wife for a Hat.*

Auditory agnosias also overlap with the syndrome of cortical deafness, resulting from bilateral lesions of the temporal cortex. Some patients with bilateral temporal lobe lesions have preserved pure tone hearing but cannot understand spoken language or repeat. As discussed earlier, this deficit is referred to as pure word deafness. Geschwind (1970) postulates that pure word deafness results from a bilateral disconnection of the input from the primary auditory cortex (Heschl gyrus) to Wernicke area in the left hemisphere. More rarely, patients show preserved auditory comprehension but impaired nonverbal auditory recognition, for example identification of animal sounds or the characteristic sounds associated with objects such as bells and whistles. This deficit is called auditory nonverbal agnosia.

In the tactile modality, parietal lesions often disrupt the identification of objects by feel, a deficit called **astereognosis**. If the patient can describe the sensory characteristics of an object but not identify it, this also can qualify as tactile agnosia. Rare patients with bilateral parietal lesions have no ability to recognize objects by touch on either side.

Dementias: Neurology of Cognition

Dementia is defined as a gradual deterioration of previously intact cognitive functions secondary to diffuse rather than focal brain disease. The *Diagnostic and Statistical Manual of Mental Disorders,* 4th edition (DSM-IV), commonly used by psychiatrists, defines dementia in terms of memory loss and at least one additional cognitive function, such as language, visuospatial functioning, apraxia, or executive function. Although the pattern of cognitive deterioration varies, memory loss is usually the first symptom, and other deficits follow. Tests of language function frequently show deficient naming, although fluency of spontaneous speech and repetition remain normal. In later stages, reading, writing, and auditory comprehension begin to deteriorate. Patients may evolve from an initial deficit of anomic aphasia to a pattern resembling Wernicke or transcortical sensory aphasia. Other cortical deficits, such as apraxia and acalculia, are frequently present.

In contrast to this common pattern of language dissolution in dementing illness, which is typical of AD, is a less common pattern in which focal deficits predominate early in the illness. For example, cases of primary progressive aphasia have apparently focal aphasic deficits that gradually progress over years. Some patients fail to show memory loss or other cognitive deficits for years after onset. Mesulam (1982) first called this syndrome primary progressive aphasia, but more recent studies have placed this presentation within a broader category of frontotemporal dementia (discussed later in this chapter). The primary progressive aphasia syndrome is also divided into nonfluent and fluent forms; one of the latter is a syndrome called semantic dementia in which the patient not only cannot think of names but does not understand the meaning of words. In most series, nonfluent aphasia in dementia usually indicates a pathology other than typical AD, whereas the pathology of semantic dementia and fluent progressive aphasia is more variable (Mesulam 2000, 2003).

Dementia can be caused by any of a multitude of diseases, which can be classed into three major groups of conditions: **systemic diseases**, primarily involving organ systems outside the central nervous system; **neurologic diseases**, marked by degeneration of other systems than the higher cortical functions; and **diseases presenting primarily with loss of cognitive faculties**.

Dementias Secondary to Systemic Diseases

Most of the dementia-causing systemic diseases are listed in Table 19-4. Because most of these conditions are treatable, identifying them is essential. For many metabolic disorders, such as disturbances of electrolytes (hyponatremia), failure of the liver or kidneys, and calcium disturbances, patients present with an acute confusional state or delirium rather than chronic dementia. Toxic disorders include the effects of chemicals, heavy metals, alcohol, and drugs. Chronic alcohol ingestion coupled with poor nutrition may cause symptoms of thiamine deficiency, Wernicke-Korsakoff syndrome. Technically, this syndrome is a pure amnesia (loss of memory) rather than a dementia, but there is evidence that chronic alcohol abusers may develop a true dementia as well. Among toxins, prescribed drugs are among the most common treatable causes of dementia. Sedative effects of multiple medications may combine to cause chronic mental impairment. A few drugs cause confusional states when used alone—for example, the anticholinergic effects of drugs, such as tricyclic antidepressants, antihistamines, and neuroleptics, may produce anticholinergic encephalopathy. A nutritional cause of dementia is vitamin B_{12} deficiency.

Infections are a relatively infrequent but important cause of dementia. The most treatable cause is infectious meningitis. Viral encephalitis is a more acute syndrome that may leave dementia in its wake. Dementia is also an aspect of AIDS. Although some patients have secondary

Table 19-4

Systemic Diseases Associated with Dementia

Metabolic disorders

    Low sodium, low calcium, high calcium, and aluminum

    Renal, hepatic, and pulmonary failure

    Dialysis dementia

Nutritional

    Vitamin B_1 and B_{12} deficiency and pellagra

Endocrine

    Hypothyroidism, hyperthyroidism, Cushing, and hyperparathyroidism

Toxic

    Heavy metals and organic compounds

    Drugs, polypharmacy, and alcoholism

Infections

    Neurosyphilis

    Chronic meningitis: bacterial, fungal, and tuberculous

    Parasitic diseases

    Sequelae of viral encephalitis

    Subacute sclerosing panencephalitis

    Progressive multifocal leukoencephalopathy

    Creutzfeldt-Jakob disease

    AIDS dementia complex

Vascular diseases

    Multi-infarct dementia and Binswanger's disease

    Multiple cholesterol emboli

    Collagen vascular diseases and vasculitis

    Arteriovenous malformations

Neoplasms

    Brain tumor and increased intracranial pressure

    Multiple metastatic tumors

    Neoplastic meningitis

    Chemotherapy and radiation toxicity

    Limbic encephalitis

infections and tumors affecting the nervous system, the HIV itself appears to cause chronic encephalitis, resulting in dementia (**AIDS dementia complex**). Multiple strokes also can cause dementia, and vascular cognitive impairment often is mixed with AD, representing the second most common cause of dementia after AD itself.

Neurologic Diseases Associated with Dementia

The second group of dementias involves neurologic diseases that lead to cognitive deterioration. Normal pressure hydrocephalus and basal ganglia diseases are the most common examples. **Normal pressure hydrocephalus** is characterized by the gradual onset of mental slowing and then frank dementia, gait difficulty, and urinary incontinence. Brain imaging studies show dilation of the cerebral ventricles out of proportion to the degree of brain atrophy. Some patients respond dramatically to shunting procedures, in which spinal fluid is rerouted from the cerebral ventricles into the abdomen, and experience return of mental function and improved gait and urinary continence.

Most other neurologic diseases associated with dementia fall under the heading of neurodegenerative diseases, in which specific populations of neurons deteriorate. Several diseases that affect the basal ganglia also produce a pattern of subcortical dementia. The most common is Parkinson disease, which is characterized by bradykinesia (slowed movement), rigidity, resting tremor, masklike or expressionless face, and dysarthric speech. Patients exhibit slowed mental processes. A variant of Parkinson disease is Lewy body dementia in which subtle motor manifestations of Parkinson disease accompany a dementing illness, often with prominent visual hallucinations and confusion. At autopsy, the Lewy bodies are present not only in the substantia nigra but in the cortex. The family of Parkinson-plus disorders—corticobasal degeneration, progressive supranuclear palsy, and multisystem atrophy—are also associated with dementia. Other diseases that combine a movement disorder with a dementing illness are Huntington disease and Wilson disease.

Another neurologic disease not considered primarily a dementia is multiple sclerosis. Recent studies that have included neuropsychological test batteries have found that most patients with chronic multiple sclerosis have significant cognitive impairments. There is some suggestion from recent studies that multiple sclerosis plaques in the deep periventricular white matter, seen frequently on **brain** MRI studies of these patients, may correlate better with cognitive and mood disturbances than with physical disability.

Primary Degenerative Dementias

A few diseases primarily cause slowly progressive dementia. AD is the most common, accounting for 50–60% of most series of autopsied cases of dementia. The disease is defined by the presence of senile plaques in the neuropil of the cerebral cortex and neurofibrillary tangles (silver-staining strands) in the neurons of the cerebral cortex, hippocampus, and nucleus basalis of Meynert. The pathology of Alzheimer disease is difficult to separate from that of normal aging of the brain, and recent studies have found that nearly 50% of people > 80 years meet the clinical criteria for dementia (Evans et al. 1989). Careful examination and testing for treatable factors, as discussed earlier, are therefore essential for diagnosing AD. Although many drug therapies are being tested in AD, the ultimate cause of the neuronal degenera-

tion and curative treatment remain to be discovered. Genetic defects have been found to underlie some early-onset cases of AD, and a gene for apolipoprotein E4 appears to increase the likelihood of development of the sporadic disease.

Recently, drugs that block acetylcholinesterase have been found to improve memory in patients with AD. The drugs tacrine (Cognex), donepezil (Aricept), rivastigmine (Exelon), and galantamine (Razadyne) are the first agents to show clear benefit to patients with AD. Another U.S. Food and Drug Administration (FDA) approved drug, memantine (Namenda), has been shown effective in patients with moderate to severe AD. This drug blocks the N-methyl-D-aspartate (NMDA) subtype of the glutamate receptor in the brain. Other promising therapies are in the experimental pipeline. Recent clinical trials have been disappointing in regard to antioxidants, such as vitamin E, and nonsteroidal anti-inflammatory drugs (NSAIDs). Estrogen hormones, previously thought to be protective against cognitive decline in older women, have been shown to be associated with dementia. Healthy diet, exercise, and treatment of vascular risk factors, such as hypertension and elevated lipids may be the most effective ways to prevent dementia in normal people.

Pick disease is a dementing disease that has a predilection for the frontal and temporal lobes, often beginning unilaterally. The findings include silver-staining intraneuronal inclusions called Pick bodies but few or no senile plaques and neurofibrillary tangles, which are seen in AD. Pick disease may be clinically indistinguishable from AD, but many cases present with focal frontal lobe syndromes or isolated aphasia before progressing to general dementia. Pick disease now is considered to be part of a family of diseases called frontotemporal dementia, in which there is selective degeneration of the frontal and temporal lobes on one or both sides of the brain. Patients may present with progressive aphasia, usually of the nonfluent type, or with behavioral disturbances similar to those discussed for frontal lobe syndromes. A minority of patients also develop motor neuron disease.

The syndrome of primary progressive aphasia, especially the nonfluent type, is rarely secondary to AD but can be considered a part of the spectrum of frontotemporal dementia. Disorders underlying this syndrome include Pick disease, nonspecific neuronal loss and gliosis, and corticobasal degeneration. Some familial cases of frontotemporal dementia are associated with a gene defect on chromosome 17.

Creutzfeldt-Jakob disease is a rapidly progressive syndrome characterized by mood changes, dementia, seizures, myoclonus, and exaggerated startle responses. The course progresses from first symptoms to death in 6–12 months or less. The disease is rare, occurring in approximately one per one million people per year worldwide. Creutzfeldt-Jakob disease is interesting because it was found to be transmitted by inoculation of tissues via contaminated surgical instruments, corneal transplants, and pituitary extracts. A proteinaceous infectious particle is thought to be the cause of the disease, not a DNA-containing virus. Early changes on MRI studies and a new spinal fluid test called the 14-3-3 protein can be helpful in diagnosis. A variant of this disease is bovine spongiform encephalopathy (BSE), or mad cow disease, which has been transmitted by beef from infected cattle.

Traumatic Brain Injury

Traumatic brain injury (TBI) is a major cause of death and disability, particularly in young people. An acute blow to the head may cause instantaneous loss of consciousness and a brief period of retrograde amnesia, such that the patient does not remember the blow that caused the loss of consciousness. The term *cerebral concussion* implies a head injury with a brief loss of consciousness and brief retrograde amnesia but no other evidence of structural disruption of the brain. A great deal of research has concentrated on these minor head injuries and the resultant postconcussive syndrome. Such patients have normal brain imaging studies, including skull radiographs, CT scans, MRI studies, and electroencephalograms. Patients frequently complain of headaches, poor concentration and memory, insomnia, irritability, mood swings, and sometimes vertigo or dizziness.

More severe brain injuries may initially cause coma and evidence of contusion or bruising of the brain, shear hemorrhages into the brain tissue, or pooling of blood in the subdural or extradural space. Such patients are more severely impaired than patients with concussive injuries, and they frequently have motor deficits as well as impaired cognition. These patients commonly require prolonged rehabilitation, first in inpatient and later outpatient settings. Impaired memory and attention are common accompaniments, as are frontal lobe syndromes, such as impulsive or agitated behavior. These patients are typically uninhibited and inappropriate in their behavior, and they frequently call attention to themselves on rehabilitation units. In terms of language, high-level impairments are frequently found, especially in the organization of discourse. Occasionally, aphasias similar to those seen in stroke patients develop after TBI, especially in patients with localized damage to the left cerebral hemisphere from subdural hematomas, intracerebral hemorrhages, or contusions.

CLINICAL CONSIDERATIONS

PATIENT ONE

This 51-year-old woman, previously healthy except for smoking and postmenopausal hormone-replacement therapy, underwent an elective total knee-replacement surgery. The evening after the surgery, she was noted to be somewhat confused, but no other specific symptoms were noted. There was a question of an irregular heart rhythm postoperatively, but she was in normal sinus

rhythm at the time of evaluation. She went to sleep uneventfully. She apparently had a stroke before sleep. The next morning, her family reported she was speaking gibberish. She did not have any facial droop, arm or leg weakness, or numbness. She was evaluated by a consulting speech language pathologists (SLP), who noted the following:

- Fluently spoken speech
- Paraphasic substitutions and meaningless jargon utterances
- Poor repetition
- Impaired auditory comprehension
- Poor processing of written language
- Substantial naming difficulty

A brain MRI study showed an acute infarction in the left temporal lobe (Fig. 19-1). The frontal and parietal lobes were not affected.

Question: Can you identify the aphasia type and lesion site and then comment on the nature of the underlying cause?

Discussion: This collection of neurolinguistic symptoms (impaired auditory comprehension, paraphasic substitutions, and jargon utterances) indicates Wernicke (fluent) aphasia in its acute stage. This stroke syndrome likely resulted from an embolism that traveled into the middle cerebral artery and selectively occluded the inferior branches.

PATIENT TWO

A 72-year-old man with a prior history of hypertension, hyperlipidemia (elevated cholesterol), and obstructive sleep apnea developed the abrupt onset of difficulty seeing out of his right visual field. He was noted to have confusion and mild memory difficulty. He was taken to the emergency room (ER) and was examined by a neurologist who noted the following:

- Well-oriented and able to speak fluently
- No ability to name colors
- Complete inability to read
- Mild short-term memory difficulty
- No motor or sensory deficits
- A faint carotid bruit

A brain MRI study showed an infarction in the left occipital lobe, within the territory of the left posterior cerebral artery (Fig. 19-2). Magnetic resonance angiography (MRA) showed reduced filling of branches of the left posterior cerebral artery.

Question: Can you explain what type of aphasia is usually associated with the lesion noted on the MRI study?

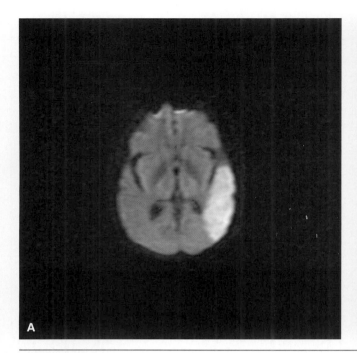

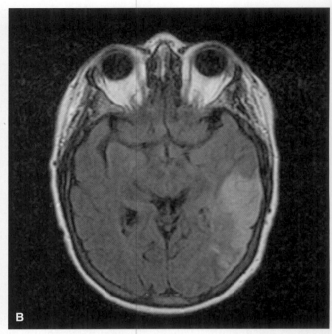

Figure 19-1 **A.** An acute infarct in the left temporal lobe on a diffusion-weighted MRI image. **B.** Verification of the infarct on fluid attenuated inversion recovery imaging (FLAIR), which is essentially a T2-weighted image with the cerebrospinal fluid signal subtracted.

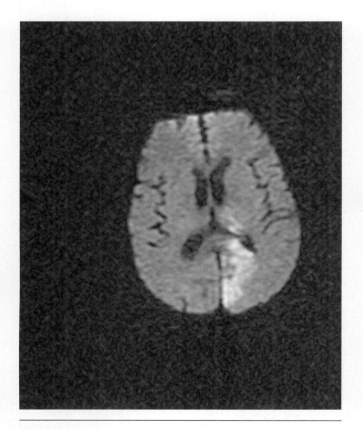

Figure 19-2 Axial diffusion-weighted MRI study showing an acute infarction in the left occipital lobe, extending into the splenium of the corpus callosum, the thalamus, and the medial temporal region.

Discussion: This is a case of pure alexia without agraphia, secondary to an infarction in the territory of the left posterior cerebral artery, which had further involved the splenium of the corpus callosum, as evident in the MRI study. According to the disconnection theory of pure alexia, the callosal lesion prevents visual information processed in the intact right occipital lobe from reaching left hemisphere language centers for reading and color naming.

PATIENT THREE

A 47-year-old HIV-positive man with an acute onset of dysarthria was taken to the ER where he presented with the following symptoms:

- Dysarthric speech marked by slowness of articulation, explosive and overarticulated syllabic stress, loudness, and pitch breaks as well as prolonged intervals between sounds
- Difficulty with swallowing
- Impaired balance with a tendency of falling to the left
- Left ptosis and a smaller pupil on the left than the right
- Left facial numbness
- Weakness of the left palate
- Numbness of the right side of the body
- Ataxia of the left limbs and the trunk
- No language and cognitive impairments

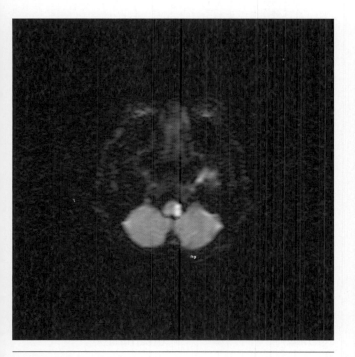

Figure 19-3 Axial diffusion-weighted MRI study showing a left lateral medullary infarction after the occlusion of the left vertebral artery.

A brainstem MRI study revealed an infarction in the left lateral medulla (Fig. 19-3).

Question: Can you explain how a left medullary lesion could relate to the observed clinical signs?

Discussion: This is a case of ataxic dysarthria subsequent to a lateral medullary lesion; the cause of the infarct was occlusion of the left vertebral artery, which gives off the branch called posterior inferior cerebellar artery. The lateral medullary lesion (Wallenberg syndrome) affects the trigeminal spinal tract nucleus, nucleus ambiguus, and lateral spinothalamic tract containing spinothalamic fibers from the contralateral half of the body. It causes a dissociated loss of sensation owing to the levels of fiber crossings. The syndrome is marked by the loss of pain sensation from the ipsilateral face (trigeminal [CN V] nerve) and the contralateral side of the body (spinothalamic tract fibers). The involvement of the nucleus ambiguus (vagus [CN X] nerve) contributed to swallowing difficulty. Many patients with this syndrome, depending on the lesion size, show involvement of the inferior cerebellar peduncle and/or have a cerebellar infarction. The affection of the inferior cerebellar peduncle in this case had contributed to the dysarthric speech.

PATIENT FOUR

This 53-year-old woman had to stop working as a secretary because of increasing difficulty in thinking of words and signs of nonfluent aphasia. Neurologic examination showed a healthy-appearing woman with nonfluent speech, poor naming, and relatively preserved comprehension. She had no other neurologic deficits. A brain MRI study showed a severe atrophy of the left temporal lobe (Fig. 19-4).

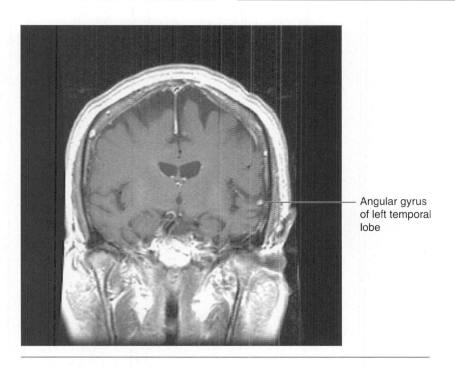

Angular gyrus
of left temporal
lobe

Figure 19-4 Coronal brain MRI study showing left temporal lobe atrophy with some frontal atrophy.

Question: Can you explain the type of aphasia that is usually associated with the lesion site revealed in the MRI study?

Discussion: This is a case of primary progressive aphasia (nonfluent type). The primary progressive aphasia has apparent focal aphasic deficits that gradually progress over years. Some patients fail to show memory loss or other cognitive deficits for years after onset; the patient cannot think of names or understand the meaning of words. The nonfluent aphasia in dementia usually indicates pathology other than typical AD, whereas the pathology of semantic dementia and fluent progressive aphasia is more variable.

*This chapter was written by Howard S. Kirshner, Department of Neurology, Vanderbilt University Medical Center, Nashville, TN.

QUIZ QUESTIONS

1. Define the following terms: acalculia, agraphia, alexia, apraxia, dementia, dysarthria, neologism, and paraphasia.

2. List at least three functional impairments associated with the pathologic involvement of the frontal, parietal, and temporal lobes.

3. Provide the behavioral definitions of dementia, aphasia, apraxia, and dysarthria.

TECHNICAL TERMS

acalculia	contusion
agnosia	dementia
agraphia	dysarthria
alexia	hemiparesis
Alzheimer disease	hippocampus
anosognosia	hyperparathyroidism
aphasia	hyponatremia
apraxia	neologisms
ataxia	neurofibrillary tangles
concussion	paraphasias

SUMMARY

This chapter discusses the functional organization of the human cerebral cortex and the principal syndromes of abnormal cortical functioning that result from brain diseases. The emphasis is on speech and language disorders, including related disorders, such as apraxia, agnosia, dementia, and TBI. These topics constitute the part of neurology increasingly known as behavioral neurology or cognitive neuroscience.

Diagnostic Techniques and Neurologic Concepts

LEARNING OBJECTIVES

After studying this chapter, students should be able to:

- Explain common brain imaging techniques

- Describe the simplified technical basics of all these imaging techniques

- Outline the clinical significance of each brain imaging technique

- Explain the mechanism of the sodium Amytal infusion technique used for assessing cerebral dominance

- Explain the mechanism of electromyography and its clinical significance

- Discuss the mechanism of electroencephalography and its clinical value

- Describe the physiology of sleep and explain associated patterns of brain activity

- Discuss the concept of the evoked potential technique

- Describe the technique and functional aspect of the dichotic listening paradigm

- Explain common neurosurgical procedures and their treatment purposes

- Discuss the neurolinguistic significance of surgical procedures, such as corticography, subcortical implant, and stereotaxic surgery

- Discuss myopathic, neuropathic, and seizure disorders

- Explain common patterns of inheritance and associated genetic disorders

An array of diagnostic techniques and medical concepts apply to the management of neurologically impaired patients. Addressing or even listing all of them is beyond the scope of this chapter; only the most relevant clinical concepts, treatment procedures, and diagnostic techniques relating to the management of patients with neurologic and neurolinguistic impairments are discussed.

BRAIN IMAGING

Brain imaging involves the use of neuroradiologic techniques to evaluate normal and abnormal brain structures. Since the beginning of the 20th century, imaging of the brain has progressed steadily; however, the most notable developments have taken place only within the past 3 decades. Examples of early imaging techniques, which incorporate the use of ionizing radiation (x-rays), are **plain radiography**, **pneumoencephalography**, and **cerebral angiography**. Newer imaging techniques, which are not limited to X-rays, include **magnetic resonance**, **radionuclide**, and **isotope** technologies. Each technique provides a different perspective of live brain tissue and differs in terms of its tissue resolution and the time it takes to visualize pathology.

Among the older techniques, pneumoencephalography (not discussed here), was particularly invasive. It not only evaluated the ventricular cavities and flow of cerebrospinal fluid (CSF) but also indirectly evaluated the cerebral morphology based on the distortion of patterns in the CSF pathways. Cerebral angiography, another older invasive technique, has been highly useful for providing morphologic evaluation of the cerebral vasculature. It is rapidly being replaced by newer new and less invasive techniques, such as computed tomography angiography and magnetic resonance angiography (MRA).

Among the newer techniques, **computed tomography (CT)** has been in use since the late 1970s. It uses X-rays to display sectional brain anatomy with the aid of computer technology. More recently, developments in **magnetic resonance technology** has spawned a number of exciting tools, such as **magnetic resonance imaging (MRI)**, **functional MRI (fMRI)**, **diffusion tensor imaging (DTI; also called tractography)**, **magnetic resonance spectroscopy (MRS)**, MRA, **diffusion-weighted imaging (DWI)**, and **perfusion MRI**. These techniques provide clearer and more detailed images of the cerebral morphology, aspects of brain functioning, and the internal physiologic environment. **Single photon emission computed tomography (SPECT)** and **positron emission tomography (PET)** employ the use of radioactive tracers or isotopes to evaluate particular aspects of brain function.

Cerebral Angiography

Among the earliest radiologic techniques, cerebral angiography is still an excellent tool for evaluating the cerebral vasculature. It is used to diagnose vascular disorders such as atherosclerotic disease, aneurysms, vasculitis, and arteriovenous malformations (AVMs) and can determine the degree of vascularity of certain tumors. This procedure is invasive and, therefore, is associated with some degree of risk, primarily stroke. When appropriately used, however, it can provide invaluable clinical information for planning medical and surgical treatment.

Cerebral angiography is performed in a dedicated angiography suite designed solely for this procedure. Arterial access first must be established, commonly via a puncture of the **common femoral artery**. However, sometimes the brachial and axillary arteries may be used for arterial access when femoral artery access is either impossible or hazardous. Historically, the carotid and vertebral arteries, and even the abdominal aorta have been used for arterial access, but this is no longer routine. The selected artery is punctured, and a catheter (tubular instrument) is inserted into the artery and guided by fluoroscopy to the arch of the aorta and then to the carotid or vertebral artery. Once the

catheter is in place, a radiopaque contrast agent is injected. This is followed by a series of high-speed radiographs taken from various angles. Images taken early in the process depict the filling of the lumens of the injected arteries, as the radiopaque material outlines the major (anterior, posterior, and middle) cerebral arteries and their divisions; smaller arteries are usually not distinguishable (Fig. 20-1). Filming is continued to distinguish the opacification by the contrast medium of the capillary bed and cerebral venous anatomy.

The ability to visualize the pattern and extent of the opacified vasculature helps identify arterial pathologies, such as thrombosis, hemorrhage, aneurysm (localized arterial dilatation), blood supply to lesions (tumors), and mass effect (irregularly displaced vessels). With thrombosis, there is little or no arterial filling beyond the blockage point, although this finding is not frequently demonstrable (Fig. 20-2). The technique can reveal poor capillary contrast staining, which indicates early draining veins or retrograde arterial filling. Unfortunately, a paucity of angiographic

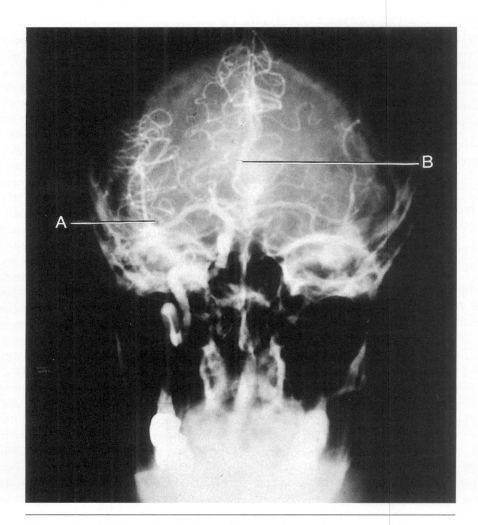

Figure 20-1 Anteroposterior view of a normal carotid angiogram showing the important arteries: middle cerebral artery branches (*A*) and anterior cerebral artery branches (*B*).

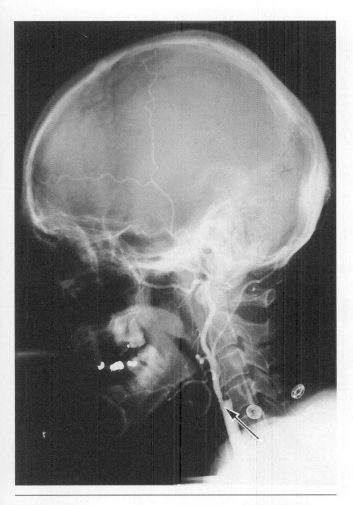

Figure 20-2 Lateral view angiogram of a left internal carotid artery thrombosis (*arrow*). Notice that there is no filling of the internal carotid artery beyond its bifurcation with the external carotid artery.

findings does not exclude the diagnosis of thrombosis, and the presence of angiographic findings are not specific for this condition.

In the case of a **hemorrhage**, contrast extravasation is seen only with massive bleeding at the time of the study, and cerebral hematomas are usually angiographically identified by their mass effect on the surrounding vessels and the relative paucity of the contrast staining. Aneurysms are local dilatations of cerebral arteries. AVMs are consistent with large feeding arteries that fill early, a tangle of abnormal vessels called a nidus, and dilated tortuous draining veins. Arterial displacement, which reflects mass effect, also can suggest a brain tumor or a process extrinsic to the brain but inside the skull, such as a subdural hematoma.

Digital subtraction is a relatively recent development in cerebral angiography. A computer is used to collect, digitize, and process the information from the radiograph, rather than simply allowing it to form a direct shadow on the film. This provides many advantages related to the ability to manipulate the accumulated data. For instance,

the contrast-filled lumen of the arteries can be rendered more conspicuous by subtracting the overlying bony structures, which would show up on routine plain radiographs. In digital subtraction, contrast medium is released into the artery through a catheter, after which a series of radiographs is taken and fed into a computer. The computer subtracts the images taken before the artery was outlined from the images taken after the introduction of contrast material.

The acquisition speed and processing of angiographic data present numerous advantages in the evaluation and display of the information, but the stunning advances are modulated by some disadvantages. For example, the improved contrast resolution of digital subtraction angiography is countered by the lower spatial resolution relative to conventional plain film angiography. Most modern-day angiography suites, however, are digital, and manufacturers continue to improve the spatial resolution. Digital substraction angiography requires a less contrast medium than the conventional version. Furthermore, it allows the evaluation of vessels in multiple projections.

Computed Tomography

Developed in the early 1970s, CT was considered a major breakthrough in brain imaging because, for the first time, clinicians were given direct and noninvasive in vivo visualization of brain structures. CT uses a narrow beam of X-rays to examine the head and brain in a series of slices, usually 1–10 mm thick. A thin, collimated X-ray beam passes through the head; on the other side, the transmitted radiation is recorded by a series of detectors, and the data are digitized on a series of volume cell elements (voxels) that form a matrix. The data of absorbed X-ray particles (photons) are processed by a computer, which creates a two-dimensional image of a particular slice of the brain based on mathematical calculations. Each image is displayed in varying shades of white, gray, and black to correlate with different areas of X-ray attenuation. A number of strategies and techniques are used by the manufacturers to create this mathematical, two-dimensional representation of the brain. British scientist G. N. Hounsfield was awarded the Nobel Prize in 1973 for helping develop this technique.

As mentioned, CT diagnosis relies on the detection of density variations from X-ray particle absorption by various brain structures (Fig. 20-3A). For example, the skull and acute blood are higher in density constructs and absorb (or attenuate) more X-ray particles; thus their computer-generated image appears mostly in the white range. White and gray matter and the fluid-filled ventricles are less dense and attenuate fewer X-ray particles, so their images are assigned a gray shade. Structures with less density—air, fat, and CSF—attenuate or stop fewer X-ray particles and thus appear black.

Based on photon absorption coefficients (Hounsfield units) on a gray scale, structures are assigned a numeric value ranging between −1000 (for air) and +1000 (for dense bone). Intracranial lesions are in general either **high-** or **low-density lesions**. High-density intracranial lesions, which

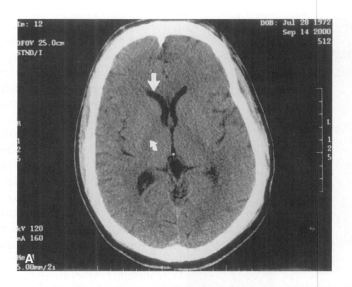

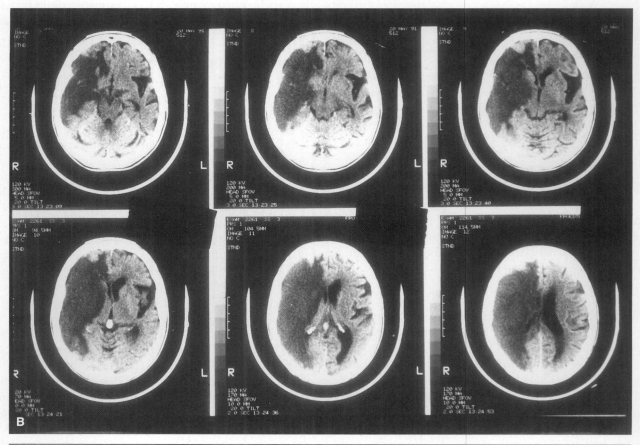

Figure 20-3 A. Axial CT scan of a normal brain. The lower density of the fluid-filled anterior horns of the lateral ventricle (*straight arrow*) can be clearly distinguished from the adjacent brain parenchyma. The basal ganglia (*curved arrow*) is also visible. B. X-ray CT series showing a massive infarct in the right hemisphere involving the frontal, parietal, and occipital lobes.

are especially significant to students in communicative disorders, are acute hemorrhages and calcified lesions. Important low-density lesions are cerebral chronic infarction, edema, and cystic lesions (Fig. 20-3B; Table 20-1). Tumors may be either high or low density.

In the early days of CT scanning, scientists hoped to characterize cerebral pathology according to density measurements alone, but this was rapidly abandoned, as almost every disease entity proved to be a dynamic process that displayed a range of X-ray attenuation profiles, depending

Table 20-1

Brain Structures Appearance on CT Images

Structure	Appearance
Acute blood and bone	Bright white
Subacute blood	Light gray
White and gray matter	Gray
Tumor	Gray to white
Fat	Light black
Air	Dark black

on the disease stage and other complicating factors. There is, however, an inaccurate but understandably persistent tendency to characterize lesions solely according to their density on CT.

Various radiopaque materials can be injected into the patient to characterize pathologic processes and demonstrate certain vascular anatomy. Contrast agents may be injected intravenously or intra-arterially and localize in the intravascular space, which becomes more conspicuous because of the greater attenuation of X-rays by the contrast. However, some pathologic conditions show contrast staining as a result of a breakdown of the blood–brain barrier, allowing seepage of contrast from the intravascular compartment into the cerebral tissues. In addition, contrast enhancement in some pathologic states occurs only during a certain stage of the disease.

Despite other advances in neuroimaging, CT scanning still remains a reliable diagnostic tool. For increased scanning times, CT remains the preferred diagnostic tool for uncooperative patients because the image is not significantly degraded by motion artifacts. It can readily detect fresh (acute and subacute) hemorrhages and can identify bone fractures. The advent of three-dimensional (3D) CT allows clinicians to create images in multiple planes from volume reconstruction.

The disadvantages of the CT technology include exposure to ionizing radiation and modest contrast resolution. Furthermore, limited differentiation between gray and white matter, the inability to identify infarcts (acute or subacute) and ischemia within the first 24 hr of onset, and poor visualization of structures in the posterior fossa owing to bony infarct further contribute to its limitations.

CT has been used extensively in neurolinguistics for studying brain–behavior relationships. In an excellent description of CT, Gado et al. (1979) provides a comprehensive framework for relating brain anatomy on CT to language regions and Brodmann areas. Naeser and Hayward (1987), Damasio (1998), and many other researchers have used CT to demonstrate anatomic correlations for classical aphasias.

Alexander et al. (1987) used CT to demonstrate the existence of subcortical aphasias.

Magnetic Resonance Imaging

MRI does not use hazardous ionizing radiation, as do CT and conventional X-ray techniques. Rather, it creates images of structures in living brains from the magnetic signal of the atomic nuclei of water, the hydrogen protons. Water is one of the main body components, and body tissues differ in their water concentrations.

Hydrogen protons, with positive and negative areas, have a north and south pole and act as spinning magnetic bars. Without any external interference, the magnetic activity of hydrogen protons is random; and, overall, they cancel each other out. The foundation of the MRI procedure is to place the body (e.g., the brain) in an artificial external magnetic field, which causes the hydrogen protons of the tissue to align in a single plane. This external magnetic field, which acts as a strong magnet, is usually ~1.5 T (teslas) and ranges from 0.3 to 5 teslas, which is about 100,000 times greater than the earth's average magnetic field of 50 μT. A radiofrequency pulse excites the hydrogen protons. The transmission of this pulse, produced in short bursts from an external radiofrequency transmitter, is absorbed by the protons. This cancels out the magnetic effect of some atoms while providing extra energy to other aligned hydrogen atoms by resonating and perturbing them to rearrange themselves in a different plane, depending on the tissue type. When the externally administered radio frequency signal ends, the relaxed hydrogen atoms return to their previous orientation; however, before doing so, they release an electromagnetic signal (called echo).

The formation of a magnetic resonance image relies on the differential relaxation of the hydrogen protons. The radiofrequency signals from hydrogen protons are collected by a computerized coil and converted into images using both their location in 3D space and various shades of gray, black, and white. These shades represent different strengths of signals and create images that correspond to differences in proton relaxation. Because bone contains limited water, it produces fewer signals relative to the other cerebral structures (Fig. 20-4).

There are two important terms used with respect to the MRI: T1 and T2. They represent the time difference (in milliseconds) between the application of the radiofrequency pulse and the peak of the signal from the relaxed hydrogen protons. The image constructed from the time constant in the canceled-out protons that slowly return to their magnetic field is called a T1-image. A T2-weighed image is an image created from the time constant of the protons that received high energy, were not canceled out and lose their energy more rapidly as they return to their previous magnetic state. The image acquisition parameters of T1 and T2 reflect the contrast properties of the image. T1, for example, delineates anatomic

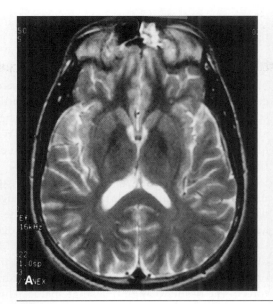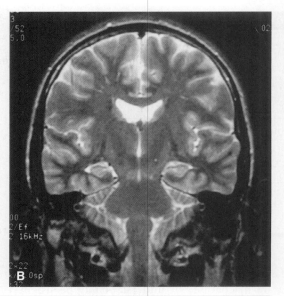

Figure 20-4 **A.** A normal T2-weighted (fast spin echo; FSE) axial MRI image of the brain. Note that an incidental small amount of left frontal sinus disease is present. **B.** A normal T2-weighted (FSE) coronal MRI image of the brain.

details well but is a poor indicator of water changes in tissue that are present in edema and stroke. T2 images are more sensitive to water changes in tissue and have proven to be a better diagnostic tool for the identification of edema and ischemia. Both sequences provide diagnostically important information by showing different degrees of contrast between normal and pathologic tissues, such as gray matter, white matter, and CSF (Table 20-2).

A relatively recently introduced T2-based MRI technique called **fluid attenuated inversion recovery** (FLAIR) can identify brain lesions better and with greater clarity. The presence of CSF in the ventricles and subarachnoid space makes it hard to see the parenchymal (cellular) hyper-

intensity. On FLAIR sequences, the CSF signal is subtracted, which allows any excess H_2O in the brain to stand out more than on T2 sequences.

The advantages of using MRI include the ability to reveal better anatomic detail of normal and abnormal structures than can CT (Fig. 20-5). MRI helps identify a variety of brain abnormalities, provides a clear differentiation between gray and white matter, separates bone from the surrounding tissue, detects ischemic infarcts early, and—most important—does not expose the patient to ionizing radiation. Among the disadvantages of MRI are its limitations in detecting acute and/or subacute hemorrhage, difficulties with claustrophobic individuals, longer imaging times than CT, and exposure to intensely loud sounds.

Table 20-2

Normal and Pathologic Structures seen on T1- and T2-Weighted MRI Studies

State of Health	Structure	T1	T2
Normal	Bone	Black (+)	Black (+)
	Gray matter	Gray (dark)	Gray
	White matter	Gray	Gray (dark)
	Cerebrospinal fluid	Black (+)	Black (+)
Pathologic	Infarct (acute and subacute)	Gray (dark)	Gray to white
	Ischemia (acute and subacute)	Gray (dark)	Gray to white
	Tumor	Gray (dark)	Gray to white
	Edema	Gray (dark)	Gray to white

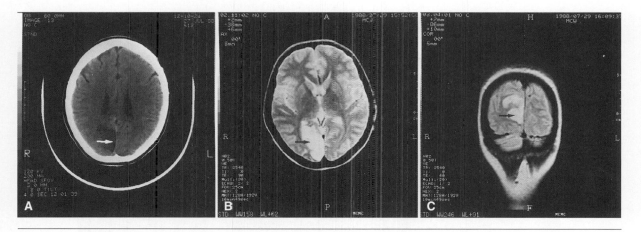

Figure 20-5 Three views of a massive right occipital infarct in a single patient. A. X-ray CT image. B. Transverse view MRI study. C. Coronal view MRI study.

ADVANCES IN MRI

Advances in MRI have provided ways to evaluate different physiologic correlates associated with brain functions; the most notable of these techniques are **fMRI** (which displays areas of cortical activity and is based on oxygenated blood flow differences in the functionally active cortex relative to the resting cortex), **DWI** (extremely important for diagnosing acute stroke and other conditions and is based on the evaluation of random intracellular molecular motion of water), **DTI** (evaluates white matter tracts based on the diffusion of water along the white matter bundles), perfusion **MRI** (evaluates blood flow, blood volume, and cerebral perfusion), **MRS** (evaluates the biochemical composition of brain tissue), and **MRA** (evaluates the vascular anatomy).

Functional MRI

fMRI displays changes in brain signals as a result of changes in neuronal brain activity. More specifically, it measures transient and small changes in blood oxygen levels and blood flow associated with cortical-neuronal events in response to a controlled (linguistic or sensorimotor) task. As an important neurolinguistic technique for students of human behavior, fMRI is used to precisely map brain areas activated through specific stimuli, such as sensorimotor, visual, linguistic, and nonlinguistic tasks (Figs. 20-6 and 20-7). This has allowed researchers to observe the differences and/or progressive physiologic changes in activated brain regions. Altered blood flow patterns are associated with a variety of pathologic states in brain tissue. fMRI not only is important for the investigation of normal or basic function in vivo but also has become a valuable source of information for guiding the treatment of pathologic conditions. The imaging technique helps clinicians monitor brain tumors, stroke, and degenerative or chronic central nervous system (CNS) disorders, such as seizures and multiple sclerosis. The localization of the sensorimotor

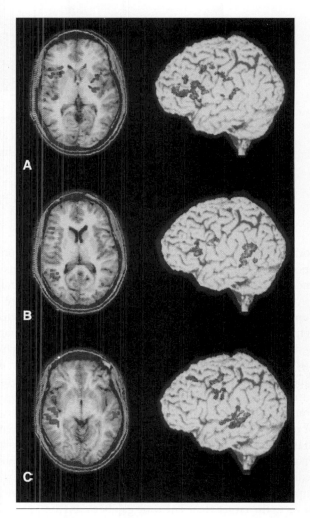

Figure 20-6 Anomalous cortical representation in a patient with demonstrated left hemispheric dominance on the Wada test. The fMRI images show bilateral cortical activation of the language areas during three tasks: *A*, lexical generation; *B*, silent sentence repetition; and *C*, listening.

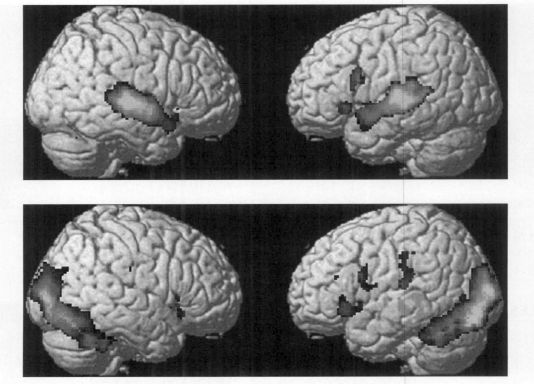

Figure 20-7 fMRI images showing bilateral cortical activation during a lexical decision task. **A.** The effect of contrasting lexical decisions when listening to real words and pseudo-words against null events. **B.** The cortical area activated during the lexical decision task when the stimuli were presented visually. The threshold of activation is significant at $p < .05$ (FWE (family wise error) corrected for multiple comparisons); activity is seen on the surface of the right and left hemispheres of the SPM2 single-subject template brain.

cortex by fMRI has proved to be extremely useful in the preoperative planning of brain surgery for tumors, **epilepsy**, and other lesions, decreasing the risk of a neurologic deficit.

Functional MRI measures **blood oxygen level–dependent** (BOLD) **effects**, which represent the differential activity of hemoglobin and deoxyhemoglobin in the magnetic environment of the MRI machine. Any eloquent part of the brain that participates in a specific linguistic or sensorimotor task exhibits greater neuronal activity in the corresponding brain region, which initiates greater oxygen consumption, subsequently causing increased amounts of released deoxygenated hemoglobin (deoxyhemoglobin) in the surrounding veins. Deoxyhemoglobin is highly paramagnetic and generates a signal that triggers a greater redistribution of blood to the target area. However, the stipulation is that there is a lag of 3–6 sec before blood flows to the target area. The time gap between the presence of deoxygenated and the return of oxygenated hemoglobin is related to the BOLD effect.

The BOLD-fMRI research paradigm involves several periods of rest alternated with periods of activation. A series of images of the brain region of interest (ROI) is taken while the patient rests. A second set of images taken while

the patient performs a controlled sensorimotor or linguistic task. In general, 30 images are acquired in a period of 90 sec. The first 10 images (30 sec) and the last 10 images (30 sec) are used as the baseline; the middle 10 images (30 sec) images are acquired when the patient is performing the specific task engaging the eloquent brain. The baseline images are subtracted from the task images, and the activated cortical areas are considered to be related to specific functions.

Although BOLD is the primary method employed for fMRI, there are other methods: **arterial spin labeling** (ASL), MRI **signal weighting** by cerebral blood flow (CBF), and **cerebral blood volume** (CBV).

Diffusion-Weighted Imaging

Diffusion is a molecular property that refers to the random, uniform, and constant movements of water molecules in all directions (Brownian motion principle); this is true of isotropic media, such as water and gases. However, the rate of water molecular movement in body tissues is related to the cellular kinetic energy, which depends on the thermal energy. Because molecular diffusion is not uniform (anisotropic) in body tissue owing to barriers placed by tissue structures (cell membrane, axons, and vascular components), it is referred to as **apparent diffusion**. **Diffusion-weighted** (DW) MRI measures the variability of Brownian uniform water in terms of an **apparent diffusion coefficient** (ADC).

In case of an infarct, the affected area in the brain undergoes cellular swelling (cytotoxic edema), which impairs water diffusion and results in an increased signal. As a diagnostic tool, DW MRI is extremely sensitive to even minute molecular motion, which makes it highly sensitive to **ischemic stroke**, a neurologic condition of great importance to students of human behavior. In ischemia, the diffusion coefficient in affected tissue attenuates by 50% or so within 3–4 min of the onset of the infarct (Fig. 20-8A and B).

The loss of blood in ischemic stroke contributes to an increased retention of intracellular water volume secondary to cytotoxic edema, resulting in restricted diffusion of water and leading to hyperintensity on DWI studies. This diminished diffusion results in a bright appearance of the diseased area so that an infarct can be identified within 15–30 min from the onset, a great improvement over standard T1- and T2-weighted MRI studies (4–6 hr) and CT scans (24–48 hr). DWI also readily differentiates subacute lesions (old infarcts, vasogenic infarcts, and deep white matter pathologies; dilated ventricular spaces; neoplasm; and demyelination), which do not become hyperintense (bright), as they do with acute stroke.

The underlying mechanism in DWI also could be related to energy failure, with a loss of Na/K pump activity and reduction of extracellular volume. With its sensitivity to molecular motion, DWI has been accepted by neuro-radiologists and neurologists as an accurate method for detecting acute stoke within minutes of onset; it is also being evaluated in a variety of other intracranial disease processes.

Perfusion MRI

Perfusion MRI uses a magnetic field to evaluate the delivery of oxygenated blood flow to cerebral tissue. Initially, vascular perfusion was measured by injecting an intravenous (IV) bolus of isotope tracers, a contrast-enhancing compound like **gadolinium**, to measure the mean transmit time and blood volume in the perfusion process. ASL, a noninvasive MRI technique that uses water as a tracer, contributes to the magnetization of the blood flowing into the brain cells to allow evaluation of cerebral perfusion. ASL not only has demonstrated altered hemodynamics of perfusion in stroke patients but also has indicated lowered mean transit time. Perfusion MRI has become the diagnostic tool of choice in the evaluation of incipient or acute stroke and is sensitive to the ischemic onset within minutes (Fig. 20.8C–E).

Diffusion Tensor Imaging

Diffusion tensor imaging (DTI), another development in MRI technology, evaluates the directionality of water molecular movements affected by tissue barriers in the body. This technique provides a way to identify normal and dysfunctioning parallel-running myelinated axonal tracts in the cortical white matter (Fig. 20-9). Molecular diffusion depends the orientation of the white matter tracks and on the integrity of the myelin. The technique is based on the understanding that nerve fibers have a typical and standard microstructure that regulates its characteristic pattern of

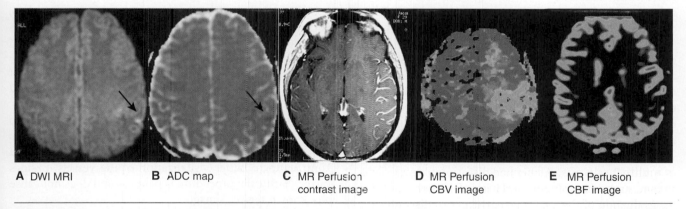

A DWI MRI   **B** ADC map   **C** MR Perfusion contrast image   **D** MR Perfusion CBV image   **E** MR Perfusion CBF image

Figure 20-8 Cerebral diffusion, perfusion and diffusion-perfusion incompatibility. **A.** Diffusion-weighted MRI image showing a hypertense area of abnormal diffusion in the motor cortical region of the posterior frontal region. **B.** Apparent diffusion coefficient image showing an area of abnormal diffusion (*dark*) in the left frontal posterior region, which is consistent with an acute ischemic lesion. **C.** Contrast-enhanced MRI perfusion image showing a contrast stagnation in the area of the left middle cerebral artery territory. **D.** Cerebral blood volume MRI perfusion image revealing a decreased blood volume in the area of injury. **E.** Cerebral blood flow MRI perfusion image showing decreased perfusion in the entire left hemisphere. This is consistent with a diffusion–perfusion mismatch in which the area of perfusion deficit is larger than the area of injury seen on diffusion imaging. This indicates a large deficit that would be damaging without successful and immediate intervention.

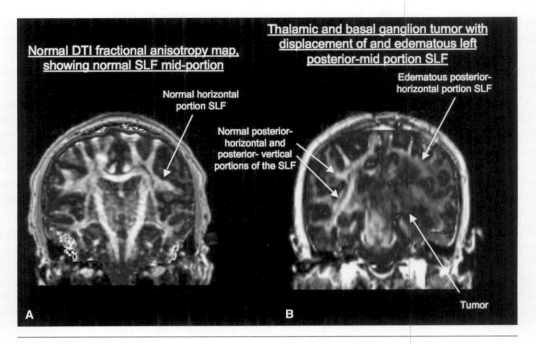

Figure 20-9 Diffusion tensor image (*DTI*) of the cortical association fiber bundle. **A.** A normal DTI fractional anisotropy map indicating a normal superior longitudinal fasciculus (*SLF*). **B.** A subcortical (thalamus and basal ganglia) tumor with displacement of an edematous SLF.

water molecule diffusion. By including diffusion gradients of water molecules in at least six noncolinear directions for a uniform sampling, directionality of water movement can be calculated by eigenvectors (a mathematical value indicating directional movement). DTI involves an analysis of the magnitude and direction of water molecules and provides an orientationally averaged measure of water diffusion, called mean diffusivity (D'), and the degree of diffusion anisotropy (differential diffusional properties in different directions), also called fractional anisotropy (FA).

From the data collected via DTI, clinicians are able to generate colored-coded maps of the diffusion anisotropy and direction of maximum diffusivity, which reflect properties of tissue microstructure. In general, water diffuses in the direction of the fiber orientation (parallel) more quickly than in other directions; this quality plays a role in clinical diagnosis. This technique is sensitive to subtle microstructural changes in white matter wiring in diseases such as multiple sclerosis, Alzheimer disease, aphasia, alexia, autism, and schizophrenia. DTI is particularly useful in the evaluation of the anatomic correlates of disconnective neurolinguistic syndromes. In its clinical applications, it has been suggested that a drop in FA reflects myelin disintegration and axonal disruption, whereas an increase in D' results from increased free water content and injury in structures that restrict water diffusion.

Magnetic Resonance Spectroscopy

MRS uses an MRI scanner to evaluate the biochemical profile of a particular area of a sampled brain. This technique is useful for both investigating brain biochemistry and

evaluating diagnostically difficult lesions in which brain morphology is normal but metabolism is abnormal. MRS is frequently used in conjunction with routine MRI studies.

Magnetic Resonance Angiography

MRA provides a method of diagnosing vascular diseases by evaluating the structural integrity of blood vessels in different projections. It has been used for detecting, diagnosing, and evaluating the treatment of heart disorders, stroke, and blood vessel disease. One MRA technique incorporates the principle of time of flight (TOF), in which the signal is obtained from the blood moving within the vessels. TOF imaging is noninvasive and requires no contrast agent. Clinically, MRA helps identify arterial stenoses and vascular conditions such as aneurysm and AVM.

Contrast bolus (gadolinium), dynamic gradient, echo MRI is another way of evaluating blood vessels. It uses intravenous contrast to enhance the signal to noise ratio and contributes to better visualization of the vessels. Besides image clarity, the procedure is painless and does not cause any known tissue damage.

Recently, **magnetic resonance venography** (MRV) has become available for imaging veins. It is useful in the diagnosis of dural sinus thrombosis.

ADDITIONAL IMAGING TECHNIQUES

Regional Cerebral Blood Flow

Regional **CBF** (rCBF) measures the flow of blood to functionally active brain areas by monitoring a radioactive tracer.

The principle underlying rCBF is that brain areas responsible for performing activities require increased blood. This elevated blood flow is needed for the additional metabolic energy required by the tissue. rCBF was the first technique that revealed the dynamics of the functional brain. The technique entails the use of **xenon**-133, a radioactive isotope. The isotope is dissolved in a sterile saline solution that is injected into an artery or inhaled. The presentation and washout (radiation attenuation) of the isotope solute are monitored using a γ-camera, which consists of multiple scintillation detectors. The camera measures attenuated radiation around the head. The information obtained from the solute is fed into a computer, which delineates different levels of blood flow with various colors and hues. Because blood flow and local metabolic activity are directly related, the images provide insights regarding which brain areas participate in various activities.

In a detailed study of specific brain function and blood flow by Lassen et al. (1978), observations of blood flow that were not uniform throughout the brain reaffirmed the conviction that there is functional localization in the brain, a belief held by classical neurologists. The study further demonstrated that there is greater blood flow to the prefrontal cortex, even during rest. Furthermore, the right nondominant hemisphere exhibited greater functional participation in speech than was previously thought, and the supplementary motor area was also important, primarily in dynamic motor activity.

Positron Emission Tomography

PET, a relative recent advancement in neuroimaging, assesses physiologic changes at the cellular level. It entails three steps:

- Tagging radioactive substances (positron isotopes) with one natural body substance (water molecules or glucose)
- Injecting the tagged radionuclide into the body
- Measuring the spatial distribution of the positron (radiation) emitting radioisotopes and their dissipated energy

PET measures glucose and metabolized oxygen distribution by looking at nerve cells and cerebral blood flow. The radionuclide fluorodeoxyglucose (FDG) has been commonly used for determining the local cerebral metabolic rate of glucose by brain cells to study cognitive, language, and speech functions. The principle underlying PET is that the collision of the injected positron with an electron leads to their mutual annihilation and results in the emission of two γ-rays (photons), which travel in opposite directions (i.e., 180° from each other). Detectors circling the brain locate these photons and feed their path into a computer, which generates the images (Fig. 20-10).

Because oxygen metabolism by cells reflects physiologic functioning, PET allows clinicians to study brain physiology that reflects mental and sensorimotor functions. Changes in types of information processing, which depend on the underlying cognitive activity, produce differential neuronal activity patterns in local regions of the brain. PET has been used to examine the physiology of brains in normal individuals and brain-damaged patients to determine the neuroanatomic correlates of different functions (Fig. 20-11). Studies of cellular glucose metabolism in aphasic patients have repudiated the belief that there is a strict localization of functions in the brain. Rather, these images demonstrated that focal brain pathology also affected the function of distant brain regions, commonly the prefrontal cortex, basal ganglia, and thalamus. For a better understanding of the application of PET to neuroanatomic pathologies in aphasic patients, consult these publications: Mazziotta et al. (1981, 1982), Metter (1987), Metter and Hanson (1985), and Metter et al. (1986).

PET is also used for detecting of abnormal brain tissue causing seizures or psychiatric disorders, in which the metabolism of glucose is different from the rest of the brain. Such localization of abnormal brain tissue provides important diagnostic information before surgery.

In addition to functional imaging, PET is also used for identifying the limit and spread of tumors in the body and the brain. Because the tumor cells are generally characterized by metabolism, the affected areas show increased cellular activity, which can be measured using deoxyglucose tagged with fluorine-18. This increased cellular metabolism provides information about tumor spread and helps in planning treatment and in determining disease outcome.

Single Photon Emission Computed Tomography

SPECT is functionally similar to PET, although it provides fewer details. Generally used for refined blood flow measurements, SPECT is performed after injection of a radiotracer substance tagged with a radiopharmaceutical. Tomographic techniques and a γ-camera are used to measure the distribution of the radiopharmaceutical. Unlike PET, which involves dual photon emission, in SPECT the radiopharmaceutical substance emits a single γ-ray. By using the point of γ-emission and its trajectory, SPECT measures rCBF. Via computer, the data can be reconstructed into three-dimensional images of blood flow in the brain (Fig. 20-12). Bhatnagar et al. (1989, 1990) and Tikofsky and Hellman (1991) used SPECT to examine cognitive and language functions in neurosurgery and neurology patients.

SODIUM AMYTAL INFUSION FOR ASSESSING CEREBRAL DOMINANCE

Sodium Amytal infusion, also known as the Wada test, involves the use of sodium amobarbital during angiography to determine hemispheric dominance. Initially introduced by Juhn Wada in the early 1940s, the technique was developed to evaluate language dominance in patients with epilepsy and psychiatric conditions who were receiving electroconvulsant therapy to the hemisphere not responsible for language. With the discovery of surgical management

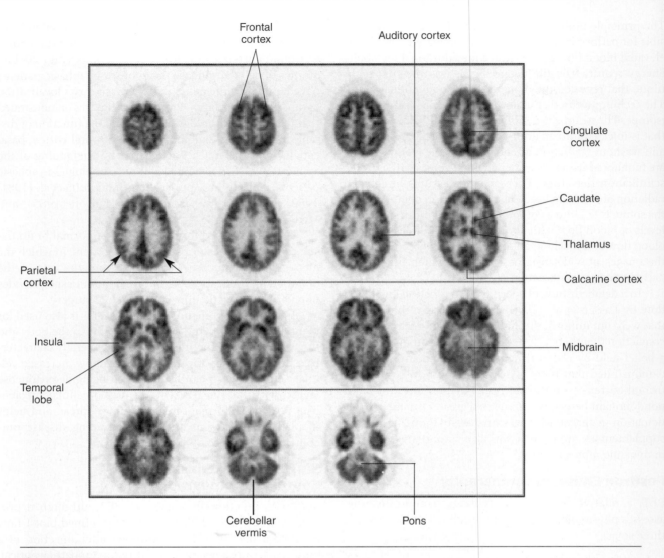

Figure 20-10 PET image of a normal brain.

of epilepsy and corticography undertaken at the Montreal Neurological Institute in 1940s, the use of sodium amobarbital became the standard tool for evaluating language dominance in patients with medically intractable epilepsy.

The intracarotid injection of sodium amobarbital induces a functional loss in the injected hemisphere lasting 2–10 min. The underlying assumption of the test is that interruption of language function after sodium Amytal infusion in either hemisphere should allow clinicians to identify the hemisphere that is dominant for language.

The procedure involves advancing a catheter from the femoral artery, under local anesthesia, into the left carotid artery. An **angiogram** is performed to determine the arterial blood supply to the hemisphere. Then a 100-mg bolus of sodium amobarbital (size of bolus depends on the medical facility) in 1 mL of water (10% solution) is injected over a 4-sec period for maximum effectiveness. The drug is injected while the patient counts and keeps the arms and fingers extended. Within seconds of the drug injection, the effect on the contralateral site of the body is observed as the patient

drops the arm and stops counting. This paralysis onset confirms successful drug infusion into the targeted hemisphere. As the drug anesthetizes one hemisphere, the contralateral arm becomes flaccid. Linguistic functions—ongoing counting and then confrontation naming—are also impaired if the injected hemisphere is dominant for language.

This procedure has been extensively used for exploring the relationship between cerebral dominance and handedness. Do left-handed individuals have left cerebral dominance similar to right-handed individuals? Or do they have a right hemispheric or bilateral language and speech representation? When used to explore this relationship, the Wada test confirmed that most right-handed individuals have left hemispheric dominance for speech (Table 20-3); however, so do most left-handed individuals. This test further revealed that a significant number of left-handed individuals also exhibit right hemisphere language or dual hemisphere language (Wada and Rasmussen 1960).

Recently, an effort was made to unravel the mental lexicon by examining the sequential unfolding of the

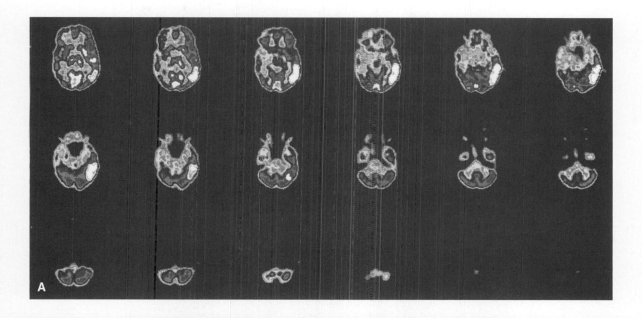

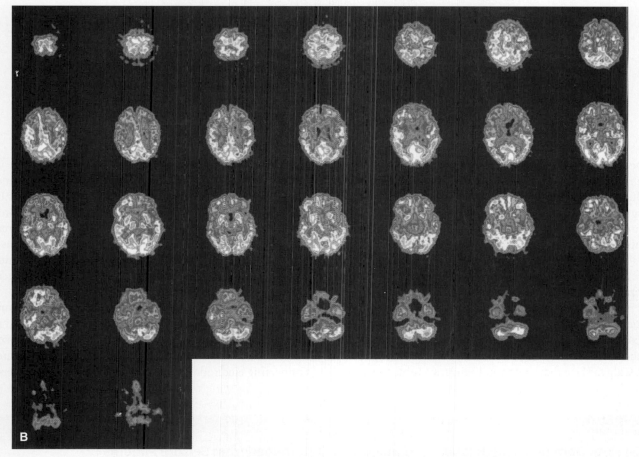

Figure 20-11 A. PET image exhibiting hyperactive metabolic activity in Wernicke area and a left inferior parietal lobule during a seizure. B. PET image indicating hypometabolism in the bifrontal and bitemporal regions in a patient diagnosed with Pick disease.

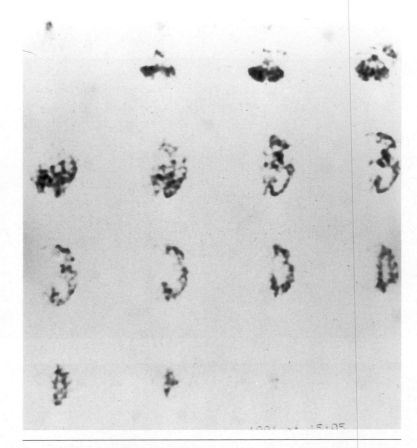

Figure 20-12 SPECT image of a stroke patient showing decreased blood flow in the right hemisphere.

processes of lexical access, retrieval, and production during the recovery of the left hemisphere from a complete drug-induced functional ablation with sodium Amytal in neurosurgical patients. It was noted that the access to the lexicon resumed in a patterned and sequential manner (Bhatnagar et al. 2006).

ELECTROENCEPHALOGRAPHY

Brain cells normally generate electrical activity. The **electroencephalogram** (EEG) provides a graphic representation of the potential differences between two separated points on the scalp surface that represent brain-transmitted electrical potentials or brain waves of the cortex below, specifically of the vertical pyramidal cells. The EEG has 8–16 channels for recording scalp-transmitted electrical activity. EEG brain wave recordings can be made simultaneously from the frontal, parietal, occipital, and temporal scalp areas. Comparisons can be made between corresponding areas of the brain hemispheres and among various areas within a single hemisphere for evaluating symmetry in wave patterns, amplitude, and duration.

Silver chloride metal electrodes (5–10 mm in diameter) are placed on the scalp for electrical recording. Eight basic points corresponding to the frontal, parietal, occipital, and temporal lobes are used. In bipolar recordings, interconnecting electrodes are paired in the sagittal, transverse,

Table 20-3				
Cerebral Dominance in Relation to Handedness, Determined from Seizure Patients				
Handedness	Total Cases	Left Hemisphere (%)	Right Hemisphere (%)	Bilateral (%)
Right	140	96	4	0
Left	122	70	15	15

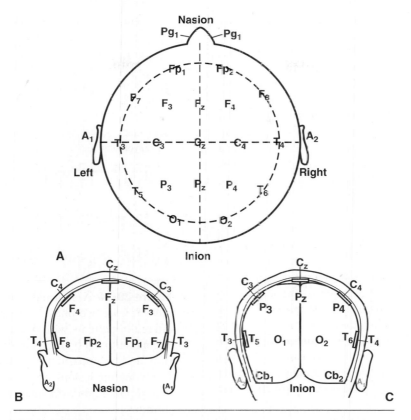

Figure 20-13 Internationally standardized 10–20 system of electrode placement for EEG recordings. **A.** Dorsal view. **B.** Anterior view. **C.** Posterior view.

and circular planes using the internationally standardized 10–20 system of electrode placement (Fig. 20-13). The earlobes and mastoid processes may be used as references for unipolar recordings.

Spontaneous cortical surface activity is generated from the fluctuating voltage differences between the apical and the basal portion of the cortical dendrites. The greatest voltages are found in areas containing masses of dendrites. EEG is an excellent diagnostic procedure for seizures. The dominant electrical brain activity appears to cluster within a few frequency ranges, represented by Greek letters (Table 20-4). There is no specific frequency for particular brain regions, although the α-frequency tends to predominate in the occipital area.

The EEG α-patterns represent normal cortical activity, predominantly in the posterior part of the brain. However, central and temporal regions may also have independent foci of α-rhythms. Eye opening and mental concentration usually suppress α-activity. The fast frequencies of β-rhythms are present in the central and frontal areas. β-Activity has relatively low voltage, usually not more than 20 μV, whereas θ- and δ-activities are not common patterns in normal adults but are seen in children. The central brain areas may contain some θ-patterns, but they do not represent dominant EEG patterns. Brain potentials are measured in microvolts (μV), and the waves may vary from 25 to 300 μV.

A seizure may display 1000-μV discharge amplitudes. Frequencies are usually 0.5–35 cycles per second.

In normal conditions, the electrical patterns in homologous parasagittal areas are similar. In contrast, patterns in the two temporal areas are usually not synchronous. Abnormal brain wave patterns are usually irregular wave combination spikes of high voltage and varied frequencies. Focal discharge areas often display spike or sharp wave reversal patterns (discussed with epilepsy). Similarly, asynchronized brain waves can be used to evaluate consciousness and reduced responsiveness of the brain (discussed with sleep).

Table 20-4

Common Brain Wave Frequencies

Type	Range (μV)
Delta (δ): generalized brain region	1–3
Theta (θ): generalized brain region	4–7
Alpha (α): posterior cortex	8–13
Beta (β): anterior cortex	>13

The EEG is an excellent diagnostic tool to examine altered levels of consciousness, such as sleep, and to evaluate seizure disorders. However, in evaluation of seizures, problems arise in deciding when to perform the test. In some cases, such as grand mal seizures, it is impossible to run an EEG when the patient is having a seizure because of movement artifacts. Routine EEG tests undertaken between seizures may be positive for the diagnosis of the condition in only 70–80% of patients. Specific techniques are used to evoke transient seizure activities for diagnostic reasons. Specific seizure-evoking methods are **hyperventilation**, **photic stimulation**, **sleep induction**, **sleep deprivation**, and **drug administration**.

Hyperventilation is used to activate the epileptic brain, which may be in a state of relative low excitability (quiescence). It is most effective for evoking abnormal discharges in patients with petit mal and psychomotor epilepsies. Photic stimulation, consisting of repeated flashes of light, can also elicit abnormal discharges in idiopathic epilepsy. An exaggerated response may occur in patients with a history of epilepsy. The response is most pronounced over the occipital and posterior parietal areas, especially in the α-frequencies. Sleep is effective for activating discharges in all forms of epilepsy and most productive in psychomotor epilepsy. In addition, sleep deprivation was found to elicit paroxysmal activity in epileptic patients.

ELECTROMYOGRAPHY

Electromyography is the visual record of muscular electrical activity during spontaneous and/or voluntary movements. During contraction, muscle fibers generate action potentials that represent the transmembrane current of muscle fibers. This electrical activity of muscles can be recorded by placing a small electrode on the skin surface over the muscle or by a needle inserted into the muscle.

Electromyography is used to diagnose diseases of the nerves or muscles (muscular atrophy, myoneural junction disorder, and denervation) when clinical evidence is absent or equivocal or must be confirmed. An examination of the quality, speed, and magnitude of electrical impulses in muscles can help detect nerve or muscle damage (Fig. 20-14). It can also differentiate among muscle disease (myopathy), atrophy of spinal motor neurons (anterior horn cell disease), disorders of the nerves (neuropathy), interruption of the nerve supply (denervation), and neuromuscular (myoneural) problems.

Muscle pathologies are determined by comparisons made with normal patterns of muscle electrical activities. For example, there is no electrical activity in a normally functioning muscle during rest. In addition, the electrical potentials that result from the nerve irritation consequent to electrode insertion do not last more than about a second in normal muscle tissues. This provides a point for the interpretation of pathologic patterns in muscles. In dener-

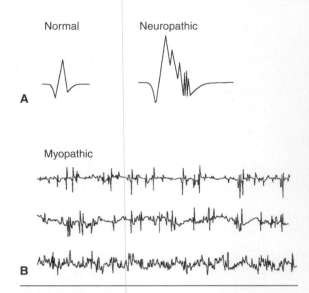

Figure 20-14 A. Normal motor action potentials have at least two phases. The phasic profile is altered in patients with neuropathic lesions and is characterized by high amplitude, long duration, and polyphasic motor unit action potentials. B. Myopathic lesions produce polyphasic motor action potentials with small amplitude and short duration.

vated (interrupted nerve) muscle fibers, for instance, there is spontaneous electrical activity and the insertional potentials can last a long time. Furthermore, denervation produces high-frequency polyphasic discharges, fibrillations, and fasciculations.

In paralyzed and atrophied muscle, there is no spontaneous electrical activity. Low-amplitude, short-lasting motor unit potentials are usually seen in cases of muscle weakness owing to myopathy (muscular disease), involvement of the roots of the peripheral nerve fibers (neuropathy), or the pathology of anterior horn nerve cells (motor neuron disease).

Fibrillation is the spontaneous action potential of a single muscle fiber, whereas fasciculation is the spontaneous discharge from an entire motor unit. Patients with neuromuscular junction disorders may exhibit one of the two following patterns: progressively increasing motor unit action potentials with repetitive stimulation of the motor nerve (as in presynaptic impairment) or gradually decreased response of muscle action potential with repetitive nerve stimulation (as in postsynaptic myoneural junction disease).

Nerve conduction studies are used to identify disorders in the transmission of impulses to muscles. A peripheral nerve along its course is stimulated, and the resultant electrical activity from the muscle is recorded. The latency of impulse, amplitude, speed, and direction of impulse conduction provide important clinical information. Measuring the amplitude of subsequent motor responses provides information about the number of muscle fibers activated, whereas recording nerve impulses at two points along the nerve helps determine the speed (velocity) of the nerve impulse and the time the impulse transmission takes. In denervating diseases, impulse transmission is slow.

EVOKED POTENTIALS

Evoked potentials are the normal electrical activities of the CNS that occur in response to specific and controlled sensory stimulation. Whether the sensory stimulus is visual, somatosensory, or auditory, evoked brain responses are recorded using electrodes placed on the scalp, usually over the respective sensory (visual, somatic, auditory) cortex. The amplitude of the evoked brain responses is quite small, ranging from <1 to 5 μV. The evoked activity can easily be obscured by larger magnitude spontaneous electrical activity in the brain and by myogenic activity. To extract the evoked potentials from non-stimulus-related background activity, signal averaging is used; multiple responses to a single repeated stimulus are amplified, summated, and averaged by a computer. Through averaging, the time-locked stimulus-related evoked activity incrementally builds; the background noise of CNS activity has a mean of 0 and thus cancels itself out in the averaging process. A careful analysis of the latency and amplitude of the evoked response peaks provides significant information about the physiology of neural pathways and possible sites of pathology in the CNS.

Visual Evoked Potential

The visual evoked potential (VEP) test, also called visual evoked response (VER), is used to evaluate electrical conduction along the optic nerve, optic tract, lateral geniculate body, optic radiations, and visual cortex. The eye is stimulated with flashes of light or black- or white-checked patterns, and electrical components of the visual response are recorded from scalp electrodes placed over the occipital area. Total time taken by impulse transmission is about 100 msec. Abnormalities of latencies, amplitudes, and wave patterns may occur in response to abnormalities at specific anatomic sites of electrical transmission. The slowed impulse latency in a VEP test is sensitive to delayed cortical responses, which are invariably affected by the presence of a white matter lesion. The VEP is an important diagnostic test for identifying optic neuritis and multiple sclerosis (probably provides a definite diagnosis).

Somatosensory Evoked Potential

Somatosensory evoked potentials (SEP) are elicited in the CNS through the electrical simulation of a peripheral nerve, such as the median nerve. The SEP wave pattern recorded from the scalp represents the functioning of the structures in the somatosensory pathway to the brain. Electric potentials that result from stimulation of the nerve are recorded from electrodes placed over the contralateral motor strip. The intensity of the stimulation used is just above that needed to elicit a motor response from a muscle group innervated by the stimulated nerve. The latency of the wave gradually increases with distance from the primary sensory area. However, delayed latency or diminished amplitude of sensory evoked potentials indicates PNS and CNS diseases. The lesion may be in the nerves, nerve roots, or spinal cord. Clinical conditions in which somatosensory evoked potentials have diagnostic value include multiple sclerosis, head injuries, brain death, and posterior column spinal cord lesions.

Auditory Evoked Potential

Auditory evoked response testing provides electrophysiologic assessment of the auditory pathways. Neural activity generated in response to the controlled presentation of acoustic stimuli (primarily clicks but also tones and speech sounds) is recorded from the scalp. Evoked response audiometry involves assessing auditory neural pathway function to estimate hearing thresholds in patients who are difficult to test. Auditory evoked potentials can also help identify the site of dysfunction in the auditory system.

The most commonly used auditory evoked potential for evoked response audiometry is the auditory brainstem response (brainstem auditory evoked response; BAER). This is a test of synchronous neural firings from the brainstem auditory pathway occurring within 10 msec of stimulus onset. Five vertex positive wave forms represent the electrical activity produced in the auditory pathway (Fig. 20-15). Wave response classes appear to represent a specific anatomic point in the auditory pathway (Table 20-5). For example, wave I appears to arise from the peripheral and distal fibers of the vestibulocochlear nerve (CN VIII); wave II, from the proximal or brainstem portion of the vestibulocochlear nerve; wave III, from the first brainstem synapse, including the cochlear complex and trapezoid body and waves IV and V, from the auditory pathway to the midbrain, including the lateral lemniscus and inferior colliculus, which besides audition, also provides a three-dimensional neurologic map of the external environment to the body (see Chapter 9). The additional wave patterns are, anatomically and clinically, undermined. The first two wave responses arise ipsilateral to the stimulus, whereas electrical activity above wave III and is thought to be generated contralaterally.

Response parameters include the absolute latencies of all of the waves, interpeak latency intervals, and to a lesser extent, the amplitudes of the waves. Abnormalities in any of these parameters suggests abnormality in the auditory periphery or CNS. BAER is a reliable tool for diagnosing tumors of the inner ear (acoustic neuroma) and auditory axonal pathology (multiple sclerosis). It can also be used to monitor brainstem function intraoperatively. Furthermore, BAER can be used as a criterion for determining brain death.

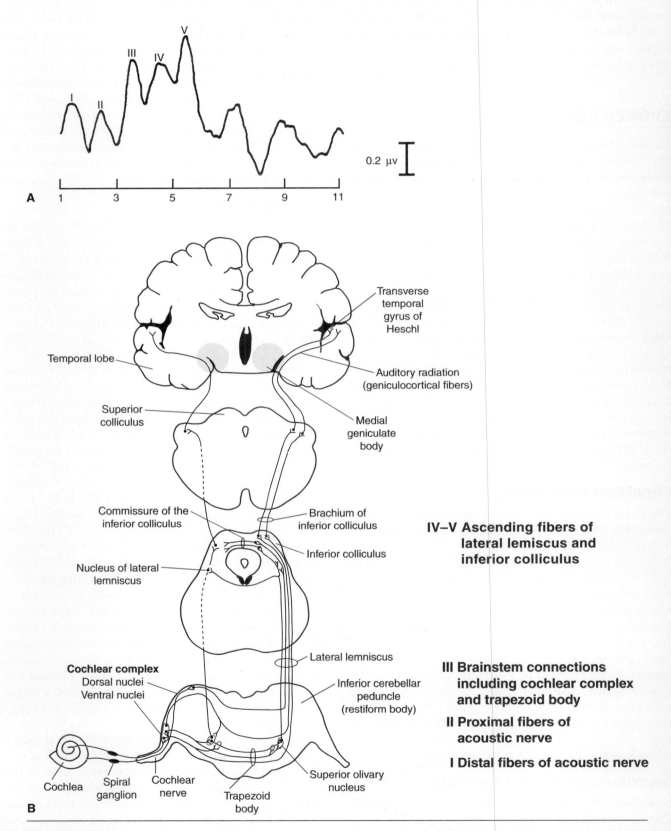

Figure 20-15 A. Normal brainstem auditory evoked responses within 10 msec from the onset of clicks. B. The relationship of the anatomic levels (*I–V*) of the auditory pathway to the brainstem response wave patterns.

Table 20-5

Wave Peaks of the Auditory Brainstem Response and Their Probable Site of Origin

Wave Number	Probable Site of Wave Pattern
I	Distal fibers of cranial nerve VIII
II	Proximal fibers of cranial nerve VIII
III	Brainstem connections, including the cochlear complex and trapezoid body
IV–V	Ascending fibers of the lateral lemniscus and inferior colliculus

The fifth peak (wave V) is the most prominent, and the threshold of this wave is found to correlate well with behavioral hearing thresholds. Latencies of waves I–V at various stimulus intensities and interwave latencies (i.e., I–V, I–II, II–V) are used to assess central conduction in the auditory brainstem. This can provide important information about the site of the lesion. Altered wave morphology and delayed peak latencies in the presence of adequate peripheral hearing indicate retrocochlear lesions. For example, a tumor in the cerebellopontine angle, affecting the vestibulocochlear nerve, may abolish waves III–V or produce a prolonged interpeak latency between waves I and III. Prolonged interpeak latencies and abnormal waveforms are commonly seen in multiple sclerosis, a demyelinating condition. However, if all wave patterns except the first are absent or abnormal, a structural brainstem abnormality is likely to be the cause.

DICHOTIC LISTENING

Commonly used for assessing cerebral dominance, **dichotic listening** is a noninvasive neuropsychologic tool that uses auditory stimuli. It involves presenting simultaneous but slightly different auditory stimuli to both ears. The atten-tion factors are minimized by requiring patients to attend to both ears simultaneously and report the stimuli they perceive. When the linguistic material presented in both ears is largely similar and spoken in the same voice, attending to the stimuli from both ears poses processing difficulties. Even though an equal number of words is presented, subjects do not demonstrate a twofold gain, which would account for each item presented to both ears. Instead, the total stimuli reported from both ears range from 125% to 150%. Loss of information has been invariably greater for stimuli presented to the left and supposedly nondominant ear by 20–25%. This results in a natural right ear advantage.

This left ear–specific loss of linguistic information and right ear superiority were investigated in the pioneering work of Kimura (1967) at the Montreal Neurological Institute in the 1960s. She attributed the right ear advantage to its direct anatomic projections to the left hemisphere, which is dominant for language and speech (Fig. 20-16). The indirect anatomic projection to the language cortex accounts for the left ear–specific information loss. The neurolinguistic implications of these findings are that right ear performance can serve as an index for determining degrees of language lateralization.

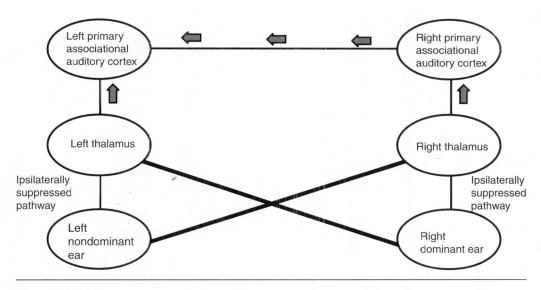

Figure 20-16 Ear projections to the auditory cortex during a dichotic listening task.

Support for the stronger contralateral auditory projections in dichotic listening came when the dichotic test results were validated by the observation of the left language lateralization by hemispheric infusion of sodium amobarbital (Milner and Branch 1967).

LUMBAR PUNCTURE

The **lumbar puncture** (spinal tap) is used for diagnosing various infections and hemorrhages of the CNS that are not observable through CT. Deviations from the normal compositional values (protein = 15–45 mg/dL, glucose = 50–70 mg/dL, and white blood cells = 1–5/mL) are considered diagnostically important. Chemical analysis of the CSF also helps in the differential diagnosis of **multiple sclerosis**, **neurosyphilis**, **Guillain-Barré syndrome**, **carcinomatous meningitis**, and **neuropathies**. Lumbar puncture is contraindicated in cases of increased intracranial pressure because of the possibility of a brainstem herniation.

In lumbar puncture, a needle is inserted into the lumbar subarachnoid space while the patient leans forward (recumbent position) or lies on his or her side. The puncture is usually made between the L3 and L4 vertebrae because spinal penetration at this point does not cause any injury to the cord or nerve roots (Fig. 2-33). Once the CSF starts flowing, the needle hub is attached to a manometer. The normal CSF pressure in an adult is 80–150 cm H_2O, which may rise to 200 cm H_2O when the person is seated. Increased intracranial pressure occurs in response to increased amounts of CSF, brain swelling, and brain tumor. A pressure level higher than normal suggests a pathologic process. Ventricular pressure can also be measured by other invasive methods, such as inserting a catheter into the lateral ventricles.

NEUROSURGICAL PROCEDURES

Craniotomy and Cortical Mapping

Craniotomy is undertaken to remove diseased brain tissue. Cortical stimulation brain mapping is used to avoid damaging sensorimotor and speech–language areas during cortical resections for seizures, tumors, and aneurysms.

Focal external electric stimulation is based on observations by Fritsch and Hitzig (1870) and Bartholow (1874), who found that electric current externally applied to the exposed brain altered sensorimotor functions in animals and humans. After the safety and reliability of focal stimulation were established, stimulation mapping became a standard part of surgical treatment for medically intractable epilepsy and was used to map the somatosensory cortex and to chart the human brain for memory and language at the Montreal Neurological Institute (Penfield and Roberts, 1959). Completed under local anesthesia while the patients remained awake, focal stimulation was used first to determine the stimulation threshold that produced after discharges and second to determine whether the diseased part of the brain was critical for language and sensorimotor functions.

Because many language functions take place around the diseased part of the brain, mapping of language in and around the area of pathology helps neurosurgeons determine whether it is safe to remove the diseased cortical tissues without any unacceptable loss, primarily of higher mental functions (speech, language, and memory) and secondarily of sensorimotor functions. This mapping also helps determine the size and extent of the tissue that can be safely resected. As a rule of thumb, no tissue resection is undertaken from the somatosensory area in the fronto-parietotemporal cortex unless there is pre-existing hemiplegia or the diseased tissue is not involved with language.

In the post-Penfield era, this technique was extensively used to treat patients with epilepsy and in surgical management of other conditions, such as tumors and AVMs. Focal stimulation acts like a reversible lesion of the brain, ranging from 4 to 8 sec; its interruption lasts only for the duration of the applied current. Furthermore, the stimulation-induced interruption provides precise details about functional localization because the lesion is only 0.5–3 mm in diameter. The technique is not known to leave any lingering effect and/or postoperative aphasia. Carefully controlled stimulation parameters pose no safety concern to patients, cause no injury to the examined brain tissue, and produce no evidence of acute inflammation to the mapped region of the brain. Multiple samples of a single behavior from a single site allow for the necessary statistical analysis and can help determine whether the evoked linguistic errors are significant.

Interpretation of the physiologic effects of focal stimulation is based on the interference it produces during ongoing activity. For example, if stimulation at a cortical site disrupts ongoing naming or speaking, the cortical area in question is considered to be functional for the task (Fig. 20-17). If the stimulation does not block or alter the naming or speaking process, the stimulated area is not considered to be involved in the ongoing activity. Although evoking distant effects of the applied stimulation remains a possibility, the low current levels (below sensorimotor threshold) rule out any distant propagation of the current. The short duration of the applied current trains to the brain, however, is the only limitation of the technique.

The operation is performed under local anesthesia to maintain a conscious patient who can participate in neurolinguistic testing. The patient answers questions while the cortex is stimulated with a bipolar electrode for a brief period. Stimulated areas that disrupt speech and/or produce motor movements are avoided during the resection of the lesion. The procedure of focal electric stimulation has been extensively used for mapping the language cortex in humans (Andy and Bhatnagar 1983; Bhatnagar et al. 2000; Ojemann 1983, 1989; Ojemann and Whitaker 1978; Penfield and Roberts, 1959).

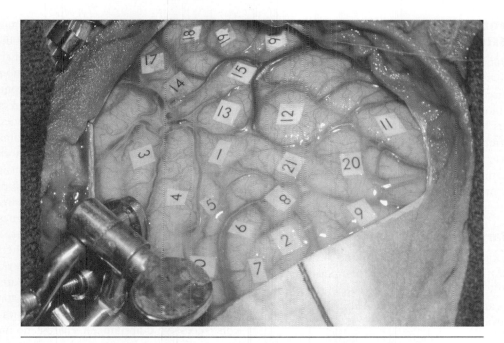

Figure 20-17 Exposed brain during electrocorticography. *Numbered tickets,* sites that were functionally mapped during intraoperative neurolinguistic testing. Many of these sites have been associated with language and memory functions.

Stereotactic Surgery and Subcortical Mapping

Stereotactic surgery involves placing a lesion or stimulus electrode at a precise subcortical location to manage involuntary movements and intractable pain. The subcortical brain structures are mapped by electrical stimulation for guidance while the patient is under local anesthesia. Mapping optimizes the beneficial results from the involvement of normal structures. Two examples of stereotactic surgery are a lesion or stimulation in the **subthalamus** or the ventrolateral nucleus of the thalamus that is used to treat Parkinsonian tremor and a lesion or stimulation in the **globus pallidus** is used to treat parkinsonian tremor and rigidity.

Investigators have examined subcortical participation in speech, language, and verbal memory by stimulating discrete subcortical areas through chronically implanted depth electrodes. Ojemann (1983) notes facilitation of verbal recall via the application of stimulation parameters below the threshold for induced language disturbance during a left thalamotomy. He attributes this effect on the registration and recall of verbal stimuli to the thalamic evoked **alerting response mechanism.** Bhatnagar et al. (1989 and 2005) note a similar facilitatory effect on verbal memory from stimulation of the left **centrum medianum,** a neurolinguistically unexplored and previously unimplicated intralaminar thalamic nucleus with rich cortical and subcortical projections. Bhatnagar et al. (1990) also report a similar, though quantitatively different, facilitatory effect on verbal

memory from the stimulation of the right centromedianus nucleus of the thalamus. These observations of facilitatory neurolinguistic effects from subcortical stimulation have opened a new avenue of research.

Cordotomy

Cordotomy, a procedure used relatively infrequently, involves sectioning the **lateral spinothalamic** tract to relieve chronic pain; it is performed when medication proves ineffective. The operation is performed under local anesthesia so that the patient can tell the surgeon when the pain is relieved and in which part of the body it is no longer felt. The ventrolateral spinothalamic tract of the cord is sectioned on the side opposite to the painful body part (see Chapter 7). The sectioning is performed three segments above the top segment level of pain. The spinal cord attachments of the **dentate ligament** are used as a reference point for sectioning the cord. They mark the plane between the overlying **pyramidal tract** and the underlying spinothalamic pain-conducting tract to be sectioned. The level of the sectioning is usually in the thoracic spinal cord for pain below the dermatomal nipple line. The cervical spinal cord is sectioned to eliminate pain in the upper extremities, shoulders, and neck.

Recently stimulation of the cord using a chronically implanted electrode has also been use to relive intractable pain. In this procedure, an electrode is placed in the spinal canal over the cord, and it is stimulated through a battery-operated unit implanted subcutaneously in the infraclavicular fossa.

Internal Carotid–External Carotid Anastomosis

A decrease in blood supply to the cortex and subcortical structures occurs when a blood vessel is occluded by a thrombosis, caused by either an embolus or a local sclerotic plaque. As the blood supply is impeded, brain tissue distal to the thrombus loses function. Restoration of the blood supply is performed by anastomosing the distal segment of the occluded artery to the superficial temporal artery. This surgery is performed through a craniotomy. At present, the benefits of this procedure are doubtful. It is used only in selected patients.

Carotid Endarterectomy

Occlusive sclerotic plaques are usually found at the region of common carotid bifurcation. Carotid endarterectomy is most frequently performed for occlusions of the **common and/or internal carotid arteries**. Carotid clamps are used for temporary occlusion of the vessel above and below the level of the thrombus. The thrombotic plaque is removed surgically through an incision overlying the thrombosed arterial site. The sclerotic plaque, which lines the inside of the vessel and occludes it, is removed by scraping it away from the inner vessel wall. The incision in the vessel wall is sutured after the plaque is removed; the temporary blood vessel clamps are released, and blood flow is re-established. Newer surgical technology involves placing a stent in the cleaned artery to prevent future plaque formation and the use of a filter to capture any dislodged plaque fragments. Development of powerful catheters has allowed surgeons to place stents in the smaller branches of the middle cerebral artery.

Aneurysm Clipping

An aneurysm is a bulging defect of the blood vessel wall that looks like a protruding nipple or balloon attached to the vessel. Aneurysms that hemorrhage or cause neurologic deficits and seizures require immediate attention. The medical management of an aneurysm involves lowering blood pressure to prevent bleeding; clipping is used to obliterate the neck or attachment of the aneurysm to the blood vessels, thus disabling it. Aneurysms are also treated without opening the skull through coiling, which involves placing a platinum coil in the aneurysm. This coil causes a blood clot to form, sealing off the aneurysm.

GENETIC INHERITANCE

The way in which an organism passes its physical attributes to its offspring is the subject of genetics. What we know about inheritance and genetic transmission can be traced to the late-19th-century work of Gregor Mendel, who observed several patterns of inherited traits by examining the crossings of different-colored flowers and pea plants.

Genes regulate the formation, distribution, and growth of cells in an embryo. The blueprint for these processes is received from both parents at the time of conception. After passing through mitotic and meiotic divisions, each parental germ cell (oogonia and spermatogonia) contains 22 somatic chromosomes and one sex chromosome (see Chapter 4). At conception, cells from the two parents combine their genetic material to form a zygote that contains 44 (22 + 22) autosomal chromosomes and either 2 X chromosomes or 1 X and 1 Y chromosomes. The genes consist of 6–7 billion base pairs of DNA arranged linearly in 23 pairs of chromosomes. Each coiled chromosome contains tens of thousands of genes. One or more pairs of genes received from the parents regulate most physical traits, such as height, hair color, body shape, aptitude, and others.

Among these thousands of genes, everyone carries a few dysfunctional genes. Some diseases are caused by one faulty gene (**dominant inheritance**), and some morbid conditions occur when a defective gene comes from both parents (**recessive inheritance**). There is no immunity against genetic illness, and large numbers of serious disorders are associated with chromosome abnormalities. Chromosomal errors occur primarily during the formation of germ cells, when meiotic processes that are supposed to reduce the chromosomes to the haploid number (23) produce a gamete cell with an extra or missing chromosome.

Most trisomies (three copies of a particular chromosome) cause severe developmental deficits and mental retardation. Three common trisomy syndromes are **Down syndrome** (trisomy 21), **Edward syndrome** (trisomy 18), and **Patau syndrome** (trisomy 13). Incidentally, most (75%) severe chromosomal malformations result in spontaneous abortion and >40% of infants born with abnormalities die. Errors of genetic inheritance also have implications for altered physiologic functions, such as metabolic, endocrine, and neurologic diseases.

Tracing the distribution of genes in the extended family is an important concept for understanding inheritance. Investigators use standard symbols to construct pedigrees, charts used in genetics to analyze inheritance and to show ancestral history (Fig. 20-18).

Mendel related his observations to the mathematical probability of inheritance. Most mathematical patterns of gene expression are calculated on the basis of gene penetration. However, if gene expression is not fully penetrated, the genetic traits may not follow the exact mathematical pattern. There are three common modes of genetic inheritance: **dominant**, **recessive**, and **X-linked**.

Dominant Inheritance

Even a single faulty gene can pass on a dominant autosomal genetic disease (Fig. 20-19). A child has a chance of receiving this kind of disease if he or she has one parent affected with the disorder. The defective gene dominates the gene from the other parent with which it is paired. In these cases, there is a 50% probability for each child to inherit the dis-

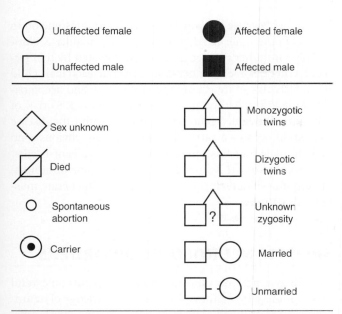

Figure 20-18 Symbols used when creating pedigree charts.

ease. At the same time, of course, there is a 50% chance that the child will not receive the faulty gene. Diseases inherited through dominant genes exhibit various degrees of symptoms, with severity ranging from mild to moderate, and most appear late in life. There are >2000 known dominant autosomal disorders, but the most pertinent to students in communicative disorders is **Huntington** chorea, a progres-

sive degenerative disease that is characterized by movement disorders and cognitive impairments.

Recessive Inheritance

Recessive inheritance requires that both parents carry the faulty gene and transmit that gene to the child (Fig. 20-20). If one parent alone is a carrier of the dysfunctional gene, this gene is not likely to be harmful because it is dominated by the normal gene that is received from the other parent. With so many genes passing from parents, it is quite rare for both parents to be affected with the same faulty gene; consequently, there is a low probability of this type of transmission. However, if both parents carry the faulty gene, a child is at risk for major birth defects. In such cases, each child has a 25% chance of inheriting the disease, a 25% chance of not inheriting the disease, and a 50% chance of receiving the faulty gene from one parent, which would make the child a carrier of the dysfunctional gene. The child's probability of getting an autosomal recessive disorder is very high if the parents have common ancestors or are close relatives. Some well-known recessive disorders are **cystic fibrosis** and **Tay-Sachs disease**.

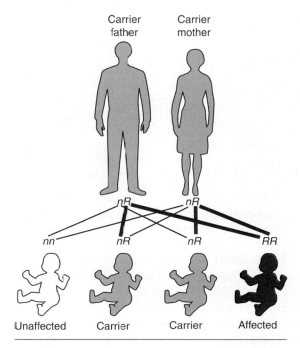

Figure 20-20 In simple recessive inheritance, both parents, usually unaffected, carry a normal gene (n) that takes precedence over its faulty counterpart (R). Each child has the following chances of inheritance: a 25% risk of inheriting two mutant R genes and thus having a serious birth defect; a 25% chance of inheriting two normal n genes and thus being an unaffected noncarrier; and a 50% chance of inheriting one n and one R gene and thus being an unaffected carrier.

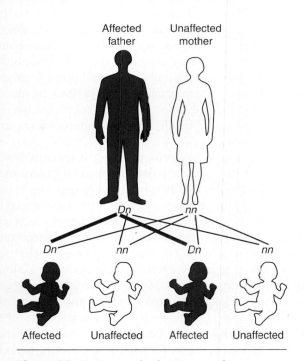

Figure 20-19 In simple dominant inheritance, one affected parent has a single faulty gene (D) that dominates its normal counterpart (n). Each child's chance of inheriting D or n from the affected parent is 50%.

X-Linked Inheritance

Males and females carry different sex chromosomes; males have one X and one Y chromosome (XY), whereas females have two X chromosomes (XX). Consequently, a female has pairs of the genes found on the X chromosome, whereas a male cannot because he has only one X chromosome. If a fertilized egg receives an X chromosome from each of the parents, the child will be female; if the fertilized egg received an X chromosome from its mother and a Y chromosome from its father, the child will be male.

X-linked inheritance involves the genes situated in the X chromosome. Generally, it is the mother who carries a faulty gene in one of her X chromosomes (Fig. 20-21). If a boy inherits a defective X-linked gene, he received it from

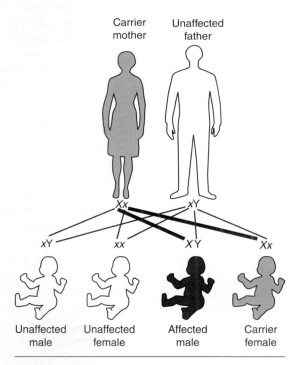

Carrier mother   Unaffected father

Xx   xY

xY   xx   X Y   Xx

Unaffected male   Unaffected female   Affected male   Carrier female

Figure 20-21 The most common form of X-linked inheritance. The unaffected, carrier mother has one faulty gene (*X*) and one normal gene (*x*), which are located on the X chromosome. The father has a normal *X* gene on the X chromosome and a normal Y chromosome. Each male child has the following chances of inheritance from his mother: a 50% risk of inheriting the faulty *X* gene and thus having the disorder and a 50% chance of inheriting the normal *x* gene and thus being normal and a noncarrier. Each female child has the following chances of inheritance from her mother: a 50% risk of inheriting one faulty *X* gene and thus being a normal carrier and a 50% chance of inheriting the normal *X* gene and thus being a normal noncarrier.

his mother because his father passes a Y chromosome on to a son. On the other hand, if a girl receives a faulty X chromosome from her mother, it will be dominated by the normal X chromosome from her father. Overall, each male child has a 50% risk of inheriting the faulty gene and accompanying disorder. Although each female has a 50% risk of inheriting the faulty gene, she will not exhibit the disease but would become a carrier like her mother. Obviously, no male-to-male transmission of a faulty X-linked gene occurs. Commonly known X-linked diseases are **color blindness**, **hemophilia** (blood clotting disorder), and **Duchenne muscular dystrophy**.

SPECIFIC NEUROLOGIC DISORDERS

Neurology is a highly clinical field that depends on careful observations of symptoms. It requires knowledge of neuroanatomy to clinically appraise co-occurring symptoms. Any alteration in neuronal functioning results in specific sensorimotor disturbances. Some of these disorders were examined in the "Clinical Concerns" section that appears in most chapters; disorders and medical concepts not previously covered are briefly discussed here.

Seizures and Epilepsy

Seizures are sensory, motor, cognitive, and affective disorders that result from abnormal electrical discharges in the brain (Fig. 20-22). Epilepsy refers to recurring seizures. Approximately 70–75% of seizures occur before age 20 and >30% of them occur before age 4 or 5. Seizures are mostly associated with high fever and may not be recurrent. The causative factors in 50% of seizure disorders are metabolic abnormalities, tumors, infarcts, infections, and physiologic disturbances. Among the remaining 50% of patients, no specific cause can be detected. Some factors that cause seizure disorders are **perinatal insult**, **trauma**, **anoxia**, **tumor**, and **metabolic disorders**.

In a normal brain, electrical activity is remarkably stable, and nerve membrane polarization and depolarization are delicately balanced. However, in epilepsy, the brain's electrical activity becomes unstable. It is characterized by a prolonged high-frequency neuronal discharge, which represents rapid and excessive depolarization of membrane potentials (Fig. 20-22). The seizures occur when electrical activity in one or more brain structures rises above a critical threshold. Epileptic discharge can recruit neighboring and functionally related neuronal elements, and thus it replicates itself while spreading from one area to another. During the course of frequently recurring epileptic discharges, some neurons remain quiescent (nonactive) for varying periods, representing excessive depolarization (fatigue) or hyperpolarization (inhibition).

Epileptic seizures are commonly divided into two types: **partial** and **generalized**. Partial seizures are further divided into **partial focal** (**simple**) and **partial complex**, and gener-

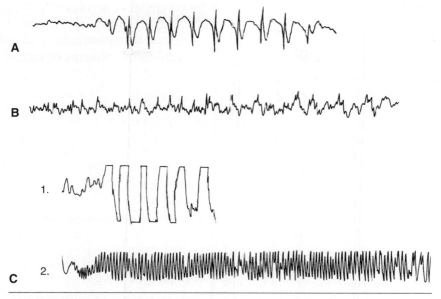

Figure 20-22 Electroencephalographic studies showing high amplitude discharges and repeated spikes representing abnormal electrical activity during a seizure. A. Petite mal (absence) epilepsy in a 15-year-old boy. B. Psychomotor epilepsy. C. Grand mal (tonic–clonic) epilepsy with two frequency patterns.

alized seizures may be either **petit mal (absence)** or **grand mal (tonic–clonic)** seizures (Table 20-6).

Partial/Focal or Simple Epilepsy

Partial focal (simple) epilepsy is usually caused by a single cortical or subcortical lesion. Symptoms are characterized by sudden onset of sensory and/or motor behaviors confined to a single body part, such as the leg, arm, or face, depending on the lesion site. For example, a lesion in the motor cortex may generate jerking of the arm. Involvement of the sensory cortex causes altered sensory perception, such as numbness or tingling. Spread of the abnormal discharge activity to adjacent cortical areas recruits other body parts into the seizure. The progressive recruitment of other body parts is called the **Jacksonian march** after the English

neurologist who first described it. For example, a Jacksonian seizure may start in the foot and spread to the lower leg, thigh, abdomen, shoulder, and arm. A jacksonian sensory spread may start as a tingling sensation in the thumb that spreads to the fingers, forearm, upper arm, and shoulder.

An aura is a focal seizure characterized by a specific sensory experience that precedes the full-blown seizure. Auras are warnings of impending seizures. Patients generally remember the aura but do not remember the automatic behavior during the temporal lobe seizure that emanates from the amygdala and hippocampus. In some cases of focal epilepsy, medication may be effective. However, in other cases, focal epilepsy responds best to localized surgical removal of the lesion and surrounding seizing brain tissue.

Table 20-6

Classification of Seizures

Partial Seizures	Focal: rhythmic spike and/or slow-wave focal discharges with sensorimotor, visceral, and/or emotional symptoms Complex: Abnormal electrical activity in amygdala, hippocampus, septum, mesodiencephalic, and association cortices with complex sensorimotor, visceral, and emotional symptoms
Generalized seizures	Petit mal: symmetrical 3-Hz spike and wave with brief episodes of automatisms Grand mal: high-voltage spike and wave activities with varied frequencies and duration, usually associated with loss of consciousness and tonic–clonic movements

Partial Complex, or Psychomotor, Seizures

Partial complex (psychomotor) seizures are the result of congenital and postnatal lesions of the medial temporal lobe structures consisting of the amygdala, hippocampus, and overlying temporal cortex. These types of seizures, occurring most frequently in adults and older age groups, are characterized by recurring episodes of automatic, irrational behavior of which there usually is no memory. The individual is cognizant of neither the actions nor the consequences of them. In addition, the patient may have episodes of aggressive behavior. There are also notable cognitive deficits characterized by inattentiveness, unclear thinking, compulsive thoughts, sensory illusions, and apathy. These types of automatic behavior occur in complex partial seizures because the discharge spreads to the cortical association areas and thereby impairs the mechanisms of thought. The automatic actions represent programmed behaviors that are released from inhibition because they no longer are under direct control of the prefrontal associational cortex. In contrast, the premotor and primary sensorimotor cortices are spared. The emotional components of automatism related to mood, sexuality, and aggression are generated in the hypothalamus and integrated with the cortically programmed behaviors at the level of the diencephalon and brainstem.

Petit Mal, or Absence, Seizures

Petit mal (absence) seizures occur in children aged 3–12, and they usually disappear after the 3rd decade of life. These seizures involve a brief loss of awareness and are often associated with staring, chewing, blinking, and occasional myoclonic jerks. A dominant familial predisposition is evident. The electrical discharge is primarily thought to involve a reverberating circuit between the cortex, thalamus, and brainstem reticular formation. The EEG brain wave pattern consists of a slow wave with spikes appearing at three per second. Drug therapy is effective in controlling this type of seizure.

Grand Mal, or Tonic–Clonic, Seizures

Grand mal (tonic–clonic) seizures usually involve the cortex, basal ganglia, diencephalon, and brainstem reticular formation. Symptoms of grand mal seizures include loss of consciousness followed by tonic convulsions consisting of repeated hyperextension of the body (tonic–clonic convulsions) and breath-holding spells resulting in cyanosis and tongue biting (Table 20-7). The average length of a tonic–clonic seizure is 1–3 min. At the end of the seizure, the patient remains tired and listless for ~1 hr. During the seizure, the EEG reveals high-frequency spikes.

A hereditary predisposition is thought to be the underlying substrate for grand mal epilepsy. The precipitating factors consist of strong emotional stimuli, hyperventilation, drugs, fever, infections, and physical stimuli such as loud noises and flashing lights. A grand mal seizure may last for several minutes before it stops completely. It is thought that two factors bring about the termination of these seizures: fatigue of the firing neurons and neuronal inhibition.

Table 20-7

General Symptoms Associated with Tonic–Clonic Phases of Grand Mal Seizures

Tonic Phase	Clonic Phase
Unconsciousness	Alternate muscle relaxation
Failing to ground	Tongue biting
Spasticity in muscles	Salivation
Transient interruption of breathing	Turning blue

Antiepileptic Drugs

Diphenylhydantoin (phenytoin, or Dilantin), **phenobarbital**, **valproate**, and **carbamazepine** (Tegretol) are the four commonly used antiepileptic drugs. With these therapeutic drugs, there usually is a marked reduction of paroxysmal discharge, and consequently the seizures are controlled. Drug combinations are often used, especially for complex syndromes made up of two or more seizure types. If drug therapy is inadequate and if it is feasible, the discharging brain tissue is surgically removed.

Sleep and Altered Consciousness

As a diagnostic tool of cortical activity, the EEG is used to differentiate between altered states of consciousness such as **stupor**, **coma**, and **brain death**; an additional term related to altered consciousness is **acute confusional state**. EEG is also used to measure brain activity during **sleep**, which is another state of mind. The cerebral cortex, which is active during periods of wakefulness, controls sensorimotor activity through a stream of impulses that diminish during sleep. The cortical activity in the awakened state is regulated by the projections of the **reticular activating system** (RAS), which is responsible for cortical activation and arousal and regulates the levels of consciousness. The RAS itself can be activated by any internal or external stimulus. Reduced activation of the RAS lowers consciousness and responsiveness (see Chapter 16). Only a massive pathology of the cerebral cortex and/or thalamus bilaterally or of the reticular formation is associated with a profound loss of consciousness.

Acute confusional state, also known as **delirium**, is the least impaired level of consciousness. It is marked by confusion, psychomotor excitability distractibility, agitation, and disorientation; additional attributes are slowed thinking, reduced processing, reduced information integration, and incoherent thinking subsequent to CNS dysfunctioning. Linguistically, this stage of confusion is marked by incomplete thoughts, paraphasia, and semantically anomalous verbal output. The patient is not clear about time and space.

Stupor is a level of significantly altered consciousness. Patients in stupor are minimally conscious and can be brought to a higher level of consciousness only through a strong stimulus, such as pain. Even after consciousness is regained, the individual may not fully participate in any activity and may lapse back into stupor. Coma, a deeper state of impaired consciousness, is a profoundly decreased level of wakefulness in which the patient remains unresponsive to painful stimuli and cannot be awakened. There is general amnesia for the duration of the coma in patients who recover.

Brain death, an irreversible form of unconsciousness, is characterized by a completely nonfunctional cerebral cortex, while the basic brainstem reflexes—breathing and heartbeat control—may be preserved. Also called persistent vegetative state, patients are incognizant of the environment, display no cognitive function, lack responsiveness to commands but breathe on their own, open eyes, and follow sleep-wake cycle. Keeping such a person alive has become a bioethical issue that has been extensively debated.

Sleep, although an active state of mind, is different from wakefulness and is characterized by diminished responsiveness. It is an important physiologic state for replenishing body energy. Deprivation of sleep has been found to affect the quality of cortical functions and has been associated with difficulty in reasoning, attending, self-monitoring, and maintaining concentration. Sleep-deprived individuals are irritable and fatigued.

Normal sleep consists of two categories: **rapid eye movement (REM)** and **non-rapid eye movement (NREM)**. NREM sleep further consists of four stages (Fig. 20-23). The EEG correlates of sleep are measured by the increased degree of the dominance of two slow waves—θ and δ—which become more and more synchronized as one enters the cycle of sleep.

One enters the REM and NREM stages many times during the sleep cycle. In the REM stage, the representative EEG pattern remains desynchronized, similar to the one seen in the awake stage (Fig. 20-24). It is characterized by mixed electric wave frequencies, with θ- and decreased α-activity (1–2 cycles/sec lower than waking). However,

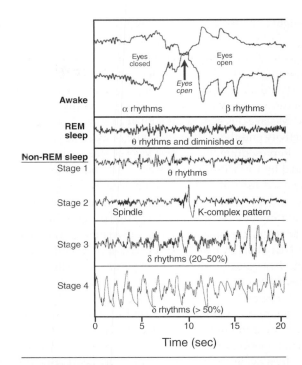

Figure 20-24 EEG rhythms during the stages of rapid eye movement (*REM*) and non-REM sleep.

there is substantial inhibition of sensory systems and the motor neurons in the spinal cord and brainstem. This immobilizes skeletal muscles except for the muscles of eye and diaphragm. On the one hand, the dominance of the parasympathetic system during REM slows down important body systems by lowering respiration, blood pressure, heartbeat, and body temperature. On the other hand, it increases gastric mobility. Disconnected from the external stimuli during this stage, the CNS becomes sensitive to internally generated signals, as seen by the imagery experiences of dreams, which are accompanied by rapid movements of the eyes. Events like dreams, nightmare, erection, and bed wetting, of which individuals may not retain any memory, are known to occur at this stage.

The rest of sleep time is spent in NREM sleep, which is marked by a greater synchronization of electroencephalographic rhythms. In NREM sleep, muscle tension is significantly reduced, and movement, though possible, is minimal. This movement is usually limited to the movements that change body position, if needed. The energy consumption of the body remains low because of the dominance of the parasympathetic system. In terms of electrical functioning, the slow EEG rhythms with large amplitude represent the synchronized neuronal activity at this stage.

During NREM sleep, a person progresses from stage 1 to stage 4; each of the stages is identified by a distinctive EEG pattern (Fig. 20-23). For example, stage 1, also called quiet wakefulness, is characterized by low-amplitude θ-EEG activity replacing the high-frequency α-wave pattern. The individual is fully relaxed, with eyes closed and fleeting

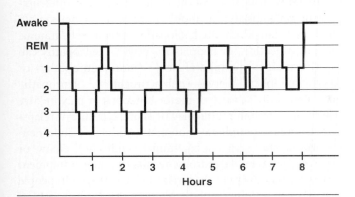

Figure 20-23 Typical time spent in the stages of rapid eye movement (*REM*) sleep.

thoughts. In terms of EEG activity, this stage is hard to distinguish from the REM stage. NREM stage 2 is marked by the emergence of short sharp bursts of α-waves, known as high-amplitude sleep spindles (12- to 14-Hz wave pattern) and K complexes in the presence of background θ-activity; the person at this stage is easily to awaken. NREM stage 3 is somewhat similar to stage 2, with 20–50% δ-activity and the sleeper in a state of extreme relaxation.

Representing the deepest level of sleep, stage 4 is dominated by >50% δ-electrical waves. The person at this stage is relaxed and difficult to awaken. Sleepwalking, sleep talking, and sleep terror are known to occur during δ-sleep, which includes stages 3 and 4. After progressing through these stages, one may reverse to different stages until reaching NREM stage 1 or REM level, completing the sleeping cycle. In a typical 7- to 8-hr sleep period, an individual alternates from NREM to REM stage every 70–120 min. This cycle repeats 3–5 times during the entire sleep period.

There are many sleep-related problems, such as disorders of initiating and maintaining sleep during normal sleeping periods, excessive daytime sleepiness, disorders of the sleep cycle, and dysfunctions associated with various stages of sleep. **Insomnia** (inability to initiate and maintain sleep during normal hours) is a common problem and is usually associated with such conditions as stress or emotional changes in life, most of which are temporary. **Hypersomnia**, or sleeping during normal waking hours, is caused by dysfunction of sleep

Narcolepsy is a common type of hypersomnia. In narcolepsy, which is inherited as an autosomal recessive trait, a person exhibits uncontrollable napping during the day. Other symptoms are cataplexy (brief loss of muscle tone with sudden emotional bursts), vivid hallucinations, and sleep paralysis, in which the patient appears awake but cannot move the limbs. One of the causes of hypersomnia is **obstructive sleep apnea**, in which excessive relaxation of the pharyngeal muscle closes the upper airway during sleep. In apnea, the person may stop breathing and awake in panic.

Toxic Encephalopathies

Encephalopathy refers to CNS dysfunctions that primarily result from impaired cellular metabolism. As discussed in Chapter 17, the metabolic functioning of the CNS depends on a consistent availability of oxygen and glucose supplied by blood. Any interruption in this supply of glucose and oxygen to the brain can cause toxic or metabolic encephalopathy. The factors affecting brain metabolism can be intrinsic or extrinsic. Degenerative brain changes in **Parkinson**, **Huntington**, and **Alzheimer** diseases are intrinsic factors, whereas externally introduced toxic agents and coagents are extrinsic factors.

The onset of toxic encephalopathy is usually gradual. Early signs include slowed cognitive processing, confusion, memory loss, impaired ability to communicate, difficulty finding words, depression, withdrawal, and indifference.

In its advanced stages, these symptoms become more pronounced and include hallucinations, agitation, communicative breakdown, inattention, seizures, and coma.

Various conditions can alter the brain's metabolism and cause toxic encephalopathy. Persistent anoxia can severely affect the brain's oxygen supply. Both vascular and pulmonary diseases contribute to anoxia. Lasting anoxia to the medulla depresses respiration and can be fatal. A depleted supply of glucose, as seen in **hypoglycemia**, and excessive concentration of blood sugar, seen in **hyperglycemia**, directly affect brain functioning.

Blood lead levels >40 mg/100 mL cause lead poisoning, a condition common in children who live in old buildings with chipping lead paint. Manifestations of lead poisoning consist of hyperactivity, behavioral problems, psychomotor (lethargy) retardation, mental retardation, epilepsy, and neuropathy. Liver diseases and renal failure are the other causes of metabolic disturbances that can affect cognitive and sensorimotor functions and personality.

Malnutrition and alcohol dependency are two of the most common causes of **thiamine deficiency**, which can be seen in **Wernicke** and **Korsakoff encephalopathy**. However, in many instances, encephalopathic manifestations are reversible if they are treated early.

Myopathies

Myopathy is a collective term referring to a group of diverse muscle diseases caused by tissue degeneration, toxicity, and inflammatory changes. The primary complaint is muscle weakness, although the muscles appear normal on clinical examination. Problems with speech and swallowing can also be found in the later stages. There are various types of muscular abnormalities. **Muscular dystrophy** is a hereditary myopathy marked by progressive weakness and atrophy. **Duchenne dystrophy** is an X-linked myopathy transmitted to male children from their mothers, who never manifest the condition. **Oculopharyngeal** and **facial dystrophies** affect extrinsic ocular and facial muscles, causing dysarthria and severe problems with ocular movements.

Peripheral Neuropathies

Neuropathy is a disease of the peripheral nerves, interrupting the transmission of impulses from motor neurons to muscles. It can be inherited; idiopathic; or caused by trauma, toxicity, infection, or neoplastic growth. Neuropathy can involve a single peripheral nerve (mononeuropathy) or several peripheral nerves (polyneuropathy). Neuropathy may affect only sensory or motor functions or may involve both; the symptom profile may be acute, chronic, or relapsing. Common peripheral mononeuropathies include neuropathy at the wrist (carpal tunnel syndrome), elbow, or knee. **Carpal tunnel syndrome** results from the entrapment of the **median nerve** at the wrist level and is seen in people whose work activity regularly requires wrist movement.

Elbow neuropathy involves the **ulnar nerve**, which is susceptible to damage at the elbow. Initial symptoms of ulnar neuropathy are numbness and tingling at the area of nerve distribution. The nerve involved in knee neuropathy is the peroneal. It is especially susceptible to damage as it passes laterally around the fibula. Sitting with the legs crossed is often a cause of this neuropathy, and foot drop and sensory and motor disturbances characterize it.

Cranial neuropathies usually involve muscles of the eye, jaw, or face. Lesions of the fibers supplying the ocular nerves can affect movements of the eye and the parasympathetic functions of the iris. Lesions of the trigeminal nerve result in sensory symptoms in the face and motor problems for the mastication muscles. Damage to the facial nucleus and its nerve results in facial paralysis (Bell palsy), and associated visceral and parasympathetic disturbances.

Neoplastic Growth

A **neoplasm** (or tumor) is uncontrolled growths of body tissue and glia cells. The underlying cause may have to do with a faulty expression of **oncogenes** (proteins involved with cellular growth) and a loss of tumor-suppressor genes as well as the growth of new blood vessels (**angiogenesis**). A tumor can be **primary** or **metastatic**. Primary tumors arise from glia or meninges within the CNS. Metastatic, also known as secondary, tumors arise elsewhere in the body and spread to the brain. Most of the spreading tumors in the brain come from cancer of the breast or lung or from melanoma (malignant cells that contain melanin and are usually found in the skin). This spread from the remote sources occurs through the lymphatics or blood vessels.

Tumors are either **malignant** or **benign**. Malignant brain tumors grow fast, invade the surrounding tissue, and are fatal. These tumorous tissues are often multifocal and microscopically undifferentiated from the surrounding unaffected tissues. Malignancy is graded on a scale I–IV. Low-grade tumors are benign; high-grade tumors are malignant.

Neoplasms (tumors) are abnormal tissue growth that is generally but not always slow and insidious. Because of the brain's ability to reorganize, patients with tumors present slowly developing and subtle clinical signs. Neoplastic growth in the brain primarily increases intracranial pressure, which slowly irritates and damages the surrounding brain tissues. Common clinical signs of brain tumors are double vision, headache, altered cognitive ability, nausea, and seizures. Most brain tumors originate from glia cells (gliomas) and include **astrocytomas**, **ependymomas**, and **oligodendrogliomas**. Other benign brain tumors are **meningiomas**, which arise from the dura mater; **acoustic neuromas or vestibular Schwannoma**, which arise from the Schwann cell sheath of the nerve; and pituitary adenoma.

Symptoms are related focally to the brain area affected by the tumor. Tumors that initially involve the silent brain regions become symptomatic in later stages. Besides focal symptoms, common clinical symptoms of a brain tumor include progressive weakness, speech or visual loss, anomia, headache, impaired concentration, forgetfulness, altered personality, and mental confusion. The most notable complications of a tumor are seizures and increased intracranial pressure. Medical treatment of tumors involves surgical excision, radiation therapy (γ-knife), and/or chemotherapy.

Cerebral Infections

Various bacteria, viruses, and other organisms can cause infection in the CNS. Generally, an infection's effect on the brain is diffuse and most commonly affects the meninges (meningitis) and cerebral cortex (encephalopathy). Infections can also be local, such as cerebral abscess, which occur in different parts of the brain. Some common infections are **viral infections**, **herpes simplex**, *Escherichia coli*, **brain abscess**, **subdural empyema**, and **syphilis**.

SUMMARY

Some commonly used and neurolinguistically pertinent neurodiagnostic techniques and medical concepts are discussed, and prevalent neurologic diseases and medical technical concepts are presented. These topics directly apply to the management of neurologic patients who are seen by professionals who have an interest in human behavior and, who work primarily in medical settings (audiologists, speech-language pathologists, and psychologists). Imaging techniques are discussed to familiarize students with the procedures, principles, and purposes underlying different contemporary neurodiagnostic and imaging techniques.

The chapter also addresses the procedural issues of sodium amytal infusion, which is used for the assessment of cerebral dominance, usually before tissue removal during craniotomy. A discussion of electroencephalography and electromyography explains how these tests are used to measure functioning of the brain cells and muscle fibers. The ways to record evoked potentials to specific and controlled sensory stimulation and their interpretation are also described.

Finally, various neurologic techniques and neurosurgical procedures, along with their neurolinguistic implications, are examined. Modes of genetic inheritance and a brief account of common neurologic diseases are presented.

QUIZ QUESTIONS

1. Define the following terms: angiography, coma, CT, dichotic listening, dominant inheritance, electroencephalography, electromyography, MRI, recessive inheritance, stupor, X-linked inheritance

2. List the four major types of brain waves and their corresponding frequencies.

3. List four subtypes of seizures.

4. What is the risk probability associated with dominant inheritance?

5. What is the risk probability associated with recessive inheritance?

6. Match each of the numbered techniques with its lettered concept.

1. electroencephalography
2. electromyography
3. sodium Amytal infusion
4. evoked potentials
5. dichotic listening
6. lumbar puncture

a. evaluation of electrical activity in muscles for diagnosing nerve and muscle diseases
b. recording electrical brain activity evoked in response to specific stimuli
c. recording of brain's electrical potentials for diagnosing seizure disorders
d. determining cerebral dominance by induced hemispheric anesthetization
e. diagnosing CNS infections and intracerebral hemorrhages
f. identifying cerebral dominance using bilateral presentation of auditory stimuli

TECHNICAL TERMS

angiogram
cordotomy
craniotomy
CT
delirium
dichotic listening
diffusion tensor imaging
dominant inheritance
electroencephalography
encephalopathy
epilepsy
evoked potential
lumbar puncture

MRI
myopathy
neuropathy
paroxysmal discharge
positron emission tomography (PET)
recessive inheritance
regional cerebral blood flow
single proton emission computed tomography (SPECT)
X-linked inheritance

abdominal muscles—Group of muscles innervated by the nerves originating from the T6–T12 spinal segments. Their contraction increases intrathoracic pressure, triggering forced expiration.

abdominal reflex—Contraction of the abdominal wall and retraction of the umbilicus toward the stimulus on stroking the skin over the abdominal quadrant. A reflex regulated by T7–T12 and the upper lumbar segments. Absence of this reflex is associated with pyramidal tract lesions (upper motor neuron).

abducens nerve—Cranial nerve VI, regulating the lateral rectus muscle, which is responsible for moving eyeball laterally. A pathologic involvement of the nerve causes the eye to rotate to the middle (medial strabismus).

abduction—Movement of the limb away from the central body axis.

abembryonic (or vegetal) pole—Pertaining to a region opposite to the implanting embryo.

abscess—Localized accumulation of pus from liquefied tissue, resulting in displacement of tissues.

absence (petit mal) seizures—Sudden and recurrent attacks of impaired consciousness secondary to bilateral cortical discharges. They are characterized by staring, blinking and twitching of cranial muscles. The underlying electroencephalograph shows an abrupt onset of a 3-sec spike.

absolute refractive period—Time immediately following the action potential in which no other action potential can be initiated.

abulia—Impaired ability to make a decision and perform voluntary actions along with reduced speech output, usually associated with bilateral prefrontal lobe pathologies.

acalculia—Impaired ability, acquired after brain damage, to perform simple arithmetic calculation.

accommodation—Parasympathetically mediated visual response that the lens undergoes to keep a near object in focus.

acetylcholine (ACh)—Neurotransmitter released by cholinergic neurons and widely distributed in body tissues. It primarily regulates the nervous system and muscular activity.

acetylcholinesterase—Enzyme that breaks (hydrolyzes) the neurotransmitter acetylcholine into choline and acetate, contributing to the termination of the postsynaptic current and signal. Much of the choline released by hydrolysis is recaptured by the presynaptic terminal.

achromatic—Without color.

acoustive nerve—Part of cranial nerve VIII that serves audition.

acromegaly—Condition characterized by thickened bones and tissue and caused by oversecretion of human growth (hGH) hormone during adulthood.

action potential—Electrical impulse representing a transient fluctuation in membrane potentials, which are propagated along axonal process to activate postsynaptic terminals.

acuity—Perceptual clarity, usually of auditory and visual stimuli.

acute—Short-term physiologic effects emerging immediately after pathophysiology and requiring immediate medical attention.

acute confusion state—Reversible altered level of consciousness of sudden onset marked by confusion, distractibility, disordered thinking, fluctuating attention, reduced memory, impaired perception (illusions and hallucinations), and agitation caused by toxicity in the brain.

adaptation—Diminished sensitivity of a receptor to continued stimulation.

adduction—Movement of limb toward the midline/central body axis. Opposite of abduction.

adenohypophysis—Anterior lobe of the pituitary gland.

adipsia—Condition marked by the absence of thirst or lack of desire to take water.

adrenal cortex—Outer portion of the adrenal gland, which releases cortisol on stimulation by pituitary gland.

adrenal gland—Located superior to each of the kidneys. It contains cells that on sympathetic stimulation secrete epinephrine and norepinephrine.

adrenaline—Catecholamine neurotransmitter also called epinephrine. Synthesized from norepinephrine.

adrenergic—Neurons responsible for synthesizing and releasing epinephrine (adrenaline) and norepinephrine (noradrenaline).

adrenocorticotropin—Hormone that stimulates growth of the adrenal (suprarenal) cortex and regulates the secretion of its hormones.

afferent—Axonal fibers that conduct impulses toward the central nervous system or nerve cell body.

afferent pathways—Axonal bundles mediating bodily perceived sensations of pain, touch, and temperature toward the central nervous system.

agnosia—Acquired impairment in recognizing objects while the primary modalities of sensation (touch, vision, hearing) are normally functioning.

agraphia—Impaired ability after brain damage to express through writing.

AIDS (acquired immunodeficiency syndrome)—Disorder of the immune system owing to infection with the human immunodeficiency virus (HIV-1) in which the antibodies attack the body's own immune system.

AIDS dementia complex—Progressive cognitive (dementia) syndrome occurring after chronic HIV-1 encephalitis.

akinesia—Slow initiation, or loss of power of voluntary movements seen in patients with basal ganglia pathology.

akinetic mutism—State of altered consciousness in which the patient appears intermittently alert but is unresponsive despite intact motor skills.

alar lamina—Alar plate zone of the embryonic neural tube dorsal to the sulcus limitans. Dorsal gray columns of the spinal cord and sensory centers of the brain develop from this region.

albinism—Genetically recessive condition involving partial or total lack of pigment in the skin, hair, and eyes. Results from the abnormalities of melanin production.

alexia—Impaired ability, acquired after brain damage, to comprehend written information.

alkalosis—Condition resulting from an increased acid (pH) level in body fluid.

allantois—One of the fetal membranes related to urinary bladder development. Not functionally important in human development.

alleles—Genes at corresponding positions (loci) in a chromosome pair.

α-*motor neuron*—Largest and rapidly conducting spinal motor neuron, which controls the activity of skeletal muscle fibers.

alpha (α)-wave (α-rhythm)—Brain wave with a frequency between 8 and 13 Hz. Occurs when the patient is relaxed with the eyes closed.

alpha rhythm—Present in the posterior brain region, this wave pattern of 8-13 Hertz represents the awaken and relaxed state of the brain.

alternating hemiplegia—Brainstem lesion characterized by cranial nerve impairments on the side ipsilateral to the lesion and hemiplegia and sensory loss on the opposite side.

Alzheimer disease—Chronic degenerative condition in the aging brain characterized by irreversible loss of memory, disorientation, impaired judgment, and disorders of language and cognition.

amnesia—Impaired ability to remember. Forgetting information preceding cortical injury is retrograde amnesia, whereas the inability to learn newer information after injury is anterograde amnesia.

amnion—Fetal membrane that encloses the embryo and fetus. Later the amniotic cavity is the sole cavity for the pregnant uterus.

ampulla—Sac-like canal dilation containing sensory receptors.

amygdala—Almond-shaped medial limbic structure associated with visceral and vegetative activities needed for self-preservation, such as mating, fighting, and eating. Also controls autonomic responses to stress. It is reciprocally connected to the hypothalamus, hippocampus, and thalamus. Functionally, it is concerned with emotional responses.

amyotrophic—Pertaining to muscular atrophy, as in amyotrophic lateral sclerosis.

amyotrophic lateral sclerosis (ALS; Lou Gehrig disease)—Progressive degenerative condition of spinal and cortical motor neurons characterized by progressive muscular weakness and atrophy.

anabolism—Building of energy and cellular metabolic substances that are needed for the body.

analgesia—Neurologic state in which painful stimuli are no longer perceived as being painful.

analgesics—Substances that are used to relieve pain sensation.

anaphase—Third stage in cell division.

anastomosis—Site of communication between two blood vessels. Usually involves large arteries.

anencephaly—Birth defect in which the forebrain and/or midbrain are diminished in size or are missing. Caused by the defective fusion of the neural tube during embryologic development.

anesthesia—Loss of touch and pain sensation either from a cortical lesion or from a drug-induced state of suppressed sensation.

aneuploid—Having an extra chromosome.

aneurysm—Localized, balloonlike dilation of a blood vessel caused by a weakened arterial wall or congenital defect.

aneurysm clipping—Surgical treatment involving the use of a clip to obliterate the neck of an aneurysm.

angiography—X-ray technique that involves injection of radiopaque substance for examining the structural architecture of blood vessels.

angular gyrus—Neurolinguistically important and highly developed parietal convolution in humans implicated with the reading function.

anlagen—See PRIMORDIUM.

annulospiral nerve endings—Specialized receptors that mediate muscle stretch.

anomia—Impaired ability to name objects and find words acquired after brain injury.

anorexia nervosa—Chronic psychological condition characterized by self-induced weight loss and distorted body image resulting from a loss of appetite.

anosmia—Loss of the ability to smell.

anosognosia—Failure to recognize one's own disease, a usual parietal syndrome.

anoxia—Related to oxygen deficiency in brain tissue.

ansa lenticularis—Axonal fiber bundle transmitting basal ganglia efferents from the globus pallidus to the thalamus.

antagonist—One of the paired muscles that acts in opposition to the mover (agonist) during a movement.

anterior cerebral artery—Supplies blood to the medial surface of the frontal lobe and part of the parietal lobe, in addition to the anterior four-fifths of the corpus callosum.

anterior commissure—Smaller commissural fiber bundle that interconnects the middle and the inferior temporal gyri in both hemispheres. Known to mediate olfaction.

anterior corticospinal tract—Descending motor fibers that do not cross the midline in the medulla oblongata.

anterior lobe—Cerebellar region responsible for muscle tone and equilibrium during locomotion.

anterior medullary velum—Cerebellar structure that forms roof of the fourth ventricle.

anterior nucleus—Thalamic nucleus mediating hypothalamic (mammillary body) projections to the cingulate gyrus of the limbic cortex. Participates in the regulation of visceral and emotional functions.

anterior (ventral) horn—ventral spinal gray region containing motor (final common pathway) nuclei.

anterior (ventral) root—Collection of motor (efferent) fibers, emerging from the anterior aspect of the spinal cord and extends laterally to join a posterior root to form a spinal nerve.

anterior spinothalamic tract—Axonal bundle mediating sensation related to diffuse touch to the thalamus.

anterograde reaction—See WALLERIAN DEGENERATION.

anterograde transmission—Forward information flow from the soma (cell body) to the synapse.

anterolateral spinothalamic system—Includes the axonal bundle mediating pain, touch, and temperature to the brain.

antibody—Defensive substance produced in response to a specific antigen in the body.

anticoagulant—Drug preventing the clotting of blood. Warfarin (Coumadin) is a common anticoagulant drug.

antidiuretic hormone (ADH)—Hormone produced by neurosecretory hypothalamic cells that stimulates water reabsorption from the kidney, reduces urine output, and causes vasoconstriction of arterioles (vasopressin).

antiepileptic drugs—Anticonvulsant medications used either to prevent or to treat seizure disorders.

antigen—Foreign substances in the body whose contact with cells triggers a response from the body's immune system.

aphagia—Impaired ability to swallow subsequent to brain injuries.

aphasia—Impaired ability to process language, resulting from brain damage.

apneustic area—Pontine respiratory center that stimulates the medullary inspiratory center.

apraxia—Impaired ability to execute skilled motor acts which is not caused by muscle paralysis or incoordination, sensory deficits, or incomprehension.

aqueduct—Narrow canal within the brainstem that connects the third and fourth ventricles.

aqueous humor—Watery substance, similar to cerebrospinal fluid, that is continuously produced and drained in the posterior chamber of the anterior ocular cavity.

arachnoid—Middle protective meningeal layer that covers the central nervous system.

arachnoid trabeculae—Fibrous tissue that maintains the subarachnoid space by serving as a ridge between the meningeal membranes of the arachnoid and the pia matter.

arachnoid villi (granulations)—Wormlike tufted structures that drain cerebrospinal fluid from the subarachnoid space into the superior sagittal sinus.

archicerebellum—Oldest part of the cerebellum. Includes the flocculus and nodulus and is related to equilibrium.

arcuate fasciculus—Fibers of the superior longitudinal fasciculus known to connect the association cortices of Broca area with Wernicke area.

Argyll Robertson pupil—Impaired pupillary reaction to light while the near vision reflex is preserved. Commonly seen with degenerative brain diseases such as Alzheimer disease and with encephalopathy and diabetes.

Arnold-Chiari malformation—Developmental malformation marked by a downward herniation of the medulla and cerebellum in the vertebral canal of the cervical region. Often associated with spinal bifida and hydrocephaly.

arteriosclerosis—Narrowing of arterial lumen owing to accumulation of lipids, fatty substances, and cholesterol along intimal walls of blood vessels. Also called atherosclerosis.

arteriovenous malformation—Congenital condition in which tangled and twisted arteries and veins are interconnected in a localized area, where the arterial blood shunts to the veins, bypassing the cortical tissue.

artery—Vessel carrying blood from the heart to body parts.

asphyxia—Brain cell anoxia secondary to a reduction in the regular exchange of oxygen and carbon dioxide.

aspiration—Inhalation of water or food into the bronchial tree.

association fibers—Short and long fibers that interconnect different regions within a cerebral hemisphere.

association (secondary) cortex—Functionally uncommitted regions of the cerebral cortex at birth that later assume integration of multimodality information and include the parietal-temporal-occipital association cortex, prefrontal association cortex, and limbic association cortex.

asthenia—Muscle weakness caused by cerebellar dysfunctioning.

astigmatism—Focusing disorder in which vertical and horizontal rays focus at two different points on the retina. Results from irregular lens and/or cornea curvature.

astrocytes—Neuroglia cells that support nerve cells and contribute to blood–brain barrier.

asynergia—Impaired ability to coordinate different muscles in the performance of a skilled movement.

ataxia—Lack of coordination in sequential voluntary muscular activities, resulting from a cerebellar pathology.

ataxic dysarthria—Acquired motor speech disorder subsequent to cerebellar pathology. Characterized by imprecise speech, articulatory breakdowns, and impaired stress applications.

atheroma—Lipid deposit that narrows the arterial wall occurring in atherosclerosis.

atherosclerosis—Process of narrowing of the arterial lumen owing to accumulation of fatty substances (cholesterol and triglycerides) and lipids along the intimal walls of the medianum and larger blood vessels. Results in the formation of an atherosclerotic plaque that decreases the size of the arterial lumen and is a common cause of hypertension.

atherosclerotic plaque—Lesion causing plaque resulting from accumulated fatty substances involving the tunica media of an artery and leading to obstruction.

athetosis—Involuntary, slow writhing (constant flexion and extension) movements of limbs subsequent to basal ganglia pathology.

atonia—Lack of muscle tone.

atrophy—Wasting away of muscle tissue, including reduction in muscle fiber diameter (weakening of the force of contraction owing to disuse atrophy) or disintegration of muscle fibers (denervation atrophy). This is associated with lower motor neuron pathologies.

atrophy of denervation (fiber wasting)—Severely reduced muscle mass with loss of muscle fibers, resulting from prolonged loss (6 months or more) of lower motor neuron innervation of these fibers

atrophy of disuse—Reduction in muscle body mass without loss of muscle fibers (cells) caused by decreased muscular activity.

attenuation reflex—Reflexive contraction of the middle ear muscles causing a decrease in auditory sensitivity.

audiogram—Graphic representation of hearing thresholds for tones at various frequencies.

audiometry—Assessment of hearing sensitivity for a range of pure tones using the decibel (dBSPL) scale.

auditory association (secondary) cortex—Brain region located around the primary auditory cortex, responsible for the elaboration of auditory information.

auditory reflexes—Protective simultaneous head and eye movements in response to loud auditory stimuli.

auditory system—Neuroanatomic system, beginning in the inner ear, passing through the brainstem, thalamus (medial geniculate body), and terminating in the auditory cortex. Responsible for auditory perception.

autoimmunity—Condition in which antibodies attack the body's own normal tissues.

autonomic dysfunctions—Neurologic disorders involving pupil dilation/constriction, sexual activity, perspiration, blood pressure, thirst, hunger, urination, and gastric function.

autonomic ganglia—Group of nuclei located in the peripheral nervous system that mediate impulses from the central nervous system to various visceral organs, cardiac muscles, smooth muscles, and glands.

autonomic nervous system—Division of the peripheral nervous system with sympathetic and parasympathetic fibers. Works subconsciously and innervates blood vessels, internal organs, and glands.

autoregulation—Autocerebral mechanism for regulating blood flow to the brain.

autosomal—Related to chromosomes other than sex chromosomes.

autosomal dominance—Genetic expression mode in which a dysfunctional allele possessed by one parent dominates the second allele from the other parent. Each offspring has a 50% probability of inheriting this dysfunctional gene and the disorder.

axial muscles—Muscles associated with the central part of the body that regulate movements of the body or trunk.

axon—Neuronal process capable of conducting neuronal impulses to other cell bodies.

axon collaterals—Small subsidiary processes attached to the main body of the axon.

axonal hillock—Site where the axon joins the cell.

axonal reaction—Retrograde chromatolytic changes in the soma marked by disintegration of the granules of the nissl bodies after damage to an axon.

axonal regeneration—Reconstitution of an injured axon. Most prevalent in the peripheral nervous system.

Babinski reflex—Dorsal flexion of the great toe and fanning of other toes on being stroked on the sole of the foot. Indicating pyramidal tract (upper motor neuron) pathology in adults. Named after French neurologist Joseph Babinski.

ballism—Violent flinging movements usually involving one side of the body. Associated with a lesion of the subthalamic nucleus.

Bárány caloric test—Clinically undertaken to evaluate vestibular functioning in cases of inner ear disease using the injection of water of different temperatures into the auditory canal. Cold water produces rotatory nystagmus toward the opposite direction. Whereas warm fluid triggers nystagmus toward the injected (ipsilateral) side.

basal ganglia—Group of subcortical nuclei (caudate, globus pallidus, and putamen) located within the white matter in each cerebral hemisphere. Important in movement regulation.

basal lamina—Basal plate zone of the embryonic neural tube ventral to the sulcus limitans. Ventral gray columns of the spinal cord and motor centers of the brain develop from this region, which is also called the basal plate.

basis pedunculi—Also called pes peduncle or crus cerebri. Includes descending motor fibers in the midbrain on each side.

basis pontis—Basal or inferior region of the pons.

Bell palsy—Facial paralysis causing paralysis on one side of the face. Paralyzed muscles are pulled toward unaffected side.

Betz cells—Large motor (pyramidal) cells located in the primary motor cortex.

bifurcate—A state of dividing into two branches or divisions.

bilaminar embryo—Human embryo in the 2nd week of gestation.

bilateral—Referring to two sides of the body.

bilateral innervation—Mostly refers to cranial nerve motor nuclei that receive innervation from both motor cortices, where each pyramidal tract provides both ipsilateral (minor) and contralateral (stronger) innervation.

binocular vision—Visual field area simultaneously processed in both eyes.

biopsy—Removal of tissue from the living body, usually for microscopic examination.

biorhythms—Circadian (with a cycle of 24 hr) biologic rhythms regulating body homeostasis such as the sleep–wake cycle.

bitemporal hemianopia—Loss of temporal visual fields for both eyes.

blast—Immature cell.

blastocyst—Stage in the 1st week of human development.

blastomere—Cell resulting from cleavage of a fertilized ovum.

blind spot—Retinal area, that contains no photoreceptors, located 15° medial to the visual axis and representing the optic disk through which optic nerve (cranial nerve II) fibers exit the retina.

blood—Oxygen-containing fluid that circulates through the heart, arteries, and capillaries.

blood–brain barrier—Physiologic barrier unique to brain arteries that prevents noxious substances in the blood from entering the brain.

blood pressure—Measurement of the force exerted by blood against the walls of blood vessels during ventricular systole (contraction of the heart, by which the blood is sent through the aorta for systemic circulation).

blood urea nitrogen (BUN)—Examination of the presence of nitrogen from urea in the blood for determining the normalcy of kidney function.

bony labyrinth—Represents a series of cavities in the petrous portion of the temporal bone, including the cochlea, semicircular canals, and vestibule.

brachial plexus—Network of spinal nerve fibers exiting the ventral rami of the C5–T1 nerves to supply the upper limb.

brachium—Arm-like fiber bundle. The brachium of the inferior colliculus is an auditory fiber bundle that connects the inferior colliculus to the thalamus. The brachium of the superior colliculus mediates visual information and bypasses the lateral geniculate body of the thalamus on its way to the pretectal region in midbrain.

brachium conjunctivum—See SUPERIOR CEREBELLAR PEDUNCLE.

brachium pontis—See MIDDLE CEREBELLAR PEDUNCLE.

bradykinesia—Slowness in the initiation of voluntary motor movements.

brain—Mass of nervous tissue located in the cranial cavity.

brainstem—Stem part of the brain, consisting of midbrain, pons, and medulla.

brainstem auditory evoked potentials—Technique used for measuring brainstem neuronal responses to controlled auditory stimuli.

brain waves—Electrical activity produced as a result of action potentials of brain cells

branchial arches—Five pairs of arched embryologic structures that develop into laryngeal, pharyngeal and facial muscles. Remnants of arches in lower vertebrates that give rise to muscles for specialized functions like articulation, phonation, and swallowing in the humans.

broad-based gait—Walking pattern characterized by placing the feet far apart. Often resulting from cerebellar injury.

Broca aphasia—Type of aphasia associated with a lesion in the lower premotor cortex (Broca Area) and characterized by impaired verbal output.

Brodmann areas—Approximately 50 or so brain areas identified and mapped by Brodmann on the basis of its cellular cytoarchitectonics.

bronchi—Branches of the respiratory passageway.

brownian motion—Physical property of water molecules, which refers to their constant motion and random movements in all directions.

Brown-Séquard syndrome—Hemi-spinal cord lesion resulting in spastic paralysis and proprioception loss in the body ipsilateral to the lesion and pain and temperature loss occurring contralateral.

bulbar lesion—Lesions mostly related to the medulla.

bulbar palsy—Limb paralysis secondary to the involvement of the motor nuclei in the medulla.

calcarine fissure—Located on the midsagittal surface of the occipital lobe. Separates the primary visual cortex into lower and upper opercula.

callosal sulcus—Midsagittally located sulcus separating the corpus callosum and cingulate gyrus.

caloric stimulation test—Test of vestibular function that involves irrigating the external auditory canal to evaluate the functioning of the labyrinth. See BÁRÁNY CALORIC TEST.

calvaria—Superior portion of the cranium, which has a domelike appearance.

canal of Schlemm—Venous duct of the eye that drains the aqueous humor from anterior chamber of the eyeball.

capillary—Terminal branches of arteries that the that supply blood to the brain.

carbamazepine (Tegretol)—Frequently used antiepileptic drug which is also used for pain management.

cardiac muscle—Striated muscle fibers (cells) that form the wall of the heart. Stimulated by an intrinsic conduction system and autonomic motor neurons

cardiac output (CO)—The measured volume of blood pumped from one ventricle of the heart in 1 min, rending about 5.2 L/min.

carotid arterial system—Also known as the anterior blood circulating system. Supplies blood to the head, face, and brain through the external and internal carotid arteries.

carotid endarterectomy—Surgical procedure to remove occlusive sclerotic plaques through an incision in the internal carotid artery.

carotid sinus—A dilated region of the internal carotid artery containing receptors of the vagus (CNX) nerve that monitor blood flow and pressure.

carotid vascular system—System formed by the internal carotid artery that supplies blood to the brain by dividing into the middle and anterior cerebral arteries.

carpal tunnel syndrome—Pain and paresthesia of the hand caused by an entrapment of the median nerve. Seen in people involved with work requiring constant wrist movement.

catabolism—Metabolic breakdown of complex substances into simpler substances, such as food digestion and oxidation of nutrient molecules for energy.

cataract—Age-induced painless formation of nontransparent fibrous protein that affects vision by clouding the lens. Medically treatable condition.

catastrophic reaction—Uncontrollable emotional behaviors and psychological reactions that generally result from traumatic experiences and shocking accidents. These behaviors are characterized by crying, screaming, and depression.

catecholamine—Group of neurotransmitters that has an amine and catechol ring and includes epinephrine, norepinephrine, and dopamine.

cauda equina—Bundle of spinal nerve roots that arise from the lumbosacral region and run through the lumbar cistern before exiting the vertebral canal.

caudal—Toward back of brain or tail of the spinal cord.

caudate nucleus—Nucleus of basal ganglia circuitry that is involved with motor functions.

central canal—Narrow duct connecting the fourth ventricle with the lumbar cistern.

central gray—Reticular core of nuclei around the cerebral aqueduct.

central nervous system—Consists of the brain and spinal cord. Integrates all incoming and outgoing information and generates appropriate responses.

central (penetrating) arteries—Smaller arteries that supply blood to the subcortical structures.

central sulcus—Obliquely descending sulcus on the lateral surface of brain, marking the boundary between the frontal and parietal lobes.

central visual pathways—Visual pathway from the retina of the eye to the primary visual cortex in the occipital lobe.

cerebellar cortex—Cellular layer of the cerebellum.

cerebellar peduncles—Three pairs of fiber tracts that connect the cerebellum with the brainstem.

cerebellar signs—Symptoms of dyssynergia, ataxia, and motion or action tremor associated with cerebellar pathologies.

cerebellum—Rhombencephalon derivative that serves as an important motor control center.

cerebral aqueduct (iter)—Narrow ventricular passage in the midbrain that connects the third and fourth ventricles. Also called the aqueduct of Sylvius.

cerebral cortex—Sheet of gray matter that covers the cerebral hemispheres and consists of six layers of cells.

cerebral dominance—Brain's ability to exercise greater influence on a function. Usually refers to left hemispheric superiority for processing language in most people irrespective of handedness.

cerebral hemispheres—Bilaterally located parts of the cerebrum connected by the corpus callosum. Each hemisphere is made up of the cerebral cortex and deep-lying structures (basal ganglia, thalamus and limbic structures).

cerebral palsy—Group of motor disorders, characterized by muscle paralysis, weakness, and incoordination, caused by damage to motor areas of the brain during fetal life, birth, or infancy.

cerebral veins—Venous network that collects circulated blood from the cortical and subcortical arteries and empties it into the sinus system.

cerebrospinal fluid—Clear fluid produced in ventricular cavity that protects the brain by forming a cushion in the subarachnoid space around the central nervous system.

cerebrovascular accident (CVA; stroke)—Interruption of the blood supply to brain tissue resulting in neurologic symptoms.

cerebrum—The cerebral hemispheres connected by the corpus callosum.

cervical flexure—Embryonic curvature at the junction of the hindbrain and spinal cord.

chemotherapy—Chemical treatment of a disease, usually cancer.

cholesterol—Fatlike substance abundantly found in food rich in animal fat and biles. Circulates in the blood plasma in various densities and plays an important role in the pathogenesis of atheroma. There are two types: high-density lipoproteins (HDLs), the good cholesterol, and low-density lipoproteins (LDLs), the bad cholesterol.

cholinergic—Pertaining to the cells that secret acetylcholine in the nervous system and in body tissues.

chordotomy—Surgical sectioning of tracts in the spinal cord, usually employed to control medically intractable pain.

chorea—Rhythmic, graceful, involuntary movements predominantly of distal extremities and muscles of the face, neck, tongue, and pharynx. Neostriatum is the suspected site of lesion.

chorion—Fetal membrane enclosing the embryo. It also forms part of the placenta and is highly active and functional.

choroid—Middle vascular coats of the eyeball that is the source of vascular supply to the sclera and outer retina.

choroid plexus—Pia-capillary network invaginated in the ventricles. Produces cerebrospinal fluid.

chromatolysis—Cellular changes marked by swelling, dissolution of cellular organelles (specifically Nissl bodies), and shifting of the nucleus from its central position to the periphery in response to injury.

chromosomal nondisjunction—Error in the separation of homologous chromosomes during anaphase of gametogenesis.

chromosome—One of the 46 small, dark-staining strands of condensed chromatin (DNA) located within the nucleus of a human diploid (2n) cell during cell division. Associated with RNA and histones.

chronic symptoms—Clinical symptoms developing and persisting over months to years.

ciliary body—Parasympathetically regulated ocular muscles controlling lens shape and thus its refractive power.

ciliary ganglion—Parasympathetic ganglion of the oculomotor nerve (cranial nerve III) responsible for regulating the ciliary muscle (for lens accommodation) and the sphincter muscle of the iris (for papillary constriction) with its postganglionic fibers.

ciliary muscle—Muscle that regulates the refractive power of the lens in visual accommodation.

cingulate gyrus—Limbic-cortical structure that serves emotional, somatic, and autonomic functions.

cingulum—Association fiber bundle of the limbic lobe that connects the medial, frontal, and parietal cortices with the temporal cortex.

circadian rhythm—Biological rhythm based on a 24-hour cycle and controlled by the internal clock mechanism.

circle of Willis—Arterial circle at the base of the brain that forms a major anastomotic point by connecting the carotid system with the vertebrobasilar system.

circumferential (cortical) arteries—Large (anterior, medial, and posterior) cerebral arteries that supply blood to the cortex.

clasp-knife spasticity—Increased resistance by the extensor muscles that melts away in face of a constant stretch. Rigidity is the result of an exaggeration of the stretch reflex. Is seen in spastic hemiplegia and is exemplified by the blade of a hunting knife.

claustrum—Subcortically located gray structure. Concerned with unconscious motor activity.

cleavage—Progressive mitotic division of the fertilized ovum.

climbing fibers—Cerebellar afferent fibers (olivocerebellar projections) that directly activate Purkinje cells.

closed head injury—Traumatic brain injury in which there is no penetration of the skull.

coagulation—Process of blood clot formation.

cochlea—Fluid-filled and spirally coiled structure that contains the organ of Corti, the sensory end organ of hearing.

coelom—Body cavity containing the visceral organs, such as the heart, lungs, and intestines.

cogwheel rigidity—Rhythmic interruption of resistance in a hypertonic muscle during passive manipulation.

colic—Painful spasmodic movement in any hollow internal tube. Occurs mostly in the abdomen.

collateral circulation—Alternate blood flow via an anastomosis to an area that has lost its blood supply.

collateral trigone—Region from which the lateral ventricles diverge into temporal and occipital horns.

color blindness—X-linked genetic condition in which perception of one or more colors is impaired.

coma—State of profound unconsciousness in which the patient does not respond to sensory stimuli. It is usually seen in patients with TBI and with cerebral toxicity.

commissural fibers—Association fibers that travel across the midline and connect the cerebral hemispheres.

computerized tomography (CT)—X-ray brain-imaging technique that provides cross-sectional images of the live brain and body in different planes.

conceptus—Developing human along with its membranes. Term can be applied to any developmental stage from zygote through birth.

concussion—Brain injury associated with brief loss of consciousness in absence of any visible structural damage of cortical tissue.

conduction aphasia—Type of aphasia associated with arcuate fasciculus lesion and characterized by disproportionately impaired verbal repetition with near-normal comprehension and comparatively good verbal expression.

conductive hearing loss—Hearing loss that results from an interrupted transmission of sound through the outer or middle ear to the cochlea.

cones—Retinal cells responsible for the highest visual acuity and color discrimination.

confused language—Linguistically vague use of language indicating cognitive impairment as a result of brain damage. Marked by slowed thinking, limited processing, and reduced integration of information mostly involving the right nondominant hemisphere or as a result of impaired consciousness.

conjugate eye movements—Simultaneous movement of the eyes in the same direction, which is important for focusing and reading. In disconjugate movements, both eyes do not move together to one direction, resulting in strabismus and double vision.

connecting stalk—Forerunner of the umbilical cord. Formed of extra-embryonic mesoderm.

consciousness—State of wakefulness with intact feedback between the cerebral cortex and reticular activating system in which an individual is fully alert, aware, and oriented.

consensual response—Pupillary contraction in one eye in response to light exposure in the other eye.

contralateral—The side opposite to the location of a lesion, to the location of a stimulus source, or to the location of a cortical motor control area.

contusion—Injury characterized by a bruise and tissue damage under unbroken skin.

conus medullaris—Terminal point of the spinal cord.

convex lens—Lens with an elevated surface used to correct refractive errors in hyperopia (farsightedness).

convolution—Elevations forming the surface of the cerebral hemispheres, also called gyrus (pl. gyri).

cordotomy—Surgical procedure used for sectioning a spinal tract.

cornea—Nonvascular, transparent outermost fibrous coat of the eye through which the iris can be seen.

coronal—Vertical section dividing the brain into front and back.

corona radiata—Crown-shaped, fanned sensorimotor fibers located above the internal capsule.

coronary artery disease (CAD)—Condition in which atherosclerotic plaque narrows the coronary arteries, reducing the blood flow to the heart muscles.

corpora quadrigemina—Tectal structure. Four egg-shaped structures (inferior and superior colliculi) in the dorsal midbrain that serve as reflex centers for vision and audition.

corpus callosum—Largest bundle of axonal fibers that interconnects the cortex of the cerebral hemispheres.

corpus striatum—See STRIATUM.

cortex—Collection of nerve cells that forms the external surface of the brain.

cortical blindness—Neurologic syndrome characterized by blindness for shapes and patterns with preserved ability to distinguish light from dark. Associated with bilateral damage to the visual cortex.

corticobulbar fibers—Short axonal projections descending from the motor cortex and synapsing on the brainstem motor cranial nerve nuclei. This tract serves motor speech functions by innervating the musculature of the face, tongue, and jaws.

corticospinal fibers—Long axonal projections fibers, also called pyramidal fibers, originating in the motor cortex and descending to terminate on spinal motor nuclei. This tract regulates the motor control of skeletal muscles.

cortisol—Steroid hormone released by the adrenal cortex that inhibits the immune system and mobilizes energy.

cranial nerves—The 12 pairs of nerves in the peripheral nervous system that innervate buccofacial muscles and mediate sensations of vision, smell, and touch from face.

craniosacral outflow—Parasympathetic preganglionic neurons with their cell bodies located in the brainstem and in the lateral gray matter of the sacral portion of the spinal cord.

craniosacral system—Parasympathetic division of the autonomic nervous system with preganglionic cell bodies located in the brainstem and in the lateral gray matter of the sacral portion of the spinal cord. Concerned with conserving bodily energy.

craniotomy—Surgical procedure used to open the skull for removing pathologic tissue from the brain.

cranium—Skeleton of the skull that protects the brain.

cranium bifidum—Embryologic malformation marked by absence of cranial bone fusion leading to herniation of the meninges and cortex.

cremasteric reflex—Retraction of the testicle on stroking the skin of the inner thigh. Absence of this reflex indicates a pyramidal tract lesion (upper motor neuron).

Creutzfeldt-Jakob disease—Neurologic disorder marked by an ataxia, abnormalities of gait and speech, mood changes, cognitive impairments, seizures, and myoclonus. Caused by an infectious agent, such as the spongiform encephalopathies of animals.

cristae—Vestibular sensory hair cells embedded in a gelatinous mass that project into the ampulla of each of the three semicircular canals.

critical period—Important developmental period when stimulation and environmental input are capable of modifying the neuronal circuitry in the brain. This period may have different durations for different brain regions.

crossed extension reflex—Withdrawal of a limb in response to painful stimuli with the extension of opposite side lower extremities.

crus cerebri (pes pedunculi)—Cortical pyramidal fiber tracts passing through the brainstem on their way to the lower motor neurons in the brainstem and spinal cord.

CT—See COMPUTERIZED TOMOGRAPHY.

cuneocerebellar tract—Spinal fibers mediating unconscious proprioception from the distal upper limbs to the cerebellum.

cuneus—Occipital lobe region on midsagittal surface.

cupula—Mass of gelatinous material covering the hair cells of a crista in the ampulla of a semicircular canal that are stimulated when the head moves.

cutaneous—General sensation from skin.

cystic cavity—Fluid-filled space outlined by astrocytes in large cortical lesions.

cytoarchitectonism—Related to the structure, organization, and arrangement of nerve cells in the brain.

cytoarchitectural map—Map of brain areas based on their cellular composition. Numbered Brodmann areas form the most widely used cytoarchitectural map of the brain.

cytokinesis—Changes occurring in the cellular cytoplasm during cell division.

cytologic—Related to cells.

cytoplasm—Substances present within the cellular plasma but external to the nucleus.

cytotrophoblast—Cellular layer developing from the trophoblast. Forms components of fetal membranes, such as amnion, chorion, and placenta.

dark adaptation—Process of the retina becoming sensitive to light in dim lighting conditions.

decerebrate rigidity—Sustained contractions of the extensor muscles that result from lesions in the brainstem reticular formation above the vestibular nucleus.

decibel (dB)—Unit used to measure sound intensity by calculating the ratio between two sound pressures.

decussation—Crossing over of fibers, illustrated by the decussation of the pyramidal tract and dorsal-column lemniscal fibers in the caudal medulla.

deep cerebellar nuclei—Nuclei embedded within the cerebellar medullary region, including the dentate, emboliform, globose, and fastigial nuclei.

deglutition (swallowing)—Reflexive action instigated by the sensory and motor components of multiple cranial nerves along with reticular participation.

déjà vu—Sensation of having experienced a feeling or been in a place before.

delirium—Altered state of consciousness of sudden onset that consists of fluctuating attention, confusion, distractibility, disorientation, disordered thinking, impaired memory, and agitation. Underlying causes include toxicity, structural damage, and metabolic disorders.

dementia—Acquired progressive impairment of cognitive functions and altered personality. Clinically it is characterized by reduced memory, disorientation, and impaired judgment, and is associated with structural brain diseases.

demyelination—Degenerative condition involving the insulating myelin sheath around the axon commonly seen in multiple sclerosis.

dendrites—Cellular processes that receive impulses from other cells.

dentate nucleus—Largest of the cerebellar nuclei. Involved with limb coordination.

denticulate ligaments—Fibrous ligaments attaching the spinal cord to surrounding dura mater.

depolarization—Changes in membrane potentials in which the cellular interior changes from negative (resting potential) to positive.

depression—An altered mental state characterized by feelings of sadness, despair, low self-esteem, and compulsive thoughts. Subjects also exhibit reduced motor activity, and social withdrawal. Altered autonomic functions include loss of appetite, diminished libido, and loss of interest in things considered to be significant before.

dermatome—Cutaneous body region receiving most of its sensory innervation from one dorsal root ganglion, brainstem segment, or spinal nerve.

diabetes insipidus—Condition of excessive thirst and urination caused by inadequate secretion of the antidiuretic hormone.

diabetes mellitus—Disease in which glucose is not adequately oxidized in the body tissue because of insufficient insulin.

diadochokinesia—Ability to make rapid alternating movements of the limbs.

diaphragm—Primary muscle of inspiration. Also forms a partition between the abdominal and the thoracic cavities.

dichotic listening—Neuropsychological testing tool that involves simultaneous presentation of auditory stimuli to both ears. It is used for evaluating cerebral dominance.

diencephalon—Inner part of the brain that lies between the cerebral hemispheres and the midbrain. Includes the thalamus and hypothalamus.

diffusion—Temperature-based movement of molecules from a region of high concentration to an area of low concentration, resulting in a balanced distribution.

diffusion tensor imaging—MRI technique that evaluates the pathology of the white matter in the CNS by measuring movement and directionality of water molecules in the axonal tract.

diffusion weighted imaging—Measures the diffusion of water in tissues (apparent diffusion, based on brownian motion).

digital subtraction angiography—Imaging technique comparing an X-ray image of an artery before and after an intravenous injection of a contrast substance.

diopter—Unit used for measuring the refractive power of the eye, which is reciprocally related to the focal distance.

diphenylhydantoin (phenytoin, Dilantin)—Commonly used drug for treating seizure disorders.

diplopia—Pathologic condition of double vision by which a single object is seen as being two objects.

disequilibrium—Impaired balance marked by unsteady gait, with the body wavering toward the site of lesion during locomotion.

disjunction—Separation of bivalent chromosomes during anaphase.

diuresis—Excessive secretion and output of urine. Commonly seen in diabetes mellitus.

diurnal—Occurring every day.

DNA *(deoxyribonucleic acid)*—Double-stranded molecular structure containing an organism's genetic information.

dominant inheritance—Genetic expression mode in which a dysfunctional allele possessed by on parent dominates the second allele from the other parent. Each offspring has a 50% probability of inheriting this dysfunctional gene and the disorder.

dopamine—One of the inhibitory neurotransmitters secreted by neurons in the brainstem. Its increased and decreased secretion is associated with schizophrenia and Parkinsonism, respectively.

dorsal—Toward the superior surface of the brain.

dorsal column—Ascending medial lemniscal spinal system fibers meditating postural position sense, fine discriminative touch, and vibration.

dorsal horn—Region of the spinal cord containing sensory cell bodies.

dorsal spinocerebellar tract—Spinal projections to the cerebellum mediating unconscious proprioception from the distal lower limbs.

Down syndrome (DS, trisomy 21)—Inherited defect characterized by mental retardation, small skull flattened from front to back, short and flat nose, short fingers, and a widened space between the first two digits. Results from an extra copy of chromosome 21.

dressing apraxia—Failure to dress the left half of the body owing to impaired spatial perception of a garment in relation to the body. Part of right parietal lobe syndrome.

Duchenne muscular dystrophy—Disease of muscular atrophy transmitted through X-linked inheritance.

dura mater—Outermost layer and toughest of the three meninges.

dural sinuses—Network of dura-covered passages for blood in and around the brain.

dynamic equilibrium—Ability to maintain balance during locomotion.

dysarthria—Disorders of motor speech that result from central or peripheral disturbances and it affects muscular control of the articulators.

dysdiadochokinesia—Impaired ability to undertake rapidly alternating movements subsequent to cerebellar pathologies.

dyskinesia—Impaired ability to perform voluntary movements.

dyslexia—Impaired ability to read and comprehend written information subsequent to brain damage.

dysmetria—Error in the judgment of a movement's range and distance to the target, which is associated with cerebellar lesions.

dysphagia—Difficulty in swallowing.

dystonia—Represents a series of abnormally sustained postures and slow jerky movements mostly involving the trunk, neck, and proximal limbs.

ectoderm—Outermost cellular layer of the three layered embryo.

Edinger Westphal nucleus—Visceral nucleus of the oculomotor nerve (cranial nerve III), which regulates ciliary muscles (lens accommodation) and iris muscle (papillary light reflex).

efferent—Axonal fibers that mediate nerve impulses away from the central nervous system and cell body.

electroencephalography—Technique that records normal and abnormal electrical activity from the brain. Also used to evaluate seizure disorders.

electromyography—Visual record of muscle electrical activity during rest and spontaneous and/or voluntary movements. It is used to determine causes of muscular weakness, paralysis, and involuntary twitching.

embolism—Blocking of an artery by a sclerotic tissue (embolus), which is detached from atherosclerotic plaque.

embryoblast—Inner cell mass that gives rise to the embryo proper.

embryonic (or animal) pole—Region of the blastocyst with inner cell mass. Opposite pole is abembryonic (vegetal) pole.

emmetropia—Normal vision in which light rays converge on the retina.

encapsulated endings—Ovoid fluid-filled receptors with multiple layers. Highly sensitive to deformation.

encephalitis—Condition of brain inflammation caused by viral or bacterial infection and characterized by fever, stiff neck, and headache.

encephalopathy—Dysfunction of the brain because of degenerative or structural changes in the brain.

endarterectomy (carotid)—Surgical procedure used for removing arterial plaque formed by an atheroma deposit along with the diseased arterial lining of the walls in the carotid artery. Performed if the artery is > 70% blocked.

endoderm—Innermost of the three primary germ layers.

endolymph—Extracellular fluid that fills the semicircular canals, utricle, and saccule.

endoneurium—Layer of connective tissue that wraps around axons in the peripheral nervous system.

endorphin—One of the peptides in the brain that is concerned with pain. Similar effects as morphine.

endothelial cells—Layer of cells lining the blood vessels.

enkephalin—Neurotransmitter with projections in the basal ganglia and associated structures participating in controlling pain.

enteric nervous system—Part of the autonomic nervous system regulating intestinal activity.

ependymal cells—Layer of cells that lines the interior surface of the ventricular cavity and the central canal.

epiblast—Embryonic germ layer on the dorsal aspect of the bilaminar disk that gives rise to ectoderm, neuroectoderm, and mesoderm.

epicritic—Fine discriminative touch. Includes two-point touch, stereognosis, and graphesthesia.

epidural space—Potential space between the dura and the bone visible in pathologic conditions.

epilepsy—Sensory, motor, cognitive, and affective disorder with some altered consciousness that results from abnormal electric discharges in the brain.

epinephrine (adrenaline)—Important reticular formation catecholamine neurotransmitter that is synthesized from norepinephrine.

epineurium—Connective tissue sheath that surrounds a nerve in the peripheral nervous system.

epithalamus—Part of the thalamus consisting of pineal gland and habenular nucleus.

equilibrium—State of body balance in space. Dynamic equilibrium maintains balance when moving. Static equilibrium maintains balance in a relatively stationary (nonmovement) state.

estrogen—Female sex hormones that promote development of sex characteristics.

etiology—Study of the causes of a disease.

euploid—Exact multiple of haploid number of chromosomes.

eustachian tube—Tube that connects the middle ear with the nasopharynx. Equalizes air pressure on both sides of tympanic membrane (eardrum).

excitatory postsynaptic potential—Impulses that activate the postsynaptic cell to generate an action potential.

expanded tips endings—Receptors with expanded tips. Slow-transmitting and moderately adapting mechanoreceptors.

expiration—Physiologic process of expelling air from the lungs. Also called exhalation.

extension—Movement that straightens a limb.

extensor—Muscle that causes limb extension when it contracts.

external capsule—Slender white fiber bundle located lateral to the putamen.

extracellular fluid (ECF)—Fluid outside body cells, similar to interstitial fluid.

extra-embryonic—Derived from a trophoblast.

extrafusal fibers—Contractile muscle fibers that make up the bulk of a skeletal muscle.

extrapyramidal pathways—Motor tract fibers that convey motor information from the brain down to the spinal cord and originate from the basal ganglia subthalamic nucleus, and substantia nigra.

extreme capsule—Slender white fiber bundle located lateral to the putamen and external capsule.

facial nerve—Cranial nerve VII, which is responsible for controlling all the muscles of facial expression, taste from the anterior two-thirds of the tongue, and secretory regulation of glands.

falx cerebelli—Triangular-shaped vertical extension from tentorial cerebelli that separates the cerebellar hemispheres.

falx cerebri—Large, sickle-shaped extension of dura between the cerebral hemispheres.

far point—Point from which light rays originate.

fasciculation—Involuntary contractions of groups (fasciculi) of muscle fibers from hyperexcitability of motor units.

fasciculus (fasciculi)—Bundle of nerve fibers that originate from a common source, terminate at a common point, and mediate a common function.

fasciculus cuneatus—Sensory fibers carrying sensations of fine discriminative touch from the upper half of the body.

fasciculus gracilis—Sensory fibers carrying sensations of fine discriminative touch from the lower half of the body.

fastigial nucleus—Cerebellar nucleus connected to the vestibular system. Plays a role in equilibrium.

fertilization—Penetration of a secondary oocyte by a sperm cell, resulting in a gamete.

fetal alcohol syndrome (FAS)—Refers to the effects of intrauterine exposure to alcohol on a fetus, resulting in retarded growth and limited cognitive skills.

fetus—Developing organism in utero from the beginning of the 3rd month to birth.

fibrillation—Spontaneous twitch of individual muscle fibers.

fibromyalgia—Syndrome of chronic musculoskeletal pain owing to undetermined etiology.

fields of Forel (H fields)—Prerubral region through which various basal ganglia projections pass before terminating in the thalamus.

filum terminale—Fibrous extension of the spinal cord attached to the coccyx.

fissure—Groove region bordering the gyri on the brain surface, also called sulcus (pl. sulci).

flaccid—Weakened muscle with less than normal tone. A lower motor neuron symptom.

flaccid dysarthria—Motor speech disorder associated with injuries of cranial nerve motor neurons.

flexion—Muscle movement that bends a limb.

flexor—Muscle that contracts to cause flexion.

flocculi (flocculonodular lobe)—Oldest portion of the cerebellum. Has a role in equilibrium.

focal length—Distance between the lens and the point where light rays converge to form a focused image.

focal point—Retinal point at which light rays converge for focusing.

foramen—Opening or aperture.

foramen magnum—Opening in the base of the skull through which the caudal end of the brainstem exits to connect with the spinal cord.

foramen of Magendie—Medial aperture that releases cerebrospinal fluid from the fourth ventricle to the subarachnoid space.

foramina of Luschka—Two laterally located apertures that release cerebrospinal fluid from the fourth ventricle to the subarachnoid space.

forebrain—Brain region derived from the rostral embryonic brain and including the telencephalon and diencephalon.

fornix—Bundle of fibers that mediates two-way connections among the hypothalamus, septum, and hippocampus. Important in visceral functions.

fourth ventricle—cerebrospinal fluid–filled cavity lying between the cerebellum and the medulla oblongata and pons.

fovea—Dipped area in the macula lutea. Site of central fixation responsible for sharp vision.

fragile X syndrome—X-linked recessive syndrome characterized by mental retardation, atypical facial features (long and narrow face with large ears, a prominent mandibular symphysis, and a high-arched palate), and macroorchidism (abnormally large testes).

free nerve endings—Small and slowly conducting mechanoreceptors. Associated with pain and temperature.

frequency—Number of complete cycles of vibrations, expressed in Hertz (Hz) per second.

Friedreich ataxia—Genetic condition of an autosomal recessive trait, involving the degeneration of the spinocerebellar tract and characterized by skeletal deformations, limb weakness, and loss of vibration and position sense.

frontal lobe syndrome (pseudopsychopathic behavior)—Disorder of executive functions characterized by impairments of cognitive functions (attention, memory, reasoning, thinking, planning, self-monitoring, and purposeful activity) and decision making.

frontotemporal dementia—Degenerative condition of the frontal and temporal lobes that results in personality changes, behavioral symptoms, and cognitive impairments. Also called Pick disease.

functional MRI—Neuroimaging technique that measures cortical neuronal activity (increased blood flow to the cortical area) in response to specific somatosensory or linguistic tasks.

functional plasticity—Capability of the brain to reorganize functionally after undergoing a pathologic condition.

GABAergic neurons—Inhibitory neurotransmitter neurons in the basal ganglia. Its deficiency leads to Huntington chorea.

gag reflex—Brainstem-mediated reflex—from the glossopharyngeal nerve (cranial nerve IX) and vagus nerve (cranial nerve X)—involving vomiting involuntarily, which is triggered by a touch on the posterior one-third of the tongue, the pharynx, or the soft palate.

gametes—Male and female sex cells.

gametogenesis—Process through which male and female sex cells develop.

γ-aminobutyric acid (GABA)—Major inhibitory neurotransmitter of the brain synthesized from glutamate. Its deficiency in the striatum is implicated with Huntington chorea.

γ-motor neurons—Slow-conducting, small spinal motor neurons that supply intrafusal muscle fibers.

ganglion (pl. ganglia)—Cluster of cell bodies in the peripheral nervous system.

gene expression—Process that converts gene-coded information into the operating of a cell and structure.

gene mutation—Any spontaneous heritable changes in the sequencing of DNA elements.

general functions—Touch, pain, and temperature information processed by general receptors.

general visceral efferent (GVE) fibers—Axonal fibers mediating autonomic commands to visceral structures.

generalized seizure—Extensive and synchronized electrical activity in nerve cells that spreads to the entire brain.

genes—Units of heredity located at a fixed position on a particular chromosome.

genetics—Concerned with the means and consequences of hereditary transmission.

geniculate bodies—Thalamic relay nuclei related to vision (lateral geniculate body) and audition (medial geniculate body).

geniculocalcarine fibers (optic radiations)—Visual fibers radiating from the geniculate body to the primary visual cortex in the occipital lobe.

genome—Complete DNA sequence containing entire genetic information of an individual or a species.

genotype—Genetic makeup of an individual.

genu—Angular rostral region of the corpus callosum.

geriatrics—Concerned with the medical problems and care of the elderly.

gland—Specialized epithelial cells functioning as a secretory or excretory organ.

glaucoma—Eye disease characterized by increased intraocular pressure in the anterior cavity caused by poor absorption of aqueous humor. If not treated causes optic nerve atrophy and blindness.

glia cells—Secondary cells (astroglia, microglia, and oligodendroglia) in the nervous system that serve as supportive connective tissue.

global aphasia—Aphasia characterized by profound impairment of language functions across all modalities.

globose nucleus—Cerebellar nucleus participating in the coordination of skilled movements.

globus pallidus—Part of the basal ganglia involved with motor activity.

glossopharyngeal nerve—Cranial nerve IX, which has sensorimotor functions involving the oral and pharyngeal cavities.

Golgi complex—Microscopic organelle in the cytoplasm of cells responsible for processing, sorting, packaging, and delivering proteins and lipids to the plasma membrane.

Golgi tendon organ—Specialized receptive endings sensitive to muscle tension and interdigitated among the extrafusal muscle fibers in muscle tendons.

gonadotropic—Hormones secreted in the anterior pituitary gland (adenohypophysis) that affect differential growth and function of sex gland cells.

grand mal (tonic–clonic) seizure—Seizure disorder characterized by loss of consciousness and tonic convulsions, electric discharges originating from the cortex, basal ganglia, brainstem and/or reticular formation, repeated hyperextension of the body, and breath-holding spells resulting in cyanosis (skin discoloration owing deficient oxygenation of the blood).

graphesthesia—Discriminative sensory ability used to recognize the outline of letters, words, or symbols written on the skin surface.

gray matter—Term used for the collection of cell bodies in the central nervous system.

gray ramus communicans—Short nerve containing postganglionic sympathetic fibers that extend by way of the gray ramus to a spinal nerve and then to the periphery to supply smooth muscle in the blood vessels, arrector pili muscles, and sweat glands.

gyrus—Elevated cortical regions between sulci and fissures.

haploid—Half of the normal number of chromosomes.

hearing impairment—Reduced responsiveness to acoustic stimuli.

hearing level (HL)—Individual threshold sensitivity to pure tone stimuli.

hearing tests—Pure tone stimuli used to evaluate hearing thresholds.

helicotrema—End region of the cochlea that connects the scala vestibuli to the scala tympani.

hematoma—Accumulated mass of extravasated blood, usually located in a potential space.

hemianesthesia—Loss of pain and touch sensation on one side of the body.

hemianopsia—Loss of pain and touch vision in half of the visual field.

hemiballism—Violent swinging movements on one side of the body associated with damage to the subthalamic nucleus.

hemiparesis—Mild weakness of one side of the body.

hemiplegia—Paralysis of one side of the body involving both the upper and the lower limbs.

hemophilia—Hereditary blood disorder characterized by deficient production of blood clotting factors and resulting in excessive bleeding.

hemorrhage—Discharging of blood from a ruptured artery.

hepatolenticular degeneration (Wilson disease)—Basal ganglia disease resulting from degenerative changes in the basal ganglia and liver owing to a metabolic disorder. Clinically characterized by dysarthria and involuntary movement.

heredity—Passage of parental characteristics to offspring via genes.

Heschl gyri—Short, oblique convolutions in the lateral sulcus that form the primary auditory cortex.

high altitude sickness—Condition characterized by headache, fatigue, insomnia, shortness of breath, nausea, and dizziness caused by decreased atmospheric levels of oxygen at high altitude.

hippocampal gyrus—Long convolution that overlies the hippocampus and covers the medial ventral surface of the temporal lobe.

hippocampus (hippocampal formation)—Limbic structure bordering the lateral ventricle inferior horns in the temporal lobe. Thought to be related to memory functions.

histology—Microscopic study of tissue structures.

homeostasis—Optimal state of bodily equilibrium involving the chemical composition of fluids and tissues that is conductive to normal body functioning.

homologous chromosomes—Two chromosomes that belong to a pair. Also called homologues.

homonymous hemianopia—Loss of vision in same visual fields for both eyes.

homonymous left inferior quadrantanopsia—Blindness involving the left inferior quarters of the visual field in both eyes.

homonymous left superior quadrantanopsia—Blindness involving the left superior quarters of the visual field in both eyes.

homozygous—Possessing a pair of similar alleles on homologous chromosomes for a particular gene.

homunculus—Representation of the body in the sensorimotor cortex.

hormones—Chemical substances that originate in an organ and regulate important body activities.

Horner syndrome—Neurologic condition characterized by ptosis (unilateral eyelid dropping), miosis (pupil contraction), and anhidrosis (diminished perspiration) on the ipsilateral side of the forehead. Associated with a lesion of the cervical sympathetic chain or its central projections.

human growth hormone (hGH)—Hormone secreted by the anterior pituitary gland that stimulates growth of body tissues, especially skeletal and muscular.

Huntington chorea—Progressive degenerative condition of dominant inheritance characterized by involuntary movements, cognitive deficits, and dysarthric speech.

hydrocele—Fluid-containing sac or tumor.

hydrocephalus—Accumulation of cerebrospinal fluid in the brain ventricles secondary to its impaired absorption.

hypalgesia—Increased threshold for pain resulting in a decreased sensitivity to pain.

hyperacusia—Abnormal hearing sensitivity where normal sounds seem very loud.

hyperalgesia—Decreased threshold for pain marked by increased response to painful stimuli.

hypercholesterolemia—Excessive amount of cholesterol in the blood.

hypermetropia (hyperopia)—Optical condition in which light rays focus behind the retina, also called farsightedness.

hyperparathyroidism—Increased level of parathyroid hormone secretion.

hyperplasia—Increase in cell number subsequent to an injury.

hyperpolarization—Increased internal negativity across a cell membrane causing changes in voltage.

hypersecretion—Overactivity of glands resulting in excessive secretion.

hypersomnia—Excessive sleep, usually during normal waking hours.

hyperthermia—Unusually high fever.

hypertrophy—Increase in the size of cells or organs.

hypoblast—Embryonic germ layer on ventral aspect of the bilaminar disk that gives rise to endoderm.

hypoglossal nerve—Cranial nerve XII, which controls tongue movements.

hypoglycemia—Abnormally low glucose concentration in the blood.

hypokinesia—Slow or limited movements.

hypokinetic dysarthria—Type of dysarthric speech characterized by limited and slow movement. Associated with Parkinson disease.

hyponatremia—Low level of serum sodium.

hyporeflexia—Diminished or reduced strength of a reflexive response of a skeletal muscle that results from pathology of the lower motor neuron or reduced lower motor neuron excitability.

hypothalamus—Diencephalic structure, located beneath the thalamus, that secretes hormones and regulates feeding, fighting, and sexual behavior.

hypothermia—Lowering of body temperature < 35°C (95°F). In medical management it involves a deliberate cooling of the body to slow down metabolism and reduce the oxygen needs of tissues.

hypotonia—Muscle with reduced tone and lessened resistance to passive movement.

hypoxemia—Low oxygen level in the arterial blood.

hypoxia—Lower than normal level of oxygen in body tissues.

ideomotor apraxia—Inability to carry on skilled purposeful movements to a verbal command secondary to a disconnection between motor and ideational centers.

idiopathic—Emergence of a disease without an apparent cause.

immunity—Body's natural power to resist the attack of disease or harmful agents.

impulse—Action potential.

incus—Middle ear bone.

inertia—Tendency of matter to resist change in motion (If matter is at rest, it remains at rest. If moving, it continues to move until acted on by an external force).

infarct—Area of damaged tissues caused by insufficient or blocked blood supply.

inferior cerebellar peduncle—Restiform body. One of the fiber bundles connecting the cerebellum with the brainstem. Mediates spinal and vestibular inputs to the cerebellar hemispheres.

inferior colliculus—Midbrain structure involved with auditory reflexes and is concerned with the transmission of auditory signals to the medial geniculate body of the thalamus.

inferior mesenteric ganglia—Prevertebral sympathetic nucleus.

inferior olivary nucleus—Medullary structure that mediates spinal and vestibular afferents to the cerebellum.

inflammation—Edematous response by tissue to an injury.

infundibular stem—Stalk of the pituitary gland.

inheritance—Acquisition of genetic information from parents.

inhibitory postsynaptic potentials—Impulses that inhibit the capacity of a postsynaptic cell to generate an action potential.

insomnia—Inability to sleep during the night for no apparent reason.

inspiration—Refers to the drawing of air into the lungs.

instinctual reflexes—Protective stereotypical motor responses occurring in response to biologic needs.

insula (isle of Reil)—Triangular cortical brain area buried within the lateral sulcus.

intensity—Amplitude of energy in sound waves that determines loudness.

intention tremor—Rhythmic pill-rolling movements of fingers associated with cerebellar pathology, which are apparent during voluntary movements.

intercostal muscles—Muscles located between the ribs.

interhemispheric—Relating to a structure common to both cerebral hemispheres or a structure located between them.

interhemispheric (longitudinal) fissure—Long vertical fissure that marks the medial boundary of the cerebral hemispheres.

internal arcuate fibers—Crossing fibers of the dorsal lemniscal system at the medulla that form the medial lemniscus.

internal capsule—Collection of ascending and descending fibers at the diencephalic level.

internal-external carotid anastomosis—Surgically created vascular channel connecting the internal and the external carotid arterial system to restore the blood circulation in the case of cerebral ischemia.

internal medullary lamina—Vertical layer of the white matter that divides the thalamus.

interneurons—Spinal association neurons that interconnect other nerve cells and function to modify the lower motor neuron response via facilitation or inhibition.

interpeduncular fossa—Area located on the inferior surface of the midbrain between the bilaterally located crus cerebri.

interstitial fluid—Extracellular fluid that fills the spaces between the cells of tissues and regulates the internal environment of the body.

interventricular foramen of Monro—Opening that connects the lateral ventricles in the forebrain with a single third ventricle in the midbrain.

intracranial pressure—Pressure located within the cranium or skull which is caused by space-occupying lesions in the brain.

intrafusal fibers—Specialized skeletal muscle fibers contained in the encapsulated muscle stretch receptor, called a muscle spindle, that extend parallel to the extrafusal fibers. Innervated by small γ-motor neurons. Contraction modifies the responsiveness of the stretch receptor endings.

intrahemispheric—Related to structures within one hemisphere.

intralaminar centromedian nucleus—Largest of the intralaminar nuclei in the thalamus and has extensive afferents and efferents to the brain and brainstem.

ion—Electrically charged atoms.

ion selectivity—Membrane permeability to selected ions.

ionic equilibrium—Electrical potential difference that regulates the ionic concentration gradient across the cell membrane.

ipsilateral—The same side of the CNS with reference to a given point; it is best illustrated by the lesion and its effects being on the same side of the body.

iris—Colored contractile fibers that regulate pupil size.

ischemia—Reduced supply or unavailability of blood for tissue oxygenation owing to hemorrhagic stroke, stenosis, or thrombosis. It causes cellular death.

isthmus—Narrow passage or tissue strip connecting two larger parts.

iter—See CEREBRAL AQUEDUCT.

karyotype—Presentation of an individual's chromosomes arranged in a standard format according to their shapes and sizes.

Kayser-Fleisher ring—Circle formed by the accumulation of copper around the cornea. Seen in Wilson disease.

kinesthesia—Internal awareness of the range and direction of limb movements.

Klinefelter syndrome—Male chromosomal disorder in which the individual has an additional X chromosome (47, XXY). Characterized by genital abnormalities and mental retardation.

Klüver-Bucy syndrome—Behavioral syndrome that results from bilateral ablation of the amygdala and surrounding temporal tissues. Characterized by indiscriminate eating, oral exploration, fearlessness, loss of aggression, psychic blindness, and hypersexuality.

Korsakoff syndrome—Disorder characterized by amnesic symptoms, confusion, and memory impairment caused by nutritional deficiency owing to chronic alcoholism. Also called Korsakoff psychosis, which evolves from untreated Wernicke encephalopathy.

labyrinth—Interconnecting and communicating bony and membranous cavities in the inner ear, including the semicircular ducts, vestibule, and cochlea.

labyrinthine disease—Inner ear dysfunctions characterized by deafness, tinnitus, vertigo, nausea, and vomiting.

labyrinthitis—Inflammatory condition of the inner ear clinically characterized by hearing impairment and vertigo.

lacrimal—Related to tears.

lacrimal gland—Secretory cells in the orbit responsible for the secretion of tears.

lacunar stroke—Small multiple strokes in the thalamus and basal ganglia as a result of hypertension.

lamina terminalis (lamina terminalis hypothalami)—Thin plate derived from telencephalon. It is the rostral end of former neural tube. Later in development, it forms the anterior wall of the third ventricle of the cerebrum.

lateral—Moving away from the midline.

lateral corticospinal tract—Represents the spinal location of the crossed fibers of the corticospinal tract.

lateral geniculate body—Thalamic nucleus responsible for the transmission of visual information to the cortex.

laterality—Hemispheric superiority for serving language.

lateral lemniscus—Fibers projecting auditory impulses between the superior olivary nucleus and the inferior colliculus.

lateral spinothalamic tract—Ascending fiber bundle that mediates the sensation of pain and temperature to the brain.

lateral (sylvian) fissure—Major cortical fissure that separates the temporal lobe from the frontal and parietal lobes.

lateral ventricle—Largest of the ventricular cavities in the cerebral hemispheres.

lemniscus—Collection of nerve fibers carrying similar information.

lens—Transparent organ constructed of proteins that refracts light rays on the retina.

lenticular fasciculus—Fiber bundle that transmits basal ganglia projections from the globus pallidus to the thalamus.

lenticular nucleus—General term for the globus pallidus and putamen.

leptomeninges—General term for the pia and arachnoid membranes.

leukemia—Malignant blood disease marked by abnormal white blood cells.

light adaptation—Physiologic process through which retinal cells gradually become less sensitive to bright light.

light reflex—Constriction of the pupil in response to light, a parasympathetic activity.

limbic lobe—Phylogenetically an older part of the brain that regulates reproductive behavior, instinctual reflexes, and vegetative activities.

limbic system—Visceral structures of the forebrain (dentate gyrus, amygdaloid body, septal nuclei, mammillary bodies, anterior thalamic nucleus, olfactory bulbs, and many bundles of myelinated axons) that regulate emotion and behavior.

limbic (visceral–emotional) brain—Mammalian portion of the brain responsible for motivation, emotional drive, and instinctual activities.

Lissauer tract—Pain- and temperature-mediating fibers of the dorsolateral fasciculus that travel up or down a few segments of the spinal cord before penetrating the dorsal gray matter.

lobe—Regional division of the brain bounded by fissures and sulci such as frontal, temporal, parietal, and occipital lobes.

locus ceruleus—Important reticular formation nucleus in the brainstem that produces norepinephrine and widely projects to different brain areas.

lower motor neuron (LMN)—Motor nucleus of the brainstem and spinal cord which extends its axons through the peripheral nerve roots to control skeletal muscles.

lower motor neuron syndrome—Clinical symptoms of flaccid paralysis, hyporeflexia, and muscular atrophy associated with a lesion involving spinal or cranial motor neurons and/or their axons.

lumbar cistern—Enclosed space at the end of the cord containing the cerebrospinal fluid.

lumbar plexus—Network of interjoined nerve fibers originating from T12–L4 and serving the abdomen, buttocks, and anterior thigh.

lumbar puncture—Diagnostic procedure that involves removing a small amount of cerebrospinal fluid from the lower lumbar section of the vertebral canal for chemical and cellular analyses.

luminosity curve—Visual representation of the spectral sensitivity of photoreceptors to light rays of various wavelengths.

macrophage—Phagocytic cell that digests and removes cellular debris in the brain.

macula—Specialized sensory structures in the vestibular apparatus that contribute to the maintenance of static equilibrium during linear acceleration and deceleration.

macula lutea—Yellowish area in the posterior retina that predominantly contains cones and mediates color vision.

magnetic resonance angiography (MRA)—Used to evaluate the structural integrity of blood vessels. An important diagnostic tool for identifying arterial stenosis, aneurysm, and arteriovenous malformation.

magnetic resonance imaging (MRI)—Imaging technique that uses magnetic activity of the tissue to create clear images of the living brain and body.

magnetic resonance spectroscopy—MRI application to evaluate the biochemical profile of nerve cells.

malignant—Spreading and fast-growing tumor that causes death.

malleus—Middle ear ossicle attached to the tympanic membrane.

mammillary bodies—Two small rounded hypothalamic structures posterior to the tuber cinereum that participate in related visceral and memory functions.

massa intermedia—Loose fibrous tissue that passes through the third ventricle interconnecting both thalami.

maturation—Developmental processes through which a cell reaches its full functional potential.

mechanoreceptors—Sensory receptor responsible for selective stimuli.

medial forebrain bundle—Important limbic fiber bundle that interconnects the forebrain, limbic structures, hypothalamus, and the midbrain tegmentum and connects to dopaminergic, noradrenergic, and serotonic neurons.

medial geniculate body—Thalamic nucleus responsible for transmitting auditory information to the primary auditory cortex.

medial lemniscus pathways—Sensory pathways located in the dorsal third of the spinal cord and mediate epicritic proprioception, discriminative touch, two-point discrimination, pressure, and vibration sensation.

medial longitudinal fasciculus—Brainstem fiber bundle that runs on each side of the midline in the brainstem beneath the fourth ventricle. It interconnects ocular cranial nerve nuclei with vestibular projections and plays an important role in coordinated head, eye, and body movements.

medulla oblongata—Most inferior part of the brainstem.

medullary reticulospinal tract—Located within the medulla. Projects to the spinal motor neurons and regulates muscle tone.

meiosis—Cell division process that occurs during the formation of sex cells in which the number of chromosomes is halved.

Meissner corpuscles—Sensory receptors with encapsulated endings mediating the sensation of deep and discriminative touch.

melanocytes—Pigment-producing cells in the choroid of the eyeball which increase the clarity of visual perception by absorbing stray light elements.

membrane—Thin sheet of tissue serving as a covering or as the lining of a cavity.

membrane potentials—Electric voltages across a cell membrane.

memory—Ability to retain and retrieve learned information.

Ménière disease—Chronic condition of the membranous labyrinth. Marked by edema due to an increase in endolymphatic pressure. Characterized by progressive hearing loss, vertigo, and tinnitus.

meninges—Three protective membranes (dura, arachnoid, and pia) that cover the central nervous system.

meningitis—Bacterial or viral infection of the central nervous system that causes inflammation in the meningeal membranes of the brain and spinal cord.

Merkel receptors—Receptors with expanded tips mediating touch and temperature.

mesencephalon (midbrain)—Midbrain region derived from the vesicle of mesencephalon.

mesoderm—Middle of the three primary germ layers.

metabolism—Cellular biochemical activities that include analytical (catabolic) and synthetic (anabolic) reactions that generate energy.

metaphase—Stage in mitotic cellular division.

metastasis—Spread of disease from a location in one part of the body to another, as is in the migration of cancerous cells through lymphatics and blood vessels.

metencephalon—Subdivision of rhombencephalon consisting of the pons and cerebellum.

Meyer loop—Optic fibers of the geniculocalcarine tract radiating through the anterior temporal lobe before reaching the occipital cortex.

microcephaly—Embryologic malformation in which the brain and skull cap are small in comparison to the face, resulting in mental retardation.

microfilaments—Protein actin that contribute to the cellular skeleton.

microglia—Small scavenger glia cells that digest and remove cellular debris from the CNS.

microtubules—Represented as straight protein tubulin that contribute to the cellular skeleton and are responsible for axoplasmic transport.

micturition—Urination.

midbrain—Part of the brainstem between the pons and the diencephalon. Also called the mesencephalon.

middle cerebellar peduncle—Brachium pontis. A bundle of fibers that connects the cerebellum with the basilar pons.

middle cerebral artery—Large intracranial vessel supplying blood to the entire lateral surface of the brain and parts of the basal ganglia structures.

middle ear—Air-filled cavity containing three bones.

midsagittal plane—Vertical plane through the midline of the brain or body, dividing it into equal left and right halves.

miosis—Condition of a permanently constricted pupillary aperture.

mitochondria—Organelle of the cellular cytoplasm containing enzymes providing the principle energy source for the cell.

mitosis—Cell division process in which the daughter cell receives the identical number and kinds of chromosomes.

modiolus—Conical bony structure around which the cochlea is wrapped.

monoamines—Subgroup of small molecular neurotransmitters derived from amino acids.

monocular vision—Visual field processed by only one eye.

monoplegia—Paralysis confined to one limb.

monosomy—Absence of one chromosome from a homologous pair.

morula—Tiny sphere of blastomeres.

mossy fibers—Afferent fibers that include all sensory projections to the cerebellum, except for the olivocerebellar fibers.

motion sickness—Vestibular syndrome characterized by the sensation of vertigo, dizziness, nausea, and vomiting. Present when an individual is in motion.

motion tremor (intention tremor)—Oscillatory movements caused by irregular muscle contraction in the case of cerebellar pathology. Present only during an action period as opposed to a resting condition.

motor cortex—Cortical region consisting of Brodmann area 4. Involved with control and regulation of voluntary movements.

motor end plate—Postsynaptic membrane at the neuromuscular junction.

motor neuron—Located in the anterior horn of the spinal cord. Controls muscle cells and causes muscle contraction.

motor unit—Forming a neuronal circuit consisting of an α–lower motor neuron, its axon, myoneural junctions, and innervated muscles. It acts as a unit in that if the lower motor neuron fires, all the muscle cells of the unit fire at the same time.

movement disorders—Tremor and chronic types of involuntary disorders commonly seen after basal ganglia pathologies.

multiple sclerosis—Disease of progressive degeneration of the neuronal myelin sheath from an autoimmune disorder in the central nervous system, causing impaired nerve conduction, paresthesia, and disorders of equilibrium, movement, sensation, and vision.

multipolar cells—Neurons containing many dendrites and one axon.

muscles of respiration—Include the diaphragm, abdomen, and intercostals that participate in inspiration and expiration and are controlled by spinal motor neurons.

muscle spindles—Intramuscular encapsulated receptor apparatus in specialized skeletal (intrafusal) muscle fibers that are sensitive to changes in muscle length.

muscle tone—Consistent contraction of portions of a skeletal or smooth muscle in response to activation of stretch receptors.

muscular dystrophy—Inherited disease of muscle degeneration, characterized by weakness and progressive atrophy of the skeletal muscle.

mutation—A spontaneous changes in a gene or chromosomal structure.

myalgia—Pain in muscles.

myasthenia gravis—Autoimmune neuromuscular disorder that results from growth of antibodies to acetylcholine receptors.

mydriasis—Dilation of the pupil.

myelencephalon—Medulla oblongata derived from the myelencephalic division of the rhombencephalon.

myelin—Sheath of lipid and cell membrane wrapped around an axon and contributes to the speed of impulse transmission.

myoneural junction—Synapse of an α–lower motor neuron axon on a single skeletal muscle fiber.

myopathy—Disease of muscles.

myopia—Refraction error in which light rays converge in front of the retina. Also called nearsightedness.

myosin—Thin filament protein of muscle fibers that contributes to the contraction of muscle fibers by chemical interactions.

myotatic reflex—Reflexive muscle contraction in response to muscle stretch.

myotome—Muscles innervated by the motor neurons of a single spinal segment.

narcolepsy—Sleeping disorder characterized by recurring episodes of excessive sleeping in the day and disrupted nocturnal sleep. Frequently accompanied by cataplexy, sleep paralysis, and hallucinations.

nasal hemianopsia—Loss of vision in the nasal field of one eye.

nausea—Sensation of impending vomiting.

necrosis—Island of dead tissues surrounded by normal areas of tissues.

neocerebellum—Newer part of the cerebellum (posterior lobe) concerned with skilled movements such as speech.

neocortex—Six-layered cerebral cortex found in mammals only.

neologisms—Unrecognizable new word formations of patient's own making found in the acute stages of Wernicke aphasia.

neoplasm—New and pathologic growth of tissue that can be benign or malignant.

neostriatum—General term for the basal ganglia referring to the caudate nucleus and putamen.

nerve(s)—One or more bundles of myelinated or unmyelinated fibers in the peripheral nervous system.

nerve cell—Specialized cell of the nervous system that conducts electrical impulses.

nerve conduction—Measure of impulse transmission between two points on a nerve for identifying peripheral nerve pathologies.

nervous system—Collectively refers to the brain, spinal cord, nerves (cranial and spinal), and autonomic ganglia that maintain the vital functions of the body in response to internal and external stimuli.

neural crest—Segmentally arranged neuroectodermal tissue that separates from the neural tube dorsally before it closes. Develops into elements of the peripheral nervous system and other specialized structures.

neuralgia—Pain sensation extending along the course of a nerve.

neural plate—Thickened midline plate of neuroectoderm that develops into the neural tube, giving rise to the central nervous system.

neural tube—Embryologic structure that results from the fusion of neural folds and develops into the brain and spinal cord.

neuraxis—Brain and spinal axis.

neurilemma—Outermost covering of axons formed by Schwann cells in the peripheral nervous system.

neurite—Thin tube-shaped process extending from a neuronal cell. Further divided into an axon and dendrite.

neuritis—Inflammation of nerves from structural irritation or infection.

neuroblast—Immature cell before cell division.

neuroembryology—Study of the embryologic origins and development of the nervous system from fertilization to the 8th gestational week of development.

neurofibrillary tangles—Age-induced twisting of fibers in the soma of nerve cells, often associated with Alzheimer disease. These are also found in the brains of Down syndrome patients.

neurofibrils—Small fibers within the cytoplasm serving as the channels for intracellular communication among the cytoplasmic organelles.

neurofilaments—Important components of the cellular skeleton. Serve as channels for intracellular communication.

neuroglia—Cells associated with the nervous system—including astrocytes, oligodendrocytes, microglia cells, ependymal cells and neurolemmal (Schwann) cells—responsible for a variety of supportive functions. Also called glial cells.

neuroleptic—Class of drugs (tranquilizers) used for treating psychoses.

neurology—Study of the nervous system and diseases that disrupt its structural and physiologic properties.

neuromuscular junction—Myoneural junction marked by the space between the neuron and the muscle.

neuron—Nerve cell with a cell body and its processes that participate in impulse transmission.

neuropathology—Study of the pathology of the nervous system.

neuropathy—Nerve disease.

neuropeptide—Naturally occurring amino acid chain in the nervous system modulating the response of or to a neurotransmitter.

neuropharmacology—Study of the effects of drugs on the nervous system.

neurophil—Mature white blood cell that is formed by the myelopoietic tissue found in the bone marrow.

neurophysiology—Study of the chemical, electrical, and metabolic functions of the nervous system.

neuroradiology—Subspecialty of diagnostic radiology focusing on the diseases of the central nervous system.

neurosurgery—Surgical intervention used for the removal and remediation of pathologic structures that impair the functional organization of the nervous system.

neurotransmitter—One of a variety of molecules within axon terminals released into the synaptic cleft in response to a nerve impulse and affects the membrane potential of the postsynaptic neuron. Also called a transmitter substance.

night blindness (nyctalopia)—Inability to see at night after a normal period of dark adaptation.

Nissl bodies—Endoplasmic structures in neuronal cell bodies that participate in protein synthesis.

nociceptors—Receptors sensitive to harmful stimuli such as pain.

node of Ranvier—Intervening space between two internodes (segments) of myelin.

nodulus—Part of the flocculonodular lobe of the cerebellum. Serves a role in equilibrium.

nondisjunction—Failure of two homologous chromosomes or two chromatids to dissociate during meiosis. Results in one cell having an extra chromosome and the other cell missing a chromosome.

non-rapid eye movement sleep—Stage in sleep characterized by slow and large waves. Marked with some muscle tone and paucity of dreams.

nonspecific nuclei—Thalamic nuclei that receives input from diffuse sources and projects to diffuse cortical areas—for example, intralaminar nuclei that mediate reticular projections to the cortex and influence the synchronization of brain electrical activity.

noradrenergic synapses—Nerve endings in which norepinephrine is released.

norepinephrine—Catecholamine neurotransmitter (noradrenalin) released by neurons primarily in the pons and medulla. Cells that produce norepinephrine are called noradrenergic cells.

normal pressure hydrocephalus—Large ventricles with impaired absorbing dynamics of the cerebrospinal fluid. Clinically characterized by dementia and gait disturbances seen in elderly patients.

notochord—Primitive, solid, skeletal structure derived from specialized mesodermal cells. Retained in the intervertebral disk as the nucleus pulposus and lies ventral to the neural tube.

nuclear bag fibers—Intrafusal sensory fibers mediating dynamic sensory responses of the spindles.

nuclear chain fibers—Intrafusal sensory fibers mediating static responses of the muscle spindles.

nucleolus—Located within the nucleus of a cell body, and it contains RNA needed for protein synthesis.

nucleus—Control center of a nerve cell.

nucleus cuneatus—Specialized nerve cells in the caudal region of the medulla oblongata responsible for mediating fine discriminative touch from the upper half of the body.

nucleus dorsalis of Clarke—Second-order spinal neurons that mediate unconscious proprioception.

nucleus gracilis—Specialized nerve cells in the caudal medullary region responsible for mediating fine discriminative touch from the lower half of the body.

nucleus pulposus—Adult remnant of the notochord in the intervertebral disk.

nystagmus—Oscillatory movement of eyeballs consisting of slow and fast components. Identified according to direction of fast component.

oblique plane—Section passing through the body or organ at an angle.

obstructive sleep apnea—Closing of the upper airway due to relaxation of the pharyngeal muscles, resulting in breathing problems during sleep.

occipital lobe—Posterior region of the cerebrum.

occlusive vascular disease—Vascular diseases characterized by arterial occlusion, such as thrombosis and embolism.

octonia—Gelatinous mass that incorporates sensory hair cells covered by a thin layer of densely packed calcium carbonate crystals.

ocular convergence—Directing both eyes to a common focal point for a clear visual perception.

oculomotor nerve—Cranial nerve III, which regulates the majority of the ocular muscles.

olfaction—Sense of smell.

olfactory bulb—Bulb-shaped brain structure that receives input from the olfactory receptor neurons.

olfactory cortex—Region of the cerebral cortex connected to the olfactory bulb. Includes the uncus, amygdaloid nucleus, and anterior region of the parahippocampal gyrus.

olfactory epithelium—Cellular sheet that lines the nasal passages and contains olfactory receptor neurons.

olfactory nerve—Cranial nerve I, which mediates smell.

olfactory receptor—Bipolar neuron with a cell body, lying in the mucous membrane of each nasal cavity, responsible for transducing odors into neural signals.

olfactory sulcus—Sulcal location for the olfactory bulb.

olfactory tract—Axonal bundle extending from the olfactory bulb to the primary olfactory cortex in the temporal lobe.

oligodendrocytes—See OLIGODENDROGLIA.

oligodendroglia—Glia cells that produce the myelin sheath around axons in the central nervous system.

olivocerebellar fibers—Medullary projection to the cerebellum mediating spinal and vestibular afferents.

oogenesis—Development of a female sex cell (ova).

oogonia—Primordial cell from which an oocyte is derived.

ophthalmic—Related to the eye.

ophthalmoplegia—Paralysis of the extrinsic or intrinsic eye muscles.

opsin—Protein found in the rhodopsin of rods.

optic chiasm—Structure in the visual pathway where part of the fibers from each nerve decussate to form the optic tracts.

optic disk (papilla)—Area through which the optic nerve (cranial nerve II) exits and arteries enter the eyeball.

optic nerve—Cranial nerve II, consisting of a bundle of ganglion cell receptors that passes from the eye to the optic chiasm.

optic radiation—Refers to a collection of axons coursing from the lateral geniculate body to the visual cortex.

optic tectum—Structure used to describe the superior colliculus.

optic tract—Collection of retinal ganglion cell axons extending from the optic chiasm to the brainstem.

optokinetic nystagmus—Abnormal rotary ocular movements activated by visual fixation or moving visual patterns.

organ of Corti—Auditory receptor organ that contains hair cells and supporting cells and is located in the scala media.

osmotic pressure—Pressure exerted by active elements in a solution.

ossicles—Three small bones in the middle ear: malleus, incus, and stapes.

otitis media—Infectious accumulation of serous fluid in the middle ear that, if untreated, causes conductive hearing loss.

otolithic membrane—Gelatinous membrane lying over the hair cells of the saccule and utricle in the vestibular sac.

oval window—Hole in the bony cochlea at which movement of the ossicles is transferred to movement of the fluids in the cochlea.

oxidation—Chemical dissolution of nutrients for energy.

oxytocin (Pitocin)—Peptide hormone released from the posterior pituitary. Stimulates uterine contractions in a pregnant uterus for inducing delivery and ejection of milk from mammary glands of breasts.

pacinian corpuscle—Mechanoreceptor in the skin sensitive to vibrations.

paleocerebellum—Anterior lobe of the cerebellum, primarily concerned with equilibrium and partial adjustments in locomotion.

pallidum—General term referring to the globus pallidus.

palsy—Muscle paralysis or paresis.

Papez circuit—Considered the neurologic base of emotional expression, pain control, and visceral motor activity. Interconnects the hypothalamus, brain, hippocampus (mammillary bodies), anterior thalamic nucleus, cingulate gyrus, and parahippocampal gyrus.

para-hippocampus—Memory-related cortical region located on the medial surface of the temporal lobe.

paralysis—Refers to a loss of voluntary control of the muscles. Spastic paralysis is associated with upper motor neuron syndrome, whereas flaccid paralysis is associated with lower motor neuron syndrome.

paraphasia—Inappropriate selection of words and phonemes commonly seen in aphasia.

paraplegia—Paralysis of both lower limbs and lower trunk.

parasagittal plane—Vertical plane parallel to the midline that divides the body into unequal left and right parts.

parasympathetic system—Division of the autonomic nervous system with nuclei in the cranial and sacral region concerned with the conservation of body energy.

parenchyma—Functionally specialized cells of an organ.

paresthesia—Abnormal sensation such as numbness, crawling, and itching.

Parkinson disease—Movement disorder of the basal ganglia characterized by resting tremor, muscular rigidity, and paucity of movements.

paroxysmal discharges—Periodic occurrence of abnormal electrical discharges in the brain.

pars compacta—Region of the substantia nigra with dopaminogenic projections to the striatum.

pars reticulata—Substantia nigra region receiving inhibitory striatal projections.

partial or focal epilepsy—Sudden onset of sensory and/or motor behavior confined to a single body part and a progressive recruitment of other body parts. Referred to as the Jacksonian march.

peduncle—Bundle of fibers that connects the cerebellum and brainstem.

peptide neurotransmitters—Large molecules consisting of two or more amino acids that can function as neurotransmitters or neuromodulators.

perfusion MRI—Neuroimaging technique that maps out the function of the cerebral cortex by measuring microscopic blood flow levels in the cerebral capillaries.

periaqueductal gray matter—Region surrounding the cerebral aqueduct in the midbrain.

perilymph—Fluid contained in the bony labyrinth (scalae vestibuli and tympani) that protects the membranous labyrinth.

peripheral nerve injuries—Injuries confined to nerves in the peripheral system, such as cranial nerves and/or spinal nerves.

peripheral nervous system (PNS)—Part of the nervous system that includes all the cranial and spinal nerves.

peripheral neuropathies—Diseased conditions of peripheral nerves, such as carpal tunnel.

peristalsis—Wavelike contracting movements in a hollow structure that propel its contents.

peritoneal cavity—Potential abdominal space between the layers of the parietal and visceral peritoneum.

periventricular zone—Hypothalamic region that medially borders the third ventricle.

permeability—Property of brain vessels that restricts the passage of selective fluids and noxious substances.

pernicious anemia—Anemic state characterized by a progressive decrease in red blood corpuscles. Can be fatal if not treated.

persistent vegetative state—Altered consciousness state in which patients are not aware of the environment and display no cognitive functions but t breath on their own, and follow the sleep-wake cycle.

PET—See POSITRON EMISSION TOMOGRAPHY.

pH—Indicates the degree of acidity and alkalinity in a solution, with 7 being the neutral value. A number less than 7 marks increased acidity, whereas a number greater than 7 indicates alkalinity.

phagocyte—Macrophagic microglia cells that ingest cellular debris.

phagocytosis—Process of digestion by cells referring to the removal of dead tissue by microglia cells.

phantom pain—Sensation of pain originating from the area of an amputated limb.

phenobarbital—Family of drugs commonly used in the treatment of epilepsy.

phenytoin (diphenylhydantoin, Dilantin)—Drugs used in the treatment of seizure activity.

phonologic agraphia—Writing disorder characterized by an impaired ability to convert phoneme to grapheme.

phonologic dyslexia—Impaired ability to convert grapheme to phoneme, resulting in poor reading ability, particularly for pronounceable pseudo-words.

photopigment—Rhodopsin or a visual pigment that absorbs light and undergoes structural changes, leading to the generation of an action potential.

photopsin—Visual pigment found in retinal cones.

photoreceptors—Specialized retinal cells that transfer light energy into action potentials.

pia mater—Inner most layer of the three meninges.

Pick disease—Dementia-causing disease of the frontotemporal degeneration marked by the presence of pathologic Pick bodies in the brain.

pineal gland—Thalamic organ important in diurnal rhythm.

pituitary gland—Hypothalamic structure of hormone synthesis in the central nervous system that is divided into a large anterior lobe (adenohypophysis) and a small posterior lobe (neurohypophysis).

planum temporale—Area of the superior temporal lobe posterior to Heschl Gyrus. It is larger in the left temporal lobe and is associated with cerebral dominance.

plaque—Abnormal patch of lipid deposition along the inner arterial wall. Also refers to demyelinated areas in multiple sclerosis.

plasticity—Brain's capability of being reorganized in the face of an injury, a property that is most evident in developing young brains, particularly before 6 years of age.

platelet-inhibiting drugs—Medications like such as acetylsalicylic acid (aspirin), dipyridamole (Persantine), clopidogrel bisulfate (Plavix), and ticlopidine (Ticlid) are commonly used to prevent platelet aggregation.

plexus—Network formed by the interconnected nerves from multiple spinal segments.

pneumotaxic area—Pontine respiratory center that limits inspiration and facilitates expiration.

poikilothermy—Condition in which the temperature of an organism is similar to the temperature of the environment.

polar bodies—Two or three cells formed during the first and the second meiotic division of oocytes that consists of almost all nuclear materials. Do not develop further and are lost.

polarization—Electrical resting state of a cell characterized by the polarity of ions inside and outside the cell.

poliomyelitis—Acute viral disease of the lower motor neurons in the spinal cord and brainstem.

polydipsia—Condition characterized by excessive fluid intake.

polyuria—Condition characterized by excessive discharge of urine.

pontine nuclei—Nuclei clusters that mediate cortical projections to the cerebellar cortex.

pontine pneumotaxic center—Automatic brainstem respiratory center consisting of several groups of scattered neurons in the reticular formation.

pontine tegmentum—Pontine area located below the fourth ventricle.

pontocerebellar fibers—Fibers arising from nuclei of the basilar pons and crossing to project to the cerebellum via the middle cerebellar peduncle.

portal system—Low-pressure vascular system that carries hypothalamic hormones to the anterior pituitary gland (adenohypophysis).

positron emission tomography (PET)—Imaging technique that measures live real-time cellular metabolism using radioactive substances (isotopes).

postcentral gyrus (somesthetic cortex or primary sensory cortex)—Cortical region (Brodmann area 3, 1, 2) behind the central sulcus that integrates sensory inputs from the body and provides sensory awareness.

posterior cerebral artery—One of the three cortical arteries originating from the circle of Willis and supplying blood to the basal surface of the occipital and temporal lobes and the midsagittal surface of the occipital lobe.

posterior column–medial lemniscus pathways—Sensory pathways located in the dorsal third of the spinal cord. Mediate epicritic proprioception, discriminative touch, two-point discrimination, pressure, and vibration sensation. First-order fibers remain ipsilateral and project to the second-order neurons in the caudal medulla. Second-order fibers cross the midline and project to the contralateral thalamus, the site of the third-order neurons. Third-order fibers project to the ipsilateral somatosensory cortex. See MEDIAL LEMNISCAL PATHWAYS.

postganglionic fibers—Sympathetic and parasympathetic fibers with cell bodies in the cells of the automatic ganglia. Project to the cells in the target muscles.

postganglionic neuron—Second visceral motor neuron in an autonomic pathway with its unmyelinated axon ending at cardiac muscle, smooth muscle, or a gland.

postsynaptic neuron—Neuronal surface located on the distal side of a synapse.

precentral gyrus—Primary motor cortex (Brodmann area 4), located rostral to the central sulcus.

prechordal plate—Region of tall hypoblastic cells anterior to the notochord. With ectoderm, forms the oropharyngeal membrane.

precuneus—Parietal lobe region located in the midsagittal surface.

prefrontal cortex—Recent addition to the frontal cortex, with connections to the dorsomedial thalamus, serving cognitive and personality functions.

preganglionic fibers—Sympathetic and parasympathetic fibers before synapsing on the additional autonomic ganglia.

preganglionic neurons—Autonomic nervous system neurons, with cell bodies in the spinal cord and brainstem, that project to the secondary ganglion.

premotor cortex—Area located anterior to the motor cortex that programs and regulates skilled movements.

preoptic area—Anterior portion of the hypothalamus located above the optic chiasm.

presbyacusis—Age-induced sensorineural hearing loss due to the degeneration of hair cells.

presbyopia—Age-induced impairment in the lens ability to accommodate the eyes for seeing near objects.

primary auditory cortex—Located on the superior surface of the first temporal gyrus and receiving auditory projections. Undertakes higher analysis of acoustic stimuli essential for the perception of sound.

primary motor area—Precentral gyrus region of the cerebral cortex that controls specific or groups of muscles.

primary somatosensory area—Postcentral gyrus area of the parietal cortex responsible for somatic sensation from the body.

primitive streak—Thickened region of epiblastic cells in the dorsal caudal midline of the embryo in the 3rd week of gestation. Epiblastic cells transform into mesoderm–mesenchymal cells through this region.

primordium—Earliest identifiable rudiment of tissue seen during development.

principal (inferior) olivary nucleus—Nucleus that projects spinal, vestibular, and reticular information to the cerebellum.

progressive bulbar palsy—Motor neuron disease characterized by a progressive degeneration of cranial nerve nuclei in the brainstem.

progressive symptoms—Symptoms that continue to get worse.

projection fibers—Descending and ascending axonal bundles of fibers mediating sensory and motor functions.

prolactin (PRL)—Hormone secreted by the anterior pituitary gland and is responsible for initiating milk secretion by the mammary glands.

pronation—Movement that turns the palm downward.

prophase—First stage in cell division.

proprioception—Internal awareness of position, posture, and movement.

prosencephalon (forebrain)—Embryonic part of the brain that develops into the cerebral hemispheres, basal ganglia, and limbic system.

prosopagnosia—Acquired impairment in the ability to recognize familiar faces. A right parietal lobe symptom.

protopathic—Primitive sensory system that includes pain, temperature, and crude touch.

protraction—Movement that projects a limb or organ forward.

pseudobulbar palsy—Pathologic condition involving bilateral supranuclear paralysis of the speech muscles—Has significant implications for spastic dysarthria.

psychomotor (partial complex) seizures—Convulsive disorders secondary to lesions involving the medial temporal lobe structures (amygdala, hippocampus, and overlying temporal cortex). Characterized by recurring episodes of automatic, irrational behavior of which there usually is no memory.

psychosis—Severe form of mental disorder characterized by a disorganization of thinking, personality, and behavior. The presence of delusions and hallucinations interfere with daily life.

psychosomatic—Refers to bodily disorders thought to be caused entirely or partly by emotional disturbances.

pterygopalatine ganglion—Parasympathetic postganglion of the facial nerve.

pulvinar—The posterior most thalamic nucleus.

pupil—Opening through which light enters the eye and strikes the retina.

pupillary accommodation—Bilateral reflexive constrictive reaction of the pupil in response to bright light. A parasympathetic activity. Involves the projection of light to the midbrain pretectal area and to the Edinger-Westphal (visceral) nucleus of the oculomotor cranial nerve, the ciliary ganglion, and the pupillary constrictor muscle.

pupillary aperture—Opening of the pupil.

pupillary light reflex—Change in diameter of the pupils in response to projected light. Mediated by the visceral fibers of the oculomotor cranial nerve from the brainstem to the iris.

pure tone audiometry—Audiologic assessment evaluating hearing thresholds to pure tone stimuli.

pure word deafness—Aphasic syndrome characterized by the isolation of the language cortex from the primary auditory cortices as a result of a bilateral lesion in the temporal lobes.

Purkinje cells—Large cerebellar nerve cells.

putamen—Anatomic structure of the basal ganglia.

pykrosis—A necrotic stage marked by a reduction in size of a cell.

pyramidal decussation—Crossing of motor fibers that takes place in the most caudal medulla and accounts for contralateral motor organization.

pyramidal fibers—Descending corticospinal fibers mediating motor impulses to spinal motor neurons.

pyramidal tract—The motor fibers of the corticospinal tract named because of their location in the medullary pyramids.

pyriform cortex—Primary olfactory cortex located on the medial rostral region of the uncus and hippocampal gyrus.

quadrant—One of four parts of the visual field.

quadrantanopsia—Blindness involving one-quarter of the visual field.

quadriplegia—Paralysis of all four limbs.

raphe nucleus—Collection of reticular cells located along the midline in the brainstem that diffusely project to all levels of the brain.

rapid eye movement (REM) sleep—Sleep stage characterized by high-frequency and low-amplitude EEG waves, vivid dreams, and rapid eye movements.

recessive inheritance—Genetic mode of inheritance in which both parents transmit the same affected alleles. It results in 25% probability of this dysfunctional gene transmission from both parents and the child being affected with the condition.

reciprocal inhibition—A neuronal circuitry in which an action potential is excitatory to motor units in an agonistic skeletal muscle and is excitatory to an inhibitory interneuron that, in turn, reduces the excitability of motor units in the paired antagonistic muscles. This ensures that when one muscle is contracting, its paired muscle is relaxing.

reciprocal innervation—Innervation of one of the paired muscles in which the response is opposite to the response of the other muscle connected to the same joint.

red nucleus—Midbrain cell cluster that relays cerebellar output to the motor cortex and spinal cord.

referred pain—The sensation of pain from a visceral organ is sensed as originating from another body part. The explanation for this false localization is that the visceral structures do not have separate afferent pathways, rather they synapse on the same neurons in the dorsal root ganglion that also receives somatic sensation from the superficial structures.

reflex—Hard-wired stereotypical response to a specific stimulus. All reflexes, except the stretch reflex, involve at least three neurons: the afferent neuron, one or more interneurons, and one or more efferent neurons.

refraction—Bending of light rays as they travel from one medium to another.

refraction errors—Focusing deviations from the optimal fixation point of the retina. Myopia (near-sightedness) and hyperopia (far-sightedness) are two common types of focusing errors.

regional cerebral blood flow (rCBF)—Neuroradiologic technique that measures blood flow to functionally active brain areas by monitoring a radioactive tracer.

Reissner membrane—Cochlear membrane that separates the scala media from the scala vestibuli.

Renshaw cells—Inhibitory neurons in the spinal cord that are connected to and inhibited by the collaterals of adjacent motor neurons.

respiration—Involves the transfer of gases among the atmosphere, blood, and body cells and is marked by inhalation and exhalation.

respiratory center—Reticular neurons in the brainstem that regulate the rate and depth of respiration.

restiform body—See INFERIOR CEREBELLAR PEDUNCLE.

resting membrane potential—Membrane potential of −70 mV. At this stage, the nerve cell is not generating action potentials.

resting state—Denotes the state when the cell is polarized.

resting tremor—Involuntary motor activity during rest. Associated with Parkinson disease.

reticular formation—Diffuse core of brainstem nuclei with parallel and serial projections that integrates the entire nervous system and is involved with cortical arousal and muscle preparedness.

reticulocerebellar pathway—Descending fibers that originate in the brainstem and mediate reticular projections to the cerebellum.

retina—Neural layer of the eye that contains photoreceptor cells-rods and cones.

retinal (visual yellow)—Light-absorbing molecule of rhodopsin in rods, an aldehyde of vitamin A.

retinotectal potentials—Axons that leave the retina and synapse on the superior colliculus.

retraction—Movement that pulls back a limb or organ.

retrocochlear auditory mechanism—Fibers of the acoustic cranial nerve and projections to the cochlear nuclei in the brainstem.

retrograde reaction (degeneration)—Changes occurring in the proximal portion of a damaged axon. Also called Wallerian degeneration.

rhodopsin—Visual purple pigment found in the outer segments of rod cells.

rhombencephalon (hindbrain)—Caudal-most of the primary vesicles of the embryonic neural tube. Divides into metencephalon and myelencephalon.

righting reflex—Postural pattern that controls the position of the neck and extremities in space.

rigidity—Stiff state of muscles involving both agonist and antagonist muscles, which is present throughout resistance (plastic pipe phenomenon). Clasp-knife is the transient increased resistance of extensors to passive muscle movement, which melts away with persisting resistance.

Rinne test—Tuning fork test used to detect the presence of conductive hearing loss. The stem of a tuning fork (usually 512 Hz) is first held against the mastoid process and the patient listens to the tuning fork by bone conduction. When the patient longer hears through bone conduction, the tuning fork is held near the opening of the external auditory meatus to determine if the patient can hear by air conduction. A patient with a conductive hearing loss will not hear the tuning fork by air conduction (negative Rinne).

rods—Retinal photoreceptors responsible for night vision.

Romberg sign—Evaluates equilibrium in the case of impaired proprioception from the lower extremities. The patient is asked to stand with the feet together with the eyes closed. A patient with the loss of proprioception is likely to fall when the eyes are closed.

rostral—Toward the front of the head.

rotational sensation—Persistent sensation of motion commonly seen in labyrinthine dysfunctioning.

round window—Opening between the middle and inner ear covered by the secondary tympanic membrane.

rubrospinal tract—Group of axons involved with motor movements that descend from the red nucleus and terminates on the motor neurons in the spinal cord.

Ruffini endings—Moderately adapting subcutaneous receptors mediating tactile and temperature information.

saccule—Membranous sac in the vestibule of the labyrinth.

sacral plexus—Formed by interjoined nerves originating from several sacral spinal segments.

sagittal—Vertical section dividing the brain into left and right halves.

saltatory conduction—Propagation of an action potential along a myelinated axon where current jumps from one node to the next.

satiety center—Group of hypothalamic nuclei that, when stimulated, bring about a reduction in desire to eat.

saturated fat—Fatty acid that is commonly associated with heart diseases and is prevalent in triglycerides of animal products, such as meat, milk, milk products, and eggs.

scala media—Endolymph-filled cochlear region lying between the scala vestibuli and the scala tympani.

scala tympani—Perilymph-filled lowermost compartment of the cochlea, which is connected to the scala vestibuli through the helicotrema.

scala vestibuli—Perilymph-filled uppermost compartment of the cochlea.

Scarpa ganglion—Bipolar vestibular ganglia projecting impulses from the hair cells in the semicircular canals to the brainstem vestibular nucleus complex.

Schwann cells—Glia cells that form myelin around the axons in the peripheral nervous system.

sclera—Outer (white) layer of the eyeball.

scotoma—Area of lost vision within the visual field.

scotopic vision—Night vision mediated by rod cells.

seizure disorders—Sensory, motor, cognitive, and affective disorders resulting from abnormal electrical discharges in the brain.

semicircular canals—Three circular ducts containing sensory organs suspended in endolymph for reflexive control of dynamic equilibrium.

semiovale center—Mass of white matter located below the cerebral cortex.

sensorineural hearing loss—Hearing loss resulting from a dysfunctioning organ of Corti or cochlear nerve (CN VIII).

sensory cortex—Postcentral gyrus area responsible for the perception of bodily experienced modalities of pain, touch, and temperature.

sensory receptors—Nerve endings that respond to environmental changes by producing receptor (graded) potentials.

septum pellucidum—Thin membrane located above the septal nuclei and anteriorly dividing the lateral ventricles.

serotonergic—Cells that secrete serotonin, a vasoconstrictor neurotransmitter in the CNS that also inhibits gastric secretion and stimulates smooth muscle.

serotonin—Important central nervous system neurotransmitter that plays a role in sleep and wakefulness.

sex chromosomes—The X and Y chromosomes that determine the sex of an individual (XY for males, XX for females).

signs—Physician made objective clinical observations.

single photon emission tomography (SPECT)—Imaging technique that measures cerebral blood flow using a radioactive substance.

sinus—Hollow channel covered with dura in the brain that receives deoxygenated blood after circulation.

skeletal muscles—Muscles that contain striated fibers that move bones around a joint.

sleep—State of partial unconsciousness characterized by a low level of activity in the reticular activating system.

sleep disorders—Irregularity in reaching, maintaining, and leaving a physiologic state of partial unconsciousness marked with inactivity of the voluntary muscles of the body.

smooth muscle—Tissue located in the walls of hollow internal organs and innervated by autonomic motor neurons.

Snellen test—Test used to evaluate visual acuity and clarity.

sodium Amytal infusion—Test used for inducing a transient anesthetization of the human brain to determine cerebral dominance.

soma—Cell body. The central region of the neuron.

somatic—Relating to structures derived from a series of mesodermal somites, including skeletal muscles, bones, and dermis.

somatic nervous system (SNS)—Division of the peripheral nervous system consisting of somatic sensory (afferent) neurons and somatic motor (efferent) neurons.

somatosensation—Bodily experienced modalities of pain, touch, and temperature.

somatosensory evoked potentials—Evoked electric responses of the central nervous system to specific sensory activity.

somatostatin—Capable of inhibiting the release of the hormone somatotropin by the anterior lobe of the pituitary gland.

somite—Segmental blocklike mass of mesoderm on either side of the notochord. Gives rise to muscles, vertebral bodies, and skin.

sound pressure—Amplitude of sound in pressure units relative to a reference pressure.

spastic dysarthria—Impaired motor speech functions secondary to bilateral interruption of corticobulbar fibers. Characterized by articulatory imprecision, monopitch, and reduced stress.

spastic hemiplegia—Paralysis of one side of the body after a lesion in the pyramidal tract.

spasticity—Hypertonic state of muscles characterized by increased muscle tone.

special functions—Vision- and audition-related information, mediated by specialized receptors.

specific nuclei—Group of thalamic nuclei that project definitive information to functionally committed specific cortical areas—for example, the lateral geniculate body is concerned with vision and projects to the primary visual cortex.

spermatogenesis—Development of a male sex cell (spermatozoon).

spermatogonia—Male germ cell or gamete, undifferentiated and arising from the seminiferous tubule, dividing into two primary spermatocytes.

spina bifida—Several types of embryonic malformation marked by an open vertebral column.

spina bifida cystica—Embryologic failure of fusion involving one or more vertebral arches, which is associated with a meningeal cyst (meningocele) or a cyst containing both meninges and spinal cord (meningomyelocele).

spina bifida occulta—Genetic spinal defect with no protrusion of the cord or its membrane.

spinal accessory nerve—Cranial nerve XI, which is responsible for raising the shoulders and turning the head contralaterally.

spinal anesthesia—Injection of liquid anesthetic into the lumbar spinal subarachnoid space to cause a temporary loss of sensation in the lower body extending up to the level of injection.

spinal nerve—Nerve of the spinal cord that innervates the body.

spinal plexuses—Network of interconnected spinal nerves.

spinal tap—Procedure used for extracting the cerebrospinal fluid for diagnostic purposes. The cerebrospinal fluid is removed from the subarachnoid space in the lumbar region. Also called lumbar puncture.

spinal trigeminal nucleus (tract)—Second-order nucleus and descending fibers that mediate pain and temperature from the face.

spinocerebellar system—Spinal projection to the cerebellum mediating unconscious proprioception from the lower and upper limbs.

spinocerebellar tract—Fiber bundle that mediates unconscious proprioception to the cerebellum.

spinothalamic pathway—Ascending bundle of fibers that mediates the sensation of pain, touch, and temperature from the spinal cord to the thalamus.

spiral ganglia—First-order auditory nerve cells that receive impulses from the cochlear hair cells and project to the cochlear complex in the brainstem.

splenium of corpus callosum—Posterior part of the corpus callosum.

stapedius—A muscle, controlled by the facial nerve (cranial nerve VII), in the middle ear that reflexively contracts to attenuate hearing sensitivity by restricting ossicular movement.

stapes—Middle ear ossicle that is attached to the oval window.

static equilibrium—Balancing during a stationary posture.

static labyrinth—Maintenance of a balanced position of the head and body in space against gravity during rest and during straight line head movements.

stenosis—Narrowing of arteries.

stereognosis—Identification of objects by tactual sensation of shape, texture, and size.

stereotaxic (stereotactic)—Precise method of localization for lesion placement in a deep-seated brain structure using three-dimensional space. The space definition is given by the imaging modality used to define the target.

strabismus—Optic disorder in which visual axes of both eyes are not directed toward the same object.

stretch reflex—Skeletal muscle contraction resulting from passive or active stretching of the same muscle. It involves two-neuron reflex circuitry.

striate cortex—Primary visual cortex, or Brodmann area 17.

striatum—General term for the basal ganglia nuclei of the putamen and caudate nucleus.

stroke—Suddenly emerging neurologic deficits that result from vascular circulatory impairment.

stupor—Unresponsiveness from which a patient can be aroused transiently with strong and repeated stimulation.

subacute combined spinal degeneration—Spinal degeneration as a result of vitamin B_{12} deficiency. Commonly seen in chronic alcoholics and characterized by impaired transmission of proprioception and kinesthesia.

subacute symptoms—Clinical features that appear after the acute phase and are of moderate duration.

subarachnoid space—Real space filled with cerebrospinal fluid located between the pia mater and the arachnoid membrane.

subcallosal gyrus—Limbic structure located beneath the rostrum of the corpus callosum.

subdural hematoma—Localized mass of extravasated blood confined in a potential space below the dura mater.

subdural space—Potential space between the dura mater and the arachnoid membrane.

substance P—Inhibitory basal ganglia neurotransmitter that causes the suppression of dopaminergic activity in the substantia nigra.

substantia gelatinosa—Neurons located in the dorsal spinal column that receive nociceptive information.

substantia nigra—Contains many dopaminergic nuclei which project to and are inhibitory to the cells of the caudate and putamen. Degeneration of its neuron is associated with Parkinson disease.

subthalamic nucleus—Located between the internal capsule and the substantia nigra, this biconvex basal ganglia nucleus is involved with hemiballism.

subthalamus—Refers to a subcortical region that includes the subthalamic nucleus, zona incerta, and field H of Forel.

sulcus—Also called fissure. Includes the groove or furrow markings on the cortical surface.

superior cerebellar peduncle—Brachium conjunctivum. One of the fiber bundles that connects the cerebellum with the brainstem and motor cortex.

superior colliculus—Midbrain structure related to visual reflexes, such as ocular accommodation and coordinated head and eye movements.

superior olivary nucleus—Nucleus in the medullary tegmentum that is the first to receive projections from both cochleae and it plays an important role in sound localization.

supination—Movement that causes the palm to turn upward.

supplementary motor cortex—Midsagitally located extension of the premotor cortex, which is involved with bilateral aspects of motor pattern control and planning.

supramarginal gyrus—Located in the inferior parietal lobule. Linguistically important parietal lobe structure.

supraoptic nucleus—Hypothalamic nucleus.

surface dyslexia—Acquired reading impairment marked by phonemically relating grapheme to phoneme with no access to meaning through the entire word directly.

Sydenham chorea—Involuntary choreic movements appearing in children several months after streptococcal infection and subsequent rheumatic fever. The choreic movements involve the distal limbs and emotionally labile behaviors.

sympathetic chain—Series of interconnected ganglia located adjacent to the vertebral column.

sympathetic system—Anatomically and functionally distinct division of the autonomic nervous system with axonal projections from the thoracic and lumbar spinal regions. Concerned with the expenditure of body energy and with the regulation of bodily responses in flight-or-fight situations.

sympathetic trunk ganglion—Cell bodies of postganglionic sympathetic neurons located lateral to the vertebral column. The ganglia chain extends inferiorly through the neck, thorax, and abdomen to the coccyx on both sides of the vertebral column.

symptom—Patient-described subjective clinical observation.

synapse—Point of contact between two neurons where the neurotransmitter is released.

synaptic cleft—Point of junction between nerve cells.

syncytiotrophoblast—Syncytial layer without cell boundaries differentiated from the trophoblast. Enters into the formation of the placenta and its membrane.

synergy—Cerebellum-mediated coordinating aspect of muscles during movement.

syringomyelia—Developmental presence of a longitudinal cavity, mostly in the cervical spinal cord, clinically marked by pain, paresthesia, and analgesia of the hands.

tactile—Related to the sense of touch.

tardive dyskinesia—Involuntary slow and stereotypical movements of facial muscles. A side effect of psychotropic drugs such as haloperidol.

Tay Sachs disease—Disorder of autosomal recessive inheritance resulting in fatal brain damage with deterioration of mental and physical functions, convulsions, and enlarged head. Common in eastern European Jews.

tectorial membrane—Membrane that tips over the hair cells in the cochlea.

tectospinal tract—Tract that originates from nuclei in the superior colliculi and terminates on the spinal motor neurons. Regulates head and neck movements.

tectum—Region of the brainstem dorsal to the cerebral aqueduct in the midbrain that serves visual and auditory reflexes and provides a map of external space.

tegmentum—Cellular region of the midbrain and pons below the cerebral aqueduct and fourth ventricle.

telencephalon—Subdivision of the prosencephalon, which develops into the cortex of the cerebral hemispheres, basal ganglia (nuclei), and limbic lobe.

telophase—Final stage in the development of a nucleus.

tendon—Nerve fiber that attaches a muscle to a bone.

tendon organ—Proprioceptive receptors, sensitive to muscle tension and force of contraction, found chiefly near the junctions of tendons and muscles. Also called a Golgi tendon organ.

tensor tympani—Muscle, regulated by the trigeminal nerve (CN V), in the middle ear that reflexively contracts to attenuate hearing sensitivity by restricting ossicular movement.

tentorium cerebelli—Dural extension that covers the cerebellum and the floor of the cranium.

teratogen—Fetotoxic drug that causes the abnormal development of structures in the embryo.

teratogenesis—Abnormal development of an embryo that results in a deformed fetus.

teratology—Concerned with the development of malformed babies.

terminal bouton—Nerve end synaptic vesicles filled with neurotransmitters.

testosterone—Male sex hormone produced by the testicle. Promotes the development of sperm and sexual characteristics.

thalamic syndrome—Symptoms of transient hemiparesis and loss of superficial and deep sensation with preservation of crude pain in the hypalgesic (reduced sensitivity to pain) limbs secondary to infarction of the posteroinferior thalamus.

thalamus—Major diencephalic structure located on either side of the third ventricle and medial to the internal capsules. Plays an important role in sensorimotor integration and projection to the cortex.

thermal anesthesia—Loss of temperature (heat and cold) sensation.

thermal hyperesthesia—Abnormally lower threshold of sensitivity to heat and cold.

thermal hypoesthesia—Diminished sensitivity to heat and cold stimuli.

thermoreceptors—Receptors with sensitivity to heat and cold.

thiamine—Essential for growth, a vitamin present in milk and grain husks. Deficiency is associated with beriberi and Wernicke-Korsakoff syndrome, characterized by progressive personality changes and amnesia.

third ventricle—Space in the diencephalon filled with cerebrospinal fluid.

thoracolumbar outflow—Sympathetic preganglionic neurons with cell bodies in the lateral gray columns of the thoracic segments and the first two or three spinal lumbar segments.

threshold—Value of membrane potential at which the ionic current change flows into the membrane, causing the cellular interior to become positive.

thrombolytic agent—Chemical agents that dissolve blood clots and restore circulation. Also included in this category is tissue plasminogen activator (t-PA).

thrombosis—Formation of a localized clot that blocks the lumen of a blood vessel.

thymus—Lymphoid structure that functions as an endocrine gland.

thyrotropin—Thyroid trophic hormone secreted by adenohypophysis.

tic—Spasmodic involuntary twitching of muscles that are usually under voluntary control.

tissue plasminogen-activating agent (tPA)—Drug used to restore blood circulation in acute cases of thromboembolic stroke by dissolving the atherosclerotic clot.

tonotopic—Systemic organization of frequency distribution in the auditory cortex.

tract—Bundle of nerve fibers in the central nervous system.

tranquilizers—Drugs used to calm emotions without sedation.

transcortical motor aphasia—Severely limited verbal skills with preserved repetition skills caused by a lesion that separates Broca area from the surrounding association cortex.

transcortical sensory aphasia—Severely limited comprehension of spoken language and unabated repetition that results from the separation of Wernicke area from an adjacent association cortex.

transient ischemic attack (TIA)—Temporary cerebral dysfunction caused by transient disruption of the blood supply to the brain.

transient symptoms—Short-lived clinical symptoms.

trapezoid body—Transverse crossing fibers of the auditory pathway located in the pons.

tremor—Rhythmic pin-rolling movements of the fingers at rest, along with akinesia and rigidity that characterizes Parkinson disease. Intention tremor occurs during movement and results from cerebellar pathology.

trigeminal nerve—Cranial nerve V, which is responsible for sensation from the face, head, and mouth. Its motor fibers regulate the muscle of mastication.

trigeminal neuralgia—Stabbing pain involving one or more of the branches of the trigeminal nerve (CN V) that has a trigger zone. Also called tic douloureux.

trilaminar embryo—Human embryo in the 3rd week.

trisomy—Abnormal addition of an extra chromosome to a normal diploid chromosomal set.

trochlear nerve—Cranial nerve IV, which innervates the superior oblique muscle and participates in looking downward and outward.

trophoblast—Outer cell mass differentiating into cytotrophoblast and syncytiotrophoblast.

tumor—Uncontrolled neoplastic growth of tissue.

Turner syndrome—Chromosomal syndrome with 1 X and no Y chromosome (45 chromosomes), characterized by short stature, webbed-neck, abnormal sexual development, and broad chest.

tympanic membrane—Soft tissue covering that separates the external ear from the middle ear.

uncus—Structure of the limbic system associated with the perception of smell.

unipolar neuron—Neuron with a single process (neurite).

upper motor neurons (UMNs)—Cell bodies in the motor cortex and their descending axonal processes that synapse on the cranial and spinal motor neurons.

utricle—Membranous dilation of the vestibular apparatus.

vagus nerve—Cranial nerve X, which controls phonation and swallowing in addition to regulating many autonomic nervous system functions.

vascular—Related to blood circulation and blood vessels.

vascular spasm—Pathologic condition resulting from contraction of the smooth muscle of a damaged blood vessel with clinical implications for normal cerebral blood flow.

vascular system—Network of carotid and vertebrobasilar vessels supplying blood to the brain.

vasoconstriction—Decreased diameter of a blood vessel.

vasodilation—Increased diameter of a blood vessel, resulting in greater blood flow.

vasomotor center—Neural network localized in the medulla that controls arterial blood pressure and pulse rate.

vasopressin—Hypothalamic hormone transported to the posterior lobe of the pituitary gland and has an antidiuretic effect.

vein—Vessel that transports circulated blood from the body to the heart.

venous sinus system—Veins and sinuses responsible for draining blood and cerebrospinal fluid.

ventral—Location below the point of reference or the bottom of a brain structure.

ventral horn—Ventral region of the spinal cord that houses motor neurons.

ventral root—Bundle of motor fibers that originates from the spinal ventral horns.

ventral spinocerebellar tract—Pathway that mediates unconscious proprioception from the lower limbs to the cerebellum.

ventricles—Interconnected brain cavities that produce, store, and circulate the cerebrospinal fluid.

vermis—Midline structure of the cerebellum.

vertebra—Segment of spinal bone.

vertebral basilar system—Vascular network that serves the brainstem and occipital lobe.

vertex—Highest point of the dorsal surface of the head.

vertigo—Sensation that one's body or outer world is rotating in space.

vesicle (brain)—Subdivisions of the embryonic neural tube, each with a wall of neuroectoderm and a cavity.

vestibular apparatus—Part of the inner ear responsible for detecting head motion.

vestibular nerve—Division of cranial nerve VIII, which serves equilibrium and, indirectly, ocular movement.

vestibular system—Brain mechanism responsible for maintaining equilibrium.

vestibule—Cavernous part of the inner ear, consisting of the utricle and saccule, which contain sensory organs needed to facilitate reflex control of static equilibrium.

vestibulocochlear nerve (vestibuloacoustic nerve)—Cranial nerve VIII, serving audition and equilibrium.

vestibulospinal tract—Fibers that descend from the vestibular nuclei to the spinal motor neurons and regulate posture.

viscera—Internal organs of the ventral body cavity.

visceral—Vital organs of the body that have nonstriated muscles, such as the larynx, pharynx, trachea, and lungs. Innervated by the autonomic nervous system and relates to respiration, phonation, and digestion.

visceral afferent system—General sensation from the inner visceral organs.

visceral efferent system—Autonomic nervous system regulating glandular secretion and visceral structure functions.

visceral functions—Activities of the muscles of respiration, digestion, swallowing, phonation, and speech.

visceral muscles—Muscles of the heart, the spleen, the great vessels, and the digestive, respiratory, urogenital, endocrine, and speech systems, which are autonomically controlled.

viscerosomatic—Related to the viscera and body.

visual acuity—Assessment of the ability to resolve the details of distant objects. Tested with Snellen chart.

visual agnosia—Impaired ability to recognize a printed object.

visual field—Area seen by both eyes when looking straight ahead.

visual field defects—Area of blindness involving the visual fields.

visual reflexes—Include pupillary constriction in response to light and lens accommodation for near vision.

vitreous humor—Jelly-like substance in the posterior cavity of the eye. Prevents the eyeball from collapsing and contributes to intraocular pressure.

Wada test—Procedure in which the cerebral cortex is transiently anesthetized with sodium amobarbital for assessing its functions.

wallerian degeneration—Structural changes in a distal portion of an axon after it is sectioned and disconnected from the cell body in result of an injury.

watershed area—Tertiary brain area located peripheral to the primary distribution areas for the anterior, posterior, and middle cerebral arteries. This area is highly susceptible to vascular insufficiency because of its vascular dependency on multiple arteries.

Weber test—Tuning fork test in which the stem of a tuning fork is placed on the midline of the forehead. Lateralization to the poorer-hearing ear suggests a conductive hearing loss. Lateralization to the better-hearing ear suggests a sensorineural hearing loss in the other ear.

Wernicke area—Language association cortex in the left temporoparietal lobe concerned with the comprehension and formulation of language.

Wernicke encephalopathy—Syndrome of nutritional deficiency largely found in chronic alcoholics and characterized by ocular motility (ophthalmology), nystagmus, gait disturbances, and mental confusion.

white matter—General term for the axonal bundles in the central nervous system.

William syndrome—Congenital disorder caused by a continuous gene deletion and marked by distinctive facial and structural features, cognitive impairments (mental retardation and attention deficits), and hypercalcemia (elevated blood calcium levels).

withdrawal reflex—Reflexive movement causing the withdrawal of a limb by flexion at more than one joint in response to a painful stimulus on the skin surface.

X-linked inheritance—Genetic inheritance mode where diseases or traits are transmitted by a gene or genes on the X (sex) chromosome.

yolk sac, primary—Transient membranous structure of the embryo that disappears completely.

yolk sac, secondary—Specialized structure that separates from the embryo early in development and may persist through birth. Its proximal stalk gives rise to ileal (Meckel) diverticulum.

Young-Helmholtz trichromic theory—Relates color perception to the activation of three different types of cone cells.

zone of Lissauer—Outermost region of the spinal dorsal horn, which receives fibers carrying pain and temperature from the body.

zygote—Fertilized ovum (first stage in human development).

Suggested Readings

GENERAL SOURCES

Adams RD, Victor M, Ropper AH. Principles of Neuroanatomy, 7th ed. New York: McGraw-Hill, 2001.

Angevine JB, Cotman CW. Principles of Neuroanatomy. New York: Oxford University Press, 1981.

Arey LB. Developmental Anatomy: A Textbook and Laboratory Manual of Embryology, 7th ed. Philadelphia: Saunders, 1974.

Bear MF, Connors BW, Paradiso MA. Neuroscience: Exploring the Brain, 3rd ed. Baltimore: Lippincott Williams & Wilkins, 2007.

Brodal P. The Central Nervous System: Structure and Function, 3rd ed. New York: Oxford University Press, 2004.

Brown AG. Nerve Cells and Nervous Systems: An Introduction to Neuroscience, 2nd ed. New York: Springer, 2001.

Carpenter MB. Core Text of Neuroanatomy, 4th ed. Baltimore: Williams & Wilkins, 1991.

Crafts RC. A Textbook of Human Anatomy, 3rd ed. New York: Wiley, 1985.

Crosby EC, Humphrey T, Lauer EW. Correlative Anatomy of the Nervous System. New York: Macmillan, 1962.

Gelb DJ. Introduction to Clinical Neurology, 3rd ed. Boston: Butterworth-Heinemann, 2005.

Gilman S, Newman SW. Manter and Gatz's Essentials of Clinical Neuroanatomy and Neurophysiology, 10th ed. Philadelphia: Davis, 2003.

Gray H, Standring S, Ellis H, Berkovitz BKB. Gray's Anatomy: The Anatomical Basis of Clinical Practice, 39th ed. Edinburgh, UK, and New York: Churchill Livingstone/Elsevier, 2005.

Guyton AC, Hall JE. Textbook of Medical Physiology, 11th ed. Philadelphia: Saunders, 2006.

Haines DE. Fundamental Neuroscience for Basic and Clinical Applications. 3rd ed. Philadelphia, Churchill Livingston/Elsevier, 2006.

Haines DE. Neuroanatomy: An Atlas of Structures, Sections, and Systems, 6th ed. Baltimore: Lippincott Williams & Wilkins, 2004.

Heimer L. The Human Brain and Spinal Cord: Functional Neuroanatomy and Dissection Guide, 2nd ed. New York: Springer-Verlag, 1996.

Heuttel SA, Song AW, McCarthy G. Functional Magnetic Resonance Imaging. Sunderland, MA: Sinauer, 2004.

Hickok G, Poeppel D. Towards a functional neuroanatomy of speech perception. Trends Cogn Sci 2000;4:131–138.

Kandel ER, Schwartz JH, Jessell TM. Principles of Neural Science. 4th ed. New York: McGraw-Hill, 2000.

Kaufman DM. Clinical Neurology for Psychiatrists, 4th ed. Philadelphia: Saunders, 1995.

Kiernan JA. Barr's the Human Nervous System: An Anatomical Viewpoint, 8th ed. Philadelphia: Lippincott Williams & Wilkins, 2005.

Marieb EN. Essentials of Human Anatomy and Physiology, 8th ed. San Francisco: Benjamin-Cummings, 2005.

Martini FH, Ober WC. Fundamentals of Anatomy and Physiology, 7th ed. San Francisco: Benjamin-Cummings, 2004.

Nadeau, SE. Medical Neuroscience. Philadelphia: Saunders, 2004.

Nauta WJH, Feirtag M. Fundamental Neuroanatomy. New York: Freeman, 1986.

Netter F. The CIBA Collection of Medical Illustrations. Vol. 1, Part I: Nervous System: Anatomy and Physiology. West Caldwell, NJ: Ciba-Geigy, 1983.

Nolte J. The Human Brain: An Introduction to Its Functional Anatomy, 5th ed. St. Louis: Mosby, 2002.

Pansky B, Allen DJ, Budd GC. Review of Neuroscience, 2nd ed. New York: McGraw-Hill Health Professions Division, 1991.

Parent A. Carpenter's Human Neuroanatomy, 9th ed. Baltimore: Lippincott Williams & Wilkins, 1996.

Rowland LP. Merritt's Neurology, 11th ed. Philadelphia: Lippincott Williams & Wilkins, 2005.

Tortora GJ, Derrickson BH. Principles of Anatomy and Physiology, 11th ed. New York: Wiley, 2005.

Weiner HL, Levitt LP, Rae-Grant A. Neurology, 6th ed. Philadelphia: Lippincott Williams & Wilkins, 2004.

Wiederholt, WC. Neurology for Non-Neurologists, 4th ed. Philadelphia: Saunders, 2000.

Wilkinson IM. Essential Neurology, 4th ed. Malden, MA: Blackwell Science, 2005.

CHAPTER 1

Broca P. (1861). Sur la faculte du language artiule. Bulletin de la Societe d'Anthropologie, 1961;6:337–393.

Brodmann K. Vergleichende Lokalisation lehre der Grosshirnrinde in ihren Prinzipien dargestellt auf Grunddes Zellenbaues. Leipzig, Germany: Barth, 1909.

Castro, AJ. Neuroscience : An Outline Approach. St. Louis, Mosby: 2002.

Donoghue JP, Sanes JN. Organization of adult motor cortex representation patterns following neonatal forelimb nerve injury in rats. J Neurosci 1988;8:3221–3232.

Dougherty DD, Rauch SL, Rosenbaum JF. Essentials of Neuroimaging for Clinical Practice. Washington DC: American Psychiatric Publishing, 2004.

Kingsley RE. Concise Text of Neuroscience, 2nd ed. Philadelphia: Lippincott Williams & Wilkins, 1999.

Wernicke K. The Symptom Complex of Aphasia. In Modern Clinical Medicine: Diseases of the Nervous System, Church, ED. ed. (1908). New York: Appleton Century Crofts, 1874.

CHAPTER 2

Sperry RW. Forebrain Commissurotomy and Conscious Awareness. The Journal of Medicine and Philosophy, 1977;2:101.

CHAPTER 4

Bailey FR, Kelly DE, Wood RL, Enders AC. Textbook of Microscopic Anatomy. Baltimore: Williams & Wilkins, 1984.

Bhatnagar KP, Smith TD. The human vemeronasal organ. III. Postnatal development from infancy to the ninth decade. J Anat 2001;199:289–302.

Brodal P. The Central Nervous System: Structure and Function, 3rd ed. New York: Oxford University Press, 2004.

Hamilton WJ, Mossman, HW. Hamilton, Boyd, and Mossman's Human Embryology: Prenatal development of form and function, 4th ed. Cambridge: Helfer, 1972.

Lander ES, Linton LM, Birren, Nusbaum C, et al. (some 50 more authors). Initial sequencing and analysis of the human genome. Nature 2001;409:860–921.

Langman J, Shimada M, Rodier P. Floxuridine and its influence on postnatal cerebellar development. Pediatr Res 1972;6: 758–764.

Luckasson R, et al. Mental retardation, Definition, classification, and systems of support. Washington, DC: American Association on Mental Retardation, 2002.

Moore KL, Persaud, TVN. The Developing Human: Clinically Oriented Embryology, 7th ed. Philadelphia: Saunders, 2003.

Sadler TW. Langman's Medical Embryology, 9th ed. Philadelphia: Lippincott Williams & Wilkins, 2004.

CHAPTER 5

Lecours AR. Myelogenetic correlates of development of speech and language. In Lenneberg EH, Lenneberg E, eds. Foundation of Language Development, Vol. 1. New York: Academic, 1975.

Lenneberg EH. Biological Foundations of Language. New York: Wiley, 1967.

Yakovlev PI, Lecours AR. The myelogenetic cycles of regional maturation of the brain. In Minkowski A, ed. Regional Development of the Brain in Early Life. Oxford: Blackwell, 1967.

CHAPTER 6

Alexander MP. Clinical anatomic correlations of aphasia following predominantly subcortical lesions. In Boller F and Grafman J, eds. Handbook of Neuropsychology, Vol. 2. Amsterdam: Elsevier, 1989.

Andy OJ, Bhatnagar SC. Inhibitory effects of thalamic stimulation on acquired stuttering: Physiological evidence from four neurosurgical subjects. Brain Lang 1992;42:385–401.

Andy OJ, Bhatnagar SC. Thalamic-induced stuttering (surgical observations). J Speech Hear Res 1991;34:796–800.

Bhatnagar SC, Andy OJ. Alleviation of acquired stuttering from thalamic stimulation. J Neurol Neurosurg Psychiatry 1989;52: 1182–1184.

Bhatnagar SC, Andy OJ, Korabic EW, et al. The effect of thalamic stimulation in processing of verbal stimuli in dichotic listening tasks: A case study. Brain Lang 1989;36:236–251.

Bhatnagar SC, Andy OJ, Korabic EW, and Tikofsky RS. Effects of bilateral thalamic stimulation on dichotic verbal processing. J Neurolinguistics 1990;5:407–425.

Bhatnagar SC, Mandybur GT. Effects of intralaminar thalamic stimulation on language functions. Brain Lang 2005;92:1–11.

Ojemann GA. Brain organization for language from the perspective of electrical stimulation mapping. Behav Brain Res 1983;6: 189–230.

Ojemann GA, Fedio P, Van Buren JM. Anomia from pulvinar and subcortical parietal stimulation. Brain 1968;91:99–116.

Penfield W, Roberts L. Speech and Brain Mechanisms. Princeton, NJ: Princeton University, 1959.

CHAPTER 7

Bhatnager SC, Andy OJ, Korabic EW, and Tikofsky RS. Effects of bilateral thalamic stimulation on dichotic verbal processing. J Neurolinguistics 1990;5:407–425.

Bhatnagar SC, Mandybur GT. Effects of intralaminar thalamic stimulation on language functions. Brain Lang 2005;92:1–11.

Bhatnagar SC, Mandybur GT, Buckingham HW, Andy OJ. Language representation in the human brain: Evidence from cortical mapping. Brain Lang 2000;74:238–259.

Penfield W, Roberts L. Speech and Brain Mechanisms. Princeton, NJ: Princeton University, 1959.

CHAPTER 9

Bhatnagar SC, Andy OJ. Tonotypic cortical representation. Presented at the annual meeting of the Pavlovian Society of North America, Orlando Florida, 1988.

Bhatnagar SC, Andy OJ, Korabic EW, et al. The effect of thalamic stimulation in processing of verbal stimuli in dichotic listening tasks: A case study. Brain Lang 1989;36:236–251.

Bhatnager SC, Andy OJ, Korabic EW, and Tikofsky RS. Effects of bilateral thalamic stimulation on dichotic verbal processing. J Neurolinguistics 1990;5:407–425.

Donoghue JP, Sanes JN. Organization of adult motor cortex representation patterns following neonatal forelimb nerve injury in rats. J Neurosci 1988;8:3221–3232.

Geschwind N, Levitsky W. Human brain: Left-right asymmetries in temporal speech region. Science 1968;161:186–187.

Kilgard MP, Merzenich MM. Plasticity of temporal information processing in the primary auditory cortex. Nature Neurosci 1998;1:727–731.

Kingsley RE. Concise Text of Neuroscience, 2nd ed. Philadelphia: Lippincott Williams & Wilkins, 1999.

CHAPTER 12

Guyton AC, Hall JE. Textbook of Medical Physiology, 11th ed. Philadelphia: Saunders, 2006.

CHAPTER 13

Battig K, Rosvold HE, Mishkin M. Comparison of the effect of frontal and caudate lesions on delayed response and attention in monkeys. J Comp Physiol Psychol 1960;53:400–404.

Bhatnagar SC, Mandybur GT. Effects of intralaminar thalamic stimulation on language functions. Brain Lang 2005;92:1–11.

Bhatnagar SC, Mandybur GT. Electrical stimulation of brain and language. In Brown K, ed. Encyclopedia of Language and Linguistics, Vol. 4. England: Elsevier, 2006:97–105.

Brunner RJ, Kornhuber HH, Seemuller E, et al. Basal ganglia participation in language pathology. Brain Lang 1982;16:281–299.

Levy R, Friedman HR, Davachi KL, Goldman-Rakic PS. Differential activation of the caudate nucleus in primates performing spatial and nonspatial working memory tasks. J Neuroscie 1997;17.

Middleton FA, trick PL. Basal ganglia output and cognition: Evidence from anatomical, behavioral, and clinical studies. Brain Cog 2000;42:183–200.

Paxinos G, Mai, JK, eds. The Human Nervous System. New York: Elsevier, 2004.

Parkinson J. An essay on the shaking palsy. London: Sherwood, Neely and Jones, 1817.

CHAPTER 16

Bhatnagar SC, Mandybur GT. Electrical stimulation of brain and language. In Brown K, ed. Encyclopedia of Language and Linguistics, Vol. 4. England: Elsevier, 2006:97–105.

Magon HW. The waking brain, 2nd ed. Springfield, IL: Thomas, 1963.

CHAPTER 19

Alexander MP, Benson DF. The aphasias and related disturbances. In Joynt RJ, ed. Clinical Neurology, Vol. 1. Philadelphia: Lippincott, 1998.

Benson DF. The third alexia. Arch Neurol 1977;34:327–331.

Benson DR, Sheremata WA, Bouchard R, et al. Conduction aphasia: A clinicopathological study. Arch Neurol 1973;28:339–346.

Bhatnagar SC, Mandybur GT, Buckingham HW, Andy OJ. Language representation in the human brain: Evidence from cortical mapping. Brain Lang 2000;74:238–259.

Blumer D, Benson BF. Personality changes with frontal and temporal lesions. In Benson DF, Blumer D, eds. Psychiatric Aspects of Neurologic Disease. New York: Grune & Stratton, 1975.

Damasio H, Damasio AR. The anatomical basis of conduction aphasia. Brain 1980;103:337–350.

Darley FL, Aronson AE, Brown JR. Motor Speech Disorders. Philadelphia: Saunders, 1975.

Déjérine J. Contribution a letude anotomo-pathologique et cliniques des differentes varietes de cicite verbale. Memories-Societe Biologie 1892;4:61–90.

Demonet JF, Chollet F, Ramsay S, et al. The anatomy of phonological and semantic processing in normal subjects. Brain 1992;115:1753–1768.

DeRenzi E, Motti F, Nichelli P. Imitating gestures: A quantitative approach to ideomotor apraxia. Arch Neurol 1980;37:6–10.

Duffy JR. Motor Speech Disorders: Substrates, Differential Diagnosis, and Management, 2nd ed. St. Louis: Elsevier Mosby, 2005.

Evans DA, Funkenstein HH, Albert MS, et al. Clinically diagnosed Alzheimer's disease: An epidemiologic study in a community population of older persons. JAMA 1989;262:2551–2556.

Gerstmann J. Zur Symptomatologie der Hirnlasionen im Bergangsgebiet der unteren Parietal und mittleren Occipitalwindung (das Syndrom: Fingeragnosie, Rechts-Links Strung, Agraphie, Akalkulie). Nervenartzt 1930:691–695. [Reprinted in Rittenberg DA, Hochberg FH, eds. Neurological Classics in Modern Translation. New York: Hafner, 1977.]

Geschwind N. The apraxias: Neural mechanisms of disorders of learned movement. Am Sci 1975;63:188–195.

Geschwind N. The organization of language and the brain. Science 1970;170:940–944.

Geschwind N, Levitsky W. Human brain: Left-right asymmetries in temporal speech region. Science 1968;161:186–187.

Geschwind N, Quadfasel F, Segarra J. Isolation of the speech area. Neuropsychologia 1968;6:327–340.

Goldman-Rakic PS. The prefrontal landscape: Implications of functional architecture for understanding human mentation and the central executive. Philos Trans R Soc Lond B Biol Sci 1996;351:1445–1453.

Heilman KM, Maher LM, Greenwald ML, Rothi L. Conceptual apraxia from lateralized lesions. Neurology 1997;49:457–464.

Heilman KM, Meador KJ, Loring DW. Hemispheric asymmetries of limb-kinetic apraxia: A loss of deftness. Neurology 2000;55:523–526.

Hickok G, Poeppel D. Towards a functional neuroanatomy of speech perception. Trends Cogn Sci 2000;4:131–138.

Kirshner HS. Apraxia of speech: A linguistic enigma. A neurologist's perspective. Semin Speech Lang 1992;13:14–24.

Kirshner HS. First exposure neurology. New York: McGraw Hill, 2007:1–429.

Kirshner HS. Behavioral neurology. Practical science of mind and brain, 2nd ed. Boston: Butterworth Heinemann (now Elsevier) 2002:1–474.

Kirshner HS, ed. Handbook of Neurological Speech and Language Disorders. New York: Marcel Dekker, 1994.

Kirshner HS, Casey PF, Henson J, Heinrich JJ. Behavioral features and lesion localization in Wernicke's aphasia. Aphasiology 1989;3:169–176.

Kirshner HS, Tanridag O, Thurman L, Whetsell WO Jr. Progressive aphasia without dementia: two cases with focal spongiform degeneration. Ann Neurol 1987;22:527–532.

Liepmann H. Apraxie. Ergbn. der ges. Med. 1920;1:516–543. [Cited in Brown, JW. Aphasia, Apraxia, and Agnosia. Springfield, IL: Thomas, 1972.]

Mesulam MM, ed. Principles of behavioral neurology, 2nd ed. New York: Oxford University Press, 2000.

Mesulam MM. Slowly progressive aphasia without generalized dementia. Ann Neurol 1982;11:592–598.

Mesulam MM. Primary progressive aphasia–a language-based dementia. N Engl J Med 2003;349:1535–1542.

Mohr JP, Pessin MS, Finklestein S, et al. Broca aphasia: Pathologic and clinical. Neurology 1978;28:311–324.

Naeser MA, Palumbo, CL, Helm-Estabrooks N, Stiassny-Eder D, Albert ML. Severe nonfluency in aphasia: Role of the medial subcallosal fasciculus plus other white matter pathology in recovery of spontaneous language. Brain 1989;112:1–38.

Neary D, Snowden J. Fronto-temporal dementia: Nosology, neuropsychology, and neuropathology. Brain Cogn 1996;31:176–187.

Ochipa C, Rothi LJG, Heilman KM. Ideational apraxia: A deficit in tool selection and use. Ann Neurol 1989;25:190–193.

Ojemann G, Ojemann J, Lettich E, Berger M. Cortical language localization in left, dominant hemisphere. An electrical stimulation mapping investigation in 117 patients. J Neurosurg 1989;71:316–326.

Sacks O. The man who mistook his wife for a hat and other clinical tales. New York: Simon and Shuster, 1998.

Shallice T, Warrington EK. Auditory-verbal short-term memory impairment and conduction aphasia. Brain Lang 1977;4:479–491.

CHAPTER 20

Alexander MP, Benson DF. The aphasias and related disturbances. In Joynt RJ, ed. Clinical Neurology, Vol. 1. Philadelphia: Lippincott, 1998.

Alexander MP, Naeser MA, Palumbo CL. Correlations of subcortical CT lesion sites and aphasia profiles. Brain 1987;110:961–991.

Andy OJ, Bhatnagar SC. Inhibitory effects of thalamic stimulation on acquired stuttering: Physiological evidence from four neurosurgical subjects. Brain Lang 1992;42:385–401.

Andy OJ, Bhatnagar SC. Right hemispheric language: Evidence from cortical stimulation. Brain Lang 1983;23:159–166.

Andy OJ, Bhatnagar SC. Thalamic-induced stuttering (surgical observations). J Speech Hear Res 1991;34:796–800.

Bartholow R. Experimental investigations into functions of the human brain. Am J Med Sci, 1874;67:305–315.

Bhatnagar SC, Andy OJ. Alleviation of acquired stuttering from thalamic stimulation. J Neurol Neurosurg Psychiatry 1989;52:1182–1184.

Bhatnagar SC, Andy OJ, Korabic EW, et al. The effect of thalamic stimulation in processing of verbal stimuli in dichotic listening tasks: A case study. Brain Lang 1989;36:236–251.

Bhatnager SC, Andy OJ, Korabic EW, and Tikofsky RS. Effects of bilateral thalamic stimulation on dichotic verbal processing. J Neurolinguistics 1990;5:407–425.

Bhatnagar SC, Mandybur GT. Effects of intralaminar thalamic stimulation on language functions. Brain Lang 2005;92:1–11.

Bhatnagar SC, Mandybur GT. Electrical stimulation of brain and language. In Brown K, ed. Encyclopedia of Language and Linguistics, Vol. 4. England: Elsevier, 2006:97–105.

Bhatnagar SC, Mandybur GT, Buckingham HW, Andy OJ. Language representation in the human brain: Evidence from cortical mapping. Brain Lang 2000;74:238–259.

Bhatnagar SC, Stuyvessant SA, Mandybur GT, Buckingham HW. On lexical organization in the human brain: Evidence from intracarotid sodium amytal injection. Acta Neuropsychologica 2005;3:107–119.

Bruxton RB. Introduction to Functional Magnetic Resonance Imaging, Principles, and Techniques. Cambridge, UK: Cambridge University Press, 2002.

Damasio H. Neuroanatomical correlates of the aphasias. In Sarno MT, ed. Acquired Aphasia, 3rd ed. San Diego: Academic, 1998.

Dougherty DD, Rauch SL, Rosenbaum JF. Essentials of Neuroimaging for Clinical Practice. Washington, DC: American Psychiatric Publishing, 2004.

Fritsch G, Hitzig E. Uber die elektrische erregbarkeit des Grosshirns. Archiv der Anatomische Physiolosische Weisenschaftliche Medizine 1870;37:300–332. [Translated into English and reprinted as: On the electrical excitability of the cerebrum. In von Bonin G, ed. Some papers on the cerebral cortex. Springfield, IL: Thomas, 1960:73–96.]

Gado M, Hanaway J, Frank R. Functional anatomy of the cerebral cortex by computed tomography. J Comput Assist Tomogr 1979;3:1–19.

Grossman CB. Magnetic Resonance Imaging and Computer Tomography of the Head and Spine, 2nd ed. Baltimore: Williams & Wilkins, 1996.

Heilman KM, Meador KJ, Loring DW. Hemispheric asymmetries of limb-kinetic apraxia: A loss of deftness. Neurology 2000;55:523–526.

Kimura D. Functional asymmetry of the brain in dichotic listening. Cortex 1967;3:163–178.

Lassen NA, Ingvar DH, Skinhoj E. Brain function and blood flow. Sci Am 1978;239:62–71.

Lesser R, Lueders H, Klem G, et al. Extraoperative cortical functional localization in patients with epilepsy. J Clin Neurophysiol 1987;4:27–53.

Lesser R, Hahn J, Lueders H, et al. The use of chronic subdural electrodes for cortical mapping of speech. Epilepsia 1981;22:240.

Mazziotta JC, Phelps ME, Carson RE, Kuhl DE. Tomographic mapping of human cerebral metabolism: Sensory deprivation. Ann Neurol 1982;12:435–444.

Mazziotta JC, Phelps ME, Miller J, Kuhl DE. Tomographic mapping of human cerebral metabolism: Normal unstimulated state. Neurology 1981;31:503–506.

Metter EJ. Neuroanatomy and physiology of aphasia: Evidence from positron emission tomography. Aphasiology 1987;1:3–33.

Metter EJ, Hanson WR. Brain imaging as related to speech and language. In Darby J, ed. Speech Evaluation in Neurology. New York: Grune & Stratton, 1985.

Metter EJ, Jackson C, Kempler D, et al. Glucose metabolic asymmetries in chronic Wernicke's, Broca's and conduction aphasias. Neurology 1986;36(suppl 1):317.

Milner B, Branch C. Experimental analysis of cerebral dominance in man. In Millikan CH, Darley FL, eds. Brain mechanism underlying speech and language. New York: Grune & Stratton, 1967:177–184.

Naeser MA, Hayward RW. Lesion localization in aphasia with cranial computed tomography and the Boston diagnostic aphasia examination. Neurology 1987;28:545–551.

Ojemann G, Ojemann J, Lettich E, Berger M. Cortical language localization in left, dominant hemisphere. An electrical stimulation mapping investigation in 117 patients. J Neurosurg 1989;71:316–326.

Ojemann GA. Brain organization for language from the perspective of electrical stimulation mapping. Behav Brain Res 1983;6:189–230.

Ojemann G, Whitaker H. The bilingual brain. Archives of Neurology 1978a;35:409–412.

Penfield W, Roberts L. Speech and Brain Mechanisms. Princeton, NJ: Princeton University, 1959.

Tikofsky RS, Heilman RS. Brain single photon emission computed tomography: New activation and intervention studies. Semn Nucl Med 1991;21:40–57

Wada J, Rasmussen T. Intracarotid injection of sodium Amytal for the lateralization of cerebral dominance. J Neurosurgery 1960;17:266–282.

Figure and Table Credits

FIGURES

Chapter 1

Figure 1-4: Modified from Williams PL, Ed. Gray's Anatomy, 38th ed. Edinburgh: Churchill Livingstone, 1995.

Figure 1-7: Reprinted with permission from Carpenter MB. Core Text of Neuroanatomy, 4th ed. Baltimore: Lippincott Williams & Wilkins, 1991.

Figure 1-9: Courtesy of George Mandibur, MD, Department of Neurosurgery, University of Cincinnati College of Medicine, Cincinnati, OH.

Chapter 2

Figure 2-1B: Modified from Guyton AC. Organ Physiology: Structure and Function of the Nervous System. Philadelphia: Saunders, 1976.

Figures 2-3, 2-5, 2-7, 2-8, 2-10, 2-11, 2-12B, 2-15A, 2-16A, 2-24C, 2-27A–B, 2-29, 2-40B, and 2-50: Reprinted with permission from Haines DE. Neuroanatomy: An Atlas of Structures, Sections, and Systems, 6th ed. Baltimore: Lippincott Williams & Wilkins, 2004.

Figures 2-6, 2-12A, 2-13, 2-19, 2-32B, 2-33, 2-36A–B, and 2-38: Modified from Parent A. Carpenter's Human Neuroanatomy, 9th ed. Baltimore: Williams & Wilkins, 1996.

Figures 2-9, 2-17, 2-18, 2-20, 2-21, 2-41B, 2-42, 2-46A, 2-47A, 2-48A–B, and 2-49: Reprinted with permission from Parent A. Carpenter's Human Neuroanatomy, 9th ed. Baltimore: Williams & Wilkins, 1996.

Figures 2-28, 2-40A, 2-43, and 2-44: Modified from Mettler FA. Mettler's Neuroanatomy, 2nd ed. St. Louis: Mosby, 1948.

Figure 2-31A: Courtesy of Duane E. Haines, PhD, Department of Anatomy, University of Mississippi Medical Center, Jackson.

Figure 2-31B: Reprinted with permission from Mettler FA. Mettler's Neuroanatomy, 2nd ed. St. Louis: Mosby, 1948; and Parent A. Carpenter's Human Neuroanatomy, 9th ed. Baltimore: Williams & Wilkins, 1996.

Figure 2-35: Modified from Kingsley RE. Concise Test of Neuroscience. Baltimore: Williams & Wilkins, 1996.

Figures 2-39 and 2-45A: Modified from Heimer L. The Human Brain and Spinal Cord: Functional Neuroanatomy and Dissection Guide. New York: Springer-Verlag, 1983.

Figure 2-45B: Modified from House EL, Pansky B. A Functional Approach to Neuroanatomy. New York: McGraw-Hill, 1967.

Figure 2-51: Modified from Barr ML and Kiernan JA. The Human Nervous System: An Anatomical Viewpoint, 7th ed. Philadelphia: Lippincott Williams & Wilkins, 1998.

Chapter 3

Figures 3-2 to 3-5, 3-7, 3-9 to 3-19, and 3-21 to 3-25: Reprinted with permission from Haines DE. Neuroanatomy: An Atlas of Structures, Sections, and Systems, 6th ed. Baltimore: Lippincott Williams & Wilkins, 2004.

Figures 3-6 and 3-20: Modified from Haines DE. Neuroanatomy: An Atlas of Structures, Sections, and Systems, 6th ed. Baltimore: Lippincott Williams & Wilkins, 2004.

Figure 3-26: Courtesy of Duane E. Haines, PhD, Department of Anatomy, University of Mississippi Medical Center, Jackson.

Chapter 4

Figure 4-1: Modified from Bailey, FR, et al. Bailey's Textbook of Microscopic Anatomy. Williams & Wilkins, 1984.

Figures 4-2 to 4-12: Reprinted with permission from Sadler TW. Langman's Medical Embryology, 9th ed. Philadelphia: Lippincott-Williams & Wilkins, 2004.

Chapter 5

Figure 5-5: Modified from Marieb EN. Essentials of Human Anatomy and Physiology, 7th ed. Menlo Park, CA: Benjamin-Cummings, 2003.

Figure 5-8: Modified from Gilman S, Newman SW. Manter and Gatz's Essentials of Clinical Neuroanatomy and Neurophysiology, 10th ed. Philadelphia: Davis, 2003.

Figure 5-9: Courtesy of Leighton P. Mark, MD, Department of Neuroradiology, Medical College of Wisconsin, Milwaukee.

Chapter 6

Figure 6-1A–B: Modified from Parent A. Carpenter's Human Neuroanatomy, 9th ed. Baltimore: Williams & Wilkins, 1996.

Chapter 7

Figures 7-5A and 7-7A: Based on material distributed at University of Rochester, College of Medicine, Rochester, NY.

Figures 7-5B, 7-6, 7-7B, 7-8, and 7-10: Modified from Parent A. Carpenter's Human Neuroanatomy, 9th ed. Baltimore: Williams & Wilkins, 1996.

Figure 7-9B: Modified from Crosby E, Humphrey T, Lauer E. Correlative Anatomy of the Nervous System. New York: Macmillan, 1962.

Chapter 8

Figure 8-1: Modified from Carpenter MB. Core Text of Neuroanatomy, 4th ed. Baltimore: Lippincott Williams & Wilkins, 1991.

Figures 8-2A–B and 8-5: Modified from Lavine RA. Neurophysiology: The Fundamentals. Lexington MA: Heath, 1983.

Figure 8-6: Modified from Eyzaguiuirre C, Fiddone S. Physiology of the Nervous System. Chicago: Yearbook, 1975.

Figures 8-8A, 8-9A and 8-14: Modified from Parent A. Carpenter's Human Neuroanatomy, 9th ed. Baltimore: Williams & Wilkins, 1996.

Chapter 9

Figure 9-2: Modified from Lavine RA. Neurophysiology: The Fundamentals. Lexington MA: Collamore Press, 1983.

Figures 9-3 and 9-4: Reprinted with permission from Parent A. Carpenter's Human Neuroanatomy, 9th ed. Baltimore: Lippincott Williams & Wilkins, 1996.

Figures 9-6, 9-7, and 9-9: Modified from Parent A. Carpenter's Human Neuroanatomy, 9th ed. Baltimore: Williams & Wilkins, 1996.

Figure 9-10: Reprinted with permission from Haines DE. Neuroanatomy: An Atlas of Structures, Sections, and Systems, 6th ed. Baltimore: Lippincott Williams & Wilkins, 2004.

Chapter 10

Figure 10-2B: Based after Kandel ER, Schwartz JH, Jessell TM. Principles of Neural Science, 4th ed. New York: McGraw-Hill, 2000.

Figure 10-3C: Modified from Curtis BA, Jacobson S, Marcus EM. An Introduction to the Neurosciences. Philadelphia: Saunders, 1972.

Figure 10-4: Modified from Parent A. Carpenter's Human Neuroanatomy, 9th ed. Baltimore: Lippincott Williams & Wilkins, 1996.

Figures 10-6 and 10-7: Modified from House EL, Pansky B. A Functional Approach to Neuroanatomy. New York: McGraw-Hill, 1967.

Chapter 11

Figures 11-3, 11-5 to 11-7, and 11-11: Modified from Parent A. Carpenter's Human Neuroanatomy, 9th ed. Baltimore: Lippincott Williams & Wilkins, 1996.

Figure 11-9A-B: Modified from Gardener E. Fundamentals of Neurology. Philadelphia: Saunders, 1975.

Chapter 12

Figures 12-1A–B, 12-2A, 12-3, and 12-4: Modified from Parent A. Carpenter's Human Neuroanatomy, 9th ed. Baltimore: Lippincott Williams & Wilkins, 1996.

Figure 12-2B: Reprinted with permission from Mettler FA. Mettler's Neuroanatomy, 2nd ed. St. Louis: Mosby, 1948.

Figure 12-5: Modified from Carpenter MB. Core Text of Neuroanatomy, 4th ed. Baltimore: Lippincott Williams & Wilkins, 1991.

Figure 12-6A: Modified from Guyton AC, Hall JE. Textbook of Medical Physiology, 11th ed. Philadelphia: Saunders, 2006.

Chapter 13

Figures 13-1B and 13-4: Modified from Carpenter MB. Core Text of Neuroanatomy, 4th ed. Baltimore: Lippincott Williams & Wilkins, 1991.

Figure 13-7: Courtesy of Madhuri Behari, MD, Department of Neuroradiology, All India Institute of Medical Sciences, New Delhi.

Figure 13-8: Courtesy of Alexandru Barboi, MD. Department of Neurology, Medical College of Wisconsin, Milwaukee.

Chapter 14

Figures 14-1A–B and 14-2: Modified from Parent A. Carpenter's Human Neuroanatomy, 9th ed. Baltimore: Lippincott Williams & Wilkins, 1996.

Chapter 15

Figure 15-1: Reprinted with permission from Mettler FA. Mettler's Neuroanatomy, 2nd ed. St. Louis: Mosby, 1948.

Figure 15-2: Modified from Moore KL, Persaud TVN. The Developing Human: Clinically Oriented Embryology, 7th ed. Philadelphia: Saunders, 2003.

Figures 15-3 and 15-4: Reprinted with permission from Parent A. Carpenter's Human Neuroanatomy, 9th ed. Baltimore: Lippincott Williams & Wilkins, 1996.

Figures 15.9A–C, 15-10, 15-12, 15-17, and 15-21: Modified from Parent A. Carpenter's Human Neuroanatomy, 9th ed. Baltimore: Lippincott Williams & Wilkins, 1996.

Figures 15-1, 15-14, 15-15, 15-18, 15-19, 15-22 to 15-26, and 15-30 to 15-32: Based on data from House EL, Pansky B. A Functional Approach to Neuroanatomy. New York: McGraw-Hill, 1967.

Figure 15-29. Modified from Van Allen MW, Rodnitzky RL. Pictorial Manual of Neurologic Tests, 2nd ed. Chicago: Yearbook, 1981.

Chapter 16

Figures 16-6, 16-7, 16-8, 16-9, and 16-10: Reprinted with permission from Parent A. Carpenter's Human Neuroanatomy, 9th ed. Baltimore: Lippincott Williams & Wilkins, 1996.

Chapter 17

Figures 17-2 17-3A, 17-4A, 17-11, 17-12A–B: Reprinted with permission from Parent A. Carpenter's Human Neuroanatomy, 9th ed. Baltimore: Lippincott Williams & Wilkins, 1996.

Figures 17-8, 17-9*B*, and 17-10*A–B*: Courtesy of Leighton P. Mark, MD, Department of Neuroradiology, Medical College of Wisconsin, Milwaukee.

Chapter 18

Figure 18-2*A*: Reprinted with permission from Parent A. Carpenter's Human Neuroanatomy, 9th ed. Baltimore: Lippincott Williams & Wilkins, 1996.

Chapter 20

Figures 20-1 and 20-2: Courtesy of Varun K. Saxena, MD, Center for Neurological Disorders, Milwaukee.

Figures 20-4*A–B* and 20-5: Courtesy of Leighton P. Mark, MD, Department of Neuroradiology, Medical College of Wisconsin, Milwaukee.

Figure 20-6: Reprinted with permission from Lehericy S, Cohen L, Bazin B, et al. Functional MR evaluation of temporal and frontal language dominance compared with the WADA test. Neurology 2000;54:1625–1633.

Figure 20-7: Courtesy of Stefan Heim, PhD, Simon B. Eickhoff, MD, Anja K. Ischebeck, PhD, et al. Institute of Medicine, Research Centre Juelich, Juelich, Germany.

Figure 20-8: Courtesy of Lotfi Hacein-Bey, MD, Department of Radiology, Loyola University Medical Center, Chicago.

Figure 20-9: Courtesy of John L. Ulmer, MD, and Leighton P. Mark, MD, Department of Neuroradiology, Medical College of Wisconsin, Milwaukee.

Figure 20-10: Courtesy of John Mazziotta, MD, Reed Institute, UCLA Medical Center, Los Angeles.

Figure 20-11*A–B*: Courtesy of Howard S. Kirshner, MD, Vanderbilt Medical Center, Nashville, TN.

Figure 20-15*B*: Reprinted with permission from Parent A. Carpenter's Human Neuroanatomy, 9th ed. Baltimore: Lippincott Williams & Wilkins, 1996.

Figure 20-16: Modified from Bhatnagar SC, Andy OJ, Korabic EW, Tikofsky RS. Effects of bilateral thalamic stimulation on dichotic verbal processing. J Neurolinguistics 1990;4:407–425.

Figures 20-19 to 20-21: Modified from Genetic Counseling [March of Dimes Birth Defects Foundation Booklet 9-0022]. White Plains, NY: 1984.

TABLES

Chapter 4

Table 4-2: Modified from Arey LB. Developmental Anatomy. Philadelphia: Saunders, 1966.

Table 4-4: Modified from Moore KL, Persaud TVN. The Developing Human, Clinically Oriented Embryology, 7th ed. Philadelphia: Saunders, 2003.

Table 4-5: Modified from Menkes JH. Textbook of Child Neurology, 5th ed. Baltimore: Lippincott Williams & Wilkins, 1995.

Chapter 10

Table 10-3: Data from Wada J, Rasmussen T. Intracarotid injection of sodium Amytal for the lateralization of cerebral dominance. J Neurosurg 1960;17:266–282.

Chapter 16

Table 16-3: Based on Castro, AJ, et al. Neuroscience: an outline approach. St. Louis, Mosby: 2002.

Index

Note: Page numbers in *italics* refer to figures; those followed by b and t refer to boxes and tables, respectively.

Abducens nerve (CN6), 73t, 74, *74*, 318–319, *321*, 321t, 322
Abduction, 10, *12*
Absence seizure, 446
Absolute refractory period, 139
Abulia, 406
Acceleration-rotation chair, *233*, 235
Accessory nerve (CN11), 73t, *74*, 75, 337–338, 339t, *340*
Accommodation, lens, 194
Accommodation reflex, 199–200, *200*, 316–317
Acetylcholine, 143–145, *144*, 145t, 252
Acetylcholinesterase, 143, 252
Achromatopsia, 204
Acoustic aphasia, 218, 222
Acoustic nerve. *See* Vestibulocochlear nerve (CN8)
Acoustic neuroma, 147, 221
Action potential, 137–139, *138*
Acute confusional state, 446
Acute symptoms, 12
Adamkiewicz artery, 385
Adduction, 10, *12*
Adenohypophysis
    development, 124
    hormones, *367*, 367–368, 368t
Adenoma, pituitary, 147
Adrenocorticotropic hormone, *367*, 367, 368t
Afferent (sensory) fibers, 9, 29, 164, *165*
Afferent pathways
    cerebellar, 263–265, *264*, 265t
    cranial nerve, 309, *312*
    hypothalamic, 365
    reticular, 369
    spinal, *168*, 168t, 242t, *243*, 244–245
Afferent thalamic nuclei projections, *155*, 155–160, *156*, 157t
Aganglionic megacolon, 129
Agnosia, 414
    apperceptive, 204
    associative, 204
    auditory, 414
    tactile, 414
    visual, 204, 414
Agraphia, 413
    alexia with, 411
    lexical, 413
    phonological, 413
AIDS dementia, 415
Akinetic mutism, 406
Alar plate, 120
Albinism, 188
Alcoholism
    cerebellar toxicity, 270
    Wernicke-Korsakoff syndrome in, 159, 415, 448
Alerting response mechanism, 441
Alexia, 411–412, 412t
    with agraphia, 411
    aphasic, 412
    without agraphia, 204, 412
Allantois, 118
α–Motor neurons, 245, *245*
Alternating hemiplegia, *294*, 294–295, 381
Alzheimer dementia, 416
Alzheimer disease, 145

Amnesic aphasia, 410
Ampulla, 227
Amygdala, 105–106, *361*, 362–363
Amygdaloid complex, 39
Amygdaloid nucleus, 44, *44*, 105
Amyotrophic lateral sclerosis, 408
Analgesia, 175
Anaphase, 116
Anastomosis
    carotid, 442
    point of, 387b
Anatomic orientation landmarks of brain, 82–83, *83*
Anatomic structures, terminology, 10, *12*
Anencephaly, 125, *128*
Anesthesia, thermal, 175
Aneuploid, 114
Aneurysm, 389, *390*
Aneurysm clipping, 442
Angiogenesis, 147
Angiography
    cerebral, 421–423, *422*, *423*
    magnetic resonance, 430
Angular gyrus, 34
Annulospiral sensory ending, 246
Anomic aphasia, 410
Anosmia, 311
Anoxia, sensitivity to, 379b, 389–390
Anterior cavity, 185–187, *187*
Anterior cerebral artery, 381–382, *383*, 384t, *385*
Anterior chamber, 185, *187*
Anterior choroidal artery, 384
Anterior commissure, 42, 64, 104–106, *107*
Anterior corticospinal tract, 243, *244*, 292–293
Anterior horn, 107, *109*
Anterior inferior cerebellar artery, 219, 381
Anterior language cortex (Broca area), 33, 406
Anterior limb of internal capsule, 101t, 102, *102*, 106–107, *108*
Anterior lobe, 52, *53*, *54*
Anterior medullary velum, 91
Anterior nucleus, 104, *106*, 155, 157t, 159
Anterior spinal artery, 380–381, 384, *386*
Anterior spinothalamic tract, *168*, 158t, 175, *176*, *243*, 244
Anterior subcortical aphasia syndrome, 411
Anterograde movement, 13
Anterolateral spinothalamic system, 84, *84*, 168, 168t, 172–175, *173*, 174t, *176*
Anteromedial arteries, 383
Antiepileptic drugs, 446
Anton syndrome, 407
Aphasia, 409–411, 409t, 411t
    acoustic, 218, 222
    anomic (amnesic), 410
    Broca, 409
        aphemia variant, 409
    conduction, 410
    global, 410
    optic, 204–205
    subcortical, 411
    thalamic, 411
    transcortical, 410–411, 411t
        isolation syndrome form, 411
        mixed, 411

    motor, 410–411
    sensory, 411
    Wernicke, 222, 409–410
Aphasic alexia, 412
Aphemia variant of Broca aphasia, 409
Apoptosis, 136
Appendicular, 13
Apperceptive agnosia, 204
Apraxia
    constructional, 413
    dressing, 413
    gait, 413
    ideational, 414
    ideomotor, 413–414
    of learned movement, 413–414
    limb-kinetic, 414
    oculomotor, 413
    of speech, 408
Aqueous humor, 185–187
Arachnoid granulations (villi), 69–70, 400–401, *401*
Arachnoid membrane
    brain, 69–70, *70*
    spinal, 52, *56*, 71
Arachnoid trabeculae, 69, 400
Archicerebellum (flocculonodular lobe), 52, *53*, *54*, 261, 263, 263t
Archicortex, 14
Arcuate fasciculus, 63, *65*
Arcuate fibers, internal, 167, *169*
Arousal, cortical, 370–371
Arteries, 378
Arterioles, 378
Arteriovenous malformation, 389, *390*
Association areas, 16, 18, 406
Association fibers, 63–64, *64*, *65*
Associative agnosia, 204
Asthenia, 269
Astigmatism, *201*, 202
Astrocytes, 134, *136*, 136t
Astrocytoma, 147
Asynergia, 269
Ataxia, 19, 269
Athermia, 175
Atherosclerosis, 387
Athetosis, 280
Atrophy
    in hydrocephalus ex vacuo, 403
    in lower motor neuron syndrome, 253
Attention, 370
Attention-deficit/hyperactivity disorder, 128
Audiometry
    auditory brainstem response, 224, 437–439, *438*, 439t
    pure tone, 223, *224*
Auditory agnosia, 414
Auditory artery, internal, 219, 228, *379*, 381
Auditory brainstem response (ABR) audiometry, 224, 437–439, *438*, 439t
Auditory cortex, 218–219, *220*, 407
    language association, 35, 218–219, *220*, 407
    lesions, 222
    plasticity, 219b
    primary, 35, 218, *220*
    secondary, 218, *220*

Auditory meatus, external, *209, 210*
Auditory nerve, 331
Auditory reflexes, 219
Auditory system, 208–226. *See also* Hearing *entries;* Vestibular system
    central pathways, *214,* 214–219, 215t
    clinical concerns, 221–224
        hearing impairments, 221–222
        hearing tests, 222–224, *223, 224*
    clinical considerations, 215t, 224–226
    distinctive properties, 219–221
        bilateral representation, 219–220
        descending projections, 220–221
        sound source localization, 220
        tonotopic representation, 216, 220
    ear anatomy and physiology, *209,* 209–213, *211, 212*
    neural coding, 213–219
    retrocochlear neural mechanism, *213,* 213–214
    sound properties and measurement, 208–209, *209*
    vascular supply, 219
Aura, 445
Autism, 128
Autonomic nervous system, *28, 29,* 75–77, 76t, 77t, *78,* 353–360
    anatomic organization, 354, *355,* 355b
    central pathways, 359
    clinical concerns, 359–360
    cranial nerves and, 306
    hypothalamic regulation, 366
    neurotransmitters, 359, 360t
    reticular formation and, 374
    versus somatic nervous system, 77, *78*
    subdivisions, 76, 76t, 354, 354b, 354t
    visceral afferent system, 358
    visceral efferent system, 355–357
        parasympathetic, 355t, 357, *359,* 360t
        sympathetic, 355–357, 355t, *356, 357,* 358t
Autonomic pathways of spinal cord, 244
Autosomal chromosomes, trisomies, 115t
Axial, 13
Axial-limbic brain, 353–377. *See also* Autonomic nervous system; Hypothalamus; Limbic system; Reticular formation
Axoaxonic synapse, 133
Axodendritic synapse, 133
Axon, 13, *13, 132,* 133
Axon hillock, 13, 133
Axonal (retrograde) reaction, brain injury, 139–140, *140,* 141t, 142t
Axonal regeneration
    central, *140,* 142–143, 142b
    peripheral, *140,* 141–142, 142b
Axonal sprouting, 142, 142b
Axosomatic synapse, 133

Babinski sign, 295–296, *296*
Ballism, 280
Bárány test, *233,* 235
Basal ganglia, 14, *14,* 15t, 42–44, *43, 44,* 44t
    amygdaloid nucleus, 44, *44*
    anatomic structures, 101t
    caudate nucleus, 44, *44*
    claustrum, *43,* 44
    globus pallidus, *43,* 44
    lesions, 35t
    motor system
        anatomy and physiology, 274–280, *276, 278, 279*
        circuitry, 275–280, *276, 278, 279*
        clinical concerns, 280–286, 281t. *See also* Basal ganglia disorders
        clinical considerations, 286–287
        innervation pattern, 275, *276*
        neurotransmitters, *279,* 280
    putamen, 42, *43,* 44
Basal ganglia disorders, 280–286, 281t
    athetosis, 280

ballism, 280
    chorea, 280–281
    cognitive impairment in, 285–286, 416
    Huntington chorea, 282, 284, *284*
    Parkinson's disease, 281–282, *283*
    progressive supranuclear palsy, 284–285
    psychiatric concomitants, 285–286
    tremors, 281
    Wilson disease, 284, *285*
Basal plate, 120
Basal temporal language area, 407
Basilar artery, 219, *379,* 380, *380,* 381t
Basis pedunculi, 49, 96
Basis pontis, 50
Bell palsy, 328, *329,* 330
Betz cells, 289
Bilaminar embryo, 118, *119*
Binocular visual field, 185, *186*
Biologic rhythms, reticular formation and, 374
Bipolar neuron, 133
Bitemporal (heteronymous) hemianopia, 203, *203, 204*
Blastocyst, 117–118, *118*
Blastomere, 117
Blind spot, 190, *191*
Blindness
    cortical (cerebral), 39
    monocular, *203,* 204
    night, 191
Blood-brain barrier, 134, 395, *395*
Blood flow, cerebral
    regional, 430–431
    regulation, 391–393, 395t
Blood oxygen level–dependent (BOLD) effects, 428
Blood supply. *See* Cerebrovascular system
Body movement. *See* Movement
Body temperature regulation, 366
BOLD-fMRI research paradigm, 428
Bony labyrinth, 210
Brachial plexus, 58, *59,* 59t
Brachium, 13, 19
Brachium conjunctivum (superior cerebellar peduncle), 52, 95, 96, *97*
Brachium pontis (middle cerebellar peduncle), 49, 52, 93, *264,* 265, 265t
Bradykinesia, 269, 280
Brain. *See also* Cerebral *entries; individual structures*
    association areas, 16, 18
    bilateral anatomic symmetry, 7
    blood supply, *379,* 379–384, *380,* 380t–382t, 391, *394*
    Brodmann areas, 16, *17,* 18, 18t
    cellular organization, *15,* 16–18, 17t
    contralateral sensorimotor control, 7, *7*
    cultural neutrality, 8
    directional orientation, 8–10, *9,* 10t
    embryological development, 120–125, *122–123,* 124t, 125t
    flexures, 120
    functionally specialized networking, 7
    gross structures, *14,* 14–15, 15t, 30–52
        brainstem, 46–52
        cerebellum, 52
        diencephalon, 44–46
        medullary centers, 61–64
            association fibers, 63–64, *64, 65*
            commissural fibers, 64, *66*
            projection fibers, 62–63, *63*
        meninges, 65, *67,* 67–70, 67t
            arachnoid membrane, 69–70, *70*
            dura mater, 65, 67–68, *67–69*
            pia mater, 70, *70*
        telencephalon, 30–44
        ventricles, 60–61
    interconnectivity, 6
    internal anatomy, anatomic orientation landmarks, 82–83, *83*

laterality, 7, *7*
    neuronal pruning and synapse establishment, 135–137, 137b
    organizational principles, 6–8, 6t
    plasticity, 8, 137
    primary divisions, 29, *29,* 30t
    sectional planes, 10, *11,* 12t
    topographical organization, 7–8
    unilateral functional differences, 7
Brain death, 447
Brain diseases. *See* Neurologic disorders
Brain imaging, 405, 421–431
    cerebral angiography, 421–423, *422, 423*
    computed tomography, 423–425, *424,* 425t
    magnetic resonance imaging, 425–430. *See also* Magnetic resonance imaging
    overview, 421
    positron emission tomography, 431, *432, 433*
    regional cerebral blood flow, 430–431
    single photon emission computed tomography, 431, *434*
Brain injury
    axonal (retrograde) reaction, 139–140, *140,* 141t, 142t
    axonal regeneration
        central, *140,* 142–143, 142b
        peripheral, *140,* 141–142, 142b
    neuroglial responses, 141
    neuronal response, 139–143, *140,* 141t, 142b, 142t
    traumatic, 417
    Wallerian (anterograde) degeneration, *140,* 141, 141t, 142t
Brain tumor, 147, 449
Brainstem, 14, *15,* 15t. *See also* Basal ganglia; Medulla oblongata; Midbrain; Pons; Reticular formation
    cranial nerve syndromes, 344–347, *345–347,* 345t
    cranial nerves on, 300–301, *302*
    directional orientation, *9,* 10t
    gross anatomy, *46–48,* 46–52
    lesion localization, 297
    lesions, 35t
    motor system
        basal ganglia anatomy and physiology, 274–280, *276, 278, 279. See also* Basal ganglia
        clinical concerns, 280–286, 281t. *See also* Basal ganglia disorders
        clinical considerations, 286–287
        reticular formation anatomy and motor functions, 272–274, *273, 274*
    respiratory centers, *371,* 372
    transverse sections, 86–101, *87–100*
Brainstem auditory evoked response, 223, 437–439, *438,* 439t
Branchial arches, speech-related muscles and, 302, 306, 306b, 306t, *307*
Broca aphasia, 409, 412
    aphemia variant, 409
Broca area, 33, 406
Brodmann areas, 16, *17,* 18, 18t
Brown-Séquard syndrome, 182, *182,* 255, 255–256

Calcarine sulcus, 37
Callosal sulcus, 41
Caloric stimulation, 236
Canal of Schlemm, 186
Capillaries, 378
Carbamazepine (Tegretol), 446
Cardiac center, 51
Cardiac muscle, 10
Cardiovascular activity regulation, 371
Carotid arterial system, *379,* 379
Carotid artery anastomosis, 442
Carotid endarterectomy, 442
Carpal tunnel syndrome, 171, 448
Cataract, 188

Cauda equina, 57
Caudal, 8, 9, *9*, 10t
Caudate head, 106–107, *108*
Caudate nucleus, 44, *44*, 102, *102*, 103, 104, *105*, *106*, 109, *112*, 275, *276*, 277, 281t
Cell body, 12–13, *13*, 131–132, *132*
Cell death, programmed, 136
Cell division
  meiosis, *116*, 116–117, *117*
  mitosis, 114, *115*, 116
Central arteries, 380, 382–384, 386t
Central canal, 54
Central nervous system. *See also* Brain; Spinal cord
  abnormal development, 125–128, 126t, 127t, *128*
  axonal regeneration, *140*, 142–143, 142b
  centrality, 6
  directional orientation, 9, 9–10, 10t
  embryological development, 119–125, *121–123*, 124t, 125t
  gross anatomy, *14*, 14–15, 15t, 27–71, *28*
    brain
      gross structures, 30–52
      medullary centers, 61–64
      meninges, 65, 67, 67–70, 67t
      primary divisions, 29, *29*, 30t
      ventricles, 60–61
    clinical considerations, 78–80
    spinal cord
      gross structures, 52–60
      meninges, 67t, 70–71, *71*
  internal anatomy, 82–113
    brain anatomic orientation landmarks, 82–83, *83*
    brainstem in transverse sections, 86–101, *87–100*
    forebrain
      coronal sections, 101–107, 101t, *102–109*
      horizontal sections, 108–113, *110–112*
    spinal cord in cross sections, 84–86, *84–86*, 84t
  lesion localization
    cortical lesion, 77–78
    subcortical lesion, 78
  neuraxis, organizational hierarchy, 6
  neuronal structures, 13, 14t
  sectional planes, 10, *11*, 12t
Central sulcus (fissure of Rolando), 30–31, *31*, *32*
Centromedianus nucleus, 157t, 159, 160, 370–371
Centromere, 114, *115*
Cerebellar arteries, 219, 381
Cerebellar cortex, *266*, 266–268, *267*
Cerebellar disorders
  alcohol toxicity, 270
  assessment, 269
  cerebrovascular accident, 270
  progressive degenerative, 270
Cerebellar hemispheres, 52, *53*, *54*, 261, *251*
Cerebellar lobes, 261, *261*, 263, 263t
Cerebellar nuclei, 262, *262*
Cerebellar peduncle
  inferior, 52, 89, 93, *264*, 264–265, 265t
  middle, 49, 52, 93, *264*, 265, 265t
  superior, 52, 95, 96, 97
Cerebellar signs, 269–270
  ataxia, 269
  disequilibrium, 270
  dysarthria, 269
  dysdiadochokinesia, 269
  dysmetria, 269
  hypotonia, 269
  intention tremor, 269
  rebounding, 269–270
Cerebellomedullary cistern, 400, *400*
Cerebellum, *14*, 15, 15t, 102, *102*
  afferent pathways, 263–265, *264*, 265t
  development, 125

efferent pathways, *264*, 265–266, 265t
  gross anatomy, 52, *53–55*
  input, 52
  lesions, 35t
  motor system, 260–271
    anatomy, *261–264*, 261–266, 263t, 265t
    cerebellar cortex, *266*, 266–268, *267*
    clinical concerns, 268–270. *See also* Cerebellar disorders; Cerebellar signs
    clinical considerations, 270–271
    innervation pattern, 261, *264*
    motor learning and, 268
  output, 52
  vestibular projections, 230, 231
Cerebral angiography, 421–423, *422*, *423*
Cerebral aqueduct, 61, 83, *83*, 95, 97
Cerebral artery
  anterior, 381–382, *383*, 384t, *385*
  middle, 382, *383*, 384t, *385*
  posterior, 382, *383*, 384t, *385*
Cerebral blood flow
  regional, 430–431
  regulation, 391–393, 395t
Cerebral concussion, 417
Cerebral cortex, 14, *14*, 15, 15t, 405–420
  Brodmann areas, 16, *17*, 18, *18*t
  cellular organization, *15*, 16–18, 17t
  clinical considerations, 417–420
  development, 121
  disorders of cortical function, 408–417. *See also* Cortical disorders
  functional localization, 405–407
  hemispheric dominance and functional specialization, 408
  methods of study, 405
Cerebral dominance, 408, 431–432, 434, 434t, *439*, 439–440
Cerebral hemispheres, 30, *31*, *32*
Cerebral infections, 449
Cerebral lesion, differential arm/leg involvement after, 293
Cerebral plasticity, 137
Cerebral veins, 391, *394*
Cerebrospinal fluid, 399–404
  absorption, 400–401, *401*
  chemical analysis, 440
  circulation, 399–400, *400–401*
  clinical concerns, 401–403
    diagnostic significance, 403
    hydrocephalus, 401–403, *402*, 402b
  clinical considerations, 403–404
Cerebrovascular accident. *See* Stroke
Cerebrovascular system, 378–398
  blood-brain barrier, 395, *395*
  clinical considerations, 396–397
  lesion localization, 395–396
  network, 378–387
    carotid system, 379, *379*
    central arteries, *380*, 382–384, 386t
    cerebrovascular supply, *379*, 379–384, *380*, 380t–382t
    circle of Willis, 379, *380*, 381–384, *383*, 384t, *385*, *386*, 386t
    collateral circulation, 385–387, 387b
    cortical arteries, 381–382, *383*, 384t, *385*, *386*
    spinal cord, 384–385, *386*
    vertebral basilar system, *379*, *380*, 380–381, 380t, 381t
  pathology, 387–391. *See also* Stroke
  venous sinus, 391
    cerebral veins, 391, *394*
    dural sinuses, 391, *393*
    spinal veins, 391
Cerebrum, 10t, *14*, 14, 15t
Cervical flexure, 120
Cervical plexus, 58, *59*, 59t
Cervical section, 86, *86*
Chiasmatic cistern, 400, *400*

Chief (principal) sensory nucleus, 177
Childhood autism, 128
Cholesterol, and stroke risk, 392b
Chorda tympani nerve, 326
Chordotomy, 174
Chorea, 19
  Huntington, 103, 105b, 281, 282, 284, *284*
  Sydenham, 280–281
Choroid plexus, 104, *106*, 134, 188, 399, *400*
Choroidal arteries, 384
Chromatids, 114, *115*, 117
Chromatin, 114
Chromatolysis, 140
Chromosome number, 114, 115t
Chronic symptoms, 12
Cilia, 212, 227
Ciliary body, 185, *187*
Ciliary ganglion, 198–199
Ciliary muscles, 188
Cingulate sulcus, 41
Cingulum (cingulate gyrus), 36, 41, 63–64, *65*, 107, *111*, 361, 363–364, 406
Circle of Willis, 379, *380*, 381–384, *383*, 384t, *385*, *386*, 386t
Circular (constrictor) fibers, 188
Circular sulcus, 41
Circulatory disorders, cerebrospinal fluid, 401–403, *402*, 402b
Cisterns, 400, *400*
Clasp-knife spasticity, 294
Claustrum, *43*, *44*, 102, *102*
Climbing fibers, 267–268
Cochlea
  function, *212*, 212–213, 212t
  structure, 210–212, *211*
Cochlear duct, 211, 212
Cochlear implant, 221
Cochlear nuclear complex, 90, *92*, *213*, *214*, 216, 222, 307
Cochlear projections, 216
Cognitive impairment, basal ganglia disorders and, 285–286. *See also* Dementia
Cogwheel muscle rigidity, 294
Collateral circulation, 385–387, 387b
Collateral sulcus, 36
Collateral trigone area, 61
Colliculus, 13
  facial, 50
  inferior, 49, 96, 97, *214*, 216–217, *217*, 222
  superior, 49, 96, 98
Color vision, 191–192
Color vision disorders, 202
Coma, 370, 447
Commissural fibers, 64, 66
Commissure, 10
  anterior, 41, 64
  posterior, 41, *100*, 101
Commissurotomy, 39–41, 64
Common carotid artery, 379, *379*
Computed tomography, 423–425, *424*, 425t
  single photon emission, 431, *434*
Concave lens, *193*, 194
Concussion, cerebral, 417
Conduction aphasia, 410
Conduction velocities, *138*, 139
Conductive hearing loss, 221
Cones, 188–190, *189*, 190t
Confusional state, acute, 446
Conjugate eye movements, vestibular control, *231*, 232
Conjugate gaze center, 342
Consciousness, altered, 370, 446–448
Consensual response, 199
Constrictor fibers, 188
Constructional apraxia, 413
Contra- (as prefix), 12
Contralateral sensorimotor control, 7, *7*
Conus medullaris, 239
Convergence, 194

Convergent circuits, 134, *135*
Convex lens, *193*, 194
Copper, in Wilson disease, 284, *285*
Cordotomy, 441
Cornea, 188
  pigmentation, 284, *285*
Corneal reflex, 338t
Corona radiata, 62, *63*, 108
Coronal plane, 10, *11*, 12t
Corpus callosum, *38–40*, 39–41, 64, *66*, 108–109, *111*, *112*
Corpus striatum, 107
Cortical arousal, 370–371
Cortical arteries, 381–382, *383*, 384t, *385*, *386*
Cortical blindness, 39
Cortical disorders, 408–417
  agnosias, 414
  agraphias, 413
  alexias, 411–412, 412t
  aphasias, 409–411, 409t, 411t
  apraxias
    of learned movement, 413–414
    of speech, 408
  clinical considerations, 417–420
  dementias, 414–417
    neurologic diseases associated with, 416
    primary degenerative, 416–417
    systemic diseases associated with, 415, 415t
  dysarthrias, 408
  hemispheric dominance and, 408
  of speech and language, 408–413
  traumatic brain injury, 417
Cortical mapping, 440, *441*
Cortical organization
  functional, 7, 406
  topographical, 7–8
Cortical surfaces, 30–39
  dorsolateral, 30–35, *32*, *33*
  midsagittal, 36–39, *38–40*
  ventral, 35–36, *36*, *37*
Cortico-olivary system, 265
Corticobulbar tract, *292*, 293
Corticospinal fibers, 82–83, *83*
Corticospinal tract, 241–243, *244*, 289–290, *291*, 291–293, *292*
  anterior, 243, *244*, 292–293
  lateral, 83, *83*, 84, *84*, 241–243, *244*, *291*, *292*
  lesions. *See* Upper motor neuron syndrome
Coughing, 374
Cranial nerves, 71–75, 300–351
  abnormal development, 129
  anatomic classification, 73t
  autonomic functions, 306
  on brainstem, 300–301, *302*
  branchial origin of speech-related muscles, 302, 306, 306b, 306t, *307*
  clinical considerations, 347–351
  development, 128–129
  evolutionary basis, 300, 301b
  function-based combinations, 342–343, *342–344*, 344t
  functional classification, 301–302, 303t–305t, 306b
  functions, 72–75, 73t
  innervation pattern, 309–310, *313*, 314b, 314t
  nomenclature, 72, 73t
  nuclei, 306–308, *308–310*
  pathway
    motor (efferent), 308–309, *311*
    sensory (afferent), 309, *312*
  reflexes, 338t
  sensorimotor functions, 310–342
    abducens nerve (CN6), 318–319, *321*, 321t, *322*
    accessory nerve (CN11), 337–338, 339t, *340*
    facial nerve (CN7), 325–330, 326t, *327*, 328t, *329*, 330b
    glossopharyngeal nerve (CN9), 331–334, 332t, *333*

hypoglossal nerve (CN12), 338–339, 340t, *341*, 341t, 342
    oculomotor nerve (CN3), 314, 316–318, 316t, *317–318*, 321t
    olfactory nerve (CN1), 310–311, *315*, 316t
    optic nerve (CN2), 311–314, 316t
    trigeminal nerve (CN5), 319–320, 322t, *323*, 323–325, *324*, 325t
    trochlear nerve (CN4), 318, *320*, 320t, 321t
    vestibulocochlear nerve (CN8), 330–331, 330t
  syndromes, 344–347, *345–347*, 345t
  upper and lower motor neuron syndromes, 343–344
Craniotomy, 440, *441*
Cranium bifidum, 126
Creutzfeldt-Jakob disease, 416–417
Cristae, 227, 233
Critical period, 8, 127t
Crossed (intrasegmental) extensor reflex, 251, 252
Crus cerebri (pes pedunculi), 46, 82, *83*, 98
Cuneocerebellar tract, *168*, 168t, 180, *181*, 181t
Cupula, 227
Cushing reflex, 392–393
Cyst, 134
Cystic cavity, 141
Cytoarchitectural map of cerebral cortex, 16, *17*, 18, 18t
Cytoplasm, 131, *132*

Dark adaptation, 192, *192*
Deafness. *See also* Hearing loss
  pure word, 222, 410
Decibel (dB), 209
Decussation, 9–10, 96, *97*
Deep brain stimulation, 280, 282
Deep dyslexia, 412
Delirium, 446
Dementia, 414–417
  neurologic diseases associated with, 416
  primary degenerative, 416–417
  systemic diseases associated with, 415, 415t
Dendrites, 12, *132*, 132–133
Dentate nucleus, 262, *262*
Denticulate ligaments, 71
Depolarization, 139
Dermatomes, 55, *58*, 58t, 174t, 240
Deuteranomaly, 202
Developmental disabilities, 127–128
Diagnostic techniques. *See also specific techniques*
  brain imaging, 421–431
  dichotic listening, *439*, 439–440
  electroencephalography, 434–436, *435*, 435t
  electromyography, *436*, 436–437
  evoked potentials, 437–439, *438*, 439t
  lumbar puncture, 440
  neurosurgery, 440–442, *441*
  sodium amytal infusion for assessing cerebral dominance, 431–432, 434, 434t
Dichotic listening, *439*, 439–440
Diencephalon, *14*, 15t, 29, 44–46, 152–163. *See also* Hypothalamus; Thalamus
  anatomic structures, 101t
  clinical considerations, 162–163
  embryological development, 121–122, *122*, *123*, 124, 124t
  epithalamus, 160
  gross anatomy, 152, *153*
  hypothalamus, *45*, 46, 161
  junction with midbrain, *100*, 100–101
  subthalamus, 160
  thalamus, *39*, 44–46, *45*, 152–160, *154–156*, 157t, 161–162
Diffusion tensor imaging, 429–430, *430*
Diffusion-weighted imaging, 428–429, *429*
Digital subtraction angiography, 423
Dilator fibers, 188
Diopter units, 193

Diphenylhydantoin (phenytoin, Dilantin), 446
Diploid, 114
Diplopia, 318, *319*, 322
Directional brain orientation, 8–10, *9*, 10t
Disequilibrium, 270
Disjunction, 117
Distal, 10
Divergent circuits, 134, *135*
DNA, 114, 131
Dominance, cerebral, 408, 431–432, 434, 434t, *439*, 439–440
Dominant inheritance, 442–443, *443*
Dopamine, *144*, 145, 145t
  basal ganglia, 279, 280
  hypothalamic, 369
  in Parkinson's disease, 282, *283*
  reticular, 374–375
Dorsal, 8, 9, *9*, 10t
Dorsal column fibers, 88, *89*
Dorsal column–medial lemniscal (epicritic) system, 166–172, *168*, 168t, 169t, *170*, *171*
  assessment, 171–172
  lesions, 169, 171
  neural pathways, 167–169, 169t, *170*
  receptors, 167
Dorsal horns, 52, 54, 239, *240*, *241*
Dorsal lemniscus, 84, *89*
Dorsal median sulcus, 54
Dorsal motor nucleus of vagus nerve, 307, *336*
Dorsal ramus, 58, *59*, 239
Dorsal root ganglion, 164, *165*, 239, *240*
Dorsal secondary ascending tract, 177
Dorsal spinocerebellar tract, *168*, 168t, 180, *181*, 181t, 261, *264*
Dorsolateral cortical surface, 30–35, *32*, *33*, *34*
Dorsomedial nucleus, 155, 157t
Double vision, 318, *319*, 322
Down syndrome, 128
Dressing apraxia, 413
Drowsiness, 370
Duchenne dystrophy, 448
Dura mater
  brain, 65, 67–68, *67–69*
    falx cerebelli, 68, *69*
    falx cerebri, 67–68, *69*
    tentorium cerebelli, 68, *69*
  spinal cord, 52, *56*, 70–71, *71*
Dural venous sinuses, 391, *393*
Dynamic motor responses, 247, *248*
Dynes, 209
Dysarthria, 269, 408
Dysdiadochokinesia, 269
Dyskinesia, 280
Dyslexia, 412
Dysmetria, 269
Dystrophy, muscular, 448

Ear
  anatomy and physiology, *209*, 209–213, *211*, *212*
  external, *209*, 209–210
  inner, *209*, 210–212, *211*, *212*, 212t
  middle, *209*, 210
Edinger-Westphal nucleus, 98, *99*, 198, 307, 314, 316
Efferent (motor) fibers, 9, 29, 164, *165*
Efferent pathways
  cerebellar, *264*, 265–266, 265t
  cranial nerves, 308–309, *311*
  hypothalamic, 365–366
  motor cortex, 291–293, *292*
  reticular, 369
  spinal, 241–244, 242t, *243*
Efferent thalamic nuclei projections, 155, 155–160, *156*, 157t
Elbow neuropathy, 448–449
Electrical brain stimulation, 280, 282, 405
Electrical gradient, 138
Electrical transduction, hair cells, 213

Electro-oculography, 234
Electrocorticography, 440, 441
Electroencephalography, 434–436, 435, 435t, 445, 447, 447–448
Electromyography, 436, 436–437
Emboliform nucleus, 262, 262
Embolism, 387t, 388, 388
Embryo
    bilaminar, 118, 119
    trilaminar, 118
Embryoblast, 117, 118
Embryological development, 114–130
    of central nervous system, 119–125, 121–123, 124t, 125t
    chromosome number and, 114, 115t
    clinical concerns, 125–128
    critical periods, 127t
    early human, 116–119, 116–121
    fertilization and, 117–118, 118
    gametogenesis, 116, 116–117, 117
    genes and, 114
    meiosis, 116, 116–117, 117
    mitosis, 114, 115, 116
    of peripheral nervous system, 128–129
    teratogenesis and, 126, 126t, 127t
    week 1, 117–118, 118
    week 2, 118, 119
    week 3, 118–119, 120, 121
Embryonic stem cell transplantation, 143b
Emmetropia, 200, 201
Encapsulated endings, 165, 166, 166t
Encephalopathies, toxic, 448
Endarterectomy, carotid, 442
Endolymph, 212, 227, 233
Endoneurium, 135, 137
Endoplasmic reticulum, 132
Endorphins, 145t, 146
Enkephalin, 145t, 146, 375
Ependymal cells, 60–61, 134, 136, 136t
Ependymoma, 147
Epicritic system
    body, 166–172, 168, 168t, 169t, 170, 171
    face, 177, 178, 179t
Epidural space, 67, 71
Epilepsy, 436, 444–446, 445, 445t, 446t
Epinephrine, 252
Epithalamus, 121–122, 160
Equilibrium. See also Vestibular system
    cerebellum and, 263, 270
    diagnostic tests
        acceleration-rotation chair, 233, 235
        caloric stimulation, 236
    dynamic, 233
    labyrinth dysfunction and, 235
    motion sickness and, 234–235
    nystagmus and, 234, 235
    physiology, 233, 233–234, 235
    rotational sensation, 233, 233–234
    static, 234
    structures important for, 229
    vertigo and, 235
Euploid, 114
Eustachian tube, 209, 210
Evoked potentials
    auditory, 437–439, 438, 439t
    somatosensory, 437
    visual, 437
Excitatory postsynaptic potentials (EPSPs), 139
Executive function, 406
Expanded tip endings, 165, 166, 166t
Extension, 10, 12
External auditory meatus, 209, 210
External capsule, 44
External carotid artery, 379, 379
External ear, 209, 209–210
Extrafusal motor fibers, 246, 247
Extrapyramidal tracts, 243–244
Extreme capsule, 44
Eye movements

conjugate, vestibular control, 231, 232
    reticular formation and, 374
    voluntary, mechanism for controlling, 232, 232–233
Eye muscles, 321t, 342, 342–343
Eyeball anatomy, 185–188, 187

Face
    diffuse touch from, 179–180
    fine discriminative touch from, 177, 178, 179t
    pain and temperature from, 177, 178, 179, 179t
Facial colliculus, 50
Facial dystrophy, 448
Facial expression muscles, 328t
Facial nerve (CN7), 73t, 74, 74, 91, 93, 325–330, 326t, 327, 328t, 329, 330b
Falx cerebelli, 68, 69
Falx cerebri, 67–68, 69
Far point, 194
Fasciculus (fasciculi, funiculi), 13, 14t
Fasciculus cuneatus, 86, 167, 168, 168t, 169, 170, 243, 244
Fasciculus gracilis, 84, 84, 167, 168, 168t, 169, 170, 243, 244
Fastigial nucleus, 262, 262
Feeding (phagic) center, 366
Fertilization, 117–118, 118
Fibrillation, in lower motor neuron syndrome, 253
Fibrous tunic, 188
Fields of Forel, 160, 277, 278
Filum terminale, 57
FLAIR sequences, 426
Flexion, 10, 12
Flexor reflex, 250–251, 251
Flexures, brain, 120
Flocculonodular lobe (archicerebellum), 52, 53, 54
Flocculus, cerebellar, 52, 54
Focal length, 194
Focal point, 193
Folia, cerebellar, 52
Foramen magnum, 52, 55
Foramen of Magendie, 61, 61, 125
Foramina of Luschka, 61, 61, 125
Foramina of Monro, interventricular, 102, 102
Forebrain, 29, 29, 30t
    coronal sections, 101–107, 101t, 102–109
    embryological development, 120–124, 122, 123, 124t
    horizontal sections, 108–113, 110–112
Fornix, 41, 103, 105, 360, 361
Fourth ventricle, 61, 62, 83, 83, 91, 399, 400
Fovea centralis, 190
Fragile X syndrome, 128
Free nerve endings, 165, 166, 166t
Friedreich ataxia, 270
Frontal gyri, 33, 34
Frontal lobe, 30, 32, 101
    dorsolateral, 31–33, 34
    functional anatomy, 406
    lesions, 35t
    medial, 36–37
    orbital, 35–36
Frontal lobe syndrome, 406
Functional magnetic resonance imaging, 427, 427–428, 428
Fundus, 189

Gag reflex, 338t
Gait apraxia, 413
Gamete (sex cell), 114
Gametogenesis, 116, 116–117, 117
γ-Aminobutyric acid (GABA), 144, 145t, 146, 279, 280, 375
γ-Motor neurons, 245, 245
Ganglion (ganglia), 13, 14t
Ganglion cells, retinal, 189
Gasserian ganglion, 177

Gated ion channels, 138
Gaze center
    conjugate, 342
    pontine horizontal, 232
Genes, 114
Genetic inheritance, 442–444
    dominant, 442–443, 443
    recessive, 443, 443
    X-linked, 444, 444
Geniculate body
    lateral, 100, 101, 103, 104, 157t, 159, 195, 197
    medial, 100, 101, 157t, 159, 214, 217, 217–218, 218
Geniculocalcarine fibers, 197
Genome, 114
Glaucoma, 186–187
Glial cells, 12, 134, 136, 136t, 141
Gliosis, replacement, 134
Global aphasia, 410
Globose nucleus, 262, 262
Globus pallidus, 43, 44, 103, 105, 275, 276, 277–278, 278, 281t
Glossopharyngeal nerve (CN9), 73t, 74, 74–75, 90, 331–334, 332, 332t, 333
Glutamate, 145t, 146, 279, 280
Golgi apparatus, 132
Golgi tendon organs, 247, 248
Golgi type I and II cells, 133
Gonadotropic hormone, 367, 367, 368t
Grand mal seizure, 446, 446t
Graphesthesia, 167, 172
Gray matter
    brain, 12
    central, 88, 96, 97
    cerebral, 17t
    periaqueductal, 172
    spinal, 52, 54, 84, 182, 239
Growth-associated protein 43 (GAP-43), 136
Growth cones, 136
Growth hormone, 367, 367–368, 368t
Gyri of Heschl, 35
Gyrus (gyri), 10, 30, 31
Gyrus rectus, 36, 36

H fields, 160, 277, 278
Habenular nucleus, 160
Hair cells, 212, 213
Handedness, 408, 432, 434t
Haploid, 114
Head injury. See Brain injury
Head movement, reticular formation and, 374
Hearing level (HL), 209
Hearing loss, 221–222, 331
    central pathology, 222
    conductive, 221
    mixed, 221
    sensorineural, 221
Hearing sensitivity thresholds, 209, 209
Hearing tests, 222–224
    auditory brainstem response audiometry, 224
    otoacoustic emissions, 224
    pure tone audiometry, 223, 224
    tuning fork, 222–223, 223
    tympanometry, 223–224
Hematoma, subdural, 389
Hemianopia
    bitemporal (heteronymous), 203, 203, 204
    homonymous, 203, 204
    nasal, 203, 204
Hemiballism, 101, 280
Hemiplegia, 10, 291
    alternating, 294, 294–295, 381
    spastic, 293–294, 294
Hemisection, spinal, 182, 182, 255, 255–256
Hemispheres
    cerebellar, 52, 53, 54, 261, 261
    cerebral, 30, 31, 32
Hemispheric dominance, 408, 431–432, 434, 434t, 439, 439–440

Hemorrhage, 423
Hemorrhagic stroke, 389, *390*
Hepatolenticular degeneration, 284, *285*
Hertz (Hz), 208
Heteronymous, definition, 203
Heteronymous (bitemporal) hemianopia, 203, *203*, 204
Hindbrain, 29, *29*, 30t, *122, 123*, 124–125, 124t
Hippocampal sulcus, 41
Hippocampus, 36, 103, *104, 112*, 113, *361*, 363
Hirschsprung disease, 129
Histones, 114
Homonymous, definition, 203
Homonymous hemianopia, *203*, 204
Homonymous quadrantanopsia, *203*, 204
Homunculus
  motor, 289, *290*, 406
  somatosensory, 8, 31, *34*
Horizontal plane, 10, *11*, 12t
Hormones, pituitary, *367*, 367–368, 368t
Horner syndrome, 199
Huntington chorea, 103, 105b, 281, 282, 284, *284*
Hydrocephalus, 62b, 127, 401–403, *402*, 402b
  normal pressure, 416
Hyperacusia, 328
Hyperalgesia, 175
Hyperesthesia, thermal, 175
Hyperglycemia, 448
Hypermetropia, *201*, 201–202
Hyperopia, *201*, 201–202
Hyperosmia, 311
Hyperpolarization, 139
Hypersensitive tangle, 174
Hypersomnia, 448
Hyperthermia, 175, 366
Hyperventilation, seizure induction and, 436
Hypesthesia, thermal, 175
Hypoalgesia, 175
Hypoglossal nerve (CN12), 73t, *74*, 75, 88–89, 338–339, 340t, *341*, 341t, 342
Hypoglossal nucleus, 307
Hypoglycemia, 448
Hypokinesia, 280
Hypophysis. *See* Pituitary gland
Hyposmia, 311
Hypothalamic sulcus, 41, 46
Hypothalamus, 14, *14*, 15t, 41, *45*, 46, 105, 161, 364–369
  anatomic structures, *364*, 364–366, *365*
    afferents, 365
    efferents, 365–366
  clinical concerns, 369
  development, 122
  functions, 161, 366–368
    autonomic innervation, 366
    body temperature regulation, 366
    feeding, 366
    pituitary gland regulation, *367*, 367–368, 368t
    punishment, 366
    water intake regulation, 366
  lesions, 35t
  neurotransmitters and behaviors, 368–369
  nuclei, 105
Hypothermia, 175
Hypotonia, 269

Ideational apraxia, 414
Ideomotor apraxia, 413–414
Imaging. *See* Brain imaging
Improving symptoms, 12
Impulse conduction, *138*, 139
Incus, *209*, 210
Infections, cerebral, 449
Inferior cerebellar peduncle (restiform body), 52, 89, 93, *264*, 264–265, 265t
Inferior colliculus, 49, 96, *97, 214*, 216–217, *217*, 222

Inferior frontal gyrus, 33, *34*
Inferior longitudinal fasciculus, 63, *65*
Inferior (principal) olivary nucleus, 51, 89, 265
Inferior parietal lobule, *33*, 34
Inferior pontine sulcus, 49
Inferior temporal gyrus, 35, 36, *36*
Infratentorial space, 68
Infundibulum, 365
Inheritance, 442–444
  dominant, 442–443, *443*
  recessive, 443, *443*
  X-linked, 444, *444*
Inhibitory postsynaptic potentials (IPSPs), 139
Inner ear, *209*, 210–212, *211, 212*, 212t
Insomnia, 448
Insular cortex (isle of Reil), 41, *42*
Insular lobe, 30, *32*, 41, *42*
Intention tremor, 269, 281
Inter- (as prefix), 12
Interconnectivity, brain, 6
Interhemispheric (longitudinal) fissure, 30, 103, *104, 110*
Internal arcuate fibers, 167, 169
Internal auditory (labyrinthine) artery, 219, 228, *379*, 381
Internal capsule, 44, 62, *63, 102*, 102
  anterior limb, 101t, 102, *102*
  posterior limb, 102, *102*, 103, *104*
Internal carotid artery, 379, *379*
Internal carotid–external carotid anastomosis, 442
Internal medullary lamina, 153–155
Interneurons, 245, *245*
Internode, 133
Interpeduncular cistern, 400, *400*
Interpeduncular fossa, 49
Interventricular foramina of Monro, 102, *102*
Intra- (as prefix), 12
Intracerebral hemorrhage, 389
Intrafusal motor fibers, 246, *247*, 248
Intralaminar nuclear complex, 155, 157t, 159–160
Intraparietal sulcus, 34
Intrasegmental extensor reflex, 251, *252*
Ion channels, 138–139
Ion concentration gradient, 138
Ipsi- (as prefix), 12
Iris, 185, *187*, 188
Isle of Reil, 41, *42*
Isolation syndrome, 411

Jacksonian march, 445

Kayser-Fleischer ring, 284, *285*
Kinesthesia, 165, 167, 172, 177
Klüver-Bucy syndrome, 363
Knee jerk, 250, *250*
Knee neuropathy, 449
Korsakoff syndrome, 155

Labyrinth
  bony, 210
  dysfunction, 235
  membranous, 210, 227, 228
Labyrinthine artery, 219, 228, *379*, 381
Lacunar stroke, 389
Lamina terminalis, 120
Language areas
  basal temporal, 407
  Broca area, 33, 406
  thalamus, 161
  Wernicke area, 35, 218–219, *220*, 407
Language disorders. *See* Speech and language disorders
Laryngeal nerve, 336, *338*
Lateral corticospinal tract, 83, *83*, 84, *84*, 241–243, *244*, *291*, 292
Lateral dorsal nucleus, 156, 157t
Lateral fissure (sylvian fissure), 30, 31, *32*

Lateral geniculate body, *100*, 101, 103, *104*, 157t, 159, *195*, 197
Lateral inhibition, 134, *135*
Lateral lemniscus, 96, 216
Lateral nuclear complex, 156, 157t, 158
Lateral plane, 10, *11*, 12t
Lateral posterior nucleus, 156, 157t
Lateral spinothalamic tract, *168*, 168t, 172, *173*, 174–175, 174t, *243*, 244
Lateral ventricles, 61, *62*, 103, *104*, 109, *112*, 399, *400*
  anterior horn, 101, *102*
  shape, 83, *83*
Laterality, brain, 7, *7*
Lead poisoning, 448
Leak ion channels, 138–139
Lemniscus, 19
  dorsal, 84, *89*
  lateral, 96, 216
  medial, 50, 167, 169. *See also* Dorsal column–medial lemniscal (epicritic) system
Lens, 185, *187*, 188
  refraction, 192–194, *193*
  types, *193*, 194
Lenticular nucleus, 43, 44t
Lenticulostriate arteries, 382, *386*
Leptomeninges, 70
Lesion localization, 21–23, 22b–23b
  brainstem, 297
  Brown-Séquard syndrome, 256
  cerebrovascular disorder, 395–396
  clinical problem-solving approach, 21, 21b
  complete spinal transection, 256
  cortical, 77–78
  peripheral or central lesion, 256
  signs, 23t
  spinal central gray, 182
  subcortical, 78
  upper or lower motor neuron syndrome, 296–297
  visual pathway, 205
Letter-by-letter reading, 412
Levator palpebrae, 74
Lewy body dementia, 416
Lexical agraphia, 413
Limb coordination, cerebellum and, 263
Limb-kinetic apraxia, 414
Limb-withdrawal reflex, 250–251, *251*
Limbic-axial brain, 353–377. *See also* Autonomic nervous system; Hypothalamus; Limbic system; Reticular formation
Limbic lobe, 36, 41–42, *42*, 360, *361*
Limbic system, 360–365
  anatomic structures, *361, 362*, 362–364, 363t
  clinical concerns, 364
  pathways, 362, *362*
Limen insula, 41
Local anesthetics, 175
Locked-in syndrome, 345t, 346, *346*
Locus ceruleus, 370
Longitudinal fasciculus, 63, *65*
Longitudinal (interhemispheric) fissure, 30, 103, *104, 110*
Loop of Meyer, 197
Lower calcarine operculum, 37
Lower motor neuron syndrome, 253, 253–254, 295b, 296–297, 296t
  of cranial nerves, 343–344
Lower motor neurons (LMNs), 240, 245, 291
Lumbar cistern, 71, *72*, 400, *400*
Lumbar plexus, 58–59, *59*, 59t
Lumbar puncture, 71, 440
Lumbar section, 84–85, *85*
Luminosity curves, 191, *192*
Luschka, foramina of, 61, *61*, 125
Lysosomes, 132

Macula lutea, 190
Magendie, foramen of, 61, *61*, 125

Magnetic resonance angiography, 430
Magnetic resonance imaging
  advances, 427–430
  advantages, 426, *427*
  diffusion tensor imaging, 429–430, *430*
  diffusion-weighted, 428–429, *429*
  disadvantages, 426, *427*
  FLAIR sequences, 426
  functional, *427*, 427–428, *428*
  in multiple sclerosis, 148, *148*
  perfusion, 429, *429*
  T1- or T2-weighted, 425–426, *426*, 426t
Magnetic resonance spectroscopy, 430
Magnetic resonance venography, 430
Malleus, *209*, 210
Mammillary body, 41
Mammillothalamic tract, 155
Mandibular branch of trigeminal nerve, 176, 323, *323*
Mapping
  cortical, 440, *441*
  subcortical, 441
Massa intermedia, 41, 103, *105*
Masticatory muscles, 323–324, 325t
Maxillary branch of trigeminal nerve, 176, 323, *323*
Mechanoreception, 164–165, 165t
Medial frontal lobe, 36–37
Medial geniculate body, *100*, 101, 157t, 159, *214*, *217*, 217–218, *218*
Medial lemniscus, 50, 167, 169. *See also* Dorsal column–medial lemniscal (epicritic) system
Medial longitudinal fasciculus, 89, 230–231, *231*, 319
Medial medullary syndrome, 345t, 346–347, *347*
Medial nuclear complex, 155–156, 157t
Medial occipital lobe, 37, *39*
Medial parietal lobe, 37, *38*
Medial plane, 10, *11*, 12t
Medial raphe nucleus, 370
Medial reticular formation, 370
Medial striate arteries, 383
Medial temporal lobe, 39, *39*
Median nerve, 171, 448
Medulla oblongata, *14*, 15, 15t, *46*, *47*, 50–52, *51*
  caudal, 87–88, *88*, *89*
  caudal (lower) third, 88–89, *90*
  cranial nerve nuclei in, 307–308, *309*
  development, 125
  lesions, 345t, 346–347, *347*
  middle third, 89–90, *91*
  rostral third, 90, *92*
  transverse sections, 87–90, 87t, *88–92*
Medullary center(s), 61–64
  association fibers, 63–64, *64*, *65*
  cardiac, 51
  commissural fibers, 64, *66*
  projection fibers, 62–63, *63*
  respiratory, 48, 51, *371*, 372
  vasomotor, 51
Medullary reticulospinal tract, 244
Megacolon, aganglionic, 129
Meiosis, *116*, 116–117, *117*
Meissner corpuscles, 165, *166*, 166t
Melanocytes, 188
Membrane potential, resting, 138, *138*
Membranous labyrinth, 210, 227, *228*
Ménière disease, 221, 235
Meninges
  brain, 65, *67*, 67–70, 67t
    arachnoid membrane, 69–70, *70*
    dura mater, 65, 67–68, *67–69*
    pia mater, 70, *70*
  spinal cord, 67t, 70–71, *71*
Meningioma, 147
Meningitis, 65, 68b
Mental function assessment, 5t
Mental lexicon, 432, 434

Mental retardation, 127–128
Merkel receptors, 165, *166*, 166t
Mesencephalic nucleus, 177, 307
Mesencephalon. *See* Midbrain
Mesocortex, 14
Mesocortical system, 145
Mesostriatal system, 145
Metaphase, 116
Metencephalon, 29, *122*, *123*, 124–125, 124t
Microcephaly, 127
Microfilaments, 132
Microglia, 134, *136*, 136t, 141
Microtubules, 131, 132, *132*
Midbrain, *14*, 15, 15t, 29, *29*, 30t
  caudal, 96, *97*
  cranial nerve nuclei in, 307
  embryological development, *122*, *123*, 124, 124t
  gross anatomy, *46*, *47*, *49*, 49–50
  high rostral, *98*, *99*, 100
  junction with diencephalon, *100*, 100–101
  junction with pons, *95*, 95–96
  lesion 345, *345*, 345t
  rostral, 96–98, *98*
  transverse sections, 96–100, 95t, *97–99*
Midbrain flexure, 29, 120
Midbrain-reticular-limbic area, 83
Middle cerebellar peduncle (brachium pontis), *49*, 52, 93, *264*, 255, 265
Middle cerebral artery, 382, 384t, *385*
Middle ear, *209*, 210
Middle frontal gyrus, 33, *34*
Middle temporal gyrus, 35
Midline nuclear complex, 155–156, 157t
Midsagittal cortical surface, 36–39, *38–40*
Midsagittal cut, 10
Millard-Gubler syndrome, 345–346, 345t, *346*
Mitochondria, 132
Mitosis, 114, *115*, 116
Modiolus, 210
Monoamines, 145–146
Monocular blindness, *203*, 204
Monocular visual field, 185, *186*
Monoplegia, 10, 291
Monro, interventricular foramina of, *102*, 102
Monroe-Kelly reflex, 392–393
Morphine, 175
Morula, 117, *118*
Mossy fibers, 265, 268
Motion sickness, 234–235
Motor aphasia, transcortical, 410–411
Motor area, supplemental, *290*, 290
Motor cortex, 289–299, 406
  anatomy, 289–290, *290*, *291*
  cerebellar projections, 266
  clinical concerns
    alternating hemiplegia, *294*, 294–295
    pseudobulbar palsy, 294
    spastic hemiplegia, 293–294, *294*
    upper motor neuron syndrome, 293b, *295*, 295–296, *296*, 296t
  clinical considerations, 297–299
  descending pathways, 291–293, *292*
  disorders, terminology, 291
  innervation pattern, 290, 292
  lesion localization, 296–297
  primary, 289–290, *290*, *291*
  voluntary respiratory center, 372
Motor examination, 5t
Motor (efferent) fibers, 9, 29, 164, *165*. *See also* Efferent pathways
  extrafusal, 246, *247*
  intrafusal, 246, *247*, 248
Motor function, reticular integration, *274*, 274, *371*, 371–374, 372b, 372t, 373b
Motor homunculus, 289, *290*, 406
Motor neuron(s)
  α–, 245, *245*
  γ–, 245, *245*

lower, 240, 245, 291
  reciprocal innervation, 251, *251*
  upper, 91, 245
Motor neuron syndrome
  of cranial nerves, 343–344
  lower, 253, *253*–254, 295b, 296–297, 296t
  upper, 253, *255*, 293b, *295*, 295–296, *296*, 296t, 297
Motor system
  ascending levels, 238, *239*
  brainstem and basal ganglia, 272–288
    basal ganglia anatomy and physiology, 274–280, *276*, *278*, *279*
    clinical concerns, 280–286, 281t. *See also* Basal ganglia disorders
    clinical considerations, 286–287
    reticular formation anatomy and motor functions, 272–274, *273*, *274*
  cerebellum, 260–271
    anatomy, *261*–264, 261–266, 263t, 265t
    cerebellar cortex, *266*, 266–268, *267*
    clinical concerns, 268–270
    clinical considerations, 270–271
    innervation pattern, 261, *264*
    motor learning and, 268
  motor cortex. *See* Motor cortex
  spinal cord, 238–259
    clinical concerns, 252–256. *See also* Spinal syndromes
    clinical considerations, 257–259
    functions, 245–248, *246–249*
    gross anatomy, 239–240, *240–242*
    innervation pattern, 238–239, *240*, *242*
    lesion localization, 256
    motor nuclei, 245, *245*
    neurotransmitters, 252
    reflexes, 248, 250–251, *250–252*, 250t
    spinal preparation, 238
    tracts, 240–245, 242t, *243*, *244*
Motor unit, 240, *240*, 242
Movement
  disorders, 280–281, 281t
  initiation, 248, *249*
  learned, apraxia of, 413–414
  terminology, 10, *12*
Multiple sclerosis, 133, 147–149, *148*, 408, 416
Multipolar neuron, 133
Muscle
  contraction, 248, *249*
  terminology, 10
  tone, 263, 274, *274*, 280
  types, 10
Muscle spindles, 246, *247*, 248
Muscle stretch reflex, 164, 246, 248, 250, *250*, 250t
Muscular dystrophy, 448
Mutism, akinetic, 406
Myasthenia gravis, 145, 149, 252
Mydriasis, 199
Myelencephalon, 29, *122*, *123*, 124t, 125
Myelin-forming cells, central versus peripheral, 134–135
Myelin sheath, 133
Myelinogenesis, 126
Myopathies, 448
Myopia, 201, 202
Myosin, 246
Myotatic (stretch) reflex, 164, 246, 248, 250, *250*, 250t
Myotome, 55, 58t, 240

Narcolepsy, 448
Narcotics, 175
Nasal hemianopia, *203*, 204
Neocerebellum, *261*, 263, 263t
Neocortex, cellular layers, 14, *15*, 16, 17t
Neoplasia, 147, 449
Neostriatum (striatum), 43, 44t, 281t
Nerve cell. *See* Neuron(s)

Nerve conduction studies, 436–437
Nerve excitability, *138,* 139
Nerve fiber, 132, 135, *137*
Nerve impulse, 137–139, *138*
Nerve plexus, 58–59, *59,* 59t
Nerves, 13, 14t
Nervous system. *See also* Autonomic nervous system; Central nervous system; Peripheral nervous system
  categories of function, 27
  functional classification, 15–16, 16t
  gross anatomy, 27–81, *28*
Nervous tunic, 188. *See also* Retina
Neural crest, 120, *121*
Neural plate, 119–120, *121*
Neural tube, 120, *121*
Neuralgia, trigeminal, 179, 183, 325, 325b
Neuraxis, organizational hierarchy, 6
Neuroanatomy, 3t, 5, 10, 12
Neuroembryology, 3t, 5–6
Neurofilaments, 132
Neuroglial cells, 12, 134, *136,* 136t, 141
Neurohypophysis
  development, 124
  hormones, *367,* 368, 368t
Neuroimaging. *See* Brain imaging
Neurologic assessment, common areas, 5t
Neurologic disorders, 2b, 444–449
  cerebral infections, 449
  dementia associated with, 416
  major, 4t
  myopathies, 448
  neoplasia, 449
  peripheral neuropathies, 448–449
  seizures and epilepsy, 444–446, *445,* 445t, 446t
  of sleep and altered consciousness, 446–448, *447*
  toxic encephalopathies, 448
Neurologic terminology, 10, 12
Neurology, 3t, 4, 405
Neuroma, acoustic, 147
Neuromuscular junction disorders, 436
Neuron(s), 12–13, *13,* 131–151. *See also* Motor neuron(s)
  central versus peripheral, 134–135, *137*
  clinical concerns, 147–149, *148*
  clinical considerations, 149–150
  first- through third-order, 165–166, *167*
  response to brain injury, 139–143, *140,* 141t, 142b, 142t
  structure, *131,* 131–133
  types, 133, *134*
Neuronal circuits, 133–134, *135*
Neuronal pruning, 135–137, 137b
Neuronal structures of nervous system, 13, 14t
Neuronal transplantation, 143b
Neuropathology, 3t, 6
Neuropathy, 60b, 448–449
Neurophysiology, 3t, 6
Neuroradiology, 3t, 5. *See also* Brain imaging
Neuroscience, 1–25
  anatomic versus clinical orientation, 19–20, *20*
  branches, 3t
  clinical considerations, 24
  domain, 2
  learning strategies, 18–23, 18t
    clinical orientation, 19–20, *20*
    clinical problem-solving approach, 21, 21b
    functional context, 21
    simplification of terminology, 18–19
    visual approach, 19
  lesion localization, 21–23, 22b–23b, 23t
  relationship to speech-language-hearing pathology, 1–3
  scope, 3–6, 3t
  terminology, 8–13. *See also* Terminology
  training in
    benefits, 3
    nature, 2–3
    need for, 2

Neurosurgical procedures, 3t, 4–5, 440–442
  aneurysm clipping, 442
  carotid endarterectomy, 442
  cordotomy, 441
  craniotomy and cortical mapping, 440, *441*
  internal carotid–external carotid anastomosis, 442
  stereotactic surgery and subcortical mapping, 441
Neurotransmitters
  autonomic nervous system, 359, 360t
  basal ganglia, *279,* 280
  drug treatment principles, 146–147
  hypothalamic, 368–369
  reticular, 374–375
  spinal, 252
  types, 143–146, *144,* 145t
Night blindness, 191
Nociception. *See also* Pain
  body, 165, 165t, 172–175
  face, 177, *178,* 179, 179t
Nodes of Ranvier, 133
Nodulus, cerebellar, 52, *54*
Nondisjunction, 117
Noradrenergic cells, 145–146
Norepinephrine, *144,* 145–146, 145t
  hypothalamic, 368–369
  reticular, 374
  spinal, 252
Notochord, 118, *121*
Nuclear bag fibers, *247,* 248
Nuclear chain fibers, *247,* 248
Nucleolus, 131–132, *132*
Nucleus (nuclei)
  cellular, 131, *132*
  definition, 13, 14t
Nucleus ambiguus, 89–90, 307, 336, *338*
Nucleus basalis of Meynert, 143, 219b
Nucleus pulposus, 118
Nucleus solitarius, 307, *335*
Nystagmus
  induced, 234, *235*
  optokinetic, 234
  vestibular, 234, *235*

Obstructive sleep apnea, 448
Occipital lobe, 30, *32*
  dorsolateral, *32, 33,* 34–35
  functional anatomy, 407
  lesions, 35t
  medial, 37, *39*
Occipital notch, 33
Occipitofrontal fasciculus, superior, 63
Occlusive stroke, 387–389, *388,* 388t, *389*
Oculomotor apraxia, 413
Oculomotor nerve (CN3), 73–74, 73t, *74,* 98, *98*
  lesions, 199
  sensorimotor functions, 314, 316–318, 316t, *317–318,* 321t
Oculomotor nucleus, 307
Oculopharyngeal dystrophy, 448
Olfactory bulb, 36, *36*
Olfactory lobe, development, 121
Olfactory nerve (CN1), 72–73, 73t, *74,* 310–311, *315,* 316t
Olfactory sulcus, 36, *36*
Olfactory tract, 36, *36*
Oligodendroglial cells, 133, 134, *136,* 136t
Oligodendroglioma, 147
Olivary nucleus
  principal (inferior), 51, 89, 265
  superior, 216
Olivocochlear fibers, 221
Oncogene, 147
Oocyte, 116–117, *117*
Oogenesis, 117
Opercular, 10
Ophthalmic branch of trigeminal nerve, 176, 323, *323*

Ophthalmoplegia
  external, 317–318, *319*
  internal, 318
Opsin, 191
Optic aphasia, 204–205
Optic chiasm, 41, 189, *195,* 197
Optic disk, 189
Optic nerve (CN2), 73, 73t, *74,* 185, 311–314, 316t
Optic radiations, 197
Optic tract, 185, *195,* 197
Optic vesicles, 120, *122*
Optokinetic nystagmus, 234
Orbital frontal lobe, 35–36
Organ of Corti, 212
Organelles, 131, *132*
Ossicles, auditory, *209,* 210
Otitis media, 221
Otoacoustic emissions testing, 224
Otolithic membrane, 227
Otosclerosis, 221
Oval window, *209,* 210
Oxytocin, *367,* 368, 368t

Pacinian corpuscles, 165, *166,* 166t
Pain. *See also* Nociception
  assessment, 175
  from face, 177, *178,* 179, 179t
  phantom limb, 174–175
  referred, 174, 174t
  tic douloureux, 179
  visceral, 174
Pain relief, 175
Paleocerebellum, *261,* 263, 263t
Pallidum, 43, 44t
Palsy
  Bell, 328, *329,* 330
  progressive supranuclear, 284–285
  pseudobulbar, 294, 343
Papez circuit, 41–42
Papilledema, 189
Parafascicular nucleus, 159
Paragrammatic syndrome (Wernicke aphasia), 222, 409–410
Parahippocampal gyrus, 36, *36,* 41
Paralysis
  soft palate, 336, *339*
  terminology, 291
  types, 10
  vocal fold, 336
Paraplegia, 291
Parasympathetic ganglia, 29, 355b
Parasympathetic nervous system, 29, 76, 76t, 77, 354, 354b, 354t
  central pathways, 359
  effects, 77t
  neurotransmitters, 359, 360t
  visceral efferents, 355t, 357, *359,* 360t
Paravermal region, 263, *263*
Paravertebral ganglia, 356
Parietal lobe, 30, *32*
  dorsolateral, *32, 33,* 33–34, *34*
  functional anatomy, 406–407
  lesions, 35t
  medial, 37, *38*
Parietal lobules, *33,* 34
Parieto-occipital sulcus, 30, 31, *32, 33,* 33, 37
Parkinson's disease, 50b, 99b, 145, 281–282, *283,* 416
Pars opercularis, 33
Pars orbitalis, 33
Pars triangularis, 33
Partial complex seizure, 446
Partial/focal epilepsy, 445
Pedigree, 442, *443*
Peduncle, 19
Peduncular groove, 46
Peptides, 145t, 146
Perfusion magnetic resonance imaging, 429, *429*

Periaqueductal gray matter, 172
Perikaryon (cell body, soma), 12–13, *13,* 131–132, *132*
Perilymph, 212
Peripheral nerve, 54–55
Peripheral nervous system, 15
  axonal regeneration, *140,* 141–142, 142b
  cranial nerves, 71–75
    anatomic classification, 73t
    functions, 72–75, 73t
    nomenclature, 72, 73t
  embryological development, 128–129
  gross anatomy, *28, 29*
  information-carrying fibers, 9
  neuronal structures, 13, 14t
Peripheral neuropathies, 60b, 448–449
Peroneal nerve, 449
Perivascular space, 70, 400
Persistent symptoms, 12
Pes pedunculi (crus cerebri), 46, 82, *83,* 98
Petit mall seizure, 446
Phagic center, 366
Phagocytosis, 140–141
Phantom limb, 174–175
Pharyngeal nerve, 336, *338*
Pharynx, sensorimotor innervation, 343, *344*
Phenobarbital, 446
Phonologic agraphia, 413
Phonologic dyslexia, 412
Photic stimulation, seizure induction and, 436
Photochemistry, retinal, 191–192
Photophobia, 188
Photopic luminosity curve, 191, *192*
Photopsin, 191
Photoreceptors, 188–190, *189,* 190t
Pia mater
  brain, 70, *70*
  spinal, 52, *56,* 71
Pick disease, 416
Piloerector muscles, 354
Pineal body, 41
Pineal gland, *100,* 101, 160
Pinna, *209,* 209–210
Pitch, 208
Pituitary adenoma, 147
Pituitary gland, 41, 365
  development, 124
  hypothalamic regulation, *367,* 367–368, 368t
Pituitary hormones, *367,* 367–368, 368t
Planes of brain sections, 10, *11,* 12t
Planum temporale, 218, *220,* 408
Plasticity
  auditory cortex, 219b
  brain, 8, 137
Pneumoencephalography, 421
Poikilothermic state, 366
Pons, *14,* 15, 15t
  cranial nerve nuclei in, 307, *309*
  gross anatomy, 49–50, *51*
  junction with midbrain, 95, 95–96
  lesions, 345–346, 345t, *346*
  lower, 90–91, 93, *93*
  middle, 93–95, *94*
  transverse sections, 90–96, 92t, *93–95*
Pontine cistern, 400, *400*
Pontine flexure, 120
Pontine horizontal gaze center, 232
Pontine pneumotaxic center, 48, *371,* 372
Pontine reticulospinal tract, 244
Pontine sulci, 49
Pontocerebellar fibers, 94
Position sense, 167
Positional vertigo, benign, 235
Positron emission tomography, 431, *432, 433*
Post- (as prefix), 12
Postcentral gyrus (primary sensory cortex), 33, *34,* 169, *171*
Posterior cavity, *187,* 187–188
Posterior cerebral artery, 382, *383,* 384t, *385*

Posterior chamber, 185, *187*
Posterior choroidal artery, 384
Posterior commissure, 41, *100,* 101
Posterior limb of internal capsule, 102, *102,* 103, *104*
Posterior lobe, 52, *53, 54*
Posterior spinal artery, 380, 384, *386*
Posterolateral arteries, 384
Postganglionic autonomic neuron, 354, *355,* 355b
Postganglionic fibers, 77
Postsynaptic neuron, 13, 133
Postsynaptic potentials, 139
Posture, 263, 280
Potassium, 138
Pre- (as prefix), 12
Precentral gyrus, 31, *31, 34,* 406
Precentral sulcus, 31, *31, 34*
Prefrontal cortex, 31–33, *34,* 406
Preganglionic autonomic neuron, 354, *355,* 355b
Preganglionic axon, 77
Premotor cortex, 31, *34,* 406
Preoccipital notch, *32,* 33, *33*
Prerubral area (fields of Forel, H fields), 160, 277, *278*
Presbycusis, 221
Presbyopia, 194, 200
Pressure, 165
Pressure equalization in middle ear, 210
Presynaptic neuron, 13
Presynaptic terminal, 133
Pretectal area, 198
Prevertebral ganglia, 356
Primary auditory cortex, 35, 215, *220*
Primary motor cortex, 289–290, *290, 291*
Primary sensory cortex, 33, *34,* 169, *171*
Primary visual cortex, *195,* 197
Primitive streak, 118, *120*
Principal (inferior) olivary nucleus, 51, 89, 265
Principal sensory nucleus, 177
Progressive supranuclear palsy, 284–285
Progressive symptoms, 12
Projection fibers, 62–63, *63*
Prolactin, *367, 367,* 368t
Prometaphase, 114
Pronation, 10, *12*
Prophase, 114
Proprioception, 167, *177*
  assessment, 172
  unconscious, 180–182, *181,* 181t
Prosencephalon. *See* Forebrain
Prosopagnosia, 204
Protanomaly, 202
Protopathic system
  body, *168,* 168t, 172–175, *173,* 174t, *176*
  face, 177, *178,* 179, 179t
Proximal, 10
Pseudobulbar palsy, 294, 343
Pseudodepressed syndrome, 406
Pseudopsychopathic behavior, 406
Psychiatric disorders, basal ganglia disorders and, 285–286
Psychomotor seizure, 446
Pulvinar, *100,* 101, 103, *104,* 157t, *158*
Punishment, hypothalamic regulation, 366
Pupil, 188
Pupillary aperture, 194
Pupillary light reflex, *198,* 198–199, *199,* 316, *318,* 318t, 338t
Pure tone audiometry, 223, *224*
Pure word deafness, 222, 410
Purkinje cell, 266
Putamen, *42, 43,* 44, 103, *105,* 275, *276,* 277, 281t
Pyramidal decussation, 86
Pyramidal neurons, 91, 245
Pyramidal tract. *See* Corticospinal tract
Pyriform cortex, 39, 311

Quadrantanopsia, *203,* 204
Quadriplegia, 10, 291

Radial (dilator) fibers, 188
Radicular arteries, 384–385, *386*
Ranvier, nodes of, 133
Raphe nuclei, 370
Reading disorders, 411–412, 412t, 413
Rebounding, 269–270
Receptors
  Merkel, 165, *166,* 166t
  photoreceptors, 188–190, *189,* 190t
  sensory, 165, *166,* 166t
  unconscious proprioceptive, 180
  vestibular, 228
Recessive inheritance, 443, *443*
Reciprocal inhibition, 251, *251*
Recognition disorders, 204, 413
Recurrent laryngeal nerve, 336, *338*
Red nucleus, 44, 97, *98*
Referred pain, 174, 174t
Reflex(es)
  accommodation, 199–200, *200,* 316–317, *318*
  auditory, 219
  cranial nerves, 338t
  Cushing, 392–393
  Monroe-Kelly, 392–393
  myotatic (stretch), 164, 246, 248, 250, *250,* 250t
  pupillary light, *198,* 198–199, *199,* 316, *318,* 318t, 338t
  spinal, 245–246, *246,* 248, 250–251, *250–252,* 250t
  startle, 234
  visual, 197–200, 316–317, *318,* 318t
  withdrawal, 250–251, *251*
Refraction, 192–194, *193*
Refraction errors, 200–202, *201*
Regional cerebral blood flow (rCBF), 430–431
Reil, isle of, 41, *42*
REM/NREM sleep, 370, 447, *447*–448
Renshaw cell, 245
Replacement gliosis, 134
Repolarization, 139
Respiratory control, 48, 60, 60t, *371,* 371–374, 372b, 372t, 373b
Respiratory muscles, 372–373, 372t, 373b
Restiform body (inferior cerebellar peduncle), 52, 89, 93, *264,* 264–265, 265t
Resting membrane potential, 138, *138*
Reticular activating system (RAS), 48, 231, 369, 370, 446
Reticular facilitary/inhibitory areas, 274, *274*
Reticular formation, 15, *48,* 48–49, 87, *88,* 369–375
  anatomic structures, 369
    afferents, 369
    efferents, 369
  anatomy, 272, *273*
  cerebellar projections, 266
  clinical concerns, 375
  functions, 369–374
    cortical arousal regulation, 370–371
    motor function integration, 274, *274, 371,* 371–374, 372b, 372t, 373b
    sensory function regulation, 371
  neurotransmitters, 374–375
  vestibular projections, 231
Reticular nucleus, 157t, 159
Reticular (periaqueductal gray matter) projections, in pain perception, 172
Reticulospinal tract, 244
Retina
  anatomy, 188–190, *189,* 190t
  image formation, *193,* 194
  optics, 194
  pathways to visual cortex, *195,* 195–197, 196t
  photochemistry, 191–192
    color vision, 191–192
    dark adaptation, 192, *192*
    spectral sensitivity, 191, *192*
  vascular supply, 190
Retinal (visual yellow), 191

Retinal field, 185
Retrocochlear neural mechanism, *213,* 213–214
Retrograde movement, 13
Reverberating circuits, 134, *135*
Rhodopsin, 191
Rhombencephalon. *See* Hindbrain
Ribosomes, 131
Rinne test, 223, *223*
Rods, 188–190, *189,* 190t
Rolando, fissure of, 30–31, *31, 32*
Romberg test, 172, 268
Rostral, 8, 9, *9,* 10t
Rotation test, *233,* 235
Rubrospinal tract, 243
Ruffini endings, 165, *166,* 166t

Saccule, 227
Sacral plexus, 59, *59,* 59t
Sacral section, 84, *84*
Sagittal plane, 10, *11,* 12t
Salivary nucleus, 307
Saltatory conduction, 133
Satellite cells, 134
Scala media (cochlear duct), 211, 212
Scala tympani, 211
Scala vestibuli, 211
Scarpa ganglia, 228
Schlemm, canal of, 186
Schwann cells, 133, 134, *136,* 136t
Schwannoma, vestibular, 147
Sclera, 188
Sclerosis
  amyotrophic lateral, 408
  atherosclerosis, 387
  multiple, 133, 147–149, *148,* 408, 416
  otosclerosis, 221
Scotopic luminosity curve, 191, *192*
Sectional planes, brain, 10, *11,* 12t
Seizures, 436, 444–446, 445, *445t, 446t*
Self-awareness, reticular formation and, 374
Semicircular ducts, 227–228, *228–230*
Semilunar (Gasserian) ganglion, 177
Semiovale center, 108, *110, 111*
Sensation, 164–165, 165t
Sensorimotor control, contralateral, 7, *7*
Sensorimotor functions of cranial nerves. *See*
  Cranial nerves, sensorimotor functions
Sensorineural hearing loss, 221
Sensory aphasia, transcortical, 411
Sensory cortex, 33, *34,* 169, *171*
Sensory examination, 5t
Sensory (afferent) fibers, 9, 29, 164, *165. See also*
  Afferent pathways
Sensory function, reticular regulation, 371
Sensory nucleus, principal, 177
Sensory receptors, 165, *166,* 166t
Septal area, 360, *361*
Septum, *361,* 364
Septum pellucidum, 41, 101, *102,* 107
Serotonin, *144,* 145t, 146
  reticular, 370b, 374
  spinal, 252
Sex cell (gamete), 114
Sex chromosomes, trisomies, 115t
Shunt, in hydrocephalus, 403
Simple epilepsy, 445
Single photon emission computed tomography,
  431, *434*
Skeletal muscle, 10
Sleep, 370, *447,* 447–448
  disorders, 448
  seizure induction and, 436
  stages, *447,* 447–448
Sleep apnea, obstructive, 448
Smooth muscle, 10
Sneeze reflex, 338t
Snellen chart, 202, *202*
Sodium amytal infusion, for assessing cerebral
  dominance, 431–432, 434, 434t

Sodium-potassium pump, 138
Soft palate
  paralysis, 336, *339*
  sensorimotor innervation, 343, *344*
Soma (cell body, perikaryon), 12–13, *13,*
  131–132, *132*
Somatic nervous system, 16, 16t, *28, 29,* 77, *78*
Somatic structures, 10, 12
Somatosensation, 164–166
  specialized receptors, 165, *166,* 166t
  types of sensation, 164–165, 165t
Somatosensory evoked potentials, 437
Somatosensory homunculus, 8, 31, *34*
Somatosensory system, 164–184
  anatomic division, 166–175
    anterolateral (protopathic) system, *168,*
      168t, 172–175, *173,* 174t, *176*
    dorsal column–medial lemniscal (epicritic)
      system, 166–172, *168,* 168t, 169t, *170,*
      171
  clinical considerations, *182,* 182–184, *183*
  innervation pattern, 166
  principles of somatosensation, 164–166, *165,*
    165t, *166*
  three-neuron organization, 165–166, *167*
  trigeminal sensory system and, 176–180, *178,*
    179t
  unconscious proprioception and, 180–182,
    181, 181t
Somatotopic organization, 164, 169, *171*
Somesthetic association cortex, 169
Somites, 10, 118
Sound, properties and measurement, 208–209,
  209
Sound pressure level, 209
Sound pressure variations, transmission, 210
Sound source localization, 220
Spastic hemiplegia, 293–294, *294*
Spasticity, in upper motor neuron syndrome, 295
Spectral sensitivity, 191, *192*
Spectroscopy, magnetic resonance, 430
Speech and language disorders, 408–413
  agraphia, 413
    lexical, 413
    phonological, 413
  alexia, 411–412, 412t
    with agraphia, 411
    aphasic, 412
    without agraphia, 204, 412
  aphasia, 409–411, 409t, 411t. *See also* Aphasia
  apraxia, 408
  domain, 2
  motor (dysarthrias), 408
  relationship to neuroscience, 1–3
Speech areas. *See* Language areas
Speech-related muscles, branchial origin, 302,
  306, 306b, 306t, *307*
Spermatocyte, 116–117, *117*
Spermatogenesis, 117
Spina bifida, 126–127
Spinal accessory nucleus, 307–308
Spinal artery
  anterior, 380–381, 384, *386*
  posterior, 380, 384, *386*
Spinal control of muscles of respiration, 60, 60t,
  373b
Spinal cord
  anatomic structures, 52, 54–57, *55–58,* 84
  blood supply, 384–385, *386*
  cerebellar projections, 265
  cervical section, 86, *86*
  directional orientation, *9,* 9–10, 10t
  embryological development, *123,* 125
  function, 15
  internal anatomy, cross sections, 84–86, *84–86,*
    84t, 239–240, *240, 241*
  lesion localization, 256
  lesions, 35t
  lumbar section, 84–85, *85*

meninges, 67t, 70–71, *71*
motor functions, 245–248, *246–249*
motor nuclei, 245, *245*
motor system, 238–259
  autonomic pathways, 244
  clinical concerns, 252–256. *See also* Spinal
    syndromes
  clinical considerations, 257–259
  gross anatomy, 239–240, *240–242*
  innervation pattern, 238–239, *240, 242*
  spinal preparation, 238
  neurotransmitters, 252
  sacral section, 84, *84*
  sectional planes, 10, *11,* 12t
  segmental organization, 240
  thoracic section, *85,* 85–86
  tracts, 240–245, 242t, *243, 244*
  vestibular projections, 231, *231*
Spinal nerves, 164, *165,* 239, *240*
  networking, 58–60, *59,* 59t
  positions, 55, *57*
Spinal plexus, 58–59, *59,* 59t, 240
Spinal preparation, 238
Spinal reflexes, 245–246, *246,* 248, 250–251,
  250–252, 250t
Spinal roots, distribution, 58t
Spinal syndromes, 254–256
  Brown-Séquard syndrome (spinal hemisec-
    tion), *182, 182,* 255, 255–256
  complete spinal transection, *254,* 254–255, *256*
  subacute combined degeneration, 256
  syringomyelia, 183, *183,* 256, *257*
Spinal tap, 440
Spinal trigeminal tract, 87, *88*
Spinal veins, 391
Spinocerebellar tract, *168,* 168t, 180, *181,* 181t,
  243, 244–245, 261, *264*
Spinothalamic system, anterolateral, 84, *84, 168,*
  168t, 172–175, *173,* 174t, *176*
Spinothalamic tract
  anterior, *168,* 168t, 175, *176, 243, 244*
  lateral, *168,* 168t, 172, *173,* 174–175, 174t,
    243, 244
Spiral ganglia, 214
Stapedius muscle, 210
Stapes, *209,* 210
Startle reflex, 234
Static motor responses, *247,* 248
Static (stationary) symptoms, 12
Stem cell transplantation, 143b
Stereocilia, 212
Stereognosis, 167
Stereotactic surgery, 282, 441
Stimulation mapping
  cortical, 440, *441*
  subcortical, 441
Strabismus, 317–318
Stretch reflex, 164, 246, 248, 250, *250,* 250t
Stria, 13
Striate, *276, 277*
Striate arteries, medial, 383
Striatum, 43, 44t, 281t
Stroke, 387–391
  anoxia during, 389–390
  in arteriovenous malformation, 389, *390*
  cerebellar pathology, 270
  hemorrhagic, 389, *390*
  lesion localization, 395–396
  occlusive (thromboembolic), 387–389, *388,*
    388t, *389*
  risk factors, 390–391, 391t, 392b
  treatment, 393, 395
  types, 387t
  warning signs, 388t
Stupor, 370, 447
Subacute symptoms, 12
Subarachnoid hemorrhage, 389
Subarachnoid space, 69, 71, 399–400, *400–401*
Subcallosal gyrus, 41, *44*

Subcortical aphasia, 411
Subcortical mapping, 441
Subcortical structures, blood supply, 386t
Subdural hematoma, 389
Subdural space, 67
Substance P, 145t, 146, 375
Substantia nigra, 44, 49, 50b, 97–98, *98*, 276, 278–279
  in Parkinson's disease, 282, *283*
Subthalamic nucleus, 44, 100, *100*, 101, 104, *106*, 160, 281t
Subthalamus, 160, *276*, 278
Sulcus (sulci), 10, 30, *31*
Superior cerebellar artery, 219, 381
Superior cerebellar peduncle (brachium conjunctivum), 52, 95, 96, *97*
Superior colliculus, 49, 96, *98*
Superior frontal gyrus, 33, *34*
Superior laryngeal nerve, 336, *338*
Superior longitudinal fasciculus, 63, *65*
Superior occipitofrontal fasciculus, 63
Superior olivary nucleus, 216
Superior parietal lobule, 33, 34
Superior pontine sulcus, 49
Superior temporal gyrus, 35
Supination, 10, *12*
Supplemental motor area, 290, *290*
Supramarginal gyrus, 34
Supratentorial space, 68
Surface dyslexia, 412
Suspensory ligaments, 185, *187*
Swallowing, 48–49, 373
Sweat glands, 354
Sydenham chorea, 280–281
Sylvian fissure, 30, 31, *32*
Sympathetic ganglia, 29, 355b, 356, *356*
Sympathetic nervous system, 29, 76–77, 76t, 354, 354b, 354t
  central pathways, 359
  effects, 77t
  neurotransmitters, 359, 360t
  visceral efferents, 355–357, 355t, *356*, *357*, 358t
Synapse, 13, *13*, 133
  establishment, neuronal pruning and, 135–137, 137b
Synaptic cleft, 13, 133
Synaptic terminals, 13, *13*
Syringomyelia, 183, *183*
Systemic diseases, dementia associated with, 415, 415t

Tactile agnosia, 414
Tardive dyskinesia, 282
Tectorial membrane, 212
Tectospinal tract, 243
Tectum, midbrain, 49, 96
Tegmentum
  midbrain, 49, 96
  pons, 50
Telencephalon, 29, 30–44, 120–121, *122*, *123*, 124t
  basal ganglia, 42–44, *43*, *44*, 44t
  cerebral hemispheres, 30, *31*, *32*
  corpus callosum, 38–40, 39–41
  cortical surfaces, 30–39
    dorsolateral, 30–35, *32*, *33*
    midsagittal, 36–39, *38–40*
    ventral, 35–36, *36*, *37*
  frontal lobe, 31–33, *34*, 36–37
  insular lobe, 41, *42*
  limbic lobe, 41–42, *42*
  occipital lobe, *32*, *33*, 34–35, 37, *39*
  parietal lobe, *32*, *33*, 33–34, *34*, 37, *38*
  temporal lobe, *32*, *33*, 35, *39*, *39*
Telophase, 116
Temperature. *See also* Thermoreception
  body, regulation, 366
Temporal gyri, 35, 36, *36*

Temporal lobe, 30, *32*
  dorsolateral, *32*, *33*, 35
  functional anatomy, 407
  lesions, 35t
  medial, 39, *39*
Temporal planum, 218, 220, 408
Tensor tympani muscle, 210
Tentorium cerebelli, 68, *69*
Teratogenesis, 126, 126t, 127t
Terminal bouton (knob), 13, *13*
Terminology
  altered consciousness, 370
  anatomic structures, 10, 12
  body movements, 10, *12*
  cells and functions, 12–13, *13*
  cortical motor dysfunction, 291
  directional brain orientation, 8–10, *9*, 10t
  muscles, 10
  neuronal structures, 13, 14t
  planes of brain sections, 10, *11*, 12t
  simplification, 18–19
Tetraploid, 114
Thalamic aphasia, 411
Thalamic nuclei
  anterior nucleus, 155, 157t, 159
  centromedianus nucleus, 157t, 159, 160
  dorsomedial nucleus, 155, 157t
  functional classification, 160
  intralaminar nuclear complex, 155, 157t, 159–160
  lateral dorsal nucleus, 156, 157t
  lateral geniculate body, 157t, 159
  lateral nuclear complex, 156, 157t, 158
  lateral posterior nucleus, 156, 157t
  medial geniculate body, 157t, 159
  medial nuclear complex, 155–156, 157t
  midline nuclear complex, 155–156, 157t
  nonspecific, 160
  parafascicular nucleus, 159
  projections and functions, *155*, 155–160, *156*, 157t
  pulvinar, 157t, 158
  reticular nucleus, 157t, 159
  specific sensory, 160
  tiers, 153–155, *154*
  ventral anterior nucleus, 157t, 158
  ventral nuclear complex, 157t, 158–159
  ventral posterior lateral nucleus, 157t, 158
  ventral posterior medial nucleus, 157t, 158–159
  ventral posterior nucleus, 157t, 158
  ventrolateral nucleus, 157t, 158
Thalamic syndrome, 161–162
Thalamocortical fibers, 172
Thalamus, 14, *14*, 15t, 39, 41, *44–45*, *45*, 109, *112*, 152–160, *154–156*, 157t
  anatomy, 152, *154*
  anterior, 101t, 103–104, *106*
  clinical considerations, 162–163
  coronal sections through, 103–104, *104–106*
  development, 121–122
  functions, 152–153
  lesions, 35t, 161–162
  mid-, 101t, 103, *105*
  nuclei. *See* Thalamic nuclei
  posterior, 98, *100*, 101, 101t, 103, *104*
  structure, 153–155, *154*
Thermal anesthesia, 175
Thermal hyperesthesia, 175
Thermal hypesthesia, 175
Thermoreception
  assessment, 175
  body, 165, 165t, 172–175
  face, 177, *178*, 179, 179t
Thiamine deficiency, 159, 415, 448
Third ventricle, 61, 62, 83, *83*, 102, *102*, 399, *400*
Thoracic section, *85*, 85–86
Thoracolumbar system. *See* Sympathetic nervous system

Thrombosis, 387t, *388*, 388–389, *389*, 422–423, *423*
Thymus, enlarged, in myasthenia gravis, 149
Thyroid-stimulating hormone, 367, *367*, 368t
Tic douloureux (trigeminal neuralgia), 179, 183, 325, 325b
Tomography, computed, 423–425, *424*, 425t
Tongue
  muscles, 341t
  sensory innervation, 343, *343*, 344t
Tonic-clonic seizure, 446, 446t
Tonotopic representation, 216, 220
Topographical organization of brain, 7–8
Touch, 165
  diffuse
    body, 165, 175
    face, 179–180
  fine discriminative
    body, 165, 167, 169t
    face, 177, *178*, 179t
Toxic encephalopathies, 448
Tract, 13, 14t
Transcortical aphasia, 410–411, 411t
  isolation syndrome form, 411
  mixed, 411
  motor, 410–411
  sensory, 411
Transcranial magnetic stimulation, 405
Transient ischemic attack (TIA), 387–388
Transient symptoms, 12
Transverse plane, 10, *11*, 12t
Traumatic brain injury, 417
Tremor, 281
  intentional (action), 269, 281
  resting, 281
Trigeminal nerve (CN5), 73t, 74, *74*, 91, 176–180
  in diffuse touch from face, 179–180
  in fine discriminative touch from face, 177, *178*, 179t
  in pain and temperature from face, 177, *178*, 179, 179t
  sensorimotor functions, 319–320, 322t, *323*, 323–325, *324*, 325t
  three-neuron organization, 177, *178*
Trigeminal neuralgia, 179, 183, 325, 325b
Trigeminal spinal nucleus, 177, 307
Trilaminar embryo, 118
Triplegia, 10, 291
Triploid, 114
Trisomies, 115t
Tritanomaly, 202
Trochlear nerve (CN4), 73t, 74, *74*, 95, 318, *320*, 320t, 321t
Trochlear nucleus, 307
Trophoblast, 117, *118*
Tuber cinereum, 365
Tumor, brain, 147, 449
Tumor necrosis factor-a, 148
Tuning fork, 222–223, *223*
Two-point discrimination test, 171–172
Tympanic membrane, *209*, 210
Tympanometry, 223–224

Ulnar neuropathy, 448–449
Unconscious proprioception, 180–182, *181*, 181t
  clinical concerns and assessment, 180, 182
  innervation pattern, 180
  neural pathways, 180, *181*, 181t
  receptors, 180
Unipolar neuron, 133
Upper calcarine operculum, 37
Upper motor neuron syndrome, 253, 255, 293b, *295*, 295–296, *296*, 296t, 297
  of cranial nerves, 343–344
Upper motor neurons (UMNs), 91, 245
Utricle, 227

Vagus nerve (CN10), 73t, 74, 75, 334–337, 334t, 335–339
Valproate, 446

Vascular system, cerebral. *See* Cerebrovascular system
Vascular tunic, 188
Vasopressin, 366, *367*, 368, 368t
Veins, 378–379
Venography, magnetic resonance, 430
Venous sinus system, cerebral, 391, *394*
Ventral, 8, 9, *9*, 10t
Ventral anterior nucleus, 157t, 158
Ventral cortical surface, 35–36, *36, 37*
Ventral horns, 54, 239, *240, 241*
Ventral median fissure, 54
Ventral nuclear complex, 157t, 158–159
Ventral posterior nucleus, 157t, 158
    lateral, 157t, 158, 169, *171*
    medial, 157t, 158–159
Ventral ramus, 58, *59*, 239–240
Ventral secondary ascending tract, 177
Ventral spinocerebellar tract, *168*, 168t, 180, *181*, 181t, 261, *264*
Ventricle(s), 60–61
    fourth, 61, *62*, 83, *83*, 91, 399, *400*
    lateral, 61, *62*, 103, *104*, 109, *112*, 399, *400*
        anterior horn, 101, *102*
        shape, 83, *83*
    third, 61, *62*, 83, *83*, 102, *102*, 399, *400*
Ventricular cavity, shape, 83, *83*
Ventricular trigone, 44
Ventrolateral nucleus, 157t, 158
Venules, 378
Vermis, cerebellar, 52, *54*, 263, *263*
Vertebral arteries, *379*, 380, *380*, 381t
Vertebral basilar system, *379, 380*, 380–381, 380t, 381t
Vertigo, 235
Vestibular eye movements, *231*, 232
    induced, 234, *235*
Vestibular (Scarpa) ganglia, 228
Vestibular nerve and nuclei, 91, 228, *230, 231*, 266, 307, 330–331
Vestibular nystagmus, 234, *235*
Vestibular receptors, 228
Vestibular sacs, 227–228, *228–230*
Vestibular schwannoma, 147, 221
Vestibular system, 227–237
    anatomy, 227–231

semicircular ducts and vestibular sacs, 227–228, *228–230*
vestibular nerve and nuclei, 228, *230, 231*
vestibular projections, 230–231, *231*
clinical concerns, 234–236
    equilibrium assessment, *233*, 235–236
    equilibrium disorders, 234–235
clinical considerations, 236–237
physiology of equilibrium, *233*, 233–234, *235*. *See also* Equilibrium
Vestibulocerebellar fibers, 264
Vestibulocerebellum, *261*, 263, 263t
Vestibulocochlear nerve (CN8), 73t, 74, *74*, 228, 330–331, 330t
Vestibulospinal tract, 244, 263
Vibratory sense, 165, 167
Viscera, 12
Visceral afferent system, 16, 16t, 358
Visceral efferent system, 16, 16t
    autonomic nervous system, 355–357
        parasympathetic, 355t, 357, *359*, 360t
        sympathetic, 355–357, 355t, *356, 357*, 358t
Visceral pain, 174
Visual acuity assessment, 202, *202*
Visual agnosia, 204, 414
Visual cortex, 407
    association, 204
    development, 197
    lesions, 204–205
    primary, *195*, 197
    retinal pathways to, *195*, 195–197, 196t
Visual evoked potentials, 437
Visual field, 185
    defects, 202–204, *203*, 203t, 313
    monocular versus binocular, 185, *186*
    retinal representation, *190, 195*, 196–197
Visual reflexes, 197–200, 316–317, *318*, 318t
    accommodation reflex, 199–200, *200*
    pupillary light reflex, *198*, 198–199, *199*
Visual system, 185–207. *See also* Vestibular system
    central pathways, *195*, 195–197, 196t
    clinical concerns, 200–205
        color vision disorders, 202
        errors of refraction, 200–202, *201*

visual acuity assessment, 202, *202*
visual field defects, 202–204, *203*, 203t
clinical considerations, 205–206
eyeball anatomy, 185–188, *187*
lesion localization, 205
optical mechanism, 192–194
    convergence, 194
    pupillary aperture, 194
    refraction, 192–194, *193*
    retinal image formation, *193*, 194
retinal anatomy, 188–190, *189*, 190t
retinal optics, 194
retinal photochemistry, 191–192
    color vision, 191–192
    dark adaptation, 192, *192*
    spectral sensitivity, 191, *192*
retinal vascular supply, 190
Vitamin A, night blindness and, 191
Vitreous humor, 187–188
Vocal fold paralysis, 336
Vomiting, 373–374

Wada test, 431–432, 434, 434t
Wallenberg syndrome, 345t, 346, *347*
Wallerian (anterograde) degeneration, *140*, 141, 141t, 142t
Water intake regulation, 366
Watershed zone, 387
Weber syndrome, 345, *345*, 345t
Weber test, 223, *223*
Wernicke aphasia, 222, 409–410
Wernicke area (language association cortex), 35, 218–219, *220*, 407
Wernicke-Korsakoff syndrome, 159, 415, 448
White matter
    brain, 12, 61–64
    spinal, 52, 84, 239
William syndrome, 128
Wilson disease, 284, *285*
Withdrawal reflex, 250–251, *251*

X-linked inheritance, 444, *444*

Zona incerta, 160
Zygote, 116, 117